Complications of CSF Shunting in Hydrocephalus

Concezio Di Rocco
Mehmet Turgut
George Jallo
Juan F. Martínez-Lage
Editors

Complications of CSF Shunting in Hydrocephalus

Prevention, Identification, and Management

Springer

Editors
Concezio Di Rocco
Pediatric Neurosurgery
Catholic University Medical School
Rome
Italy

George Jallo
Division of Pediatric Neurosurgery
Johns Hopkins Hospital
Baltimore, MD
USA

Mehmet Turgut
Department of Neurosurgery
Adnan Menderes University School of Medicine
Aydın
Turkey

Juan F. Martínez-Lage
Regional Service of Neurosurgery and Unit of Pediatric Neurosurgery
Virgen de la Arrixaca University Hospital
Murcia, Spain

ISBN 978-3-319-09960-6 ISBN 978-3-319-09961-3 (eBook)
DOI 10.1007/978-3-319-09961-3
Springer Cham Heidelberg Dordrecht London New York

Library of Congress Control Number: 2014955606

Printed on acid-free paper

Springer is part of Springer Science+Business Media (www.springer.com)

Preface

Hydrocephalus constitutes a large proportion of the daily work of neurosurgeons all over the world. It is not only an infantile condition as it can occur at all ages of life. Hydrocephalus is the end stage of a multiplicity of causes, congenital or acquired. Many causes can lead to the development of hydrocephalus, and each one of these etiologies explains its own presentation and peculiarities, especially those concerning its appropriate management. There exists the belief that the incidence of hydrocephalus is decreasing; perhaps this could be true in cases of pediatric hydrocephalus, but, in contrast, acquired forms of the condition seem to be presently more prevalent, as happens with posthaemorrhagic hydrocephalus. Thus, the importance of hydrocephalus seems to be often underestimated.

When Ass. Professor Mehmet Turgut conceived the idea of writing a book on complications of CSF shunts, it became evident that this project was really timely taking into account the endless list of adverse events related to the treatment of hydrocephalus that almost continuously appear in the current literature. A book on these complications could fulfill an existing gap on the bibliography on the management of hydrocephalus. On the other hand, the work should also deal with the increasing utilization of neuroendoscopic techniques and with the newly appearing complications of its use.

The interest of our book should rest not only on describing the complications that may result from CSF shunting or from endoscopic procedures but also in issues concerning management and, more importantly, prevention. We agree with the aphorism that "the best shunt is no shunt" and, at the same time, we share the opinion that many complications are unavoidable but that, at large, many of them are preventable. A better understanding of the mechanisms involved in CSF shunt infection has undoubtedly led to a decrease in its occurrence. The same can be said regarding mechanical complications. However, in spite of a better awareness of CSF overdrainage syndromes and of their management, little has been achieved from the point of view of prevention. It is obvious that anatomical and physiological properties of the growing brain are dissimilar to those of the adult, with the subsequent influence on choosing the most adequate treatment. At present, no valve design has proved to fulfill the needs for CSF derivation for both infants and adults.

The first principle to avoid CSF shunt complications is to establish a solid indication for the initial treatment of hydrocephalus. Alternative methods, such as endoscopic methods or removal of the obstructing mass, must be considered at the start. Regarding election of the shunt, the superiority of one type of valve over the others has never been scientifically proven , although each specialist uses his/her preferred valve. Most neurosurgeons use the shunt that they are more familiarized with or the one that is customarily implanted in their department. In addition, for prevention of complications, special attention should be paid to all details during shunt insertion or revision, even if they appear to be insignificant.

Moreover, the resurgence of neuroendoscopic techniques for management of hydrocephalus seen in the last two decades has also evoked much debate about indications, age, and outcomes of the procedure, and they will be discussed on this work.

With these ideas in mind, we undertook the task of producing a multiauthored book and, for this end, chose a group of experts on the field. The book is divided into 24 chapters written by 46 specialists from many countries of Europe, America, Asia, and Africa. The book highlights the diagnosis, management, and prevention of complications arising from both CSF shunting and neuroendoscopy by updating the literature on hydrocephalus complications and also by including the authors' personal thoughts. Inevitably, there will be some repetitions along the text that will allow the reader to consult the chapters individually. The Editors wish that this book be useful for neurosurgeons, neurosurgical residents, neurologists, pediatricians, pediatric neurologists, radiologists, and physicians of the pediatric and general Emergency Departments.

To end, we would like to acknowledge the efforts and collaboration of Springer and of Springer personnel, Gabriele Schröder, Antonia von Saint-Paul, Sushil Kumar, Ms. G. Meena, and especially Rosemarie C. Unger (Project Coordinator), for their patience and experienced advice in the production of this book. We also would like to thank our families for their support and tolerance. Last but not least, our gratitude goes to our patients and their families for having given us their confidence and affection and for forgiving us the unavoidable "friendly fire" arising during their care that has led us to gain experience on CSF shunt complications and that has triggered our research on their management and prevention.

Hannover, Germany	Concezio Di Rocco, MD
Aydın, Turkey	Mehmet Turgut, MD, PhD
Baltimore, MD, USA	George I. Jallo, MD
Murcia, Spain	Juan F. Martínez-Lage, MD

Contents

Part I Introduction

1 **General Introduction: Why They Exist, Incidence, Social and Economic Costs, and Quality of Life** 3
George M. Ibrahim and Abhaya V. Kulkarni

2 **Clinical Manifestations of CSF Shunt Complications** 13
Juan F. Martínez-Lage, Antonio L. López-Guerrero, and María-José Almagro

3 **Neuroimaging in CSF Shunt Complications** 33
Ernesto Domenech, Cristina Serrano, and Carmen María Fernández-Hernández

Part II Complications of Extrathecal CSF Shunts

4 **Introduction: The Use of Extrathecal CSF Shunts, Optional vs Mandatory, Unavoidable Complications** 75
Rizwan A. Khan

5 **Iatrogenic Complications of CSF Shunting** 81
Juan F. Martínez-Lage, Miguel Angel Pérez-Espejo, and Ahmet Tuncay Turgut

6 **Complications Related to the Choice of the CSF Shunt Device** 109
Kevin Tsang, William Singleton, and Ian Pople

7 **Functional Complications: Hyperdrainage** 119
Erdal Kalkan, Bülent Kaya, Fatih Erdi, and Ahmet Tuncay Turgut

8 **Mechanical Complications of Shunts** 129
Vasilios Tsitouras and Spyros Sgouros

9 **Infective Complications** 141
Ali Akhaddar

10 **Posthemorrhagic and Postinflammatory Complications** 149
Joanna Y. Wang and Edward S. Ahn

11 **Complications Related to the Type of Hydrocephalus: Normal Pressure Hydrocephalus** 159
María Antonia Poca and Juan Sahuquillo

12 **Complications Specific to the Type of CSF Shunt: Atrial Shunt** 177
Luca Massimi and Concezio Di Rocco

13 **Complications of Peritoneal Shunts** 187
José Hinojosa

14 **Complications Specific to Lumboperitoneal Shunt** 203
Ignacio Jusué-Torres, Jamie B. Hoffberger, and Daniele Rigamonti

15 **Complications Specific to Pleural Type of CSF Shunt** 213
Marcelo Galarza and Patricia Martínez

16 **Complications Specific to Rare Type Procedures of CSF Shunting** 227
Bernard Trench Lyngdoh

17 **Cranio-cerebral Disproportion as a Late Complication** 233
Concezio Di Rocco and Paolo Frassanito

18 **Epilepsy as a Late Complication** 247
Mehmet Turgut and Ahmet Tuncay Turgut

Part III Complications of Intrathecal Shunts-Endoscopic Treatment

19 **Introduction: The Changed Epidemiology of CSF Shunt Complications, Failures Versus Complications** 263
Mehmet Saim Kazan and Ethem Taner Göksu

20 **Iatrogenic and Infectious Complications** 269
David A. Chesler and George I. Jallo

21 **CSF Fistulae as a Complication Due to Insufficient Correction of Altered CSF Dynamics** 277
Jogi V. Pattisapu

22 **Subdural Collections: Hygroma and Haematoma** 285
Miguel Gelabert-González, Eduardo Aran-Echabe, and Ramón Serramito-García

23 **Complications Related to Endoscopic Fenestration in Loculated Hydrocephalus** 301
Yoshua Esquenazi and David I. Sandberg

24 **Late Failures** 307
Federico Di Rocco

Index 313

Contributors

Edward S. Ahn, MD Division of Pediatric Neurosurgery, The Johns Hopkins Hospital, Baltimore, MD, USA

Ali Akhaddar, MD Department of Neurosurgery, Avicenne Military Hospital of Marrakech, University of Mohammed V Souissi, Rabat, Morocco

María-José Almagro, MD Pediatric Neurosurgery Section and Regional Service of Neurosurgery, Virgen de la Arrixaca University Hospital, El Palmar, Murcia, Spain

Eduardo Aran-Echabe, MD Department of Surgery (Neurosurgery), University of Santiago de Compostela, Santiago de Compostela, Spain

Neurosurgical Service, Clinic Hospital of Santiago de Compostela, Santiago de Compostela, Spain

David A. Chesler, MD, PhD Division of Pediatric Neurosurgery, The Johns Hopkins Hospital, Baltimore, MD, USA

Ernesto Domenech, MD Section of Pediatric Radiology, Service of Diagnostic Radiology, Virgen de la Arrixaca University Hospital, El Palmar, Murcia, Spain

Concezio Di Rocco, MD Pediatric Neurosurgery, Institute of Neurosurgery, Catholic University Medical School, Rome, Italy

Pediatric Neurosurgery, International Neuroscience Institute, Hannover, Germany

Federico Di Rocco, MD, PhD Pediatric Neurosurgery, Necker Hospital, Paris, France

Fatih Erdi, MD Department of Neurosurgery, Necmettin Erbakan University, Meram Faculty of Medicine, Konya, Akyokus/Meram, Turkey

Yoshua Esquenazi, MD Departments of Neurosurgery and Pediatric Surgery, Children's Memorial Hermann Hospital, and Mischer Neuroscience Institute, University of Texas Health Science Center at Houston, Houston, TX, USA

Carmen María Fernández-Hernández, MD Section of Pediatric Radiology, Service of Diagnostic Radiology, Virgen de la Arrixaca University Hospital, El Palmar, Murcia, Spain

Paolo Frassanito, MD Pediatric Neurosurgery, Institute of Neurosurgery, Catholic University Medical School, Rome, Italy

Marcelo Galarza, MD, MSc Regional Department of Neurosurgery, "Virgen de la Arrixaca" University Hospital, Murcia, Spain

Regional Service of Neurosurgery, Hospital Universitario Virgen de la Arrixaca, El Palmar, Murcia, Spain

Miguel Gelabert-González, MD Department of Surgery (Neurosurgery), University of Santiago de Compostela, Santiago de Compostela, Spain

Neurosurgical Service, Clinic Hospital of Santiago de Compostela, Santiago de Compostela, Spain

Ethem Taner Göksu, MD Department of Neurosurgery, Akdeniz University Faculty of Medicine, Antalya, Turkey

José Hinojosa, MD Pediatric Neurosurgical Unit, Hospital Universitario 12 de Octubre, Madrid, Spain

Jamie B. Hoffberger, MD Department of Neurosurgery, The Johns Hopkins University School of Medicine, Baltimore, MD, USA

George M. Ibrahim, MD Division of Neurosurgery, Department of Surgery, Hospital for Sick Children, Toronto, ON, Canada

George I. Jallo, MD Division of Pediatric Neurosurgery, The Johns Hopkins Hospital, Baltimore, MD, USA

Ignacio Jusué-Torres, MD Department of Neurosurgery, The Johns Hopkins University School of Medicine, Baltimore, MD, USA

Erdal Kalkan, MD Department of Neurosurgery, Necmettin Erbakan University, Meram Faculty of Medicine, Konya, Akyokus/Meram, Turkey

Bülent Kaya, MD Department of Neurosurgery, Necmettin Erbakan University, Meram Faculty of Medicine, Konya, Akyokus/Meram, Turkey

Mehmet Saim Kazan, MD Department of Neurosurgery, Akdeniz University Faculty of Medicine, Antalya, Turkey

Rizwan A. Khan, MD, MS, MCh Department of Pediatric Surgery, JNMC, AMU, Aligarh, India

Abhaya V. Kulkarni, MD, PhD, FRCSC Division of Neurosurgery, Department of Surgery, Hospital for Sick Children, Toronto, ON, Canada

Antonio L. López-Guerrero, MD Pediatric Neurosurgery Section and Regional Service of Neurosurgery, Virgen de la Arrixaca University Hospital, El Palmar, Murcia, Spain

Bernard Trench Lyngdoh, MD Department of Neurosurgery, Woodland Hospital, Shillong, Meghalaya, India

Patricia Martínez, MD Department of Thoracic Surgery, "Virgen de la Arrixaca" University Hospital, Murcia, Spain

Juan F. Martínez-Lage, MD Pediatric Neurosurgery Section and Regional Service of Neurosurgery, Virgen de la Arrixaca University Hospital, El Palmar, Murcia, Spain

Luca Massimi, MD, PhD Pediatric Neurosurgery, A. Gemelli Hospital, Institute of Neurosurgery, Catholic University Medical School, Rome, Italy

Jogi V. Pattisapu, MD, FAAP, FACS, FAANS (L) Pediatric Neurosurgery, University of Central Florida, College of Medicine, Orlando, FL, USA

Miguel Angel Pérez-Espejo, MD Pediatric Neurosurgery Section and Regional Service of Neurosurgery, Virgen de la Arrixaca University Hospital, El Palmar, Murcia, Spain

María Antonia Poca, MD, PhD Department of Neurosurgery and Neurotraumatology Research Unit, Vall d'Hebron University Hospital and Vall d'Hebron Research Institute, Universitat Autònoma de Barcelona, Barcelona, Spain

Ian Pople, MD Department of Neurosurgery, North Bristol NHS Trust, Bristol, UK

Daniele Rigamonti, MD Department of Neurosurgery, The Johns Hopkins University School of Medicine, Baltimore, MD, USA

Juan Sahuquillo, MD, PhD Department of Neurosurgery and Neurotraumatology Research Unit, Vall d'Hebron University Hospital and Vall d'Hebron Research Institute, Universitat Autònoma de Barcelona, Barcelona, Spain

David I. Sandberg, MD Departments of Neurosurgery and Pediatric Surgery, Children's Memorial Hermann Hospital, and Mischer Neuroscience Institute, University of Texas Health Science Center at Houston, Houston, TX, USA

Ramón Serramito-García, MD Department of Surgery (Neurosurgery), University of Santiago de Compostela, Santiago de Compostela, Spain

Neurosurgical Service, Clinic Hospital of Santiago de Compostela, Santiago de Compostela, Spain

Cristina Serrano, MD Section of Pediatric Radiology, Service of Diagnostic Radiology, Virgen de la Arrixaca University Hospital, El Palmar, Murcia, Spain

Spyros Sgouros, MD Department of Neurosurgery, "Mitera" Childrens Hospital, Athens, Greece

Department of Neurosurgery, University of Athens, Athens, Greece

William Singleton, MD Department of Neurosurgery, North Bristol NHS Trust, Bristol, UK

Kevin Tsang, MD Department of Neurosurgery, North Bristol NHS Trust, Bristol, UK

Vasilios Tsitouras, MD Department of Neurosurgery, "Mitera" Childrens Hospital, Athens, Greece

Ahmet Tuncay Turgut, MD Department of Radiology, Ankara Training and Research Hospital, Ankara, Turkey

Mehmet Turgut, MD, PhD Department of Neurosurgery, Adnan Menderes University School of Medicine, Aydın, Turkey

Joanna Y. Wang Division of Pediatric Neurosurgery, The Johns Hopkins Hospital, Baltimore, MD, USA

Part I

Introduction

1 General Introduction: Why They Exist, Incidence, Social and Economic Costs, and Quality of Life

George M. Ibrahim and Abhaya V. Kulkarni

Contents

1.1 **Introduction** ... 3

1.2 **Heterogeneity in Practice and Complications** ... 4

1.3 **Impact on the Individual** ... 5
1.3.1 Mortality and Hospital Length of Stay ... 5
1.3.2 Quality of Life ... 6
1.3.3 Cognitive Outcome ... 7

1.4 **Societal Impact** ... 7
1.4.1 Societal Impact in the Developed World ... 8
1.4.2 Societal Impact in the Developing World ... 9

Conclusions ... 9

References ... 10

G.M. Ibrahim, MD
Division of Neurosurgery, Department of Surgery, Hospital for Sick Children, 555 University Avenue, MG5 1X8 Toronto, ON, Canada
e-mail: george.m.ibrahim@gmail.com

A.V. Kulkarni, MD, PhD, FRCSC (✉)
Division of Neurosurgery, Department of Surgery, Hospital for Sick Children, Room 1503, 555 University Avenue, M5G 1X8 Toronto, ON, Canada
e-mail: abhaya.kulkarni@sickkids.ca

Abbreviations

CSF	Cerebrospinal fluid
ETV	Endoscopic third ventriculostomy
HOQ	Hydrocephalus Outcome Questionnaire
LOS	Length of stay
NPH	Normal pressure hydrocephalus
QOL	Quality of life
VP	Ventriculoperitoneal

1.1 Introduction

Cerebrospinal fluid (CSF) diversion procedures are among the most common neurosurgical interventions performed worldwide. The majority of these procedures are comprised of ventriculoperitoneal (VP) shunt insertions. In the United States, the annual incidence of VP shunt placement is 5.5 per 100,000 [52] with approximately 30,000 procedures performed each year amounting to $95 million of medical expenditures [1, 3, 37]. Undoubtedly, shunts have dramatically reduced the mortality and morbidity of hydrocephalus, and as such, they represent a valuable tool in the neurosurgeon's armamentarium. Nearly half of shunt-related procedures, however, are revisions of previous insertions [37], highlighting the persistent shortcomings in the use of these devices in the treatment of hydrocephalus.

Despite their necessity and ubiquitous usage, it is well established that shunts are prone to various complications that may occur throughout the

C. Di Rocco et al. (eds.), *Complications of CSF Shunting in Hydrocephalus: Prevention, Identification, and Management*, DOI 10.1007/978-3-319-09961-3_1,

Table 1.1 Selected causes of shunt failure

Hardware-related complications
Obstruction, raised intracranial pressure
Breakage
Malposition
Migration
Infection
Fluid dynamic-related complications
Overdrainage
Slit ventricles/slit ventricle syndrome
Subdural collections
Intra-abdominal complications
Infection, peritonitis, abscess
CSF pseudocyst
Visceral complications (bowel obstruction, perforation)

patient's lifetime (Table 1.1). At 5 years following shunt insertion, the cumulative complication rate was reported in one large population-based study to be 32 % [52]. Complications may include malfunctions due to obstruction, mechanical disconnection or breakage, infection, and overdrainage. In pediatric populations, 14 % of shunts will fail within 1 month of insertion [35], and within the first year, 35–50 % of shunts placed will require revision [27, 34, 45]. Twenty-nine percent of adults will also experience a shunt failure within the first year. Over the course of their lives, the vast majority of individuals with shunted hydrocephalus will require a shunt revision [38]. Factors associated with shunt complications include male sex, low socioeconomic status, younger age, repeated shunt failures, obstructive (rather than communicating) hydrocephalus, and low gestational age at the time of first shunt insertion [35, 45, 52].

The impact of these complications on affected individuals and societies is tremendous. The current introductory chapter explores the effects of shunt-related complications on patients and healthcare systems. For individuals, shunt-related complications may lead to disability or mortality. Furthermore, a greater impetus has been placed in recent years on understanding the effects of hydrocephalus and procedure-related complications on the quality of life of affected patients. The societal impact of shunt-related complications is also important to consider. We review the relevant literature in the context of both developing and developed countries. We underscore that prevention, early identification, and treatment are necessary to mitigate the personal and social costs of shunt-related complications.

1.2 Heterogeneity in Practice and Complications

In order to appreciate the impact of shunt-related complications on the individual and society, it is important to recognize that considerable heterogeneity exists in surgical decision-making concerning the management of hydrocephalus [43]. There is no consensus on the optimal methods of CSF diversion, much less the specific devices, procedures, and protocols that should be adopted uniformly to decrease the risk of shunt-related complications. In order to mitigate the burden of complications on individuals and societies, rigor must be applied in identifying modifiable patterns that result in subsequent shunt dysfunction. Indeed, this remains the mission of many organizations and consortia worldwide.

In patients who require insertion of a VP shunt, it is known that various non-modifiable factors may predispose to subsequent complications. For example, premature neonates are more likely develop shunt infections than term equivalents [24]. Furthermore, the underlying etiology of the hydrocephalus has been associated with complications, with obstructive hydrocephalus associated with a disproportionately greater incidence of complications than communicating hydrocephalus [35, 45, 52]. The few studies that have examined novel ways to mitigate shunt complications have largely yielded disappointing results; therefore, there is little evidence on the basis of which surgical decision-making can be standardized. For instance, studies have failed to demonstrate superiority of more complex or expensive shunt device over simpler alternatives [39]. Treatment decisions are often at the discretion of the attending surgeon and tailored towards the specific clinical and radiographic phenotypes of individual patients.

There is some evidence, however, to suggest that procedure-related changes may mitigate certain complications [21]. For example, it has been shown that performing shunt insertions at the beginning of the day, limiting personnel in the operating theater, and administration of periprocedural antibiotics result in considerably lower rates of shunt infections [20]. More recently, intrathecal antibiotics, minimizing exposure of shunt tubing to breached surgical gloves [24], and antibiotic-impregnated shunts [13] have been shown or suggested to decrease complications. It remains imperative for clinicians to be cognizant of heterogeneity in practice and to strive to identify best practices to mitigate shunt-related complications.

1.3 Impact on the Individual

Heterogeneity also exists in the underlying pathological conditions leading to shunt-dependent hydrocephalus. They may range from congenital malformations such as aqueductal stenosis and myelomeningocele to acquired conditions such as post-infectious or post-subarachnoid hemorrhage hydrocephalus. Importantly the underlying etiologies of hydrocephalus may be independently associated with poor outcome or poorer health-related quality of life (QOL), and indeed, disentangling the effects of shunt-related complications from other putative factors often proves difficult.

Evaluating the effects of shunt-related complications on an individual's health is furthermore complicated by the fact that numerous external factors moderate his/her well-being when faced with medical or surgical complications. For example, lower socioeconomic status, worse family functioning, and lower parental education have been shown to correlate with lower quality of life in studies of childhood hydrocephalus [22]. The multifaceted interplay between multiple variables must therefore be considered when evaluating the impact of shunt-related complications.

Concrete data on mortality, disability, and time lost provide less biased estimates of the impact of shunt-related complications on the lives of patients. More robust measures such as QOL indices may, however, provide a more in-depth picture of ways in which shunt complications affect different dimensions of a patient's well-being. In the subsequent sections, we provide a summary of various indicators used to index the effects of procedure-related complications on a patient's well-being. Namely, we review data on mortality, disability, and time lost as well as QOL and cognitive function.

1.3.1 Mortality and Hospital Length of Stay

Perhaps the most succinct ways to quantify the impact of shunt complications are to review data on mortality, disability, and length of stay in a hospital. These metrics are important as they represent salient endpoints for outcomes and often inform system-level decision-making regarding the allocation of resources. They are also useful summary statistics to measure the effect of interventions and policies in a longitudinal manner. They are, however, limited in that they do not adequately describe how shunt-related complications affect individuals and do not attempt to explain the cascade of events that lead to poor outcomes. For example, mortality due to shunt-related complications may be a result of delayed diagnosis or delayed transfer to a neurosurgical center. These endpoints also represent a summary of aggregate population-based data; therefore, it is imperative for individual neurosurgeons to record and monitor the rates of complications and adverse events in their own practice in order to strive to improve patient care.

Shunt failure may lead to raised intracranial pressure, herniation syndromes, and sudden death [17]. A large population-based study determined that among all admissions primarily involving a shunt-related procedure, in-patient mortality was 2.7 % [37]. In the same series, the most common diagnosis was shunt malfunction (40.7 %) with 42.8 % of admissions resulting in shunt replacement, suggesting that shunt-related complications are responsible for a considerable proportion of hydrocephalus-associated mortality. Indeed, a 20-year longitudinal study of 138 children with shunted hydrocephalus identified 4 deaths (2.9 %) that were directly attributable to shunt failure [38]. Furthermore, shunt infection has been shown to be significantly associated with a higher likelihood of death following CSF diversion [46]. In the literature, comparable shunt-related mortality rates of 2–5 % have been published on long-term follow-up of shunted patients [3, 16, 17, 18]. Importantly, while some deaths related to shunt malfunction occur suddenly, a considerable proportion of patients also have symptoms for hours or weeks prior to death, highlighting the importance of vigilance and education of patients and front-line healthcare workers [17].

Patients with shunt-related procedures also often have a protracted stay in an in-patient hospital unit. Nearly 50 % of patients admitted for shunt insertions had a length of stay greater than 5 days in hospital [37]. A Spanish study also showed that the mean ICU stay for shunt insertion was 8.2 days [11]. It has been shown that patients admitted with shunt-related complications have a disproportionately longer length of stay in hospital compared to those undergoing primary shunt insertion. For example, patients undergoing shunt revisions due to infection, it has been estimated that the mean duration of hospital stay adjusted for days attributable to CSF infection was 16.3 days [50]. Undoubtedly, prolonged in-patient hospital stays have a profound impact on individuals, as well as societies given the lost productivity as well as the associated healthcare costs.

1.3.2 Quality of Life

In order to adequately discuss, quantify, and ultimately mitigate the impact of shunt-related complications on the individual patient, clinically meaningful and measureable outcomes must be defined beyond standard measures, such as mortality and length of stay in hospital. Quality of life (QOL) is a multidimensional concept that describes the perceived quality of an individual's daily life, which encompasses their emotional, social, and physical states. Health-related QOL is an evaluation of how an individual's well-being may be affected over time by a disease, disability, or disorder. As previously described, one difficulty that is encountered in benchmarking the impact of shunt-related complications is that the QOL with hydrocephalus is already diminished, for example, by underlying etiologies of hydrocephalus. When evaluating how shunt-related complications further depress this baseline level, one may encounter a "floor effect," whereby depressions below the baseline become difficult to measure.

When evaluating an individual's QOL, it is also important to consider the lens from which this measurement is captured. In some studies, QOL may refer to an assessment of an individual's abilities by an external rater. For example, a physician may evaluate a patient's ability to perform a specific task and make inferences about their QOL as a result, or a parent may speak on behalf of a child and describe what they may or may not be capable of doing. Increasingly, the perspective of the patient themselves is considered valuable in evaluating their QOL. The importance of the patient's perspective is underscored by studies demonstrating the prevalence and morbidity of depression, dependence, substance abuse, unemployment, and inability to drive in this patient population [14].

QOL can be summarized into two separate categories, generic instruments (i.e., SF-36; short form with 36 questions) and disease-specific questionnaires. While the former aims to measure generalizable effects of illness on the individual, the latter focuses on issues that are most important for a given patient population. Using the generic SF-36 instrument, patients with shunted hydrocephalus reported poorer perceived health in 2 of 8 SF-36 domains, physical functioning (covering walking, self-care ability, and strenuous activity), and general health [38]. It is unclear from the literature whether shunt-related complications, such as the number of shunt revisions, are associated with worse perceived QOL on the SF-36.

Kulkarni and colleagues have developed a 51-item questionnaire to specifically quantify the physical, cognitive, and social-emotional health of children with hydrocephalus, the Hydrocephalus Outcome Questionnaire (HOQ) [25, 26]. This instrument has been assessed for validity (i.e., the degree to which it measures what it claims to measure) and reliability (the reproducibility of responses on multiple occasions). The HOQ also shows good correlations with several independent measures of health, including the Strengths and Difficulties Questionnaire [12] and Functional Independence Measure for Children [36]. Interestingly, data from QOL studies using this instrument have demonstrated considerable heterogeneity in the distribution of QOL scores [25]. For instance, 5 % of children with shunted hydrocephalus had QOL scores, which could be interpreted as worse than dead, whereas 20 % were within the normal ranges for the population.

From such disease-specific measures of QOL, which may better capture a patient's subjective experience with the illness, the impact of shunt-related complications on the individual also becomes more apparent. On multivariate analysis of QOL data from a large cohort of 346 children, increased length of stay in hospital for shunt infection and shunt overdrainage, as well as the number of proximal shunt catheters in situ were significantly associated with worse QOL [25]. Furthermore, more recent studies suggest that more severe shunt infections are associated with poorer QOL than less severe infections [28, 22].

1.3.3 Cognitive Outcome

Disorders involving the central nervous system are unique from those affecting other organs due to the premium placed on the brain, which is the substrate of identity, agency, and cognitive faculties. It is not therefore surprising that cognitive deficits in patients with hydrocephalus significantly impair their QOL [25]. Cognitive function in children with hydrocephalus, for instance, is considerably lower than other dimensions of well-being. Cognition may be impaired to varying extents in upwards of 60 % of affected individuals [44] and may encompass numerous neuropsychological domains, including language, memory, and learning.

The majority of studies evaluating cognitive function in shunted patients have focused on pediatric populations [44]. Indeed, the effects of hydrocephalus on the developing brain are an issue of importance and active scientific inquiry. As many as half of children with hydrocephalus have intelligence quotients (IQ) lower than 70 [16, 29, 32], and an equivalent proportion of infants with hydrocephalus also had severe cognitive impairment [10]. Furthermore, even individuals with IQ scores greater than 70 may possess poor learning, memory, and executive function [33]. While it remains controversial whether shunt complications contribute to cognitive impairment [29], some studies have suggested that central nervous system infections may be associated with worse intelligence outcomes [7]. Further research is, however, required to determine whether a causal relationship exists between cognitive dysfunction and shunt-related complications.

Epilepsy is also an important predictor of poor cognitive outcome, particularly in children with shunted hydrocephalus [2, 32]. The incidence of seizures in shunted patients ranges from 20 to 50 % [40]. The frequency of seizure activity has also been associated with worse QOL in patients with shunted hydrocephalus [28, 22]. It remains unclear whether seizure activity is a marker of worse underlying brain function (and therefore worse outcomes), a result of the etiology of hydrocephalus, or due to the shunt insertion. Data from one study suggest that the position of the ventricular catheter may be associated with the incidence of epilepsy, with patients implanted with frontal catheters more prone to seizures than those with parietal catheters [4]. The number of ventricular catheter revisions may also be associated with increased incidence of seizures [4], although these finding have not been corroborated by other studies.

1.4 Societal Impact

Shunt-related complications are also associated with an enormous social burden. The true impact of shunt complications on society is difficult to glean from the literature. Patients with shunted hydrocephalus are less likely to access higher education and often possess poorer social functioning and employment prospects than their peers [38], resulting in an enormous loss of productivity. It is expected that shunt-related complications exacerbate these challenges by extending time lost from work, extended lengths of hospital stay, and health-related economic costs. The effect of complications on families and communities is also substantial. The extent of the social impact of shunt-related complications is also related to the degree in which they result in impairments for the individual. For example, cognitive impairments, childhood onset, and protracted disease course may be associated with a greater cost to society [15].

There are several ways in which the societal impact of hydrocephalus and shunt-related complications may be measured. One salient measure is the cost of intervention for shunting and revisions. Healthcare costs in general comprise a large proportion of any nation's budget and have repercussions for societies, particularly with socialized healthcare systems [15]. More importantly, disease and disability associated with hydrocephalus and shunt-related complications exact a high societal price, which may be more difficult to quantify. Metrics such as years of potential life lost (YPLL), valued years of potential life lost (VYPLL), years of potential productivity lost (YPPL), and lifetime years of potential life lost (LYPLL) may be used to attempt to quantify this impact [30]. Measures such as quality-adjusted life years (QALY) also take into account the quality of life affected by the disease burden. These are often used in cost-utility analyses to evaluate the impact of a particular intervention on mitigating the cost of a disease on society. Unfortunately, there is a paucity of studies that have examined how shunt-related complications affect these metrics. Given that health economics is a burgeoning field of research, it is expected that greater emphasis will be placed on understanding the impact of shunt-related complications on these measures of society in the future.

1.4.1 Societal Impact in the Developed World

Hydrocephalus and shunt-related complications are also associated with unique social costs in developed and developing countries. In the developed world, the magnitude of the societal impact may be measured in terms of the cost associated with treating shunt complications. The cost of treating an individual with a shunt procedure was estimated in one study to be $35,816, amounting to a healthcare burden of approximately one billion dollars per year [37]. A similar study conducted in the pediatric population found that each year, total hospital charges ranged from $1.4–2.0 billion for pediatric hydrocephalus in the United States [42]. While accounting for only 0.6 % of hospital admissions, the treatment of hydrocephalus consumed 1.8 % of pediatric hospital days and 3.1 % of all hospital charges. A smaller, community-based Canadian study also corroborated the magnitude of the cost [5]. The primary payer of healthcare costs in the United States are private insurance providers (43.8 %) followed by Medicare (26 %) and Medicaid (24.5 %) [37].

Patwardhan and Nanda found that the top primary diagnosis treated was shunt malfunction at 40.7 % followed by non-communicating (16.6 %) and communicating (13.2 %) hydrocephalus, again suggesting that the complications account for a large proportion of the healthcare costs associated with hydrocephalus [37]. The contribution of shunt-related complications to the staggering economic cost of hydrocephalus is perhaps emphasized by studies that have shown a cost benefit for devices that reduce shunt infections, such as antibiotic-impregnated ventricular catheters [8, 9]. Compared to controls, patients shunted with antibiotic-impregnated shunts had lower costs of treatment, which was attributable to reduced infections in that cohort. Furthermore, one study showed that the median costs of a single admission for shunt failure were $3,964 and $23,541 for obstruction and infection, respectively [41]. Of these, the caregiver out-of-pocket expenses were $361 and $472, respectively.

Germane to the discussion of the societal costs of shunt-related complications are the societal costs associated with not placing shunts in patients who may benefit from the procedure, namely, elderly patients with normal pressure hydrocephalus (NPH). This patient group continues to face barriers in the diagnosis and treatment of hydrocephalus. It is estimated that treating individuals older than 65 years of age can lower 5-year Medicare costs by as much as $25,477 per patient or $184.3 million dollars annually [51]. Furthermore, placement of shunts in patients with symptomatic NPH has also been shown to reduce caregiver burden in one study [19]. It is, therefore, important to remember that while shunt-related complications exact a high societal burden, they are eclipsed by the cost of untreated hydrocephalus.

Table 1.2 Selected measures that may index the impact of shunt-related complications on individuals and societies

Impact on the individual
Mortality
Morbidity
Subjective or objective disability
Hospital length of stay
Quality of life
General health
Physical health
Cognitive health
Social-emotional health
Other dimensions
Important comorbidities
Epilepsy
Developmental delay
Socioeconomic impact
Impact on society
Healthcare costs
Personal costs
Years of potential life lost
Valued years of potential life lost
Years of potential productivity lost
Lifetime years of potential life lost
Quality-adjusted life years

1.4.2 Societal Impact in the Developing World

There are no reliable estimates for the incidence or prevalence of hydrocephalus in the developing world, though it is likely higher than reported in developed countries due to the prevalence of untreated or poorly treated central nervous system infections and nutritional deficiencies [31, 48]. The burden of hydrocephalus is strongly felt in the developing world where inaccessibility to surgical care and operative technologies remains a persistent challenge. In regions where CSF diversion procedures are performed, complications exert a disproportionate effect since the safety net for urgent treatment of shunt malfunctions is absent [49]. In these countries, there is a prolonged latency to presentation [47], and financial, geographic, and logistic factors often impede travel to a center capable of diagnosing and treating shunt complications.

While greater emphasis in general needs to be placed on the treatment of hydrocephalus in the developing world [49], mitigating the impact of shunt complications is expected to translate into more lives saved. One strategy to avoid shunt complications altogether is to perform endoscopic third ventriculostomies (ETV), which have been shown in combination with choroid plexus cauterization to prevent shunt dependence in the majority of African children at the Cure Children's Hospital of Uganda. Such a strategy in the management of childhood hydrocephalus is also favorable since more failures occur within 6 months, where they may be better tolerated by patients and more easily diagnosed by non-experienced observers [49]. In appropriately selected cohorts of patients, ETV may be advantageous over shunting [6, 23] and may represent one alternative to mitigate the impact of shunt complications.

Conclusions

Patients with shunted hydrocephalus are likely to encounter complications such as shunt failure throughout their lives. The magnitude of the impact of shunt complications on these individuals as well as societies is enormous (Table 1.2). Complications may be associated with mortality, a protracted length of stay in hospital, decreased quality of life as well as substantial healthcare costs and lost productivity. While shunts have undoubtedly decreased the mortality and morbidity associated with hydrocephalus, further research and inquiry is required to mitigate the impact of their complications on individuals and society.

References

1. Bondurant CP, Jimenez DF (1995) Epidemiology of cerebrospinal fluid shunting. Pediatr Neurosurg 23:254–258; discussion 259
2. Bourgeois M, Sainte-Rose C, Cinalli G et al (1999) Epilepsy in children with shunted hydrocephalus. J Neurosurg 90:274–281
3. Casey AT, Kimmings EJ, Kleinlugtebeld AD et al (1997) The long-term outlook for hydrocephalus in childhood. A ten-year cohort study of 155 patients. Pediatr Neurosurg 27:63–70
4. Dan NG, Wade MJ (1986) The incidence of epilepsy after ventricular shunting procedures. J Neurosurg 65:19–21
5. Del Bigio MR (1998) Epidemiology and direct economic impact of hydrocephalus: a community based study. Can J Neurol Sci 25:123–126
6. Di Rocco C, Massimi L, Tamburrini G (2006) Shunts vs endoscopic third ventriculostomy in infants: are there different types and/or rates of complications? A review. Childs Nerv Syst 22:1573–1589
7. Donders J, Canady AI, Rourke BP (1990) Psychometric intelligence after infantile hydrocephalus. A critical review and reinterpretation. Childs Nerv Syst 6:148–154
8. Eymann R, Chehab S, Strowitzki M et al (2008) Clinical and economic consequences of antibiotic-impregnated cerebrospinal fluid shunt catheters. J Neurosurg Pediatr 1:444–450
9. Farber SH, Parker SL, Adogwa O et al (2010) Cost analysis of antibiotic-impregnated catheters in the treatment of hydrocephalus in adult patients. World Neurosurg 74:528–531
10. Fernell E, Hagberg G, Hagberg B (1994) Infantile hydrocephalus epidemiology: an indicator of enhanced survival. Arch Dis Child Fetal Neonatal Ed 70:F123–F128
11. Gomez Lopez L, Luaces Cubells C, Costa Clara JM et al (1998) Complications of cerebrospinal fluid shunt. An Esp Pediatr 48:368–370
12. Goodman R, Meltzer H, Bailey V (1998) The strengths and difficulties questionnaire: a pilot study on the validity of the self-report version. Eur Child Adolesc Psychiatry 7:125–130
13. Govender ST, Nathoo N, van Dellen JR (2003) Evaluation of an antibiotic-impregnated shunt system for the treatment of hydrocephalus. J Neurosurg 99:831–839
14. Gupta N, Park J, Solomon C et al (2007) Long-term outcomes in patients with treated childhood hydrocephalus. J Neurosurg 106:334–339
15. Hewer RL (1997) The economic impact of neurological illness on the health and wealth of the nation and of individuals. J Neurol Neurosurg Psychiatry 63(Suppl 1):S19–S23
16. Hoppe-Hirsch E, Laroussinie F, Brunet L et al (1998) Late outcome of the surgical treatment of hydrocephalus. Childs Nerv Syst 14:97–99
17. Iskandar BJ, Tubbs S, Mapstone TB et al (1998) Death in shunted hydrocephalic children in the 1990s. Pediatr Neurosurg 28:173–176
18. Jansen J, Jorgensen M (1986) Prognostic significance of signs and symptoms in hydrocephalus. Analysis of survival. Acta Neurol Scand 73:55–65
19. Kazui H, Mori E, Hashimoto M et al (2011) Effect of shunt operation on idiopathic normal pressure hydrocephalus patients in reducing caregiver burden: evidence from SINPHONI. Dement Geriatr Cogn Disord 31:363–370
20. Kestle JR, Hoffman HJ, Soloniuk D et al (1993) A concerted effort to prevent shunt infection. Childs Nerv Syst 9:163–165
21. Kestle JR, Riva-Cambrin J, Wellons JC 3rd et al (2011) A standardized protocol to reduce cerebrospinal fluid shunt infection: the hydrocephalus clinical research network quality improvement initiative. J Neurosurg Pediatr 8:22–29
22. Kulkarni AV, Cochrane DD, McNeely PD et al (2008) Medical, social, and economic factors associated with health-related quality of life in Canadian children with hydrocephalus. J Pediatr 153:689–695
23. Kulkarni AV, Drake JM, Kestle JR et al (2010) Endoscopic third ventriculostomy vs cerebrospinal fluid shunt in the treatment of hydrocephalus in children: a propensity score-adjusted analysis. Neurosurgery 67:588–593
24. Kulkarni AV, Drake JM, Lamberti-Pasculli M (2001) Cerebrospinal fluid shunt infection: a prospective study of risk factors. J Neurosurg 94:195–201
25. Kulkarni AV, Drake JM, Rabin D et al (2004) Measuring the health status of children with hydrocephalus by using a new outcome measure. J Neurosurg 101:141–146
26. Kulkarni AV, Rabin D, Drake JM (2004) An instrument to measure the health status in children with hydrocephalus: the hydrocephalus outcome questionnaire. J Neurosurg 101:134–140
27. Kulkarni AV, Riva-Cambrin J, Butler J et al (2013) Outcomes of CSF shunting in children: comparison of hydrocephalus clinical research network cohort with historical controls: clinical article. J Neurosurg Pediatr 12:334–338
28. Kulkarni AV, Shams I (2007) Quality of life in children with hydrocephalus: results from the hospital for sick children, Toronto. J Neurosurg 107:358–364
29. Lacy M, Pyykkonen BA, Hunter SJ et al (2008) Intellectual functioning in children with early shunted posthemorrhagic hydrocephalus. Pediatr Neurosurg 44:376–381
30. Lee WC (1997) Quantifying the future impact of disease on society: life table-based measures of potential life lost. Am J Public Health 87:1456–1460

31. Li L, Padhi A, Ranjeva SL et al (2011) Association of bacteria with hydrocephalus in Ugandan infants. J Neurosurg Pediatr 7:73–87
32. Lindquist B, Carlsson G, Persson EK et al (2005) Learning disabilities in a population-based group of children with hydrocephalus. Acta Paediatr 94:878–883
33. Lindquist B, Persson EK, Uvebrant P et al (2008) Learning, memory and executive functions in children with hydrocephalus. Acta Paediatr 97:596–601
34. Liptak GS, McDonald JV (1985) Ventriculoperitoneal shunts in children: factors affecting shunt survival. Pediatr Neurosci 12:289–293
35. McGirt MJ, Leveque JC, Wellons JC 3rd et al (2002) Cerebrospinal fluid shunt survival and etiology of failures: a seven-year institutional experience. Pediatr Neurosurg 36:248–255
36. Msall ME, DiGaudio K, Rogers BT et al (1994) The functional independence measure for children (WeeFIM). Conceptual basis and pilot use in children with developmental disabilities. Clin Pediatr (Phila) 33:421–430
37. Patwardhan RV, Nanda A (2005) Implanted ventricular shunts in the United States: the billion-dollar-a-year cost of hydrocephalus treatment. Neurosurgery 56:139–144; discussion 144–5
38. Paulsen AH, Lundar T, Lindegaard KF (2010) Twenty-year outcome in young adults with childhood hydrocephalus: assessment of surgical outcome, work participation, and health-related quality of life. J Neurosurg Pediatr 6:527–535
39. Pollack IF, Albright AL, Adelson PD (1999) A randomized, controlled study of a programmable shunt valve versus a conventional valve for patients with hydrocephalus. hakim-medos investigator group. Neurosurgery 45:1399–1408; discussion 1408–11
40. Sato O, Yamguchi T, Kittaka M et al (2001) Hydrocephalus and epilepsy. Childs Nerv Syst 17:76–86
41. Shannon CN, Simon TD, Reed GT et al (2011) The economic impact of ventriculoperitoneal shunt failure. J Neurosurg Pediatr 8:593–599
42. Simon TD, Riva-Cambrin J, Srivastava R et al (2008) Hospital care for children with hydrocephalus in the United States: utilization, charges, comorbidities, and deaths. J Neurosurg Pediatr 1:131–137
43. Stagno V, Navarrete EA, Mirone G et al (2013) Management of hydrocephalus around the world. World Neurosurg 79:S23.e17–S23.e20
44. Topczewska-Lach E, Lenkiewicz T, Olanski W et al (2005) Quality of life and psychomotor development after surgical treatment of hydrocephalus. Eur J Pediatr Surg 15:2–5
45. Tuli S, Drake J, Lawless J et al (2000) Risk factors for repeated cerebrospinal shunt failures in pediatric patients with hydrocephalus. J Neurosurg 92:31–38
46. Tuli S, Tuli J, Drake J et al (2004) Predictors of death in pediatric patients requiring cerebrospinal fluid shunts. J Neurosurg 100:442–446
47. Upadhyaya P, Bhargava S, Dube S et al (1982) Results of ventriculoatrial shunt surgery for hydrocephalus using Indian shunt valve: evaluation of intellectual performance with particular reference to computerized axial tomography. Prog Pediatr Surg 15:209–222
48. Warf BC (2005) Hydrocephalus in Uganda: the predominance of infectious origin and primary management with endoscopic third ventriculostomy. J Neurosurg 102:1–15
49. Warf BC, East African Neurosurgical Research Collaboration (2010) Pediatric hydrocephalus in east Africa: prevalence, causes, treatments, and strategies for the future. World Neurosurg 73:296–300
50. Wilkie MD, Hanson MF, Statham PF et al (2013) Infections of cerebrospinal fluid diversion devices in adults: the role of intraventricular antimicrobial therapy. J Infect 66:239–246
51. Williams MA, Sharkey P, van Doren D et al (2007) Influence of shunt surgery on healthcare expenditures of elderly fee-for-service medicare beneficiaries with hydrocephalus. J Neurosurg 107:21–28
52. Wu Y, Green NL, Wrensch MR et al (2007) Ventriculoperitoneal shunt complications in California: 1990 to 2000. Neurosurgery 61:557–562; discussion 562–3

Clinical Manifestations of CSF Shunt Complications

2

Juan F. Martínez-Lage, Antonio L. López-Guerrero, and María-José Almagro

Contents

2.1 **Introduction: Hydrocephalus and Shunt Problems** 13
2.2 **General Scope of Hydrocephalus and CSF Shunt Revisions** 14
2.3 **Terms, Concepts, and Definitions** 14
2.3.1 Shunt Structure 15
2.3.2 Types of CSF Draining Systems 16
2.3.3 Shunt Failure, Shunt Malfunction, and Complications 16
2.4 **Clinical Manifestations of Shunt Failure** 16
2.4.1 General Clinical Features of Shunt Failure 16
2.4.2 Clinical Features of Mechanical Failures 17
2.4.3 Age as a Risk Factor for Shunt Dysfunction 18
2.4.4 Early vs. Late Shunt Failures 20
2.4.5 Role of Hydrocephalus Etiology in Shunt Failure 20
2.4.6 Malfunction in Different Draining Spaces 22
2.5 **How Does Shunt Infection Manifest?** 23
2.6 **Functional Complications** 24
2.6.1 Clinical Manifestations of Underdrainage 24
2.6.2 Clinical Features in Overdrainage 25
2.7 **Hemorrhage as a Complication of CSF Shunting** 25
2.8 **Epilepsy Related to CSF Shunting** 27
2.9 **Making the Diagnosis of Shunt Failure** 27
Conclusions 29
References 29

J.F. Martínez-Lage, MD (✉)
A.L. López-Guerrero, MD • M.-J. Almagro, MD
Pediatric Neurosurgery Section and Regional Service of Neurosurgery, Virgen de la Arrixaca University Hospital, 30120 El Palmar, Murcia, Spain
e-mail: juanf.martinezlage@gmail.com; lopezlopezguerrero@yahoo.es; mjalmagronavarro@yahoo.es

2.1 Introduction: Hydrocephalus and Shunt Problems

CSF shunts constitute the mainstay of treatment for hydrocephalus of diverse etiologies and are among the most common procedures performed in pediatric neurosurgery [88]. For practical purposes, hydrocephalus can be classified into two main groups: obstructive and communicating (nonobstructive) aimed at indicating the two most popular techniques for its treatment, CSF shunting or endoscopic third ventriculostomy (ETV). Most cases of obstructive hydrocephalus are now treated with neuroendoscopic procedures, mainly ETV, while CSF shunts continue to be utilized for treatment of many cases of both obstructive and nonobstructive hydrocephalus.

At present, the use of shunting procedures is questioned due to the large number of complications with which they are plagued. However, shunts have saved the life of a considerable number of patients, have decreased morbidity and mortality, and have improved the quality of life of many individuals with hydrocephalus.

C. Di Rocco et al. (eds.), *Complications of CSF Shunting in Hydrocephalus: Prevention, Identification, and Management*, DOI 10.1007/978-3-319-09961-3_2,

Accordingly, the continued use of CSF shunting procedures and the increasing use of ETV justify an account of the symptoms and signs with which complications are apt of manifesting in this setting.

2.2 General Scope of Hydrocephalus and CSF Shunt Revisions

According to Bondurant and Jimenez, there are approximately 125,000 hospital discharges with the diagnosis of hydrocephalus each year in the USA, comprising 36,000 shunt-related procedures and 33,000 placement of shunts with an economic cost of 100 millions of USA $ a year. Nearly half of this amount is spent on shunt revisions [7]. Massimi et al. noted a recent change in the epidemiology of hydrocephalus [54]. These authors observed a decrease in the incidence of hydrocephalus related to myelomeningocele, aqueduct stenosis, CNS infections, craniocerebral malformations, and head injuries. The rate of posthemorrhagic hydrocephalus remains stable, while the incidence of tumor-associated hydrocephalus is on the rise [54]. In our mean, approximately 40 % of pediatric neurosurgical operations have to do with hydrocephalus and its complications. We have also observed a steady decrease in the number of new cases of infantile hydrocephalus attributable to better prevention measures, to prenatal diagnosis, and to improvement in neonatal care. There is also a diminution in the rate of surgical revisions probably related to the reduction in the global incidence of hydrocephalus, to the generalized use in our mean of programmable valves, and to the introduction of ETV. We have not appreciated significant changes in the incidence of operations for normal pressure hydrocephalus (NPH).

Wong et al. have recently reported the patterns of neurosurgical adverse events of CSF shunt surgery [88]. Shunt failure constitutes a serious problem with a cost of 1.4–2 billion dollars in hospital charges a year. Wong et al. analyzed 14,683 new ventricular shunts implanted in pediatric and adult patients. Failures during the first year may have an incidence as high as 50–70 % and an estimated rate of 5 % yearly thereafter [87]. Table 2.1 summarizes the distribution of the commonest reported complications of hydrocephalus treatment. Briefly, adverse events of surgical treatment of hydrocephalus can be classified into three groups: (a) mechanical, (b) infectious, and (c) functional. Iatrogenic failures will be dealt with in a separate chapter.

Table 2.1 Incidence of CSF shunt complications

Type of complication	%
Mechanical complications: proximal catheter, valve, or distal catheter obstruction, disconnection, fracture, migration, etc.	8–64
Functional complications (under- and overdrainage)	3–50
Shunt infection	3–12
Intra-abdominal complications (only in peritoneal shunts)	1–24
Intracranial hemorrhage	4
Epilepsy	20–30

2.3 Terms, Concepts, and Definitions

Hydrocephalus consists of an excessive accumulation of cerebrospinal fluid (CSF) within the cavities of the brain or around it. Concerning *etiology*, the causes of hydrocephalus are often grouped into congenital or acquired and may result from a variety of pathological processes such as congenital and malformative conditions, intracranial hemorrhage, infection, trauma, and brain tumors or cysts (Table 2.2). Regarding *pathophysiology*, hydrocephalus is the result of excessive production, flow obstruction, or impaired reabsorption of CSF. Hydrocephalus may involve different cranial cavities and is often described, mainly by neuroradiologists, as mono-, bi-, tri-, or tetraventricular referring to the number of dilated ventricles proximal to the site of obstruction. *External hydrocephalus* consists of the extra-axial accumulation of fluid probably by impaired absorption. *Arachnoid cysts* have also been considered as localized forms of hydrocephalus and communicating hydromyelia as a

Table 2.2 Etiology of hydrocephalus

Origin	Cause of hydrocephalus
Congenital	Sylvian aqueduct stenosis
	Antenatal communicating of undetermined cause
	Stenosis/atresia of ventricular foramina
	Dandy-Walker malformation
	Intracranial cysts
	Chiari malformations I and II
	Craniofacial anomalies
	Vein of Galen aneurysm
	Antenatal CNS infection
	Storage diseases
Acquired	Posthemorrhagic (prematurity)
	Posthemorrhagic (adults)
	Tumoral (obstructive or areabsortive)
	Postinfectious and parasitic (obstructive or areabsortive)
	Posttraumatic
Normal pressure hydrocephalus	

form of intramedullary hydrocephalus [44, 52]. *Normal pressure hydrocephalus* (NPH) is a condition of poorly known origin and is now also termed chronic hydrocephalus of the adult [64].

In relation to *temporal occurrence*, hydrocephalus may present in acute, subacute, or chronic forms. Hydrocephalus may be *active* or *passive* and has to be differentiated from brain *atrophy*. This is particularly true in the case of children afflicted with destructive brain diseases as infections, hemorrhage, or trauma to the central nervous system (CNS). Elderly patients or those with arterial hypertension, atherosclerosis, diabetes mellitus, previous cerebrovascular accidents, or small ischemic brain lesions may also show brain atrophy in imaging studies.

Arrested hydrocephalus means adequately treated (shunted) hydrocephalus. *Compensated hydrocephalus* refers to all other forms of hydrocephalus at various levels of compensation that often entails some cost to the patient. *Uncompensated hydrocephalus* in children refers to progressive ventricular enlargement, usually accompanied by macrocephaly. The term uncompensated hydrocephalus is also applied to a situation of stable ventricles associated with developmental delay, cognitive impairment, impaired consciousness, or progressive neurological deficit. The concept of "cure" is rarely applied for shunted hydrocephalus given the current uncertainty for diagnosis even when intracranial pressure (ICP) monitoring or hydrodynamic tests are utilized. According to Rekate, children with communicating hydrocephalus have a probability as high as 50 % of becoming shunt independent at a later age [67]. Patients with doubtful diagnosis of hydrocephalus usually give equivocal results on current tests that justify the exceptional use of the term cure referring to hydrocephalus. Therefore, it seems reasonable to review children with ventriculomegaly if they are neurologically stable and if psychomotor development remains on time. Patients in this situation should be followed up closely even with serial ophthalmologic and psychometric studies.

2.3.1 Shunt Structure

CSF shunts divert the excess of fluid from the ventricles (or other fluid-filled spaces, as subdural collections and intracranial cysts) to another body cavity. Basically, a shunt is composed of three components: a proximal (ventricular) catheter, the valve, and a distal catheter. These pieces can be manufactured in separated parts that are assembled at the time of insertion or be manufactured in a single kit called *unishunt*. Most shunts may also contain accessories such as integrated *pumping devices* or *reservoirs*, and they may also be supplied with an independent *antisiphon device* or with a siphon-controlling device integrated in the valve.

Most valves are of differential pressure type, flow regulated, or anti-gravitational. Valves may also be of fixed pressure (low, medium, or high pressure), or they may be externally adjustable (programmable valves). The internal mechanism that regulates CSF flow and pressure of the valve may consist of slits, diaphragm, ball and spring, or miter mechanisms. The components of the shunt are made up of silicone, complemented with other polypropylene or hardened plastic parts or with metallic connectors. Some silicone tubing is cured with silver for increasing resistance to stretching or kinking, while barium impregnation of the tubes is commonly utilized for radiologic identification of the integrity of the shunt.

2.3.2 Types of CSF Draining Systems

The most popular type of shunting device is the ventriculoperitoneal shunt (VP), followed by ventriculopleural, ventriculoatrial (VA), lumboperitoneal (LP), and more rarely ventriculo-gallbladder (VGB) shunt. Other types of CSF shunt systems are presently considered only of historic interest. External ventricular drainage (EVD) consists of a temporary device endowed with a ventricular (or subdural) catheter that connects with a collecting bag. A variety of CSF drainage is the ventriculo-subgaleal shunt that drains the ventricular CSF to the subgaleal space and is commonly used as a temporizing measure for controlling ICP especially following ventricular hemorrhage or infection. In addition, ETV is a form of internal derivation of CSF that communicates the floor of the third ventricle with the basal cisterns. At present, ETV is more and more utilized for avoiding the innumerable complications of CSF shunting.

2.3.3 Shunt Failure, Shunt Malfunction, and Complications

The term *shunt failure* is not well defined in the current literature. The most accepted view is that shunt failure consists of the inability to reach the goal of surgery. In CSF shunting, failure refers to the incapability of accomplishing an appropriate control of hydrocephalus (as opposed to success) indicated by revision, replacement, or removal of the shunt. The term *complication* refers to any adverse event that interferes with the expected success of the procedure including new insertions, revisions, or replacements of the valve. Complications may or may not be related with the surgical technique or the valve, and may or may not end with shunt revision or replacement. Complications may derive from problems related to the valve, the patient, or the surgery. In many occasions, the terms failure and complication are interchangeably used in the literature. The variety of devices and accessories employed for shunting of CSF attests for the lack of a rigorous knowledge of the mechanisms involved in the pathophysiology of hydrocephalus and the lack of established guidelines for its treatment. In addition, no CSF shunt has demonstrated its superiority over other shunt type.

2.4 Clinical Manifestations of Shunt Failure

As stated before, shunt failure refers to any condition that ends in revision, replacement, or removal of a CSF valve or even in the patient's death. Failure may be related to (a) mechanical malfunction, (b) infection, or (c) over- or underdrainage.

2.4.1 General Clinical Features of Shunt Failure

Shunt failure can show up in several ways and may proceed with a rapid or slow onset and variable evolution. Shunt malfunction may appear *acutely*, with alarming signs of brain herniation, i.e., rapidly declining level of consciousness, pupillary changes, posturing, apneic spells, and bradycardia, indicating that we are facing an emergent situation [1, 25, 40]. Patients arriving in hospital in this way let little time for reflection and need emergent management. More often, *subacute* shunt failure appears in a less stressful scenario that permits calm assessment and allows time for planning the appropriate (medical or surgical) management. Shunt malfunction can also present with *chronic* manifestations such as mild psychomotor retardation, decreased vision, impaired ocular motility, unsteady gait and falls, mood changes, decreased school performance, increased tone and reflexes in the lower limbs, or symptoms and signs of brain stem involvement or of hydromyelia [51, 57]. In patients operated on for NPH, shunt failure is proclaimed by return to their presurgical situation. Patients show slow mental deterioration, urinary urgency or incontinence, and a worsening gait. Headaches, dizziness, and focal symptoms or signs appear exceptionally in NPH patients with shunt malfunction.

2.4.2 Clinical Features of Mechanical Failures

Mechanical malfunction is the most frequent cause of CSF shunt failure. Its incidence may be as high as 50 % in children [4]. Shunt malfunction may be due to proximal catheter obstruction (the most common), valve obstruction, distal catheter occlusion, disconnections of shunt parts, fracture of the tubing, or migration of the proximal or distal catheters. Brain debris, choroid plexus, blood, or tissue reactions often occlude proximal catheters. Slit ventricles and faulty placement of the catheter within the ventricle may also interfere with the flow through the catheter.

On the contrary, the valve itself appears as the most dependable part of the shunt system. Obstruction of the valve is very rare and, in our experience, it happened in very few cases, and it was almost always produced by blood clots [42]. Breakage of the valve itself may occur without any apparent cause or may follow a cranial traumatism. Obstruction of the distal catheter generally occurs in systems with distal slit valves and very rarely in open-ended catheters [15]. In exceptional occasions, the distal tube may be occluded by fecal contents indicating bowel perforation. In the abdomen, distal catheters may be occluded by ingrowth of mesothelial cells and fibroblasts [17]. Kinking of the tube is also of very rare occurrence and is always due to a defective placement.

Detachment of ventricular catheters is almost exclusively due to a loose ligature or to using absorbable sutures. Separations of distal catheters generally occur at the site of connection to the valve, even in systems with soldered components. Stress rupture of the shunt tubing, in one or several pieces, usually takes place on the anterior neck or upper part of the chest wall and is favored by sustained or repeated stretching or friction. Notable deterioration of drainage systems usually occurs in shunts implanted for more than 5 years [20]. Rupture and disconnections mainly happen when there exist biodegradation and calcification of the outer surface of the tubes (Fig. 2.1) caused by aging of the device [6, 17, 20, 21, 76]. Resistance to rupture perhaps might be improved by incorporating tubes to the shunt device with a greater cross-sectional area [79].

Proximal catheters, reservoirs, and even the entire shunt may migrate into the brain, the ventricle, the scalp, or the subgaleal space. In occasions, catheter migration is accompanied by the valve (Fig. 2.2) or reservoir itself [12, 24, 42, 72]. Hydrogel-coated (BioGlide) catheters (devised to decrease cell adhesion aimed at reducing shunt obstruction and infection) seem to be more prone to disconnection and intracranial migration than standard devices [12]. In the same way, the proximal catheter (and its accompanying reservoir or valve) may be pulled out of the ventricle and be displaced down toward the subcutaneous tract. The distal catheter may be stretched out of the peritoneum too, migrating to the subcutaneous abdominal or thoracic tract or into the pleural space, or it may even follow an upward course and penetrate the skull, ventricle, etc. [43, 78]. Detached or broken distal catheters may totally migrate and lodge into the peritoneal cavity.

There are anecdotal reports on perforations and migrations of the distal tubing into the bowel, stomach, liver and gallbladder, scrotum, urinary bladder, pleural space, bronchi, and heart. Bowel perforation seems to be the most severe form of this complication [16]. Extrusion of shunts may take place through the anus, umbilicus, mouth, vagina, operation scars, midlumbar region, etc. [16, 19, 29].

Distal catheters of VA valves may also break or disconnect and stay in situ or migrate to the right heart ventricle, right atrium, pulmonary arteries, or cava vein [36]. All these mechanical complications habitually show the signs and symptoms reported above and are intimately related to the body cavity where the shunt drains (peritoneum, pleura, heart, lumbar spine, etc.).

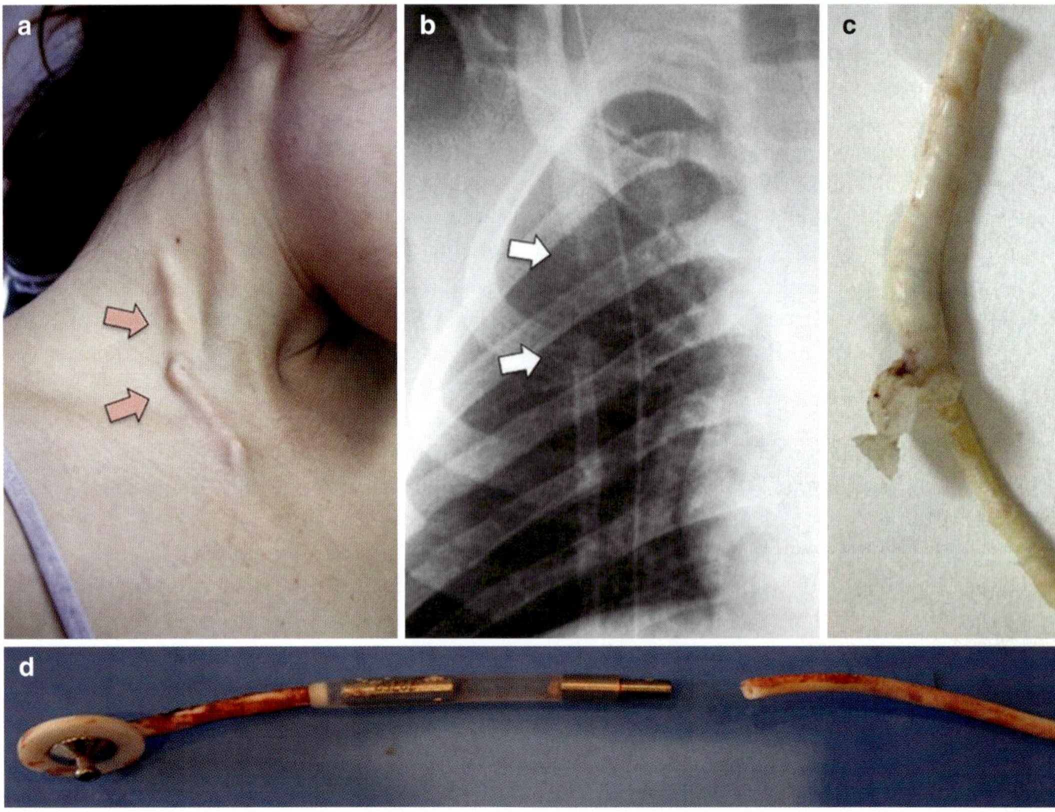

Fig. 2.1 (**a**) Photograph of a 20-year-old patient showing calcified subcutaneous shunt tubing (*arrows*), (**b**) radiograph illustrating the calcified tube (*arrows*), (**c**) photograph of the removed catheter, (**d**) photograph of a removed broken and calcified shunt

2.4.3 Age as a Risk Factor for Shunt Dysfunction

Complications of CSF shunting are more prevalent in *neonates and infants* due to the special characteristics these patients possess [18, 19, 48]. There is an increased incidence of both shunt malfunction and shunt infection in this age group in comparison with older children and adults. This vulnerability is due to brain immaturity, skull flexibility, skin fragility (Fig. 2.3a), and compromised immunity. In neonates and infants, irritability, vomiting, decreased appetite, and lethargy, together with bradycardia and apneic episodes, indicate shunt malfunction. Bradycardia and apnea constitute a very reliable indication of shunt failure [40]. Clinical examination findings include abnormal growth of head circumference, bulging of the anterior fontanel (Fig. 2.3a), suture diastasis, sunsetting eyes, and dilated scalp veins (Table 2.3). Palpation of the anterior fontanel may give a reliable estimate of intracranial pressure and is a very dependable sign in children with open skull bones (Fig. 2.3b).

Shunt failure in *older children* and *adults* manifests itself with an almost constant *triad* that consists of headaches, vomiting, and somnolence [4]. Other complaints include blurred or failing vision, squint, loss of appetite, mood changes, and new onset or increase in the number of seizures. Table 2.4 shows some frequent (and less frequent) symptoms and signs of shunt malfunction in older children and adults. Differential diagnosis in children who present with vague symptoms must be made against common infantile diseases, especially gastrointestinal viral diseases or mild upper respiratory tract infections. Children are also prone to experience otitis

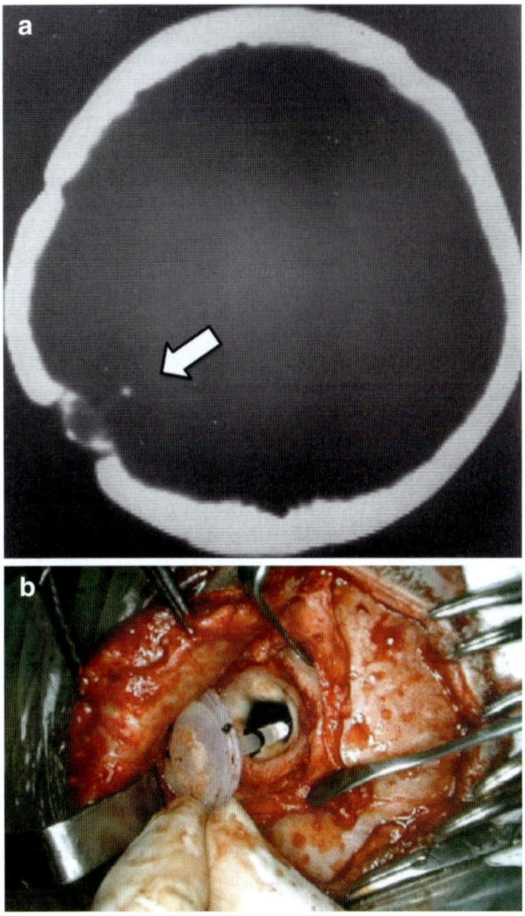

Fig. 2.2 (**a**) CT scan depicting partial intracranial migration of a valve reservoir (*arrow*), (**b**) intraoperative photograph during replacement of the reservoir. Note the enlarged cerebral orifice

media, and individuals with myelomeningocele often suffer from repeated urinary infections that may resemble (or mask) those of shunt failure.

Less often, shunt malfunction evolves with chronic and subtle clinical features as failing vision, mood and behavioral changes, gait clumsiness, frequent falls, regression or stagnation of developmental milestones, or even with deficient schooling progression. Clinical examination may show papilledema, spastic paraparesis, hypertonus, hyperreflexia, uni- or bilateral sixth cranial nerve palsy, cervical defense, spinal rigidity, erythema, palpable pseudotumors, or fluid collections along the shunt tract (Fig. 2.4a, b). Rupture or disconnection of the distal catheter can be diagnosed by palpating the entire shunt along the trajectory through the subcutaneous tissue. Partial calcification of distal catheters indicates tube degradation and should raise the suspicion of catheter breakage with or without intra-abdominal migration (Fig. 2.1). In peritoneal shunts, features of shunt malfunction referred to the abdominal cavity are usually the most striking (Table 2.4).

There is a group of pediatric patients who are admitted repeatedly to hospital with repeated shunt failure ("poor-shunt patients") [81]. The main cause for recurring malfunction is proximal catheter obstruction. Known causative factors for this complication are a younger age at insertion, overdrainage, concurrent other surgeries, and certain causes of hydrocephalus [81].

Bergsneider et al. and Vinchon et al. [5, 84] reported several forms of shunt dysfunction in adults with pediatric-onset hydrocephalus and have also given an account of other related conditions such as *adult slit ventricle* syndrome, multi-compartmental hydrocephalus, newly diagnosed noncommunicating hydrocephalus, and non-NPH and NPH hydrocephalus [5]. Risk factors for shunt malfunction in adults has been especially described in VA shunts especially after previous multiple external drainages [32]. Adult NPH patients with shunt malfunction often return to hospital with the complaints of deterioration in comparison with the amelioration noted immediately after shunting. Clinical features in this group of patients consist of worsening gait, aggravation of urinary problems, and failing memory. Rarely these patients complain of headaches, mental dullness, dizziness, or seizures. Physical examination shows increased reflexes and Babinski sign, gait ataxia, parkinsonism, and signs of frontal release as sucking and grasping reflexes. Muscle strength is normal and there is no sensory loss. However, the appearance of focal signs, as hemiparesis, should raise the suspicion of a subdural hematoma. In an extensive series of chronic subdural hematomas, six instances (0.6 %) were associated with shunted hydrocephalus and presented with behavioral disturbances or headaches [26].

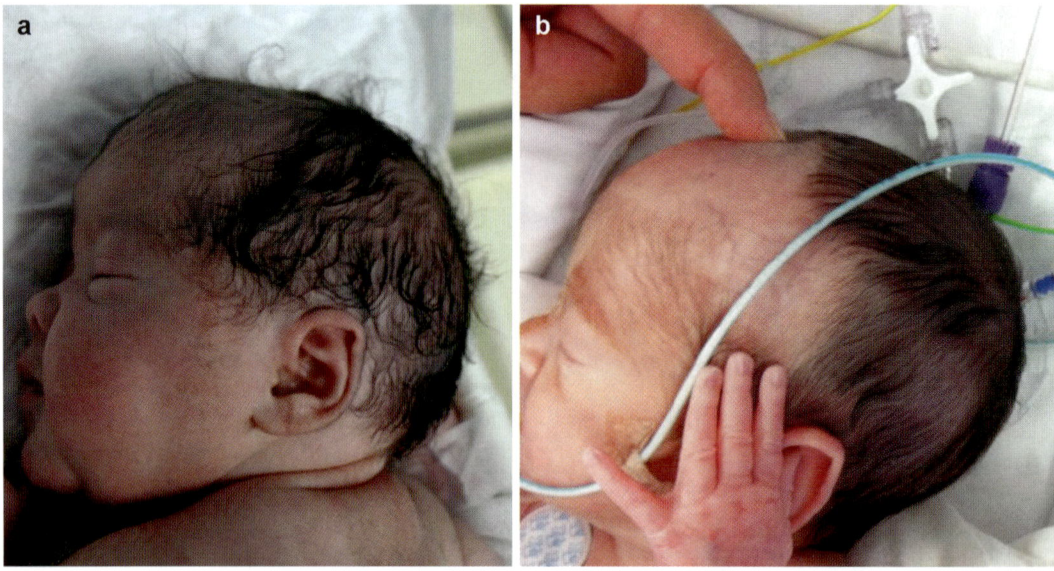

Fig. 2.3 (**a**) Photograph of an infant with a bulging fontanel soon after valve revision, (**b**) photograph showing the technique of fontanel palpation

Table 2.3 Symptoms and signs of shunt malfunction in infants

Symptom	Sign
Irritability	Increasing head circumference
Vomiting	Bulging fontanel
Somnolence	Suture diastasis
	Dilated scalp veins
Poor feeding	Sunsetting eyes
Decreased activity	Axial hypotonus, limb hypertonus/hyperreflexia
Unspecific symptoms	Bradycardia
	Apneic episodes
	Fluid collections around reservoir, valve, or shunt tract
	Swelling/erythema along shunt tract
	Skin breakdown, skin erosion, CSF leakage
Most reliable: irritability, vomiting, bulging fontanel, and sunsetting eyes	

2.4.4 Early vs. Late Shunt Failures

The majority of early complications occurs in the first year after shunt insertion and is in relation with patient age and condition, the surgical technique, and the function of the shunt itself. The most frequent reasons for early failure both in children and adults are proximal catheter obstruction and shunt infection [23]. In our experience, technical problems related to valve placement and inadequate selection of valve's characteristics (pressure and size) may cause early shunt failure too. Late shunt dysfunction is almost exclusively due to proximal or distal catheter block or to fracture or disconnection in relation with problems pertaining to aging of the implanted material and to late infection. The hazard of shunt failure decreases as a function of time in both newly placed and revised shunts: "the longer a shunt functions, the less likely it is to fail" [53]. The rate of shunt infection decreases as a function of time too. Mc Girt reported a 14 % rate of failures for all shunts during the first month after shunt implant and only a 5 % rate beyond 4 years [53]. Obviously, shortening of the distal catheter due to the child's growth is also a late age-related cause of shunt failure.

2.4.5 Role of Hydrocephalus Etiology in Shunt Failure

There is no agreement in different studies as to the role played by etiology of hydrocephalus in the rate of subsequent shunt complications.

Table 2.4 Symptoms and signs of shunt malfunction in older children and adults

Symptom	Sign
Headaches	Papilledema
Vomiting	Decreased level of consciousness
Somnolence	Fluid collection along shunt tract
Drowsiness	Hyperreflexia
Blurred vision/diplopia	Limb hypertonus
Loss of vision	Spastic paraparesis
Neck/back pain	Bradycardia/Tachycardia
"Shuntalgia"	Macrocephaly
Instability/ataxic gait/falls	Sixth cranial nerve palsy/squint
Vague symptoms	Upward gaze palsy
Increase in seizures	Palpable gap in the shunt tract
Worsening psychomotor development	Pseudotumoral mass around shunt tubing/calcified tubing
Ataxia	Apneic spells/respiratory arrest
Syncope	Tetraparesis
Schooling difficulties	Abdominal guarding/distension
Abdominal pain/constipation	Chest pain/cough
Dyspnea	
In NPH: failure to improve/return to presurgical condition	
Most common: headaches, vomiting, somnolence, and papilledema	

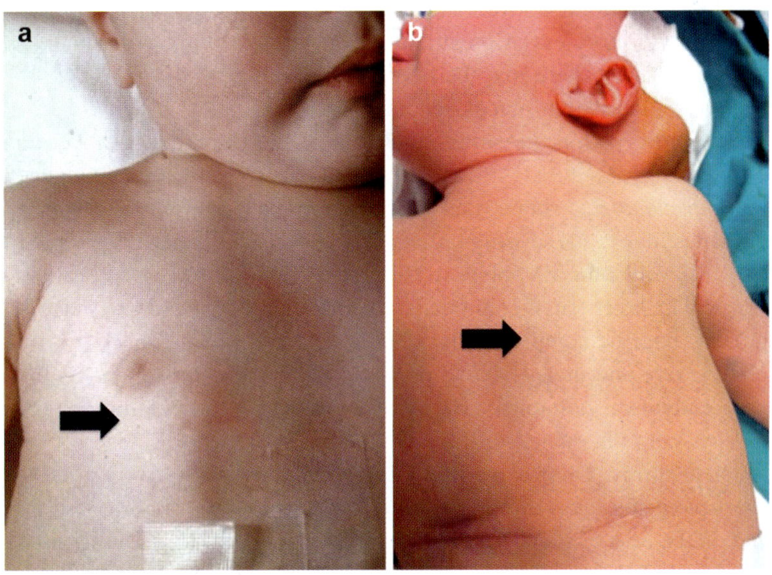

Fig. 2.4 (**a**) Photograph illustrating skin reddening along the thoracic wall in a child with shunt infection (*arrow*), (**b**) photograph of the thoracic tract of a VP shunt showing subcutaneous accumulation of fluid (*arrow*)

Some find no differences between the diverse causes of hydrocephalus in the occurrence of shunt failures [28, 63]. However, others report an increased rate of shunt malfunction in patients with intraventricular hemorrhage, meningitis, or tumors [37, 39, 63]. Reported risk factors in tumoral hydrocephalus comprise age, tumor histology, and concurrent or prior surgical procedures (external ventricular drains, craniotomy, etc.) [66]. There is a higher rate of severe complications in myelomeningocele patients with the Chiari II malformation at the time of shunt malfunction. These patients may suffer early damage to the brain stem and upper cervical cord that causes breathing problems and quadriparesis [25, 51, 57].

2.4.6 Malfunction in Different Draining Spaces

Ventriculoperitoneal shunts may fail due to numerous causes as ascites (Fig. 2.5a), hernias, hydrocele, ileus, intussusception, torsion of omental cyst, peritonitis, peritoneal pseudocyst, volvulus, perforation of viscus, peritoneal pseudotumor, and catheter extrusion through several places (umbilicus, rectum, vagina, scrotum, mouth, gastrostomy wound, etc.). Most of these complications usually evolve with features of shunt malfunction and/or with those of infection [16]. An often overlooked cause of shunt malfunction is severe constipation (Fig. 2.5b) that causes increased intra-abdominal pressure thus impairing CSF drainage from the ventricles [49, 54, 71].

Malfunction of *ventriculopleural* valves is generally due to accumulation of fluid in the pleura (aseptic hydrothorax), pneumothorax, and rarely to pleural empyema or fibrothorax [45, 80]. Symptoms of thoracic involvement include chest pain, cough, shortness of breath, and tachypnea. On examination there may be decreased breath sounds, dullness on percussion, subcutaneous emphysema, pallor, sweating, tachypnea, and cyanosis.

Ventriculoatrial shunts are at present rarely implanted due to the severity of the problems that they may originate. VA valves in children require frequent catheter lengthening due to the patients' growth. Specific complications of VA valves are often severe and include bland or septic pulmonary embolism, pulmonary hypertension, endocarditis, cor pulmonale, cardiac arrhythmias, and shunt nephritis. Clinical manifestations include chest pain, shortness of breath, low-grade fever, and, in the case of shunt nephritis sepsis, hepatosplenomegaly, arterial hypertension, hematuria, and proteinuria [61, 83].

Lumboperitoneal shunts are used in communicating hydrocephalus, NPH, pseudotumor cerebri, CSF fistulas, and postsurgical pseudomeningocele. LP valves have a high rate of complications [14, 85]. One of their main drawbacks of LP shunts is the difficulty they present for assessing their function. Morbidity of LP shunts may be due to mechanical complications (block,

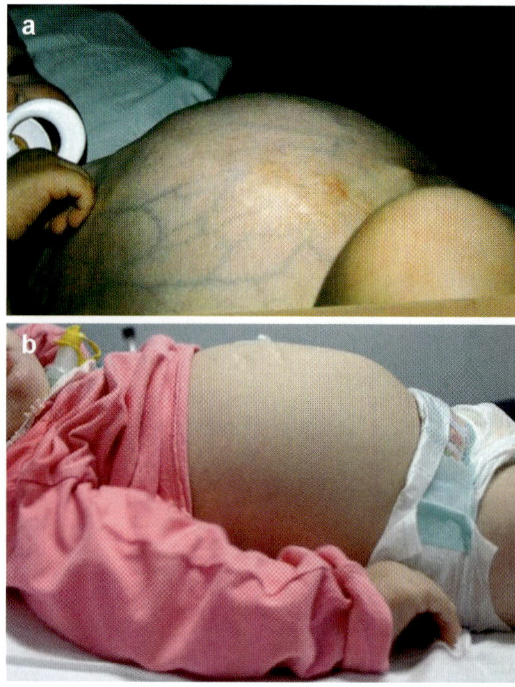

Fig. 2.5 Photographs of two patients: (**a**) one with ascites due to infection, (**b**) the other with abdominal distention due to chronic constipation

migration), overdrainage (subdural collections), infection, and development of acquired Chiari malformation. Acquired tonsillar herniation is the most feared complication, and it is thought to be more prevalent following the placement of valveless systems. Clinical features include back pain, back stiffness, sciatica, neurological involvement in the lower limbs, scoliosis, and those pertaining to symptomatic tonsillar herniation [14, 85].

Ventriculo-gallbladder shunts are indicated after failure of previously placed VP, VA, or ventriculopleural shunts. Complications comprise malfunction, disconnection, infection, gallbladder atony, gallbladder calculi, peritonitis, and bilious ventriculitis [27, 77].

Subdural-peritoneal shunts are used for draining subdural collections of fluid. Their main complications are blockage, infection, disconnection, migration (including intracranial migration of the entire system), CSF leakage, and skin ulceration, together with overdrainage that may produce cranioencephalic disproportion and proximal catheter adherence to brain surface at removal [22, 34].

Ventriculo-subgaleal shunts are currently used for temporary control of hydrocephalus of intraventricular hemorrhage in premature neonates. These shunts may present with infection, blockage, CSF leakage from the wound, and intracranial hemorrhage and with pressure-related head molding caused by compression from the subgaleal collection of fluid.

2.5 How Does Shunt Infection Manifest?

Ventricular shunt infection is a common complication of CSF shunting that causes high morbidity and mortality. A recent study on infection after initial CSF shunting in children, comprising 7,071 children, reported 825 shunt infections that produced 4,434 shunt revisions [74]. During a 24-month follow-up, CSF shunt infection rates were 11.7 % per patient and 7.2 % per procedure. Significant risk factors for infection ($p<0.05$) included young age, female sex, Afro-American race, public insurance, intraventricular hemorrhage, respiratory complex chronic conditions, subsequent revisions, hospital volume, and surgeon case volume [74]. Predictors of infection in a cohort of 979 shunted patients, 130 (13 %) comprised bacterial growth in CSF, of which 58 (5.9 %) had a final diagnosis of shunt infection [70]. Risk factors for shunt contamination comprise recent (<90 days) shunt surgery, fever, abdominal pain, CSF leak, and erythema or swelling along the shunt tract [70]. For these authors, an important feature discriminating between shunt failure and shunt infection after new placement or valve revision is the presence of fever and leukocytosis (>15,000) [70].

Risk factors for shunt infection in adults include previous CSF leaks, revisions for dysfunction, operation performed late in the day, and longer surgical time [32]. Most clinical manifestations of shunt failure cannot conclusively distinguish between malfunction and infection, except for cases in which clinical features and laboratory tests of shunt infection are clearly identifiable (Table 2.5).

Table 2.5 Symptoms and signs of shunt infection

Symptoms	Signs
Headache	Fever
Nausea/vomiting	Fluid collection along shunt tract
Feeding problems	Erythema along shun tract
Lethargy	Cellulitis
Irritability	Incisional wound infection/ frank pus discharge
Changes in sensorium	Nuchal rigidity/meningeal signs
Neck/back pain	
Abdominal pain	Abdominal distention/ guarding
Diarrhea/constipation	Palpable intra-abdominal mass
Respiratory symptoms: chest pain, cough, dyspnea	Respiratory insufficiency signs/hypoventilation/ tachypnea

Common symptoms of shunt infection include those of shunt malfunction (headaches, vomiting, etc.) plus those of infection such as feeding problems, fever, malaise, fatigue, and lethargy. Signs include neck rigidity, swelling, erythema or cellulitis around the shunt tract (Fig. 2.4), leakage of CSF, or frank discharge of pus from the surgical incision. Prevention of skin ulceration over the valve involves choosing an adequate cranial site for valve placement and avoiding prominent zones of the head, especially in infants (Fig. 2.6a) and in debilitated or bedridden patients [33]. A scar over the valve reservoir (or other shunt component) suggests the probable infection of the device (Fig. 2.6b). However frank features corresponding to wound or tract contamination are seldom present. Low-grade infections by coagulase-negative staphylococci or other skin microorganisms account for the majority of shunt contamination, but in these cases obvious clinical features of infection, even hyperthermia, are usually lacking.

In peritoneal shunts (VP or LP), symptoms and signs of infection related to the abdomen usually are most prominent. The patients often complain of abdominal pain and distention, nausea and vomiting, or constipation. On examination, there may be abdominal tenderness, guarding and distention in peritonitis or ascites (Fig. 2.5a), or a

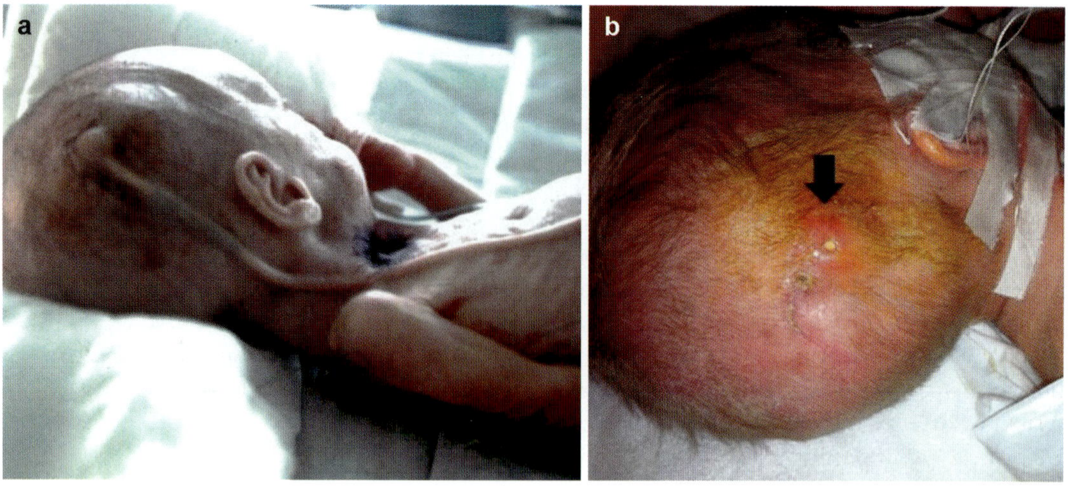

Fig. 2.6 (**a**) The image shows the extremely thin skin of a premature infant. The entire trajectory of the shunt can be easily viewed. (**b**) The photograph shows an exposed part of a valve reservoir (*arrow*)

palpable mass in the case of a pseudocyst. In VA shunts, early or late features of systemic infection, sepsis, or endocarditis may be the hallmark of the presence of valve infection. Shunt nephritis, a late form of VA shunt infection, usually evolves with sepsis, arterial hypertension, hematuria, and proteinuria. In ventriculopleural shunts, infection usually shows up with pleuritic pain, fever, tachypnea, dyspnea, or other features of respiratory tract involvement.

Meticulous surgical technique and extreme measures of asepsis are regarded as crucial for the prevention of shunt contamination [13, 82]. Modifications of surgical techniques include reduced personnel in the operating room, shunting as first case in the day, use of adhesive drapes on the skin, double gloving, no-touching technique, bathing the valve components with an antibiotic solution, meticulous wound closure to prevent CSF leakage, etc. There is some controversy on the role played by hair shaving on the incidence of shunt contamination, but the results are not conclusive [9]. Similarly, there are also unresolved discrepancies about the role played by the factor "experience of the surgeon" (trainees vs. experienced surgeons) on the infection rate [41, 74].

Regarding infection prophylaxis, we consider that the preparation of the surgical field is one of the most important actions to be taken for preventing shunt contamination. We customarily follow Venes's recommendations for preventing infections [81]. Patients are shaved immediately before operation. The skin is scrubbed with povidone iodine (Betadine) solution for 10 min and then covered with adhesive drapes. We also submerge the shunt components in a solution of vancomycin prior to insertion and use three doses of intravenous prophylactic antibiotics [48]. In a systematic literature review on the subject comprising 5,613 pediatric and adult shunting procedures, antibiotic-impregnated shunts resulted in a significant reduction of shunt infection over standard shunts and in no increase in microbial resistance to antibiotics [60].

2.6 Functional Complications

In this section of the chapter, we will briefly comment on the clinical features pertaining to diverse syndromes that produce intracranial hypotension or hypertension related with the use of CSF shunting and that are referred to as under- or overdrainage.

2.6.1 Clinical Manifestations of Underdrainage

Symptoms and signs of CSF underdrainage are those related to intracranial hypertension and that we have been already described (Tables 2.3

and 2.4). Underdrainage is most usually due to using a valve of a higher pressure than the one needed for the patient. Using siphoning-retarding devices or flow-controlled valves, especially in infants and young children, may cause decreased drainage too. Situations with increased pressure at the draining cavity can also lead to underdrainage, for example, increased peritoneal (or pleural) pressure as seen in obesity, pregnancy [87], abdominal tumors, constipation, etc. [49, 55, 71]. The drainage may also be affected by an inadequate absorption of hyperproteic CSF by the peritoneum resulting in ascites as happens with optic-chiasmatic tumors [86]. Multi-compartmental hydrocephalus drained by multiple catheters may lead to symptoms and signs of malfunction by an asymmetrical distribution of forces within the diverse cavities of the CNS.

Isolated fourth ventricle may present one or more of the following clinical features: involvement of cranial nerves sixth and seventh, hoarseness, dysphagia, dysarthria, bradycardia, diplopia, nystagmus, ataxia, irregular breathing, neck pain and rigidity, and hemiparesis as a result of pressure on the brain stem and high spinal cord. Occasionally, these symptoms are produced by a direct injury to the brain stem by a too long catheter [38, 59]. Increased CSF pressure in enlarged and trapped fourth ventricle may contribute to development of cervical spinal cord edema (presyrinx state) or of communicating hydromyelia with symptoms of brain stem involvement and quadriparesis [51, 57].

2.6.2 Clinical Features in Overdrainage

The most frequent symptom of CSF hyperdrainage is *orthostatic headaches* that are typically relieved by lying down in horizontal position. Many times orthostatic headaches are seen shortly after shunt insertion or revision and subside with time needing no further treatment. In neonates and infants with excessive drainage of CSF, the fontanel may be sunken and the sutures overlap (Fig. 2.7). The babies may also show decreased appetite and trunk hypotonus. Symptomatic subdural hematomas are exceptional in this age.

Most often, overdrainage in older children and adults induces the formation of subdural collections of fluid or chronic subdural hematomas by excessive drainage of CSF. These extra-axial collections may be asymptomatic or may cause focal neurological deficits. CSF overdrainage is also thought to be the origin of recurring episodes of proximal catheter obstruction with associated shunt malfunction. Enophthalmos may be a late sign of intracranial hypotension related to CSF overshunting [31].

Slit ventricle and *slit-ventricle syndrome* (SVS) have been the subject of many studies regarding pathogenesis and management [3, 11, 46, 68]. Slit ventricles, often found in routine imaging, are usually asymptomatic and do not require surgical treatment. On the contrary, the SVS produces severe symptoms as incapacitating headaches, vomiting, mood changes, failing vision, syncope, and mental confusion with variable changes in the state of consciousness. In severe cases, there may be impending signs of coma, brain herniation with bradycardia, apnea, fixed pupils, and posturing. SVS has been reported as being exclusive of patients of pediatric age, but features of this condition may also be found in adults [5]. SVS has not been reported in the presence of brain atrophy [19]. SVS may also occur in arachnoid cyst treated with cyst-peritoneal shunts [47, 52]. Another manifestation of CSF shunt overdrainage has been named *craniocerebral disproportion* and refers to a special form of functional or structural skull synostosis that results in brain compression [47]. Diagnosis and management of overdrainage syndromes will be discussed in a separate chapter.

2.7 Hemorrhage as a Complication of CSF Shunting

Intraventricular hemorrhage can be produced at the moment of puncturing the ventricle with the proximal catheter. Irrigation of the ventricle with warm saline usually clears the fluid in a few

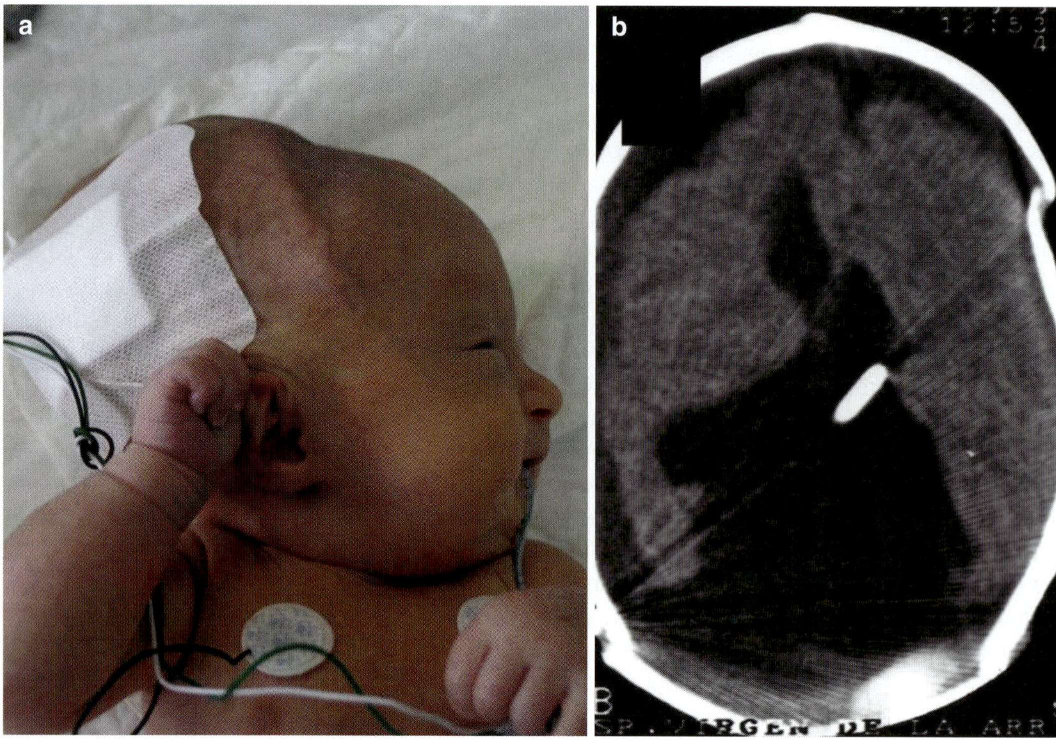

Fig. 2.7 (**a**) Photograph of a child's head showing a sunken fontanel and overriding skull bones due to overdrainage early after initial shunting that was resolved by upgrading the pressure of an externally adjustable valve, (**b**) CT scan of the same patient before valve pressure readjustment

minutes, as CSF fluid clearance usually requires only time and patience. If the hemorrhage does not subside, an EVD is left in place and maintained as long as necessary. Ventricular bleeding constitutes the most dreaded surgical adverse event during proximal catheter revisions. These catheters usually stick to the choroid plexus or to the ventricular walls. Utmost care must be taken at the time of pulling the catheter out of the ventricle. However several maneuvers are apt of decreasing the eventuality of intraventricular bleeding as are gentle rotation of the catheter while slowly pulling it off. Others recommend washing the internal lumen of the tube with saline for disrupting the adhesions or using intraluminal coagulation with a metallic stylet or with a flexible coagulating electrode as those used in neuroendoscopy [50]. A second ventricular catheter must be readily available if clots or cerebral debris would plug again the one that is being implanted. The catheter may also be left in situ if one feels that it is firmly adhered within the ventricle. Others prefer to coagulate with diathermy or laser using through an endoscope. During all the maneuvers for proximal catheter removal, we tightly held its outermost orifice with a straight baby-mosquito forceps to avoid the inadvertent intraventricular migration (a frequent cause of retained ventricular catheters). In case of serious ventricular hemorrhage, the new catheter may become blocked causing a sudden neurological deterioration that usually manifests early after surgery requiring a repeat shunt revision. *Gross intraventricular hematomas* constitute an extremely infrequent complication of CSF shunting [35] that requires EVD and probably intraventricular injections of urokinase for accelerating the lysis of the clots [50].

Cortical bleeding may also occur during the opening of the dura mater. This hemorrhage can be easily controlled with mono- or bipolar coagulation. However, in some occasions, it requires enlarging the bone orifice of the burr hole to reach the bleeding artery. These superficial hemorrhages usually have no clinical consequences, and the patients remain symptom-free.

Subdural hematomas may be found in patients with large heads and thin parenchyma after shunting as occurs in children with macrocephaly and large ventricles or in the elderly with brain atrophy [2]. Its occurrence is more frequent in adults (4–23 %) than in children (2.8–5.4 %) and in patients with NPH (20–46 %). The proposed mechanism for the development of a subdural hematoma is the stretching and ruptures of bridging veins as a consequence of excessive drainage of CSF. In this context, chronic subdural hematomas are more prevalent than acute subdural hematomas. The clinical picture of subdural hematoma ranges from absence of symptoms to manifestations of shunt failure or of a mass lesion. Treatment is reserved for patients with clinical symptoms or for those who show midline displacement on imaging studies.

Epidural hematomas exceptionally complicate CSF shunt procedures [2, 65]. They predominantly occur in young patients and in those with macrocephaly and large ventricles. They develop as the result of vascular stretching in the presence of a dura mater that is less adherent to the skull than that of older adults. Patients may be asymptomatic or present features of shunt failure or of a mass lesion. Small epidural hematomas are best left untreated as is usually done in epidurals found in accidental trauma. As expected, symptomatic epidurals require craniotomy and valve upgrading.

2.8 Epilepsy Related to CSF Shunting

Children with hydrocephalus and CSF shunts have a higher incidence of epilepsy than the general population (6–59 %) [8]. Excluding patients with tumoral hydrocephalus, the incidence of seizures in a large series of shunted patients was as high as 30 % [8]. Reported risk factors for epilepsy in this population are the etiology of hydrocephalus (especially congenital causes and brain malformations), antecedent shunt revision, previous valve infection, site of proximal catheter insertion, and perhaps the presence of the shunt by itself that is considered to represent an epileptic focus [8]. This view is supported by the abnormalities found in EEG recordings that show slow waves and epileptic discharges in the hemisphere that harbors the shunt and at especially at the site of catheter insertion. However, this opinion is not generally shared. Epilepsy in hydrocephalic children is associated with a poor intellectual outcome and with problems in behavior. In our experience, seizures are especially seen in association with slit ventricles.

2.9 Making the Diagnosis of Shunt Failure

As in other neurosurgical conditions, diagnosis of shunt failure must be based on a careful *clinical history* that includes etiology of hydrocephalus, personal antecedents, age at shunt placement, type of initial valve, prior infections and their outcome, history of previous shunt malfunctions and symptoms when it occurred, and identification of the type and pressure of the last valve. History should record present complaints if any, level of schooling and socialization, concurrent diseases, and present treatments and allergies (latex allergy is frequent in spina bifida patients). Baseline neuroimaging studies must be routinely performed for comparison if shunt malfunction would occur.

Physical examination starts with a complete neurological assessment (including fundoscopy) and with serial measurement of the head circumference, checking that it follows an appropriate growth curve. In neonates and infants, it is followed by inspection of the head, estimating the *tension of the fontanel* by digital palpation (Fig. 2.3b) and checking the separation of the cranial sutures if any. The position of the eyes (sunsetting eyes, squint) and the size of the epicranial veins are also observed. Then, the integrity of the whole shunt system is ascertained by palpation of its entire trajectory, looking for gaps in the tube, for fluid collections along the tube, and for pseudotumoral masses or calcified zones.

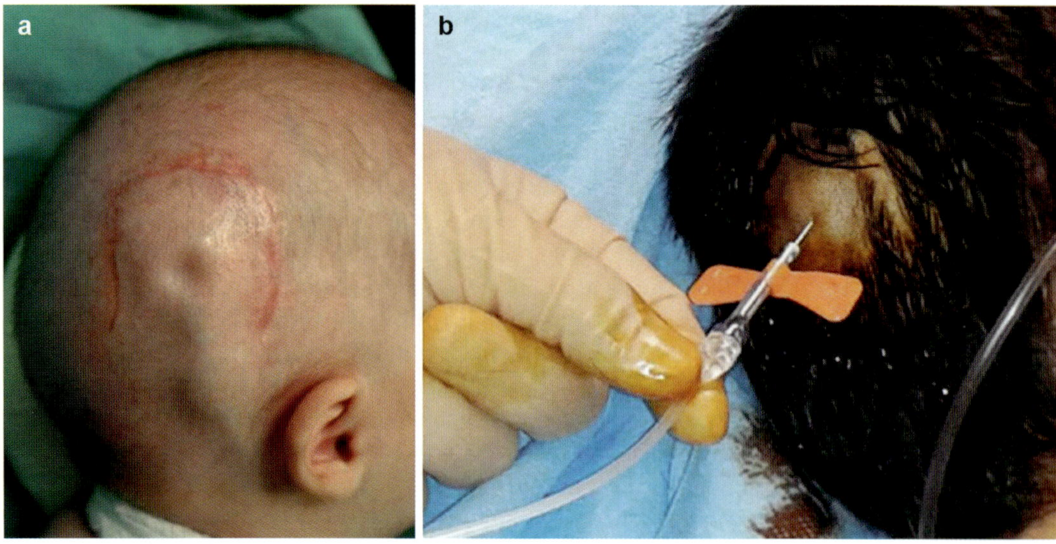

Fig. 2.8 (**a**) Photograph of an umbilicated reservoir. At operation the ventricular catheter was completely occluded by choroid plexus. (**b**) Image illustrating the technique of shunt tapping

In our experience, *pumping of the valve reservoir* is a useful adjunct for the diagnosis of shunt failure [69]. When there is no shunt malfunction, the reservoir empties and refills easily. In experienced hands, pumping the reservoir three or four times is sufficient for testing patency of the system. If the reservoir is felt hard to palpation, probably there exists occlusion of the valve or of the distal catheter. When there is a proximal catheter obstruction, the reservoir empties but refills slowly or does not refill at all and remains depressed ("umbilicated") (Fig. 2.8a). The reliability of this test has been also questioned [62, 67, 69]. Some authors warned on the intracranial hypotension that can be produced by this maneuver and recommend that parents should not be allowed to pumping the chamber [10].

Another valuable tool for testing the valve function is the *shunt tap* [75]. Under stringent sterile conditions, the reservoir is punctured with a 23G or 25G butterfly system (Fig. 2.8b), and then the pressure is measured. If there is no spontaneous drip, gentle aspiration with a small syringe for encouraging fluid leak can be attempted. When the proximal catheter is obstructed, no fluid will come out either spontaneously of after aspiration. The intraventricular pressure can also be measured attaching a plastic manometer to the needle. Samples of CSF are routinely obtained and sent for biochemical and cytological study and for microbiological culture. Another method for estimating shunt function consists of connecting the needle to a recording system thus obtaining a *continuous monitoring of the intracranial pressure* from the reservoir (Fig. 2.9). The shunt tap is inexpensive, easy to perform, and repeatable [75]. The shunt puncture has scarce risks of shunt contamination and even less risks of damaging the valve or the reservoir and of causing an intracranial hemorrhage [56, 58]. ICP measurements are also used for diagnosis in doubtful cases of shunt failure [30, 73].

Obviously, neuroimaging studies are customarily utilized for the diagnosis of CSF shunt failure. The commonest methods include transfontanelar ultrasonography, shunt series, computerized tomography, cranial magnetic resonance imaging, and Doppler studies. The shuntogram consists of assessing the flow of CSF along the tube after injection of a radioopaque contrast medium in the reservoir. Isotopic CSF flow studies are presently utilized in only special occasions.

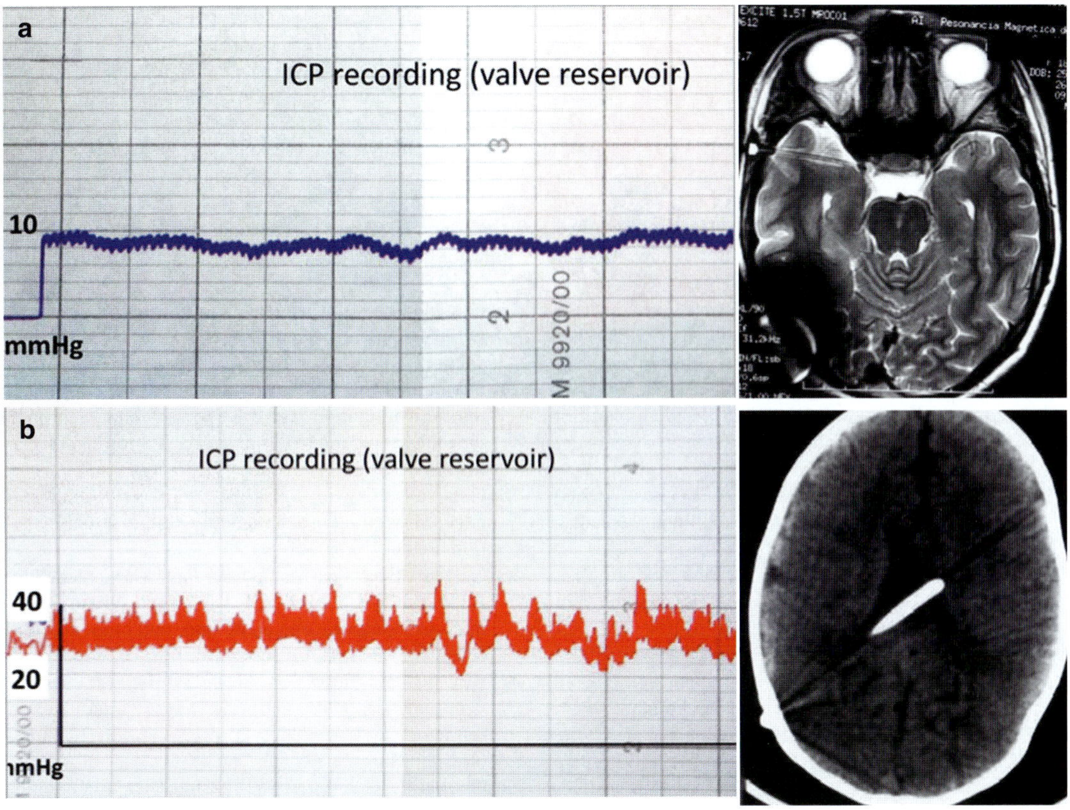

Fig. 2.9 (**a**) Ventricular pressure recording through the valve reservoir in suspected shunt malfunction. Ventricular pressures were within the ranges of the valve. On the right MRI of the patient depicting the proximal catheter within a middle fossa arachnoid cyst. (**b**) Distal catheter malfunction: recording during the shunt tap, showing basal pressures of 20 mmHg with waves of up to 40 mmHg. On the right, CT of the same patient showing incipient dilatation of previously collapsed ventricles

Conclusions

The most frequent complications of CSF shunting are mechanical, infectious, or functional. It is not always easy to distinguish which type of complication is causing the shunt dysfunction. Complications may present with a variety of symptoms and signs that must be carefully ascertained before proceeding to surgical revision. These clinical manifestations vary according to the patients' age, etiology of hydrocephalus, cavity of CSF drainage, and type of valve and according to its occurrence early or late after initial shunt insertion or previous surgical revision.

To conclude, it is very important to bear in mind that the objectives of CSF shunting are (1) to provide control of the raised ICP, (2) to avoid mechanical and functional complications, (3) to prevent infection, and (4) to delay as much as possible shunt revision or replacement.

Appropriate knowledge of the mechanisms that contribute in the production of CSF shunt failures, preventive measures to avoid them, together with forthcoming improvements in shunts' constructs will doubtless contribute to decrease the number and the severity of these complications.

References

1. Adderley R (2010) Acute respiratory failure following shunt disconnection. Cerebrospinal Fluid Res 7(Suppl 1):552
2. Aguiar HA, Shu EBS, Freitas ABR et al (2000) Causes and treatment of intracranial hemorrhage

complicating shunting for pediatric hydrocephalus. Childs Nerv Syst 16:218–221
3. Albright AL, Tyler-Kabara E (2001) Slit-ventricle syndrome secondary to shunt-induced suture ossification. Neurosurgery 48:764–770
4. Barnes NP, Jones SJ, Hayward RD et al (2002) Ventriculoperitoneal shunt block: what are the best predictive clinical indicators? Arch Dis Child 87:198–201
5. Bergsneider M, Miller C, Vespa PM, Hu X (2008) Surgical management of adult hydrocephalus. Neurosurgery 62(SHC Suppl 2):SHC643–SHC660
6. Boch AL, Hermelin E, Sainte-Rose C, Sgouros S (1998) Mechanical dysfunction of ventriculoperitoneal shunts caused by calcification of the silicone rubber catheter. J Neurosurg 88:975–982
7. Bondurant CP, Jimenez DF (1995) Epidemiology of cerebrospinal fluid shunting. Pediatr Neurosurg 23:254–258
8. Bourgeois M, Sainte-Rose C, Cinalli G et al (1999) Epilepsy in children with shunted hydrocephalus. J Neurosurg 90:274–281
9. Broekman MLD, Van Beijnum J, Peul WC, Regli L (2011) Neurosurgery and shaving: what's the evidence? J Neurosurg 115:670–678
10. Bromby A, Czosnykya Z, Allin D et al (2007) Laboratory study on intracranial hypotension created by pumping the chamber of a hydrocephalus shunt. Cerebrospinal Fluid Res 4:2
11. Caldarelli M, Novegno F, Di Rocco C (2009) A late complication of CSF shunting: acquired Chiari I malformation. Childs Nerv Syst 25:443–452
12. Chen HH, Riva-Cambrin J, Brockmeyer DL et al (2011) Shunt failure due to intracranial migration of Bioglide ventricular catheters. J Neurosurg Pediatr 7:408–412
13. Choux M, Genitori L, Lang D, Lena G (1992) Shunt implantation: reducing the incidence of shunt infection. J Neurosurg 77:875–880
14. Chumas PD, Kulkarni AV, Drake JM et al (1993) Lumboperitoneal shunting: a retrospective study in the pediatric population. Neurosurgery 32:376–383
15. Cozens JW, Chandler J (1997) Increased risk of distal ventriculoperitoneal shunt obstruction associated with slit valves or distal slits in the peritoneal catheter. J Neurosurg 87:682–686
16. Davidson RI (1976) Peritoneal bypass in the treatment of hydrocephalus: historical review and abdominal complications. J Neurol Neurosurg Psychiatry 39:640–646
17. Del Bigio MR (1998) Biological reactions to cerebrospinal fluid shunt devices: a review of cellular pathology. Neurosurgery 42:319–326
18. Di Rocco C, Marchese E, Velardi F (1994) A survey of the first complication of newly implanted CSF shunt devices for the treatment of nontumoral hydrocephalus. Cooperative survey of the 1991–1992 Education Committee of the ISPN. Childs Nerv Syst 10:321–327
19. Di Rocco C, Massimi L, Tamburrini G (2006) Shunts vs. endoscopic third ventriculostomy in infants: are there different types and/or rates of complications. Childs Nerv Syst 22:1573–1589
20. Echizenya K, Satoh M, Ueno H et al (1987) Mineralization and biodegradation of CSF shunting systems. J Neurosurg 67:584–591
21. Elisevich K, Mattar AG, Cheeseman F (1994) Biodegradation of distal shunt catheters. Pediatr Neurosurg 21:71–76
22. Ersahin Y, Tabur E, Kocaman S, Mutluer S (2000) Complications of subduroperitoneal shunts. Childs Nerv Syst 16:433–436
23. Ferguson SD, Michael N, Frimm DM (2007) Observations regarding failure of cerebrospinal fluid shunts early after surgery. Neurosurg Focus 22(4):E7
24. Fukuhara T, Namba Y, Kuyama H (2004) Ventricular reservoir-migration into the lateral ventricle through the endoscopic tract after unsuccessful third ventriculostomy. Pediatr Neurosurg 40:186–189
25. Galarza M, Gravori T, Lazareff JA (2001) Acute spinal cord swelling in a child with a Chiari II malformation. Pediatr Neurosurg 35:145–148
26. Gelabert-Gonzalez M, Iglesias Pais M, García-Allut A, Martínez-Rumbo R (2005) Chronic subdural haematoma: surgical treatment and outcome in 1000 cases. Clin Neurol Neurosurg 107:223–229
27. Girotti ME, Singh RR, Rodgers BM (2009) The ventriculo-gallbladder shunt in the treatment of refractory hydrocephalus: a review of current literature. Am Surg 75:734737
28. Griebel R, Khan M, Tan L (1985) CSF shunt complications: an analysis of contributory failure. Childs Nerv Syst 1:77–80
29. Gupta A, Ahmad FU, Kumar A et al (2006) Umbilical CSF fistula: a rare complication of ventriculoperitoneal shunt. Acta Neurochir (Wien) 148:1205–1207
30. Hanlo PW, Gooskens RHJ, Faber JAJ et al (1996) Relationship between anterior fontanelle pressure measurements and clinical signs in infantile hydrocephalus. Childs Nerv Syst 12:200–209
31. Hwang TN, Rofagha S, McDermontt MW et al (2011) Sunken eyes, sagging brain syndrome: bilateral enophthalmos from chronic intracranial hypotension. Ophthalmology 118:2286–2295
32. Korinek AM, Fulla-Oler L, Boch AL et al (2011) Morbidity of ventricular cerebrospinal fluid shunt surgery in adults: an 8-year study. Neurosurgery 68:985–995
33. Kouyialis AT, Stranjalis G, Boviatsis EJ (2005) Selection of cranial site for shunting debilitated patients. Acta Neurochir (Wien) 147:763–765
34. Kurschel S, Puget S, Borgeois M et al (2007) Factors influencing the complication rate of subduroperitoneal placement for the treatment of subdural hematomas in children. J Neurosurg 106(3 Suppl):172–178
35. Kuwamura K, Kokunai T (1982) Intraventricular hematoma secondary to a ventriculoperitoneal shunt. Neurosurgery 10:384–386
36. Langmoen IA, Lundar T, Vatne K, Hovind KH (1992) Occurrence and management of fractured peripheral catheters in CSF shunts. Childs Nerv Syst 8:222–225

37. Lazareff JA, Peacock W, Holly L et al (1998) Multiple shunt failures: an analysis of relevant factors. Childs Nerv Syst 14:271–275
38. Lee M, Leahu D, Weiner HL et al (1995) Complications of fourth-ventricular shunts. Pediatr Neurosurg 22:309–314
39. Liptak GS, McDonald JV (1985) Ventriculoperitoneal shunts in children: factors affecting shunt survival. Pediatr Neurosci 12:289–293
40. Livingston JH, McCullagh HG, Kooner G et al (2011) Bradycardia without associated hypertension: a common sign of ventriculo-peritoneal shunt malfunction. Childs Nerv Syst 27:729–733
41. Lund-Johansen M, Svendsen F, Wester K (1994) Shunt failures and complications in adults as related to shunt type, diagnosis, and the experience of the surgeon. Neurosurgery 35:839–844
42. Martinez-Lage JF, Poza M, Esteban JA (1992) Mechanical complications of the reservoirs and pumping devices in ventricular shunt hydrocephalus. Br J Neurosurg 6:321–325
43. Martínez-Lage JF, Poza M, Izura V (1993) Retrograde migration of the abdominal catheter as a complication of ventriculoperitoneal shunts: the fishhook sign. Childs Nerv Syst 9:425–427
44. Martínez-Lage JF, Ruíz-Maciá D, Valentí JA, Poza M (1999) Development of a middle fossa arachnoid cyst. A theory on its pathogenesis. Childs Nerv Syst 15:94–97
45. Martínez-Lage JF, Torres J, Campillo H et al (2000) Ventriculopleural shunts with new technology valves. Childs Nerv Syst 16:867–871
46. Martínez-Lage JF, Pérez-Espejo MA, Almagro MJ et al (2005) Síndromes de hiperdrenaje de las válvulas en hidrocefalia infantil. Neurocirugia (Astur) 16:124–133
47. Martínez-Lage JF, Ruiz-Espejo Vilar A, Pérez-Espejo MA et al (2006) Shunt-related craniocerebral disproportion: treatment with cranial vault expanding procedures. Neurosurg Rev 29:229–235
48. Martínez-Lage JF, Almagro MJ, Del Rincón IS et al (2008) Management of neonatal hydrocephalus: feasibility of use and safety of two programmable (Sophy and Polaris) valves. Childs Nerv Syst 24:549–556
49. Martínez-Lage JF, Martos-Tello JM, Ros-de-San Pedro J, Almagro MJ (2008) Severe constipation: an under-appreciated cause of VP shunt malfunction: a case-based update. Childs Nerv Syst 24:431–435
50. Martínez-Lage JF, Almagro MJ, Ruíz-Espejo A et al (2009) Keeping CSF valve function with urokinase in children with intra-ventricular haemorrhage and CSF shunts. Childs Nerv Syst 25:981–986
51. Martínez-Lage JF, Alarcón F, López-Guerrero AL et al (2010) Syringomyelia with quadriparesis in CSF shunt malfunction: a case illustration. Childs Nerv Syst 26:1229–1231
52. Martínez-Lage JF, Pérez-Espejo MA, Almagro MJ, López-Guerrero AL (2011) Hydrocephalus and arachnoid cysts. Childs Nerv Syst 27:1643–1652
53. McGirt MJ, Leveque JC, Wellons JC 3rd (2003) Cerebrospinal shunt survival and etiology of failures: a seven-year institutional experience. Pediatr Neurosurg 38:34–40
54. Massimi L, Paternoster G, Fasano T, Di Rocco C (2009) On the changing epidemiology of hydrocephalus. Childs Nerv Syst 25:795–800
55. Mirzayan MJ, Koenig K, Bastuerk M, Krauss JK (2006) Coma due to meteorism and increased intraabdominal pressure subsequent to ventriculoperitoneal shunt dysfunction. Lancet 368:2032
56. Moghal NE, Quinn MW, Levene MI, Puntis JWL (1992) Intraventricular hemorrhage after aspiration of ventricular reservoirs. Arch Dis Child 67:448–449
57. Muthukumar N (2012) Syringomyelia as a presenting feature of shunt dysjunction: implications for the pathogenesis of syringomyelia. J Craniovertebr Junction Spine 3:6
58. Noetzel MJ, Baker RP (1984) Shunt fluid examination: risks and benefits in the evaluation of shunt malfunction and infection. J Neurosurg 61:328–332
59. O'Hare AE, Brown JK, Minss RA (1987) Specific enlargement of the fourth ventricle after ventriculoperitoneal shunt for posthemorrhagic hydrocephalus. Arch Dis Child 62:1025–1029
60. Parker SL, Anderson WN, Lilienffeld S et al (2011) Cerebrospinal fluid shunt infection in patients receiving antibiotic-impregnated versus standard shunts. J Neurosurg Pediatr 8:259–265
61. Piatt JH Jr, Hoffman HJ (1989) Cor pulmonale: a lethal complication of ventriculoperitoneal CSF diversion. Childs Nerv Syst 5:29–31
62. Piatt JH (1992) Physical examination of patients with cerebrospinal fluid shunts: is there useful information in pumping the shunt? Pediatrics 89:470–473
63. Piatt JH Jr, Carlson CV (1993) A search for determinant of cerebrospinal fluid survival: retrospective analysis of a 14-year institutional experience. Pediatr Neurosurg 19:233–242
64. Poca MA, Sahuquillo J, Mataró M (2001) Actualizaciones en el diagnostico y tratamiento de la hidrocefalia "normotensive" (hidrocefalia crónica del adulto). Neurologia 16:353–369
65. Power D, Ali-Khan F, Drage M (1999) Contralateral extradural haematoma after insertion of a programmable-valve ventriculoperitoneal shunt. J R Soc Med 92:360–361
66. Reddy GK, Bollam P, Caldito G et al (2011) Ventriculoperitoneal shunt complications in hydrocephalus patients with intracranial tumors: an analysis of relevant risk factors. J Neurooncol 103:333–342
67. Rekate HL (1991–1992) Shunt revision: complications and their prevention. Pediatr Neurosurg 17:155–162
68. Rekate HL (2004) The slit ventricle syndrome: advances based on technology and understanding. Pediatr Neurosurg 40:259–263
69. Rocque BG, Lapsiwala S, Iskandar BJ (2008) Ventricular shunt tap as a predictor of proximal shunt malfunction in children: a prospective study. J Neurosurg Pediatr 1:439–443
70. Rogers EA, Kimia A, Madsen JR et al (2012) Predictors of ventricular shunt infection among

children presenting to a Pediatric Emergency Department. Pediatr Emerg Care 28:405–407
71. Sahuquillo J, Arikan F, Poca MA et al (2008) Intra-abdominal pressure: the neglected variable in selecting the ventriculoperitoneal shunt for treating hydrocephalus. Neurosurgery 62:143–150
72. Schueler WB, Mapstone TB, Gross NL (2010) Migration of a ventricular tapping reservoir unto the third ventricle. J Neurosurg Pediatr 6:550–552
73. Schumann M, Sood S, McAllister JP et al (2008) Value of overnight monitoring of intracranial pressure in hydrocephalic children. Pediatr Neurosurg 44:269–279
74. Simon TD, Hall M, Riva-Cambrin J et al (2009) Infection rates following initial cerebrospinal fluid shunt placement across pediatric hospitals in the United States. J Neurosurg Pediatr 4:156–165
75. Sood S, Kim S, Ham SD et al (1993) Useful components of the shunt tap test for evaluation of shun malfunction. Childs Nerv Syst 9:157–162
76. Stannard MW, Rollins NK (1995) Subcutaneous catheter calcification in ventriculoperitoneal shunts. AJNR Am J Neuroradiol 16:1276–1278
77. Stringel G, Turner M, Crase T (1993) Ventriculo-gallbladder shunts in children. Childs Nerv Syst 9:331–333
78. Taub E, Lavyne MH (1994) Thoracic complications of ventriculoperitoneal shunts: case report and review of the literature. Neurosurgery 34:181–184
79. Tomes DJ, Hellbusch LC, Albert LR (2003) Stretching and breaking characteristics of cerebrospinal fluid shunt tubing. J Neurosurg 98:578–583
80. Torres-Lanzas J, Ríos-Zambudio A, Martínez-Lage JF et al (2002) Ventriculopleural shunts to treat hydrocephalus. Arch Bronconeumol 38:511–514
81. Tuli S, Drake J, Lawless J et al (2000) Risk factors for repeated cerebrospinal shunt failures in pediatric patients with hydrocephalus. J Neurosurg 92: 31–38
82. Venes JL (1976) Control of shunt infection. J Neurosurg 45:311–314
83. Vernet O, Campiche R, de Tribolet N (1995) Long-term results after ventriculo-atrial shunting in children. Childs Nerv Syst 11:176–179
84. Vinchon M, Boroncini M, Delestret I (2012) Adult outcome of pediatric hydrocephalus. Childs Nerv Syst 28:847–854
85. Wang VY, Barbaro NM, Lawton MT et al (2007) Complications of lumboperitoneal shunts. Neurosurgery 60:1045–1049
86. West GA, Berger MS, Geyer JR (1994) Childhood optic pathway tumors associated with ascites following ventriculoperitoneal shunt placement. Pediatr Neurosurg 1:254–259
87. Wisoff JH, Kratzert KJ, Handweker SM et al (1991) Pregnancy in patients with cerebrospinal fluid shunts: report of a series and review of the literature. Neurosurgery 29:827–831
88. Wong JM, Ziewacz JE, Ho AL et al (2012) Patterns in neurosurgical adverse events: cerebrospinal fluid shunt surgery. Neurosurg Focus 33(5):E13

Neuroimaging in CSF Shunt Complications

3

Ernesto Domenech, Cristina Serrano, and Carmen María Fernández-Hernández

Contents

3.1 **Introduction** 33

3.2 **Imaging Techniques** 34
3.2.1 Conventional Radiography (Shunt Series) 34
3.2.2 Ultrasounds 36
3.2.3 Computerized Tomography............ 37
3.2.4 Magnetic Resonance Imaging.......... 37
3.2.5 Radionuclide Shunt Studies 41

3.3 **Normal Imaging Appearance of CSF Shunts** 41
3.3.1 Ventricular Shunts.................... 41
3.3.2 Endoscopic Third Ventriculostomy....... 42

3.4 **Postoperative Complications After Shunt Placement** 43
3.4.1 Intraventricular Hemorrhage........... 43
3.4.2 Parenchymal Hemorrhage.............. 43
3.4.3 Subdural Hematomas or Hygromas 43
3.4.4 Pneumocephalus 43
3.4.5 Other Complications.................. 45

3.5 **Intracranial Complications of CSF Shunts** 45
3.5.1 Acute–Subacute Complications 45
3.5.2 Chronic Complications 55

3.6 **Extracranial Complications of CSF Shunts** 59
3.6.1 Shunt Misplacement 59
3.6.2 Disconnection and Fracture of the Shunt .. 60
3.6.3 Distal Obstruction.................... 61
3.6.4 Pneumothorax and Subcutaneous Emphysema......................... 62
3.6.5 Hydrothorax (Pleural Effusion) 62
3.6.6 Fibrothorax 64
3.6.7 Complications Related to Shunt Variants .. 64
3.6.8 Tricuspid Valve Pathology 65
3.6.9 Thromboembolic Disease and Pulmonary Arterial Hypertension........ 65
3.6.10 Abdominal Complications 65

Conclusions 68

References 68

3.1 Introduction

Ventricular shunts are commonly used to treat hydrocephalus. The placement of cerebrospinal fluid (CSF) shunts has become one of the most common procedures performed by neurosurgeons. Despite significant improvements in shunt procedures, shunt malfunction and complications remain common [1, 2]. Shunt failure occurs in 40–50 % of patients during the first 2 years after shunt surgery [3]. The incidence of ventriculo-peritoneal (VP) shunt failure ranges from 25 to 40 % at 1 year and 63–70 % at 10 years. Failure rates with ventriculoatrial and ventriculopleural shunts are slightly higher [4].

Often malfunctions are due to complications such as obstruction, breakage, migration, or infection. CSF shunt complications necessitate a systematic approach for diagnosing the etiology of shunt failure [5]. This evaluation should

E. Domenech, MD (✉) • C. Serrano, MD
C.M. Fernández-Hernández, MD
Section of Pediatric Radiology, Service of Diagnostic Radiology, Virgen de la Arrixaca University Hospital, El Palmar, Murcia 30120, Spain
e-mail: domenech-rx@hotmail.com; serrano5977@gmail.com; cm_fh@hotmail.com

C. Di Rocco et al. (eds.), *Complications of CSF Shunting in Hydrocephalus: Prevention, Identification, and Management*, DOI 10.1007/978-3-319-09961-3_3,

begin with an appraisal of the patient's symptoms [5]. Shunt malfunction manifests clinically with headaches, nausea, abdominal pain, pain at the site of myelomeningocele repair, vomiting, lethargy, irritability, fever, increasing head size, persistent bulging of the anterior fontanel, and seizures [2].

Imaging often confirms the diagnosis and reveals the underlying cause [4]. So, a multimodality approach is typically required for the diagnosis of shunt malfunction including plain radiographs, ultrasound (US), computerized tomography (CT), magnetic resonance imaging (MRI), radionuclide studies (isotopic shuntogram), CSF pressure studies, and cultures that provide complementary information [5]. Radiologists should be familiar with all the potential causes of shunt failure and with the diagnostic yield of the different imaging modalities [2].

3.2 Imaging Techniques

The entire course of the shunt can be initially examined with plain radiography for disconnections, kinks, breaks, or migration of the shunt tubing, which may be confirmed afterwards with other imaging modalities. Additional examinations include brain CT searching for ventricular size changes or other signs of increased intracranial pressure (ICP), abdominal sonography to evaluate the peritoneal end of the shunt, MRI to look for central nervous system (CNS) infection or hemorrhage, and injection of contrast material into the shunt system to help in confirming CSF leaks and disconnections and in locating the site of obstruction [2, 6].

3.2.1 Conventional Radiography (Shunt Series)

Conventional radiographs are mainly performed to search for breaks, disconnections, or catheter migration [4]. The radiographic "shunt series" typically consist of anteroposterior and lateral views of the head, chest, and abdomen to examine the entire course of the CSF shunt device [6, 7] (Fig. 3.1). Visualization of the intraperitoneal catheter may be difficult in obese patients in whom image contrast is degraded both by photon scatter and by the increased peak kilovoltage required to traverse the soft tissues. Image quality may be further degraded by longer exposure times that increase the likelihood of motion artifact. A potential solution is to obtain separate radiographs of each abdominal quadrant if required [4].

To facilitate radiographic evaluation, the catheter and distal tubing are manufactured with either barium impregnation, which allows visualization of the entire tube, or they may be endowed with intermittent radiopaque markers along their course or tips. The valve itself is almost always entirely radiopaque [7]. Disconnections of VP shunt mechanism are a recognized complication and occur most commonly at the level of the valve, where the proximal and distal tubing meet [8]. Similarly, actual breaks in the catheter tubing are more likely to occur in the neck, likely owing to its increased mobility [7].

Other plain radiographic findings include the ectopic position of the shunt catheters. The tubing may also be coiled, causing shunt malfunction, which is a readily detectable plain radiographic finding. Occasionally, development of an abdominal pseudocyst or abdominal catheter adhesions might be suspected on plain radiography by the observation of a fixed, static position of the distal catheter tip on subsequent studies [3, 7].

Briefly, catheter obstruction may not produce any findings on plain radiographs; consequently, the value of shunt series is further limited to demonstrating disruptions of the system, including disconnections and kinks [7]. Some authors have demonstrated that the shunt series have a sensitivity lower than 19.4 %, while others suggest that the true sensitivity is not higher than 31 %. Plain radiographic examination has a low sensitivity and significant false-negative rates for detecting shunt abnormalities. In addition, the existence of many possible causes of shunt failure, together with the use of ionizing radiation, limits the role of the shunt series to identifying potential mechanical causes [2, 7].

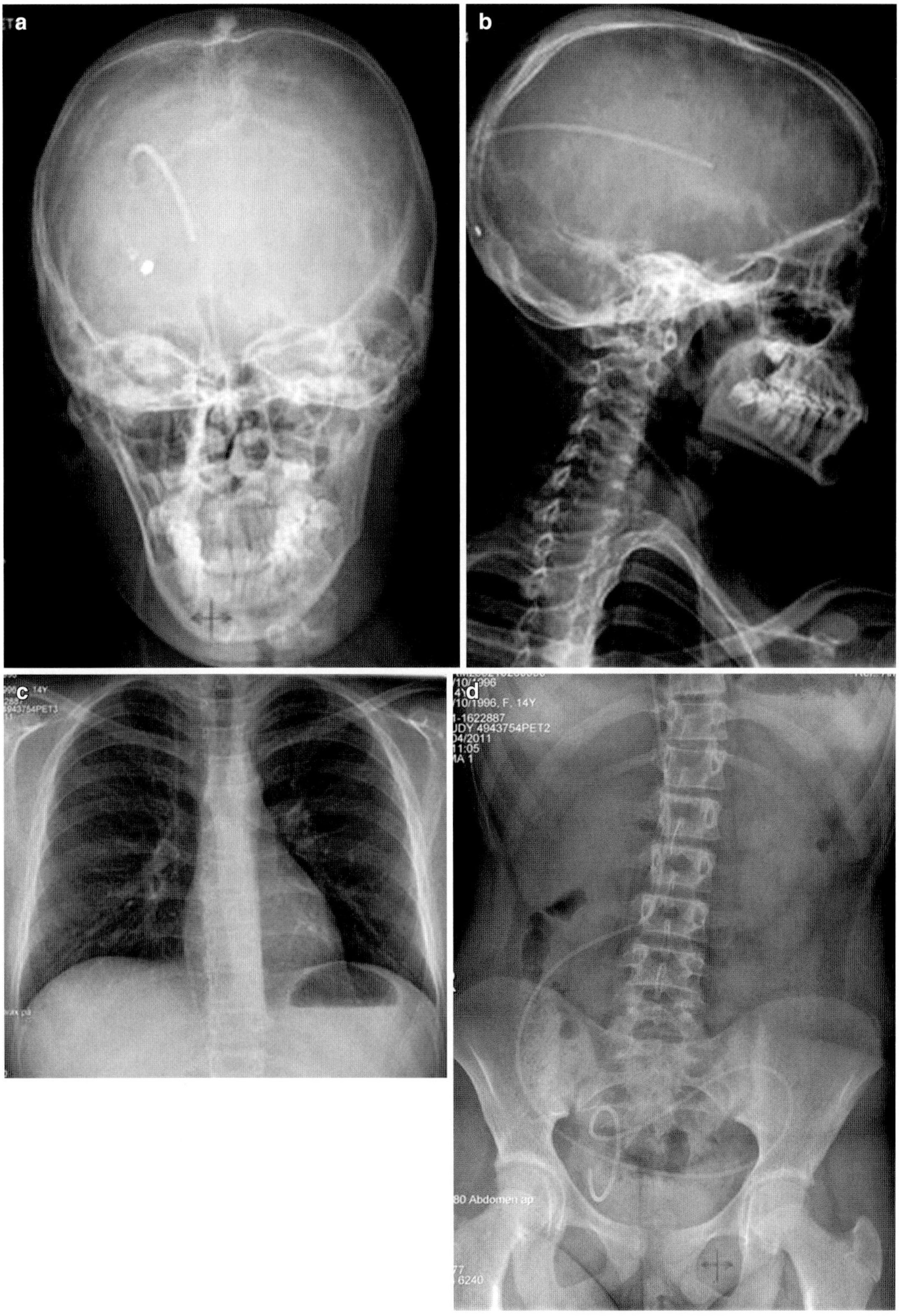

Fig. 3.1 Shunt series in a 14-year-old patient with a Strata VP shunt: (**a, b**) skull, (**c**) chest, and (**d**) abdomen radiographs showing the integrity of the shunt

The estimated radiation dose from a plain skull, chest, and abdomen radiograph is 525 millirem (5.28 mSv). This radiation dose is approximately equivalent to 2 years of background radiation. If a mechanical cause of failure is suspected, it might be possible to obtain plain radiographs using lower mA settings, without losing diagnostic information for evaluating the catheter components [7]. The radiographic shunt series provides critical information for operative planning, and some authors propose that this study may be better employed after the decision of a surgical revision of the shunt has been taken, based on clinical grounds, CT, MR, and/or nuclear imaging [6].

3.2.2 Ultrasounds

Transfontanelar US are used to explore the brain and the ventricles, but its use is limited to the first 12–18 months of life when the anterior fontanel is still open (Fig. 3.2). Ultrasonography can be used as a bedside screening test. The size and shape of the lateral ventricles are easily visualized, but the size of the third and fourth ventricles sometimes is difficult to assess by this technique. Therefore, the precise diagnosis and cause of hydrocephalus are rarely made by US alone. Furthermore, US are usually unable to show details of the posterior fossa, the aqueduct, the third ventricle floor, and the foramen magnum. Besides, the quality of the

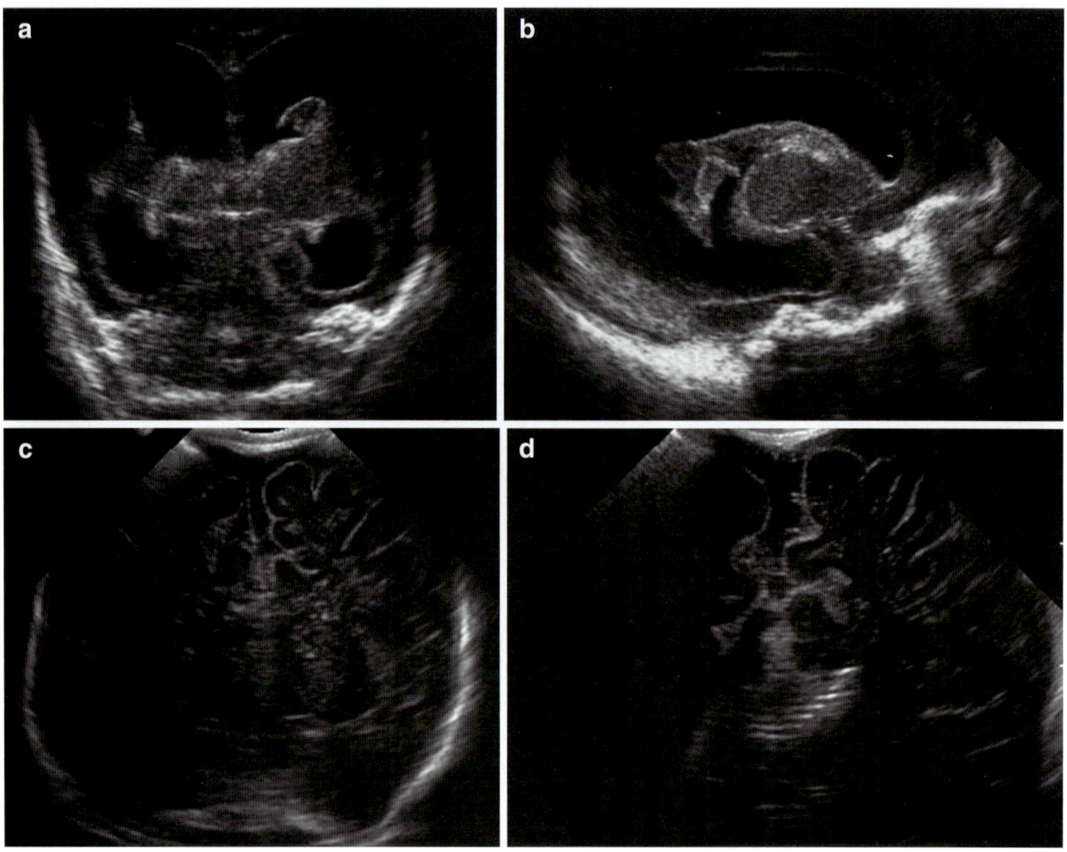

Fig. 3.2 Transfontanelar US in post-hemorrhagic hydrocephalus: (**a**, **b**) a 29-gestational-week newborn with grade III hemorrhage. (**c**) Coronal and (**b**) sagittal cuts showing hydrocephalus with a left intraventricular clot. (**c**, **d**) A 27-gestational-week neonate given a Polaris valve for progressive hydrocephalus illustrating suture straddling and clinical suspicion of overdrainage. Coronal views demonstrating (**c**) ventricular collapse and (**d**) the intraventricular valve

US image is user dependent, and its reproducibility is not high. Accordingly, the best indication for US is the follow-up of ventricular dilatation, before or after surgical treatment, limiting its use to the first 2 years of life. In case that surgical treatment of ventriculomegaly is indicated, other means of brain imaging are ordinarily obtained [5, 8, 9].

Abdominal US is frequently used to assess the peritoneal end in VP shunts and to demonstrate its complications as are an abnormal position of the distal catheter, CSF pseudocysts, etc. Thoracic US can also be indicated in the evaluation of pleural fluid in ventriculopleural shunts (though they are rarely used because of frequent pleural effusions) [2, 10].

3.2.3 Computerized Tomography

CT is the best method for imaging the brain as it is easily available, reliable, and compatible with standard life support devices [8]. CT is often the preferred technique (especially in emergencies) because of its wide availability, ease of use, and brief imaging time [11]. CT of the head is also commonly utilized for follow-up examinations as subsequent CT studies can be easily compared. Children often do not necessitate to be sedated. In the case of shunt obstruction, the nature and site of the occlusion can be easily viewed with CT that shows ventricular dilatation proximal to the block, accompanied by normal-sized or compressed ventricles distal to it, although not with sufficient detail. CT is also very useful in the follow-up of patients after initial shunt placement (Fig. 3.3). The ventricular size usually decreases gradually from the time of shunt insertion up to 12 months, and then it often remains stable. Most authors consider that the 1-year follow-up CT head scan is the most useful baseline study for long-term follow-up [5].

However, taking into account that most CSF shunt failures appear soon after initial shunting and that they are more common during the first year, some authors recommend to obtain a 3-month scan. In addition, young children need a lifelong follow-up, and also they often require frequent CT studies for assessment during episodes of suspected shunt malfunction [9, 12]. The most important concern about CT follow-up studies in shunted children is the repeated use of ionizing radiation and its consequent potential cumulative risk for developing cancer later in life [5]. Steps to minimize the risk for possible long-term complications of ionizing radiation are, therefore, particularly relevant in children undergoing multiple follow-up CT scans. Low-dose CT protocols are being designed to balance image quality and radiation dose [11].

3.2.4 Magnetic Resonance Imaging

MRI achieves similar structural findings than CT and is being increasingly used to reduce radiation exposure [4]. MRI is the examination of choice for showing ventricular dilatation, being capable of differentiating ventriculomegaly from hydrocephalus, and can also reveal its underlying cause [8].

Significant MRI-induced heating has not been shown to be a problem in recent models of shunt valves. An external magnet can adjust pressure settings of modern programmable valves. Changes in valve pressure settings often occur after exposure of these valves to MRI magnetic fields [13]. Before performing a MRI examination to a patient harboring a programmable valve, the radiologist must confirm if the shunt is or is not resistant to reprogramming by the magnetic field strength of the scanner. After scanning, the neurosurgeon will usually check whether the valve pressure setting has changed using a compass provided by the valve's manufacturer [4, 14]. Newer valves, such as the Polaris and Pro-GAV, are resistant to accidental reprogramming even at 3-T magnetic fields, and do not require adjustments of the pressure settings of the device after a MRI study. In case of having to perform a MRI to a patient with an unfamiliar valve, the radiologist must check the patient's written clinical report about the type of valve or contact the manufacturer (or representative) for specific MRI safety guidelines.

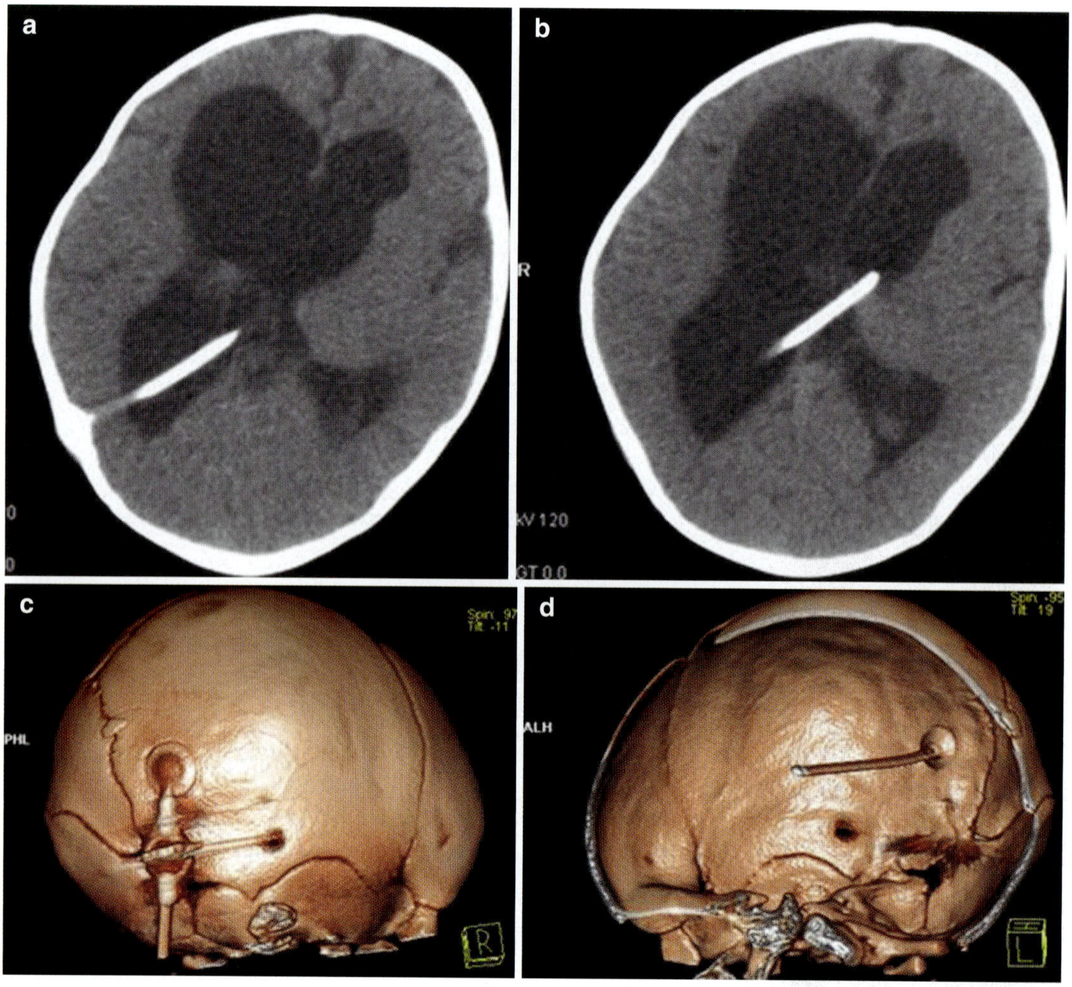

Fig. 3.3 Post-hemorrhagic hydrocephalus patient with Polaris valve. Simple cranial CT in the axial plane shows hydrocephalus and the intraventricular catheter well positioned in left frontal horn (**a**,**b**). In 3D Volumen Rendering reconstruction (VR) (**c**,**d**) the intraventricular catheter, reservoir, valve and distal catheter are seen

At present, the normal anatomy of CSF pathways, and the function of CSF drainage systems, demands a detailed study. For this purpose, new MRI sequences, either alone or in combination, are obtained in addition to conventional T1- and T2-weighted images. Although various MR cisternography and motion-sensitive MRI techniques are utilized, 3D CISS or its equivalent, TSE or FSE, and cine PC have gained wide acceptance in evaluating CSF flow and in depicting the anatomy of the cisterns [15, 16].

3.2.4.1 Conventional Sequences

T1- and T2-weighted are the sequences routinely used. Both are quite informative for demonstrating pathologic signal intensities within the brain parenchyma and for the assessment of ventricular shape and size. In addition, these sequences show most of the space-occupying lesions in both intra- and extra-axial locations (Fig. 3.4) [8]. Conventional MRI also provides useful information about the etiology of the hydrocephalus. Nevertheless, these criteria depend on a subjective evaluation by the neuroradiologist that may render the images difficult to assess in some instances, and thus they may be hardly comparable in postsurgical studies [17, 18]. The demonstration of the presence or absence of hemorrhage and of related membranes in the cisterns by using hemosiderin-sensitive sequences under the age of 2 years is also essential. Gradient echo (GRE) T2* or susceptibility weighted imaging (SWI) easily detects previous hemorrhage in the ventricles and cisterns.

3.2.4.2 Three-Dimensional Constructive Interference in the Steady State

Three-dimensional constructive interference in the steady state (3D-CISS) is a gradient-echo imaging

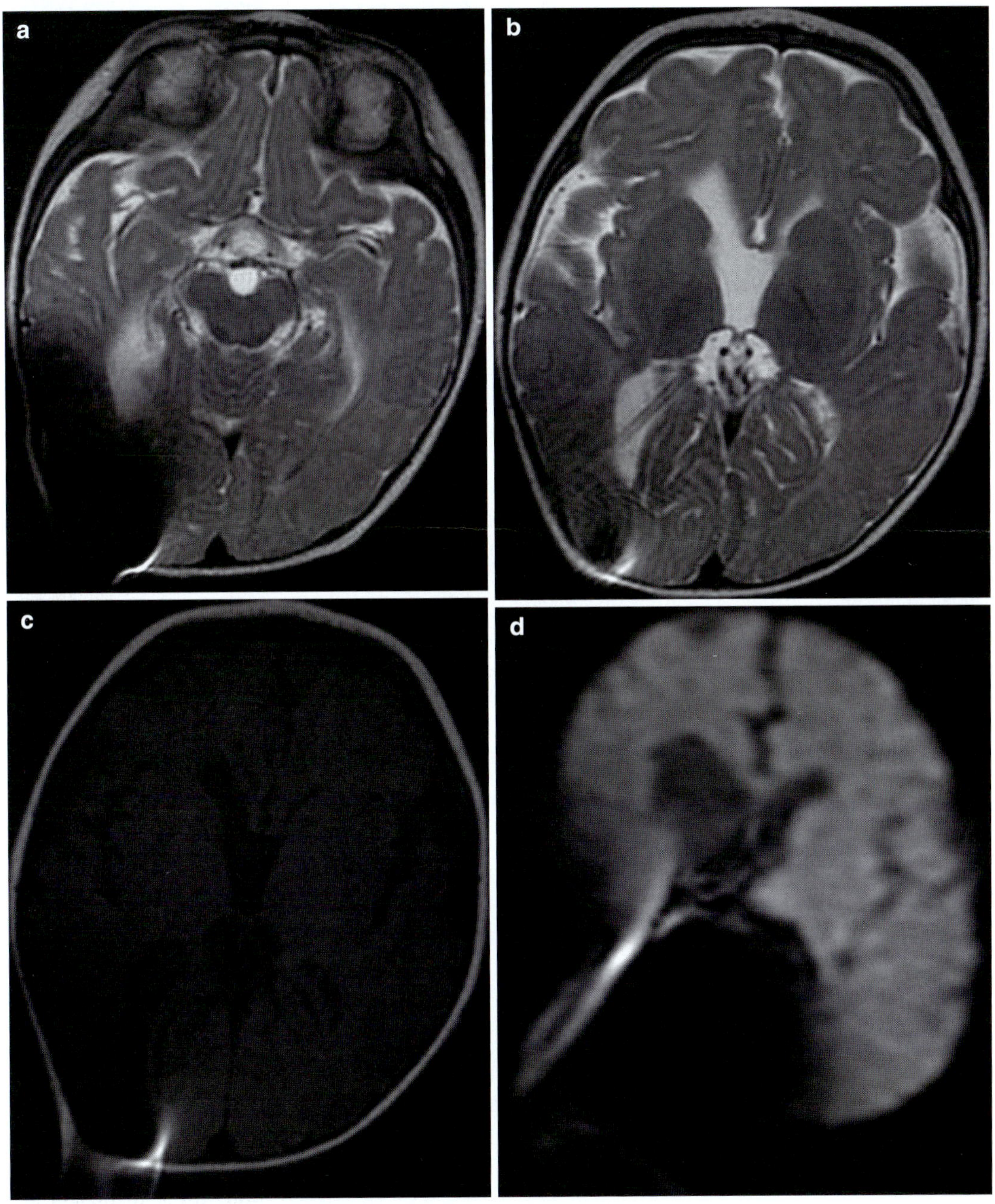

Fig. 3.4 Control cranial MR of a 7-month-old patient with a Polaris valve showing an artifact caused by the intraventricular catheter in axial FSE T2 (**a**), FSE T1 (**c**), b1500 DWI (**d**), and gradient-echo (**e**) sequences. Axial T2 plane shows the intraventricular catheter (**b**)

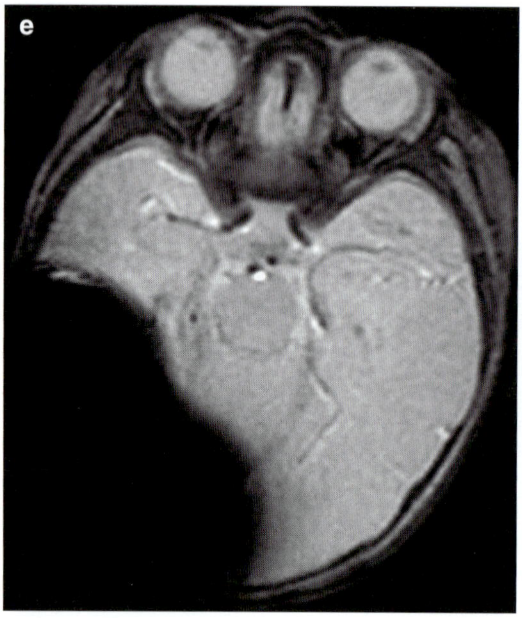

Fig. 3.4 (continued)

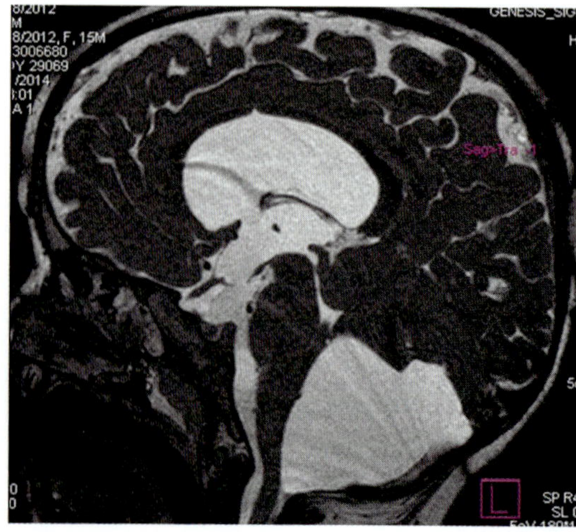

Fig. 3.5 Sagittal 3D-CISS performed in the midsagittal plane in a 15-month-old patient with a fourth ventricle giant cyst, secondary hydrocephalus given an ETV. All the midline structures, ETV stoma, and basal cisterns can be evaluated in this sequence

technique with high resolution that remains sensitive to flow and provides fine anatomic details of the CSF pathways. 3D-CISS enables locating the obstruction and determining the upstream impact. It provides anatomical information about third ventricle morphology and its relationships, details that are extremely useful before performing an ETV. These sequences also allow for a good visualization of the cerebral aqueduct and for the diagnosis of the cause of obstruction, sometimes better than with classical sequences [8, 15, 16, 19, 20]. The value of 3D-CISS has been already demonstrated in hydrocephalus, and its advantage has been shown not only for demonstrating anatomical details but also for depicting the presence, location, and extension of membranes within the cisterns, which are of help for guiding ETV [16, 21]. Membranes in the foramen of Monro, superior velum medullaris, fourth ventricle outlets, and even intraventricular cystic masses may not visible in conventional T1- and T2-weighted images but are depicted with these sequences [16]. We routinely obtain sagittal 3D-CISS images in the midsagittal plane covering midline structures, basal cisterns, and fourth ventricle outlets with an extremely high resolution that allows reconstructions in any plane without losing data (Fig. 3.5).

3.2.4.3 Cine Phase Contrast

Cardiac-gated cine phase-contrast (PC) MRI is the only technique currently available to noninvasively detect CSF flow. It is a rapid, simple, and noninvasive technique that is sensitive to CSF flow [8, 15, 22, 23]. The PC-MRI generates signal contrast between flowing and stationary nuclei by sensitizing the phase of the transverse magnetization to the velocity of motion [24]. The technique provides "to-and-fro" CSF flow velocity and direction during a single cardiac cycle with a specially designed flow-sensitive GRE sequence. CSF flow is pulsatile and synchronous with the cardiac cycle; therefore, cardiac gating can be used to provide increased sensitivity [24, 25]. The cardiac-gated phase-sensitive technique is based on the subtraction of two similar GRE images, one with flow-encoding activated gradients and another with identical parameters but without these activated gradients. The difference in phase between the subtracted images is due to motion along the particular gradient axis. In this way, the signal from the stationary tissues is almost completely eliminated. Two series of PC imaging techniques are applied in the evaluation of CSF flow, one in the axial plane, with through-plane velocity encoding in craniocaudal direction for flow quantification, and another in the sagittal plane with in-plane velocity encoding in the craniocaudal direction for qualitative assessment [24].

The sensitivity of the flow-encoding gradients must be prospectively set to prevent aliasing. Qualitative midline sagittal and quantitative axial images perpendicular to the imaging plane, mostly the aqueduct, must be acquired. It takes a maximum of 10 min to get both sequences with gating [15, 16]. Flow in craniocaudal direction is encoded in shades of white, while flow in caudocranial direction is encoded in shades of black.

CSF flow MRI can be used to distinguish communicating and non-communicating hydrocephalus, to localize the level of obstruction in obstructive hydrocephalus, to detect communication of arachnoid cysts with the subarachnoid space, to differentiate between arachnoid pouches and subarachnoid space, to discriminate between syringomyelia and cystic myelomalacia, and to evaluate flow patterns in posterior fossa cystic malformations. This imaging method can also provide significant information in the preoperative evaluation of the Chiari 1 anomaly and of normal pressure hydrocephalus (NPH) and also in the postoperative follow-up of patients given an ETV or a VP shunt [24].

But cine PC has several disadvantages. To prevent aliasing artifact, which could affect the quality of both qualitative and quantitative assessments of cine PC, the strength of the velocity-encoding gradient needs to be set properly before scanning. On the other hand, cine PC demonstrates only bidirectional flow in a selected direction [16]. Whereas cine PC shows CSF flow, it is unable to demonstrate cisternal anatomic details and should be used in conjunction with 3D-CISS. Furthermore, this technique is limited because of poor visualization of turbulent flow and of its inability to measure bulk flow [8, 23].

3.2.5 Radionuclide Shunt Studies

Radionuclide CSF shunt studies can evaluate shunt patency and differentiate proximal versus distal shunt obstruction, and, in some cases, it may show the site of obstruction by indicating where isotopic activity fails to progress. In fact, the combination of CT and radionuclide imaging is more sensitive than CT alone in the diagnosis of shunt malfunction. The technique consists of injecting 99 mTc-pentetate or pertechnetate (0.25–1.5 mCi) into the valve reservoir with the patient supine. Care must be taken to ensure that the radiopharmaceutical is suitable for intrathecal injection because the sensitivity to endotoxin effects is higher for intrathecal injections than for the intravenous route. Immediately after the injection, dynamic imaging is performed for up to 30 min, typically using 30 s per frame. Activity progressively accumulates along the shunt tract and disperses quickly at the distal site of drainage. Radionuclide may also reflux into the ventricular system in certain models of valve. When the activity remains localized at the injection site, it indicates either obstruction or isotope extravasation. The latter is excluded by imaging the chest and abdomen for evidence of systemic absorption [4].

3.3 Normal Imaging Appearance of CSF Shunts

3.3.1 Ventricular Shunts

Hydrocephalus can be treated by CSF diversion or by endoscopic third ETV [26]. Ventricular shunting represents the traditional treatment for hydrocephalus. The anatomy of a ventricular shunt consists of three parts: the proximal catheter, the valve (with or without a reservoir), and the distal catheter. The catheters are typically made of silicone and have a diameter of 2–3 mm. Catheters are hypointense on T1- and T2-weighted MRI images and hyperdense on CT. The reservoir and valve are normally radiolucent, but they have radiopaque markers to allow for visualization (Fig. 3.1). The tip of the proximal catheter is placed at the widest part of frontal horn of the lateral ventricle, away from the choroid plexus and in front of the foramen of Monro [5]. The proximal catheter may be inserted either into the frontal or occipital regions through a small burr hole in the skull [26]. The catheter exits via the burr hole and connects to a reservoir that allows CSF fluid sampling and intraventricular pressure measurements. The reservoir is connected to the inflow port of a one-way valve, while the distal catheter is joined to the outflow port of the valve and is tunneled subcutaneously to end in the drainage cavity. The valve regulates the amount of CSF drainage and plays an essential role in the successful treatment of hydrocephalus [5]. In programmable shunts, the valve contains magnets that enable transcutaneous adjustments of the valve's opening pressure [2, 4]. Shunts are commonly placed in the peritoneum, right atrium, or pleural space. VP shunting is the preferred method for CSF shunting by most neurosurgeons due to fewer complications and to the relative ease of peritoneal access [27]. Intra-abdominal pathology, such as peritoneal adhesions or recurrent peritonitis, necessitates placement or relocation into an alternative drainage site [4]. VA shunts are generally chosen when VP shunting has already failed or is contraindicated. The right atrium may be accessed percutaneously via the facial, subclavian, or internal jugular vein [28], and proper placement of the distal VA catheter may be ensured by real-time transesophageal echocardiography. The primary disadvantage of VA shunts is their risk of serious intravascular complications. On the other hand, ventriculopleural shunts have been rarely used for long-term shunting because of the high incidence of hydrothorax. Some authors have reported using ventriculopleural shunts for temporary CSF drainage in cases of VP or VA shunt infection and of tumoral hydrocephalus [4].

Radiologists are usually asked to assess shunt function by determining the position of the shunt tubing and for estimating the ventricular size. Decrease in ventricular size after shunting depends on several factors among them the cause of hydrocephalus. A prompt reduction as shown by a 24-h after shunting CT is expected in uncomplicated cases. CT scan will depict a normal or slit-like appearance of the ventricles in 60–80 % of shunted children [5]. If the ventricular size remains unchanged after 1–3 days, the patency of the shunt system should be questioned [26].

3.3.2 Endoscopic Third Ventriculostomy

ETV is an increasingly popular treatment of hydrocephalus since it avoids many of shunt-related complications, especially those of shunt dependence and overdrainage [21]. The main indication for performing an ETV is obstructive hydrocephalus, for example, in cases of aqueduct stenosis or tumors at its vicinity [26]. Age is the main determinant of outcome after ETV, with younger children, especially neonates, having a poorer prognosis [29]. Specifically, ETV resolves hydrocephalus in 80 % of children older than 2 years of age, but is not as effective in children younger than 2 years due to immaturity of the arachnoid granulations [21, 30, 31]. In ETV, an endoscope is used to create a hole in the floor of the third ventricle, immediately anterior to the mammillary bodies. It allows the passage of intraventricular CSF to the interpeduncular and suprasellar cisterns, from where it can flow laterally and upwards over the cerebral convexities to sites of CSF resorption [26]. If ETV does not result in adequate resolution of hydrocephalus, a ventricular shunt can still be placed.

Endoscopic management must also be considered before shunt replacement in cases of CSF shunt malfunction to avoid shunt-related complications. Some cases require staged endoscopic procedures to adequately communicate cavities in loculated hydrocephalus [32]. Decrease in ventricular size following ETV, in contrast with shunting, may be more gradual and occurs over several weeks [31]. MR is the study of choice for the assessment of the success of an ETV (Fig. 3.5) as only MR can assess the patency of the surgically created stoma in the floor of the third ventricle and observe the CSF pulsating through it [26].

3.4 Postoperative Complications After Shunt Placement (Table 3.1)

3.4.1 Intraventricular Hemorrhage

Intraventricular hemorrhage during shunt revision in shunted patients is a potentially serious complication due to the almost constant adhesions of the proximal catheter tip to the choroid plexus and/or to ventricular walls [5, 33, 40]. Hemorrhage complicating shunt failure is a known predictor of future ETV failure. Intraventricular bleeding arises from subependymal vessels or from the choroid plexus when these vascular structures are injured by the ventriculoscope or by the endoscopic instruments. Generally, the blood loss is stopped by means of a continuous irrigation with Ringer's solution to clear the clots or even one has to resort to placing an EVD if the hemorrhage continues [5, 33–35]. Postoperative neuroimaging may demonstrate a subependymal hematoma (Fig. 3.6) that might require an adjunctive surgical procedure for its management [33, 36].

The reported incidence of intraventricular hemorrhage ranges around 1–3 % of the cases [34, 37], although some authors indicate a higher incidence ranging between 3.5 and 6 % in infants [38, 39]. This higher rate could be explained in part by taking into account the less favorable ventricular anatomy in this age group, such as smaller Monro's foramina and larger interthalamic adhesions, which would increase the risk of surgical damage during the surgical procedure [33].

Hemorrhages within the ventricles, which many times evolve in an urgent scenery, are usually assessed by CT.

Table 3.1 Postoperative complications after CSF shunting

Complications
Intraventricular hemorrhage
Parenchymal hemorrhage
Subdural hematomas or hygromas
Pneumocephalus
Ventricular collapse/mantle inversion
Subarachnoid hemorrhage

3.4.2 Parenchymal Hemorrhage

The occurrence of intracerebral hematoma due to damage to the brain vessels during the introduction of the proximal catheter or the ventriculoscope, although possible, is rather uncommon but possesses an important potential morbidity [5, 33, 35, 41]. Large intraparenchymal and intraventricular hemorrhages are disastrous complications, especially in patients who have coagulopathies or are receiving anticoagulants (Fig. 3.6) [2]. These hemorrhages are well delineated in CT studies, and the smallest one does not require further surgical treatment.

3.4.3 Subdural Hematomas or Hygromas

Subdural hematomas or hygromas usually follow a benign course [5, 42]. In acute subdural hematomas, excessive loss of CSF during the endoscopic procedure is probably the main pathogenetic mechanism [33]. Post-shunting subdural collections have been reported to be more frequent in patients with long-standing macrocrania and subsequent craniocerebral disproportion characterized by a remarkably decreased intracranial compliance [33, 43]. On the contrary, subdural fluid collections after EVT have been only occasionally described (an overall rate of 0.5–1.5 % was reported in a large series) [35].

Neuroimaging studies (CT or MRI) contribute to the diagnosis of these subdural collections and are used to follow-up their evolution and to monitor the results of treatments. In general, the appearance of these collections does not differ from the normal images of subdural hygromas and hematomas found in other conditions.

3.4.4 Pneumocephalus

The presence of intracranial air following CSF shunting or endoscopic procedures is usually unimportant. However, tension pneumocephalus represents infrequent but dangerous complication [44]. Intracranial air (Fig. 3.6) results

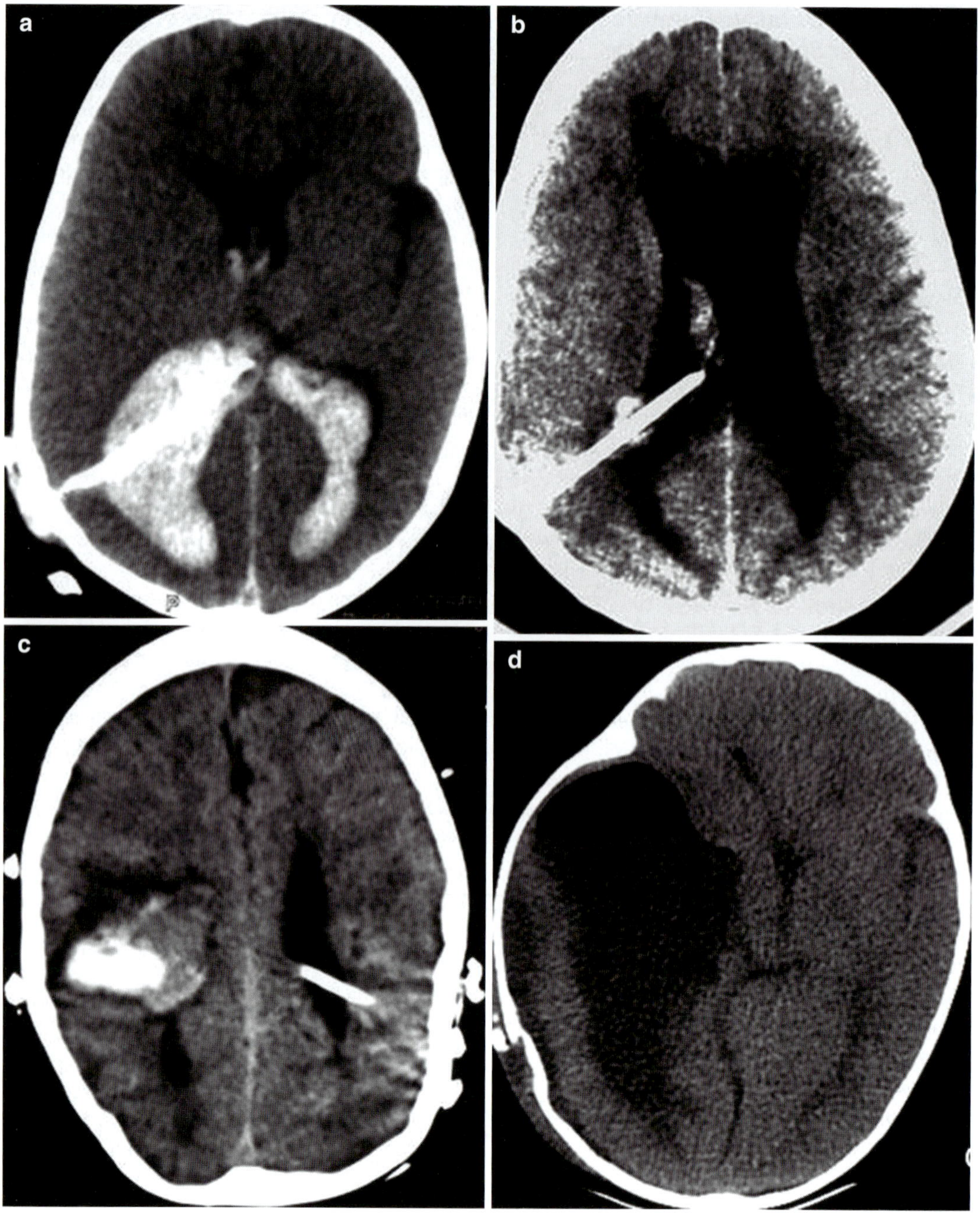

Fig. 3.6 Postsurgical complications. (**a**) Axial CT with intraventricular hemorrhage in occipital horns after catheter placement. (**b**) Non-contrast cranial CT with intraventricular hemorrhage and clot around intraventricular catheter. (**c**) Postsurgical CT that shows parenchymal hemorrhage in right frontal lobe adjacent to the lateral ventricle. (**d**) CT in a patient with loculated hydrocephalus and pneumocephalus in temporal horn after shunt placement. (**e**) b1500 DWI MRI performed after urgent catheter replacement illustrating subacute ischemic infarction in left occipital lobe. (**f**) Axial cranial CT after ETV procedure with hematoma in the anterior limb of internal capsule and pneumoventriculus in the right frontal horn

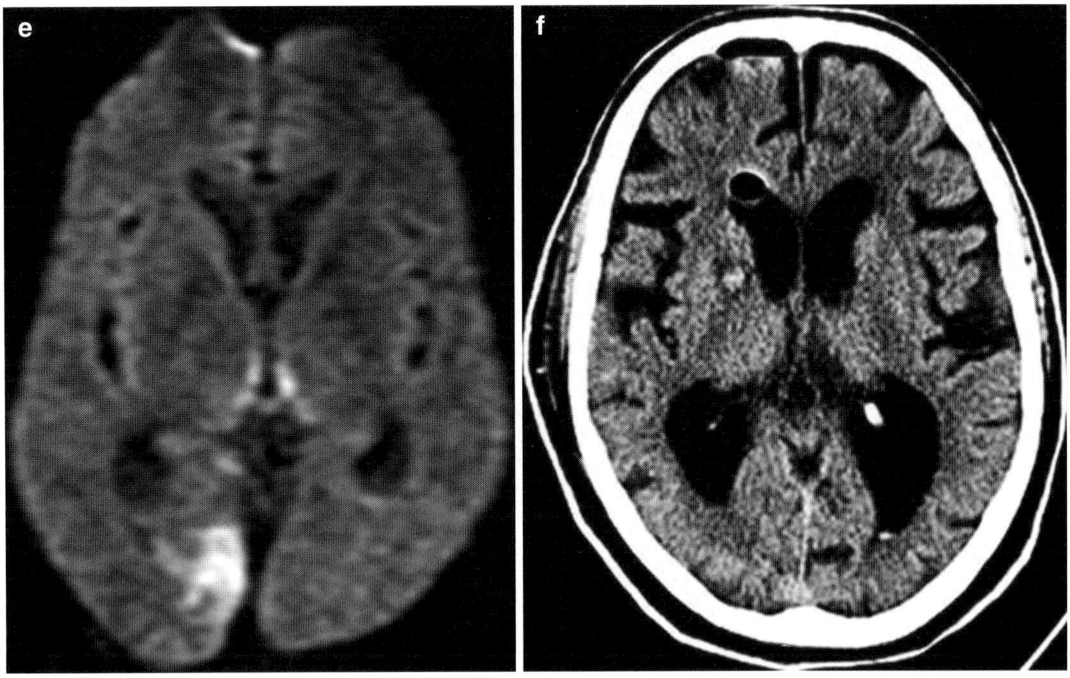

Fig. 3.6 (continued)

from the reduction in volume of the brain due to perioperative CSF leaks during the extrathecal CSF shunt implant or during the procedure of ETV [33, 45]. The presence of pneumocephalus, its volume, and distribution is clearly depicted with the current neuroimaging procedures (CT, MRI, and even with plain skull radiographs).

3.4.5 Other Complications

Another extremely rare complication of CSF overdrainage is the appearance of ventricular collapse and associated cerebral mantle inversion that are clearly depicted by CT or MRI studies [96]. They may require shunt replacement with flow-regulated valves, valve pressure upgrading, or addition of siphoning retarding [5]. Another unusual complication of CSF shunting is the occurrence of subarachnoid hemorrhage that is also well delineated by CT or MRI studies.

3.5 Intracranial Complications of CSF Shunts (Table 3.2)

3.5.1 Acute–Subacute Complications

3.5.1.1 Shunt Infection

Infection is a common etiology of shunt failure and represents the second cause of shunt dysfunction after mechanical malfunction [5, 33]. The reported incidence of shunt infection ranges from 1 to 40 % and average 8.5–15 % [33, 46, 47]. The majority of shunt infections occur in the postoperative period (70 % within 1 month, 85 % within 9 months) and are thought to be mainly due to contamination during the surgery [5, 27, 33, 50]. Intraoperative contamination by skin flora is the primary mode of infection, while other sources of shunt infection are proximal seeding from meningitis and distal seeding from peritonitis and wound infections [5]. Skin bacteria, such as *S. epidermidis* (50–90 % of the cases) and *S. aureus* (15–40 %), are most commonly

Table 3.2 Intracranial complications of CSF shunts

Type of intracranial complication
Acute–subacute complications
Shunt infection
Obstruction
Disconnection/fracture
Catheter malpositions/migrations
Overdrainage and slit ventricle syndrome
Loculations
Subcutaneous CSF collections and CSF fistula
Complications of ETV
Chronic complications
Craniosynostosis
Cranioencephalic disproportion
Meningeal fibrosis
Perishunt porencephaly and periventricular leukomalacia
Trapped fourth ventricle
Pneumocephalus

found in early infectious complications [33, 51]. Other causative agents are gram-negative rods (15 %) and *Propionibacterium acnes* [5]. Shunt contamination may primarily originate from the skin incision proper and has been related to insufficient asepsis, defective surgical material, and long-lasting operations [33, 52].

Late infections are less common. In fact, only 10–15 % of overall infectious complications occur 1 year after the shunt implantation and are attributed to contamination of the distal catheter by the visceral content or infiltration of germs through superficial skin wounds [33, 50]. The involved pathogens in late infection (*P. acnes*, *Enterococcus faecalis*, *Streptococcus faecalis*) arise from the hair follicles or from the colonic contents and are capable of contaminating the catheter and even of reaching the cerebral ventricles [33, 50].

Infection in VP shunts may be evidenced by wound infection, fever, shunt malfunction, or peritonitis. VA shunts are associated with a similar incidence of infection; however, endocarditis and septic emboli result in higher morbidity and mortality. Similarly, infection of ventriculopleural shunts may result in empyema [4].

In comparison with extrathecal CSF shunts, infections in the context of ETV are not so problematic. The absence of the foreign body represented by the shunt apparatus limits the infection rate to 1–5 % of the cases [33–35, 48]. The incidence of infection seems to depend more on a history of previously infected shunts or external drainages than on the actual ETV procedure [33, 35, 37, 49].

The clinical signs of shunt infection are nausea, headache, and lethargy. Fever may or may not be present. Meningeal symptoms may also be absent because there is little communication between the infected ventricles and meningeal CSF. Lumbar and ventricular punctures are routinely performed to isolate these bacteria, but cultures are usually sterile. Instead, CSF obtained from the shunt reservoir typically allows for isolation of the causative organism [5]. Regarding management of shunt infection, several variants of treatments may be utilized [2, 5]. These will be discussed in detail in the corresponding chapter or the book.

CT and MRI may show irregular leptomeningeal and ventricular ependymal enhancement consistent with meningitis and ventriculitis, respectively [4]. Ventriculitis may be seen on contrast-enhanced CT or MRI as an irregular enhancement of the ependymal lining of the ventricles or of the cerebral cortical sulci [2, 5]. Debris within the ventricles, especially on diffusion-weighted imaging, are shown by differences in intensity between infected and normal fluid constituting the best neuroimaging sign of ventriculitis. Contrast-enhanced sequences demonstrate ependymal lineal contrast uptake. Pachymeningeal enhancement not due to infection can also be seen due to overshunting that can persist postoperatively for months [4, 5].

3.5.1.2 Shunt Obstruction

A shunt can be occluded at three points: the proximal catheter, the valve, and the distal catheter. The two most likely sites of obstruction are the ventricular catheter tip, which can be blocked by in-growing choroid plexus, and the shunt valve, which can be blocked by blood and debris [5].

In general, the postoperative period has the highest risk for shunt obstruction originated by debris and blood products. However, obstruction can occur at any time after shunt placement approaching a rate of 0.5 % per month [4, 5]. Ventricular catheter obstruction was found as the main cause of mechanical failure (63.2 %) followed by distal catheter occlusion (23.5 %), migration (8.8 %), disconnection (1.4 %), and breaking (1.4 %) [33].

Proximal catheter block accounts for 50 % of all failures within the first 2 years after shunt placement [4]. Proximal catheter obstruction frequently results from choroidal and ependymal reactions around the tip of the ventricular catheter. Actually, the proximity of the choroid plexus and the catheter tip is recognized as the most common cause of proximal shunt malfunction [33].

Whatever the site of obstruction, the symptoms are related to the secondary pathological increase in ICP [33]. The clinical presentation of shunt obstruction varies with age. Infants often present with nausea, vomiting, and irritability. Older children and adults, however, present with symptoms such as headache, nausea, vomiting, cranial nerve palsies, and ataxia [5, 27].

Imaging can reveal the position of the proximal catheter, normal connections, and ventricular enlargement (Fig. 3.7). Comparison of the last scan with preexisting or baseline studies is critical for demonstrating signs of either overt or subtle ventricular enlargement. When ventricular size is equivocal, blurring of the margins of the ventricles due to transependymal spread of CSF, perishunt edema, and subgaleal fluid collections suggests the presence of acute obstruction [5]. The proximal catheter can also migrate within the ventricle causing faulty CSF drainage. Outer migration of the proximal catheter is most commonly caused by traction of the distal catheter by scar tissue along the chest wall or the peritoneal entry site [27]. Diagnosis of shunt block is aided by comparing postoperative catheter placement on CT and conventional radiographs with images obtained when the patient becomes symptomatic [4].

3.5.1.3 Disconnection and Breakage

Disconnections most commonly occur shortly after shunt placement [2, 4]. They represent the second most common cause of shunt failure in children and most often occur in the neck that constitutes an area with greater mobility [2, 5]. Detachment of shunt components can occur at the connection of the shunt tubing to the reservoir or at the level of Y-shaped connectors, which are sometimes used to drain two ventricular cavities simultaneously (Fig. 3.8) [2]. Shunt disconnections became rare after the introduction of the one-piece or soldered shunts. Nowadays, disconnection is usually due to the stretching of junctions of the proximal or distal catheter to the valve or to fracture of the shunt tubing [33, 40].

Material failures and surgical errors are often primary causes of shunt detachment [27]. Factors predisposing to disconnection include shunt aging, restricted mobility, repetitive trauma, and the presence of catheter connections and valve junctions. As shunts age, they undergo calcification and biodegradation rendering them more susceptible to breakage. The fibrous tissue that develops along the tubing also anchors the catheter leading to disconnection or fracture as the child grows [5].

Neuroimaging diagnosis of shunt disconnection is mainly made by the "shunt series" (Fig. 3.9) [27]. This diagnostic method reveals radiolucent gaps between segments and, in occasions, zones of calcification. It is important to remember that certain shunt components may also be radiolucent and should not be mistaken for disconnection (a common diagnostic pitfall). Comparison of these images with previous radiographs is mandatory as many shunting devices have sections of radiolucent tubing or valves [2, 4, 5]. Small collections of CSF can develop at the site of rupture or disconnection and are visualized on CT slices. CT can demonstrate subgaleal collections and enlarged ventricles too [2, 5, 33].

3.5.1.4 Catheter Malposition and Migration

Malposition of the proximal or distal limbs of shunts can result in malfunction. In certain cases, however, malfunction may not occur if the lateral apertures of the catheter remain within the ventricle as occurs when the position of the shunt tip is unchanged respect to prior studies. Shunt

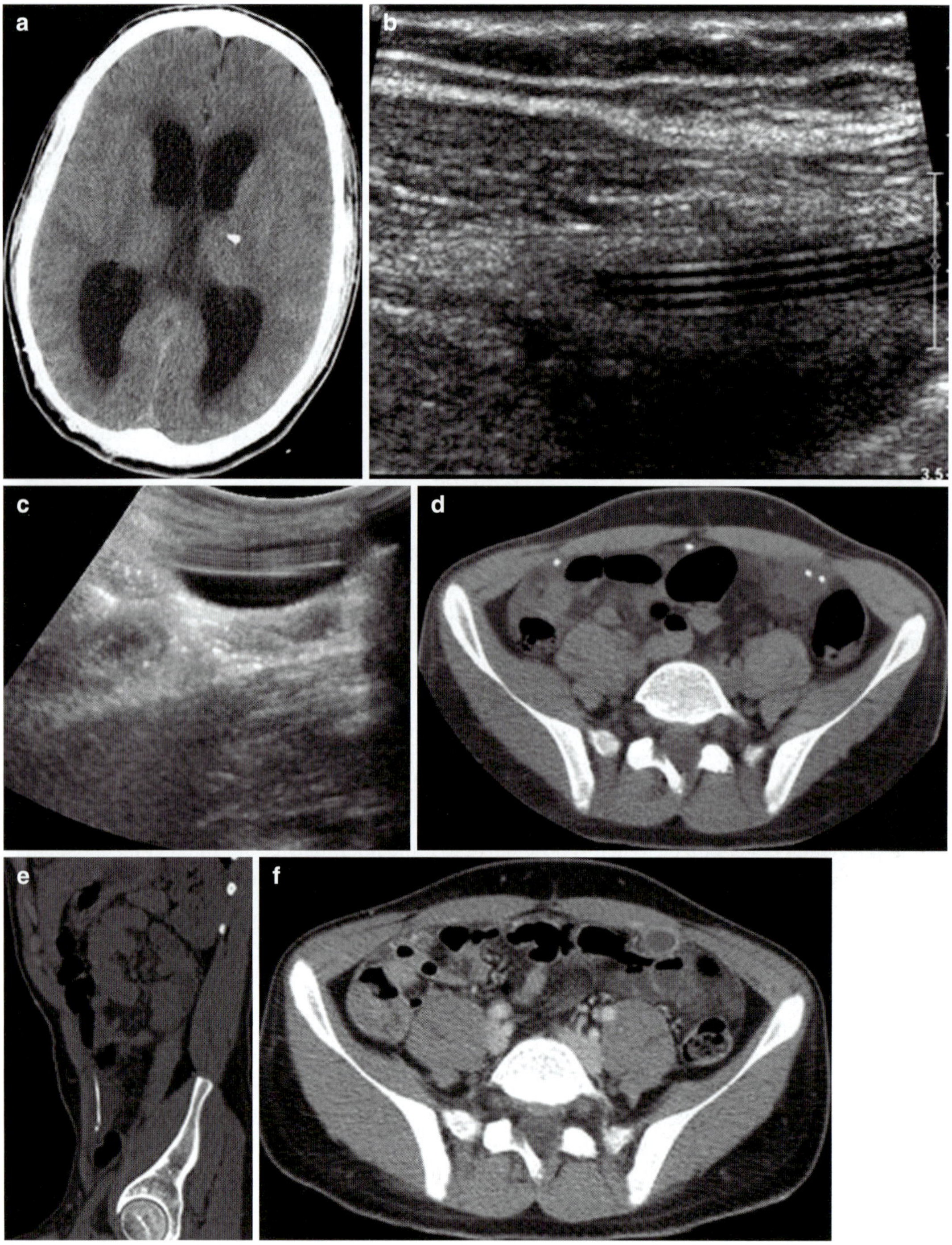

Fig. 3.7 A 20-year-old-man given a VP shunt who presented with altered mental status. (**a**) Transaxial CT depicting diffuse hydrocephalus and transependymal CSF by distal shunt obstruction. (**b**, **c**) Abdominal US showing intraperitoneal fluid collection surrounding catheter tip. (**d**) Transaxial CT image and (**e**) sagittal reconstruction revealing intraperitoneal fluid collection surrounding the catheter tip in the left paracolic gutter. (**f**) Transaxial CT image 1 month later that demonstrates improvement in the left pseudocyst

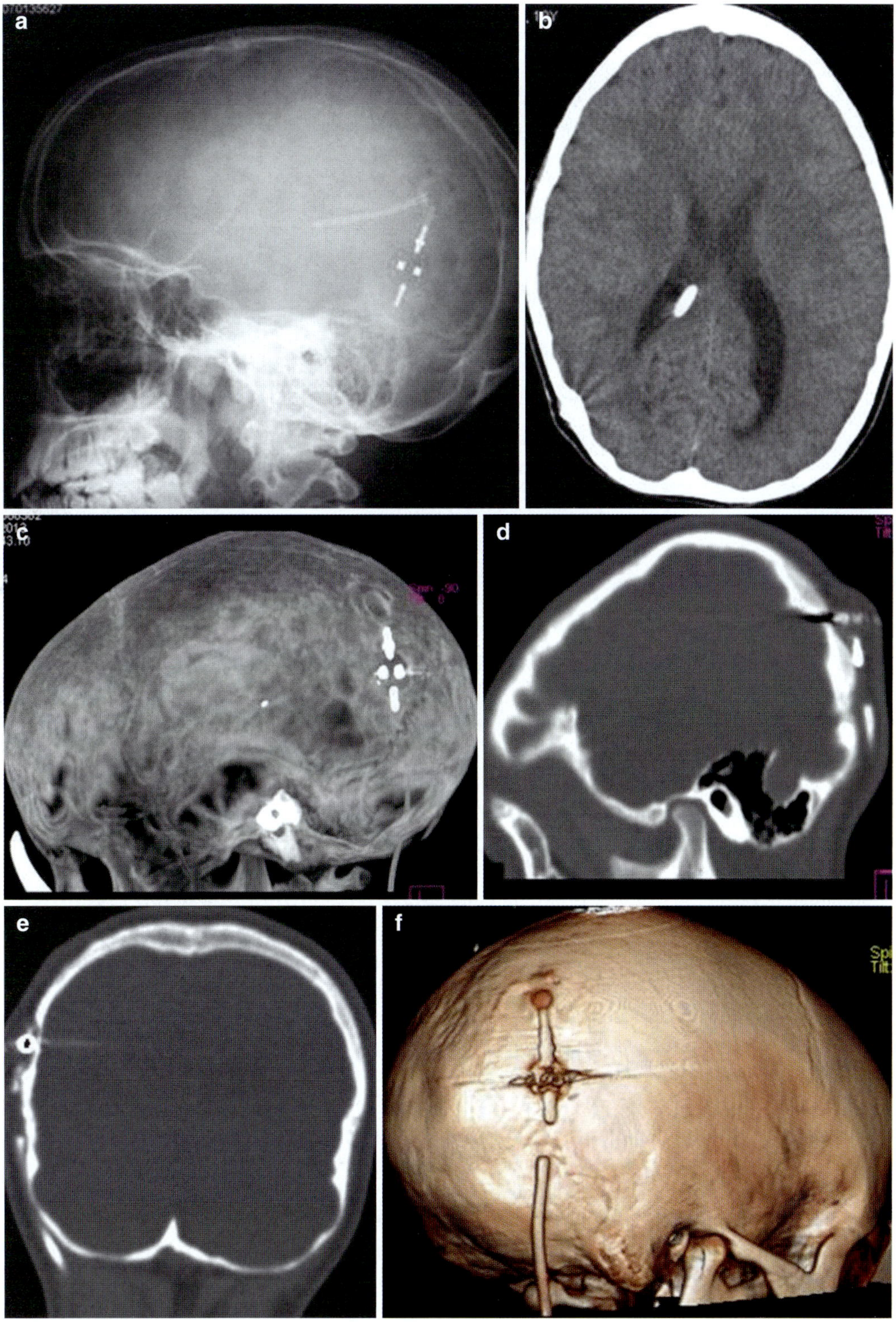

Fig. 3.8 Distal catheter disconnection in a 10-year-old-patient with a Sophy valve and clinical suspicion of shunt malfunction. A disconnection of the distal catheter next to the valve is demonstrated in lateral cranial view of SS (**a**), sagittal (**d**), and coronal (**e**) 2D multiplanar reconstruction (MPR), 3D maximum intensity projection (MIP), (**c**) and VR reconstruction of cranial CT (**f**). Axial plane of cranial CT shows slightly enlarged ventricles and intraventricular catheter (**b**)

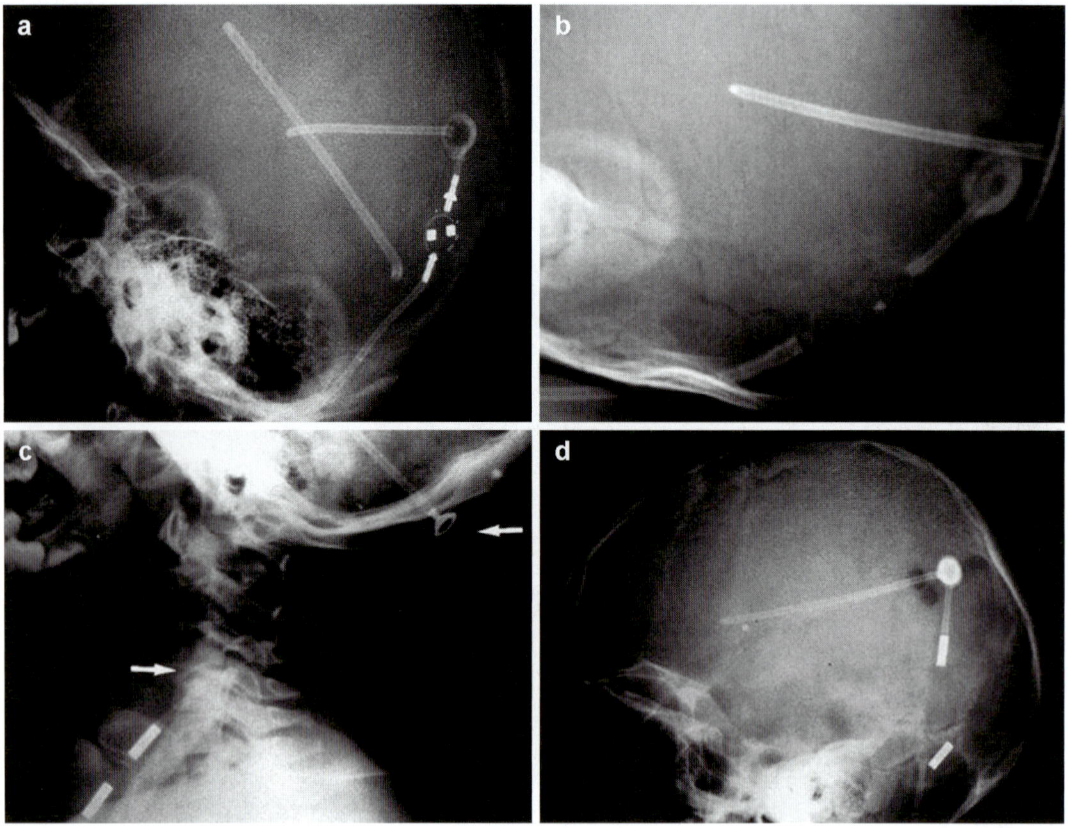

Fig. 3.9 Disconnection and breakage in lateral cranial SS. (**a**) Intraventricular retained catheter; note the presence of another valve (Sophy). (**b**) Reservoir detachment. (**c**) Disconnection and migration (*arrows*) of the reservoir. (**d**) Valve fracture after a head trauma

migration can occur at the distal or proximal end of the shunt (Fig. 3.10). Once the catheter is fixed to the subcutaneous tissues by fibrous tissue, the continued growth of the child results in traction and catheter migration. The proximal catheter can migrate to a non-draining area, such as the choroid, or to an extraventricular location in the parenchyma [5].

Flexion–extension of the head facilitates upward movement of the peritoneal catheter. In addition, the positive abdominal pressure against the negative suction from the intraventricular pressure, the loss of subcutaneous tissue, and the use of shunts with spring coils [53] might also contribute to the proximal migration of the catheter inside the ventricles, the subarachnoid, and subdural space or into the subgaleal scalp tissue [33, 54].

3.5.1.5 Overdrainage and Slit Ventricle Syndrome

Placement of CSF ventricular shunts may be complicated by overdrainage in variable proportions [55]. Diverse manifestations of excessive CSF drainage occurred in approximately 18 % of hydrocephalic children in one of our series [56]. Ventricular size returns to normal within 24 h after shunt placement with a subsequent more gradual reduction that depends on the cause and chronicity of hydrocephalus. However, if the lateral ventricles collapse too rapidly, the brain may not be elastic enough to fill the space. The resulting disparity between the brain size and skull (Fig. 3.11) leads to formation of subdural hygromas or hematomas [4, 5].

Chronic overdrainage is relatively common and is shown as small-sized or slit-like ventri-

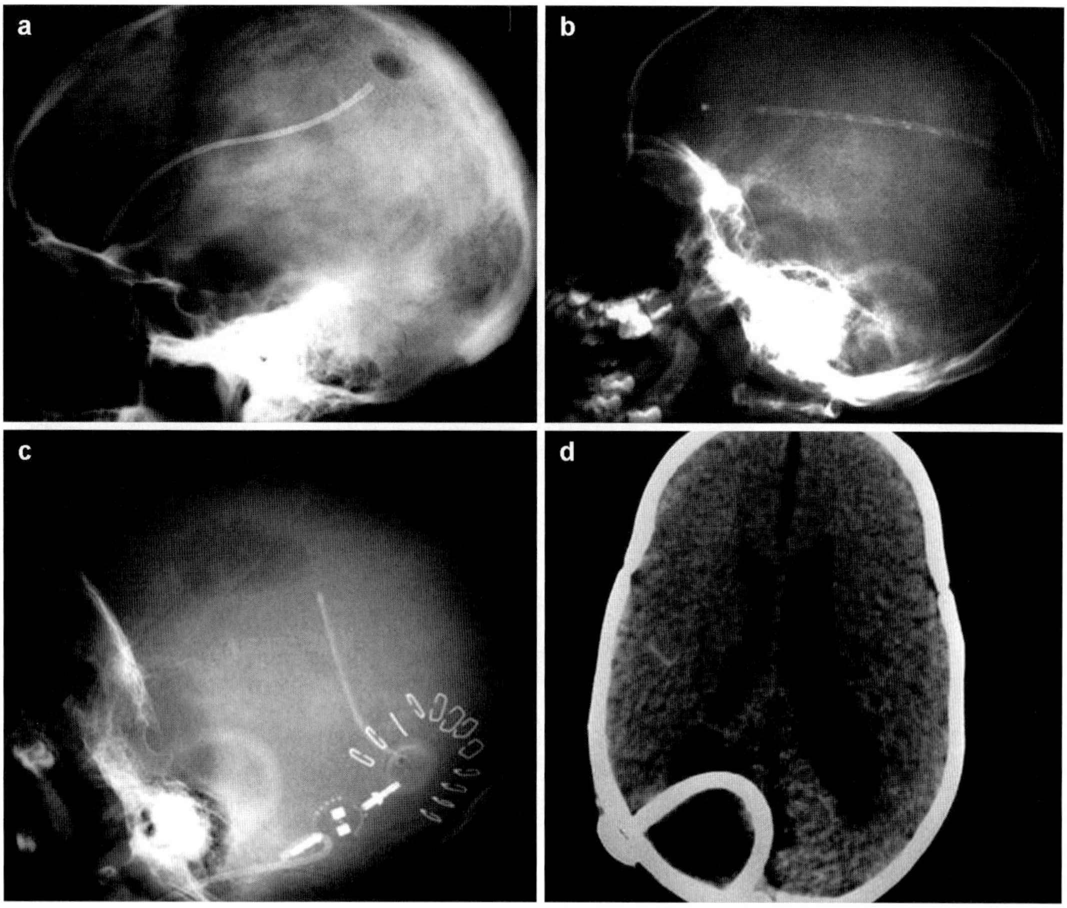

Fig. 3.10 Catheter misplacements. (**a**, **b**) Cranial lateral views of SS that show excessive length of the ventricular catheter. (**c**) Postoperative skull X-ray film depicting pneumocephalus and kinking of the distal catheter just at the back of the valve. (**d**) Axial CT depicting a curved intraventricular catheter and surrounding porencephaly

cles on neuroimaging studies in up to 50 % of shunted children [4]. Slit-like ventricles are non-significant clinically in the majority of cases. The interest of this finding rests on the association of slit-like ventricles to its symptomatic counterpart called "slit ventricle syndrome" (SVS). This syndrome is defined as the presence of intermittent symptoms of raised ICP associated with the slit-like appearance of the ventricles on neuroimaging studies [33].

Only 0.9–3.3 % of shunted children present the clinical manifestations of the SVS. The majority of patients with small ventricles do not develop the syndrome, and their ventricles will dilate in the event of shunt malfunction [2]. However, up to 11 % of children with symptoms of shunt failure can have slit-like ventricles as well due to the presence of the SVS. This syndrome is uncommon, but it may be responsible for an important number of shunt revisions [5, 57]. SVS usually develops during the first decade [33] being at increased risk children with a shunt placed before 1 year of age [5, 58].

The most accepted pathogenic mechanism for the appearance of slit ventricles would be an excessive reduction in ventricular size due to CSF overdrainage, causing intermittent obstructions of the catheter by the ventricular walls with subsequent reopening when the cerebral ventricle enlarges as a result of the secondary increase in ventricular pressure [33]. On the contrary, chronic overdrainage causes noncompliant ventricles due

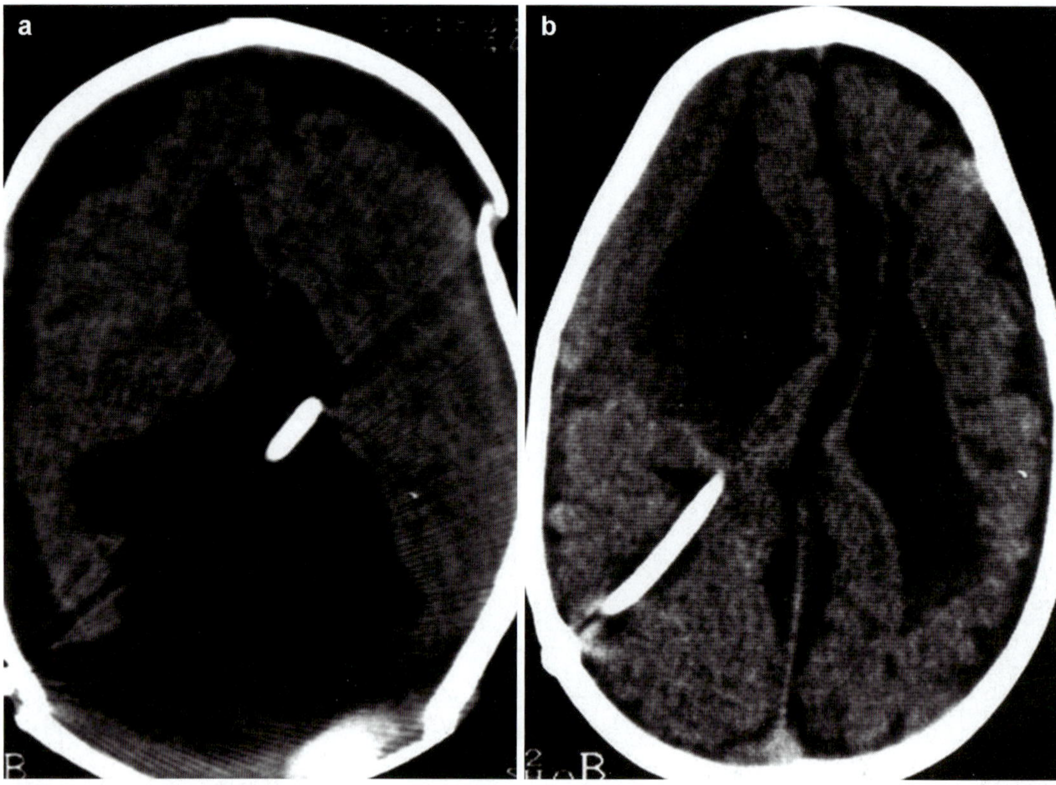

Fig. 3.11 CT of overdrainage. (**a**) Intraventricular catheter with dysmorphic ventricles, bilateral subdural hygromas and sclerosis of the coronal suture. (**b**) Intraventricular catheter with frontal subacute subdural hematoma, right frontal arachnoid cyst, and cerebral collapse

to a combination of venous congestion, subependymal gliosis, and microcephaly or craniostenosis. As a result, the ventricles remain collapsed around the catheter despite dangerous intraventricular pressure rises.

Diagnosis is made clinically by showing elevated ICP that correlates with patient symptoms in the absence of ventriculomegaly. There are no imaging criteria for the diagnosis of SVS [4]. Patients with this syndrome have small ventricles at CT or MR [2] (Fig. 3.12). Other neuroimaging manifestations of overshunting include lateral ventricular collapse around the proximal catheter tip or even cortical mantle collapse and subdural hematoma formation [5].

3.5.1.6 Loculation

This occurs when separate, non-communicating, fluid pouches develop within the ventricles. Children with a history of hemorrhage or ventriculitis are at increased risk for developing septae. At the time of initial shunt placement, loculations may not be noted as they may be masked by the ventricular dilatation. The loculations may develop progressively resulting in isolated segments of the ventricular system that are not adequately drained. These CSF compartments may enlarge causing symptomatic compression of the surrounding brain [3]. Management consists of communicating the loculated compartments with the rest of the ventricular system, which is best achieved with neuroendoscopic methods aimed at leaving the child with a single shunt [3]. MRI delineates best the anatomy of these loculated compartments (Fig. 3.13) and may also show transependymal flow adjacent to the isolated cavities [4].

3.5.1.7 Subcutaneous CSF Collections and CSF Fistulas

They have been described as manifestations of mechanical shunt malfunctions. However, they can even be observed in patients with patent

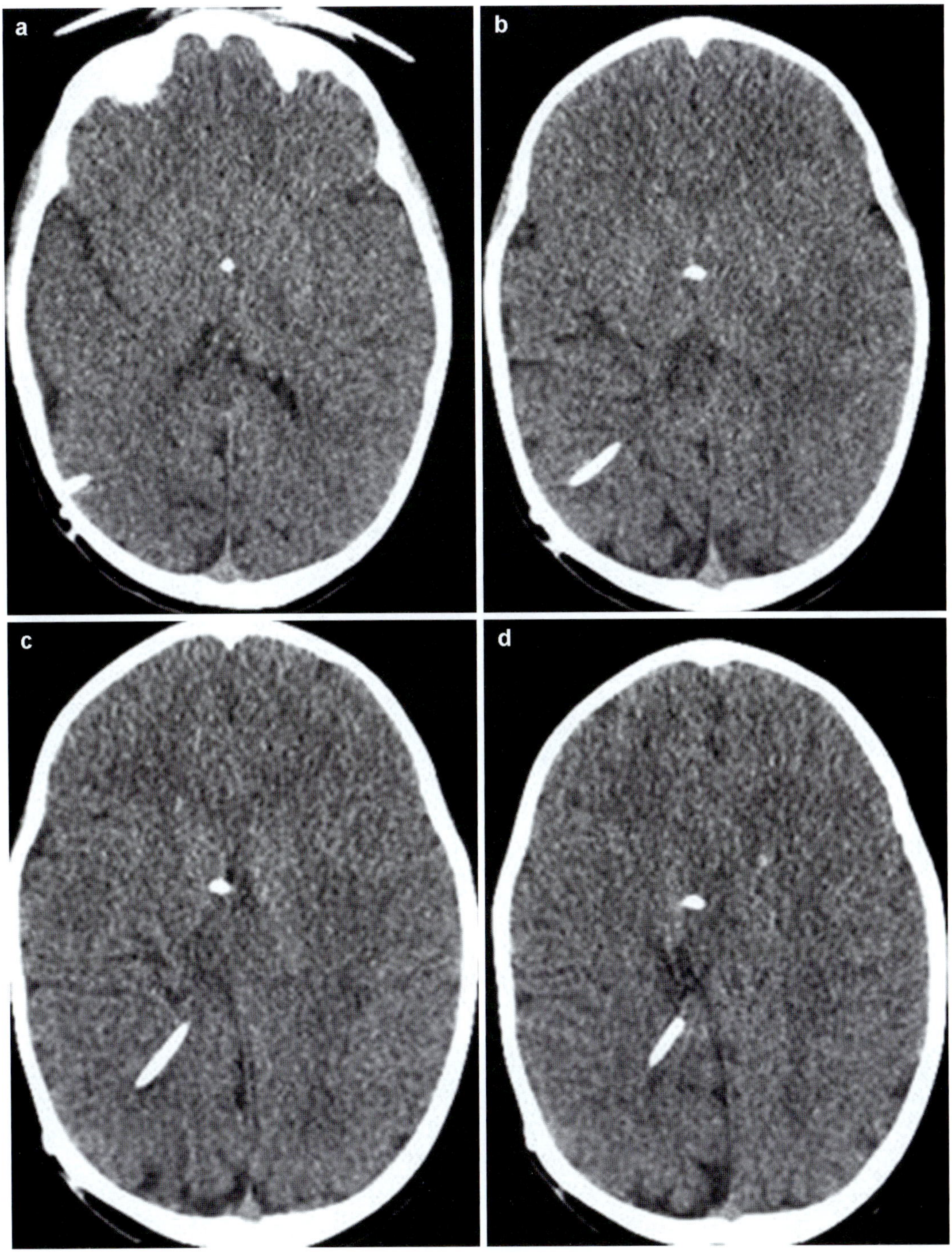

Fig. 3.12 Slit ventricle syndrome. Post-hemorrhagic hydrocephalus treated with a Miethke valve in a patient with headache and seizures. Cranial CT showing the proximal catheter and slit-like ventricles (**a–d**)

shunts. The incidence of subcutaneous CSF collections and CSF leakage in patients with normally functioning shunts varies between 0.1 and 5.5 % [59]. CT or MRI may reveal the persistence of ventricular dilatation that reflects the existence of CSF underdrainage. Subgaleal CSF collections

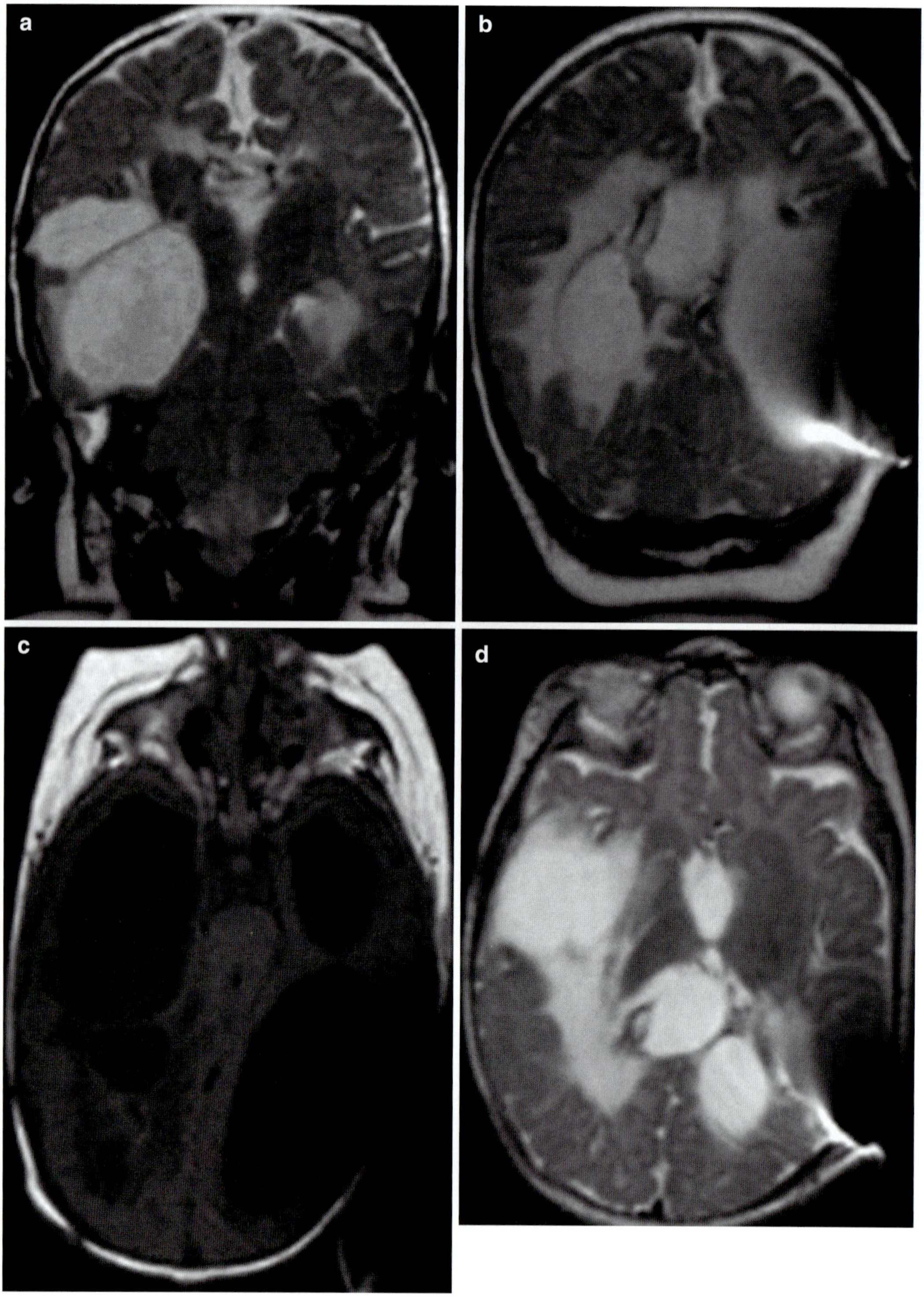

Fig. 3.13 Loculations. Patient with ventriculitis, septated hydrocephalus and VP shunt (Polaris). Cranial MR with coronal T2 (**a**, **b**), axial T1 (**c**) and axial T2 sequences (**d**, **e**, **f**) shows septated hydrocephalus with transependymal edema

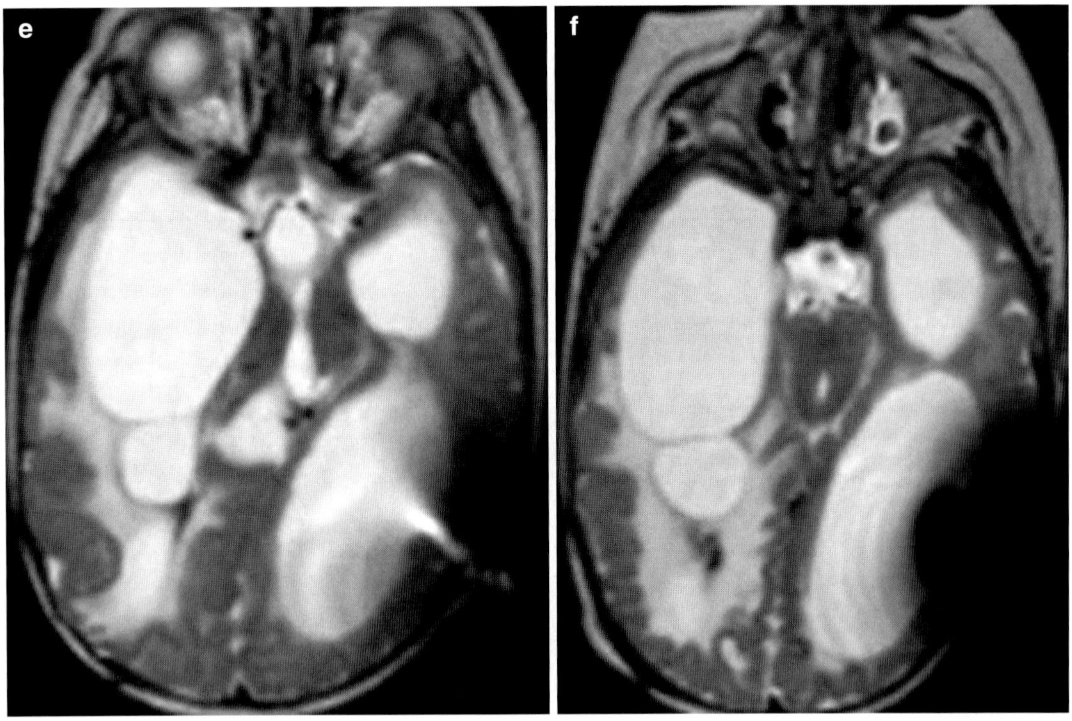

Fig. 3.13 (continued)

and CSF leakages may also occur after ETV, with an overall incidence of 2–18 %, and usually indicate failure of the procedure [35, 60].

3.5.1.8 Complications in ETV

Vascular injuries. Injury to the basilar artery or to its branches is a rare but extremely severe complication of ETV. The most frequently injured vessels are those located within the interpeduncular cistern that contains the basilar artery, the P1 segment of the posterior cerebral arteries, and the posterior choroidal arteries; the posterior compartment contains the perforating branches of the basilar and of the posterior cerebral arteries. The damage to these vessels usually manifests with cisternal or ventricular hemorrhage that are appropriately documented by performing an emergent CT study. MRI and angio-MRI best document late complications of vascular rupture. The suspicion of the development of a pseudoaneurysm calls for an angiographic study.

Neurological damage results from an injury to the nervous structures caused by the endoscopic instrumentation. The anatomical structures most frequently damaged during ETV are the walls of the third ventricle and those delimiting the foramen of Monro. Short-term complications are commonly represented by contusions of the thalamus, the fornix, or the mammillary bodies, secondary to the incorrect manipulation of the ventriculoscope or of the endoscopic instruments (Fig. 3.6) [35].

3.5.2 Chronic Complications

Chronic overdrainage causes noncompliant ventricles due to a combination of venous congestion, subependymal gliosis, microcephaly, and craniosynostosis [60–63]. The ventricles may remain collapsed around the catheter even after extreme increases of the ICP [64]. Diagnosis is made purely based on clinical manifestations with elevated intracranial pressure that correlates with patients' symptoms in the absence of ventriculomegaly as seen in CT or MRI studies [33].

3.5.2.1 Craniosynostosis

Craniosynostosis secondary to the placement of a CSF shunt device is reported with an incidence of about 10–15 % and is often associated with the SVS. The phenomenon arises from the osteoblastic/osteoclastic activity following the relief of raised ICP that leads to remodeling and lamination of the skull with formation of new bone along the inner skull table. Infants are particularly prone to this complication. In fact, some of the predisposing factors are exclusive for this age group, such as sunken fontanelle, overlapping of previously diastatic bones, and premature closure of the sutures. Other recognized predisposing factors are dense parasutural bone, early appearance of definable diploe, widened diploic spaces, few convolutional or endocranial vascular landmarks, and low cranium-to-face ratio [63]. In these situations, craniectomies and skull reshaping procedures may be required for allowing for future brain growth and for relief of intracranial hypertension (Fig. 3.14). Craniosynostosis features

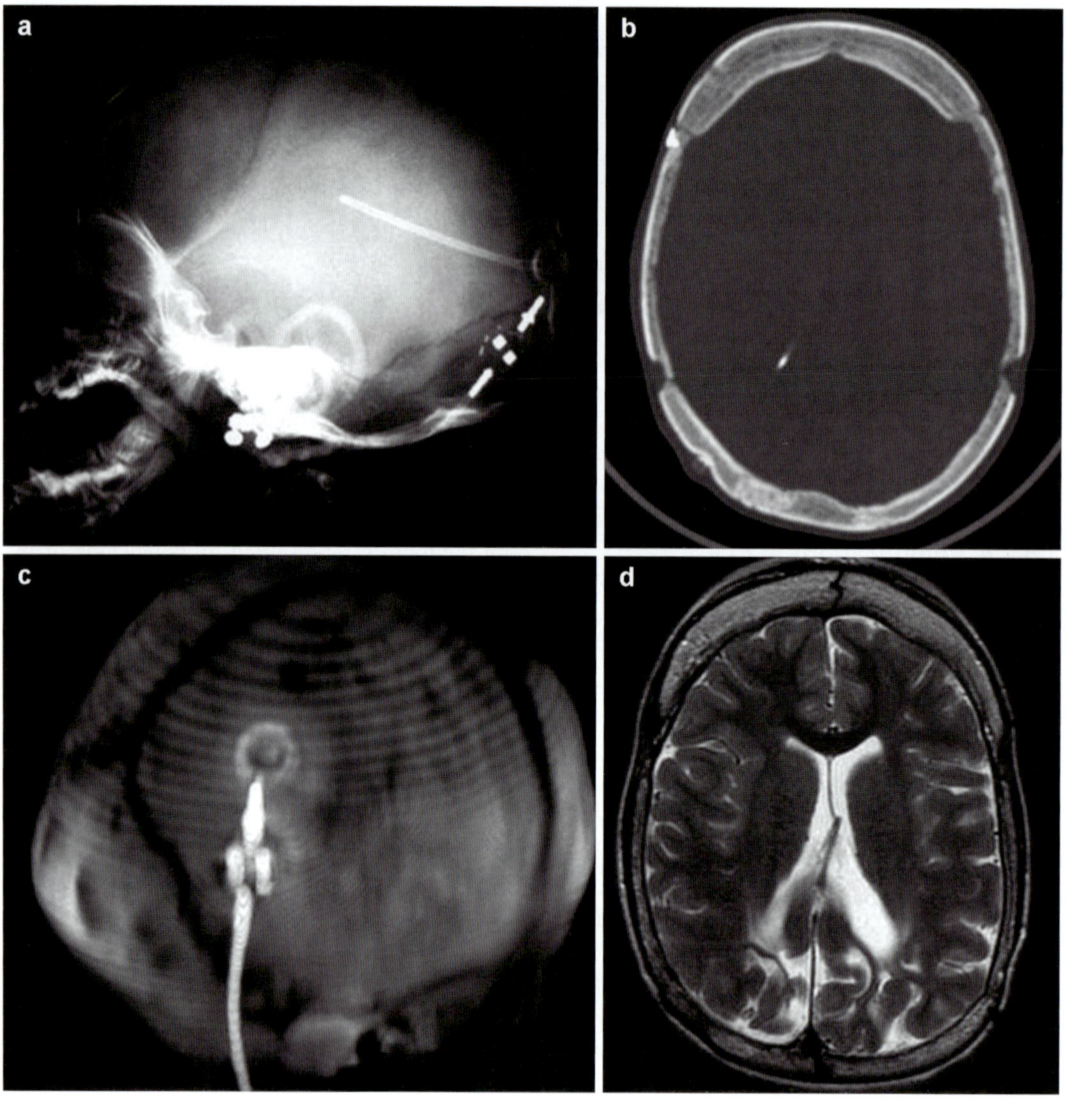

Fig. 3.14 Suture diastasis and cranial hyperostosis. (**a**) Cranial lateral view of SS and (**c**) VR CT reconstruction that show the shunt and suture diastasis. (**b**) Axial cranial CT and (**d**) cranial MR with axial T2 sequence demonstrating a widened diploe

are closely related to those of cranioencephalic disproportion. Demonstration of sutural closure requires performing CT with bone-window settings and with 3D-CT reconstructions. Structural brain changes secondary to craniostenosis are best delineated by MRI that may show indirect signs of brain compression and even secondary descent of the cerebellar tonsils.

3.5.2.2 Acquired Cranioencephalic Disproportion

Acquired cranioencephalic disproportion is a further late complication of extrathecal CSF shunts observed almost exclusively in patients operated on during infancy. Characteristically, such a complication is often associated with a caudal herniation of the cerebellar tonsils into the upper cervical canal (acquired Chiari type I malformation) together with an upward dislocation of the superior cerebellar vermis into the great Galen's vein cistern [65, 66]. The neuroimaging demonstration of this clinical picture requires using CT and MRI studies (Fig. 3.14).

3.5.2.3 Meningeal Fibrosis

Meningeal fibrosis is another manifestation of excessive or long-lasting CSF drainage, or it may originate from chronic subdural fluid collections. Its development is related with depositions of collagen and vascular granulation tissue resulting in intense enhancement on postcontrast MRI or CT.

3.5.2.4 Perishunt Encephalomalacia and Periventricular Leukomalacia

CT and MRI studies may show perishunt porencephaly (especially during episodes of shunt failure) and periventricular leukomalacia that are commonly seen in chronically shunted patients (Fig. 3.15).

3.5.2.5 Trapping of the Fourth Ventricle

Compartmentalization of the ventricular system in myelodysplastic children may result from some anatomical anomalies, such as an enlarged massa intermedia, an eccentric bulge from the head of the caudate nucleus, prominent commissural fibers, and anterior pointing of the frontal horns that contribute to narrowing of the foramina of Monro [67]. Further risk factors for isolation of the ventricles are the development of inflammatory membranes in postinfective or posthemorrhagic hydrocephalus or those that follow chemical- or radiation-induced ventriculitis. Overdrainage is also involved in the pathogenesis of isolated ventricles in SVS and trapped fourth ventricle [68]. In the first instance, distortion of the cerebral structures results in blockage of CSF circulation. In the second one, the pressure gradient between the supratentorial (lower pressure) and infratentorial ventricular system (higher) created by the shunt leads to the upward displacement of midline cerebellar structures into the tentorial incisura with subsequent distortion of the aqueduct and secondary impairment of CSF circulation.

Trapping of the fourth ventricle is particularly common in case of arachnoid adhesions that impair the egress of CSF through the foramina of Magendie and Luschka. The incidence of the isolated fourth ventricle (nearly 2.5 %) is higher than that of the supratentorial ventricular system (0.5–1 %) [67–69]. A trapped fourth ventricle occurs when loculations isolate the fourth ventricle from the supratentorial ventricles. These changes are caused by scarring at the cerebral aqueduct and the foramina of Luschka and Magendie and by the secondary closure of the aqueduct induced by the shunt itself. A second ventriculostomy catheter placed in the fourth ventricle is usually used for relieving the symptoms of raised ICP and brain stem compression produced by the expansion of the fourth ventricle (Fig. 3.15).

The above-described changes can be displayed by neuroimaging studies, especially by MRI. Imaging shows normal or small lateral ventricles and an enlarged fourth ventricle that compresses the brain stem. Sagittal MRI is particularly useful for showing occlusion or distortion of the cerebral aqueduct [5].

3.5.2.6 Pneumocephalus

Pneumocephalus is a rare late complication that can occur months to years after intraventricular

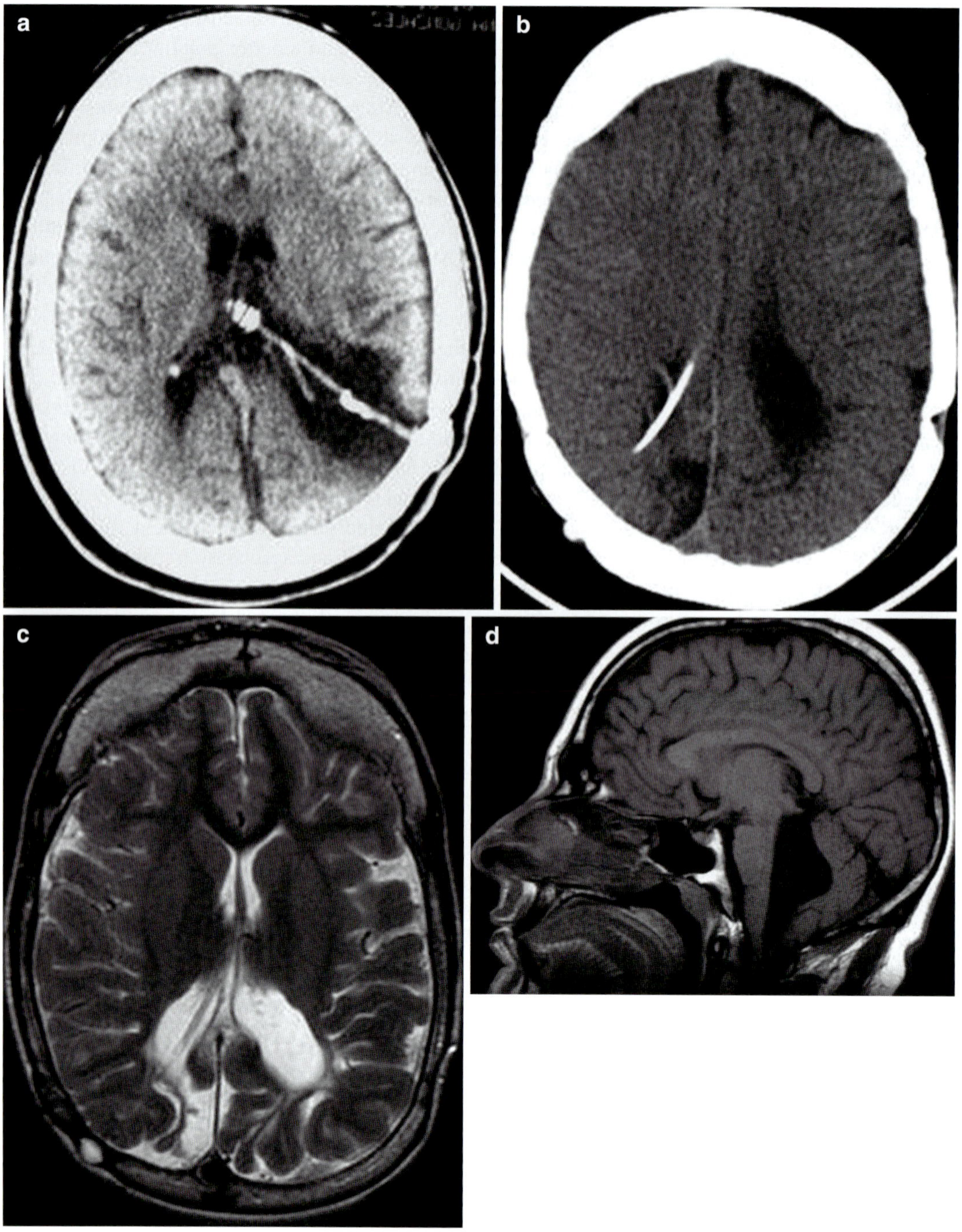

Fig. 3.15 Perishunt porencephaly and trapped fourth ventricle. (**a**) Transaxial CT image shows perishunt encephalomalacia left parietal. (**b**) Transaxial CT image and (**c**) cranial MR with axial T2 sequences showing perishunt encephalomalacia and right occipital and ventricular dysmorphia, (**d**) cranial MR with sagittal T1 sequence depicting marked dilatation of a trapped fourth ventricle. (**e**) Spinal MR with sagittal T2 sequence revealing cervical hydromyelia

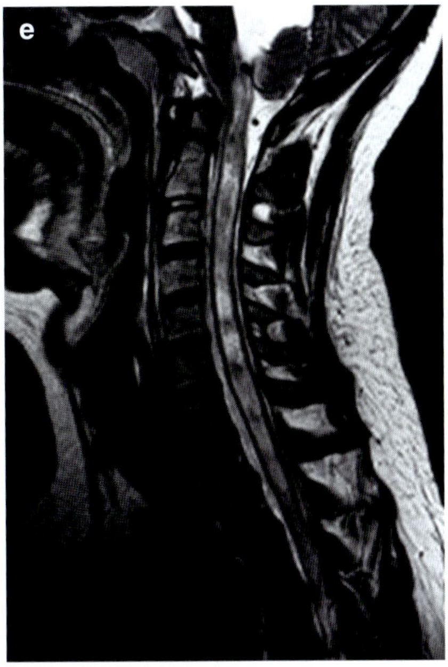

Fig. 3.15 (continued)

shunt placement. Siphoning at the catheter tip produces negative intracranial pressure that draws the air into the brain [70]. Air can also enter the skull through congenital or acquired bone orifices at the skull base in the presence of an intracranial negative pressure. Pneumocephalus may also occur in intracranial infections (colonic perforation). CT and MRI studies depict the neuroimaging of intracranial air and can help to ascertain the cause of the pneumocephalus.

3.6 Extracranial Complications of CSF Shunts (Table 3.3)

The typical shunt device involves the placement of a catheter placed within the ventricles, while the location of the distal catheter can be more variable. VP shunting is the most frequently used system for drainage of CSF given the large surface and high reabsorption capability of the peritoneum. Other sites for distal catheter placement include the superior vena cava, the right atrium of the heart, and the pleural space. Lumboperitoneal and ventriculo-gallbladder shunts are also presently utilized. Other shunts, as those ending in the ureter, fallopian tubes, etc., are now considered only of historical interest.

Table 3.3 Extracranial complications of CSF shunting

Type of complication
Shunt misplacement
Disconnection/fracture
Distal obstruction
Pneumothorax/subcutaneous emphysema
Hydrothorax/pleural effusion
Fibrothorax
Complications related to shunt variants (VA shunt)
Tricuspid valve pathology
Thromboembolic disease/pulmonary hypertension
Abdominal complications
Pseudocysts
Ascites
Inguinal hernia/hydrocele
Viscus perforation

VP shunts are however prone to experience diverse complications, with failure rates as high as 40 % within the first year after placement and 50 % within 2 years [8]. Shunt failure may result from mechanical and functional causes or may occur as a consequence of infection [71]. Noninfectious causes of shunt failure include obstruction, disconnection, and fracture. In addition, specific intra-abdominal causes of mechanical failure have been well documented, including the development of peritoneal pseudocysts, ascites, spontaneous knot formation, and migrations through the anus or to other places as the subgaleal space [3, 54, 72]. Occasionally, development of an abdominal pseudocyst or abdominal catheter adhesion might be suspected on plain radiography by the observation of a fixed, static position of the distal catheter tip on subsequent studies [3].

3.6.1 Shunt Misplacement

Shunt misplacement can also occur at the distal end of the catheter, including the abdomen, atrium, or pleura. Patients present with abdominal discomfort and eventually may develop headache, nausea, or vomiting. When the peritoneal distal tubing is misplaced, a

CT scan often discloses ventricular dilatation after some delay [8]. A common place for distal catheter misplacement is the preperitoneal space commonly revealed by a subcutaneous fluid collection under the abdominal incision. A lateral radiograph of the abdomen usually depicts the catheter coiling under the anterior abdominal wall.

Migration or extrusion of VP shunts is less common than the aforementioned complications. In infants, migration may be favored by a loose fixation of the catheter to the abdominal wall or by its high mobility within the peritoneal cavity [54]. On the other hand, an increase in the abdominal pressure associated with an unobliterated processus vaginalis [73] or with the patency of the umbilical end of the vitello-intestinal duct may be responsible for migration of the distal catheter into the scrotum or to extrusion through the umbilicus, respectively.

An intrathoracic migration of the distal VP catheter into the pleural space, heart, and pulmonary arteries is a rare but well-documented complication. The course of the catheter into the pleural space may be supradiaphragmatic because of incorrect subcutaneous tunneling or transdiaphragmatic, via a congenital diaphragmatic defect, foramen of Bochdalek, foramen of Morgagni, and esophageal hiatus or via a diaphragmatic perforation [76, 77]. Complications of the intrathoracic migration of VP shunts include tension CSF hydrothorax or pneumothorax, bronchial perforation, or pneumonia [78]. Proposed mechanisms of intracardiac migration include unintentional transvenous placement of the shunt [74, 75] and suction of the catheter into the heart by negative inspiratory pressures. The erosion of the diaphragm by the shunt tip may result from the respiratory movements and/or from the presence of congenital diaphragmatic hiatuses, such as the foramen of Morgagni and the foramen of Bochdalek, and might explain shunt migration into the mediastinum or the pleural cavity [79–81]. Subcutaneous fluid collections over the shunt tract may be caused by disconnections or ruptures (by stress fracture) of the distal catheter (Fig. 3.16) [40]. Disconnections are not seen with the one-piece shunts. These complications and those related to odd positions of distal catheters are readily shown on plain radiographs or in CT [74, 75].

3.6.2 Disconnection and Fracture of the Shunt

Disconnection commonly occurs shortly after shunt placement and is considered as an *early complication* although it also may occur exceptionally as a late complication too [2]. CSF accumulation under the skin at the site of disconnection may be visible on CT. Shunt radiographs readily show a gap between the proximal catheter and the reservoir or the valve and the distal catheter. It is important to remember that some valves and connectors have radiolucent zones that can be mistaken for disconnection. The tubing proximal and distal to a radiolucent connector is linearly aligned, whereas the tubing proximal and distal to a disconnection may be angulated. Comparison with previous radiographs is also helpful in making the distinction [5].

On the contrary, shunt fracture occurs as a *late complication* being related with mechanical stress, degradation, and calcification of the tube and with the normal growth of the patients. Accordingly, shunt fracture is almost exclusively seen in older children and adolescents [82, 83]. The distal tubing, that is initially free to slide trough the subcutaneous tract, becomes fixed to the subcutaneous tissue or to the abdominal scar and is subjected to shear forces that promote its breakage [5]. Fractures most commonly occur in the neck or upper chest where the catheter is most mobile. Common presentation consists of symptoms of raised ICP accompanied by pain, mild erythema, or swelling along the shunt tract, often in a location close to the shunt fracture [8]. Patients may be asymptomatic because the fibrotic scar tissue that surrounds the tube temporarily acts as a conduit that continues draining CSF [8]. As with disconnection, a palpable subcutaneous collection of CSF may form at the fracture site. Plain shunt radiographs are most sensitive for showing the discontinuity of the catheter and

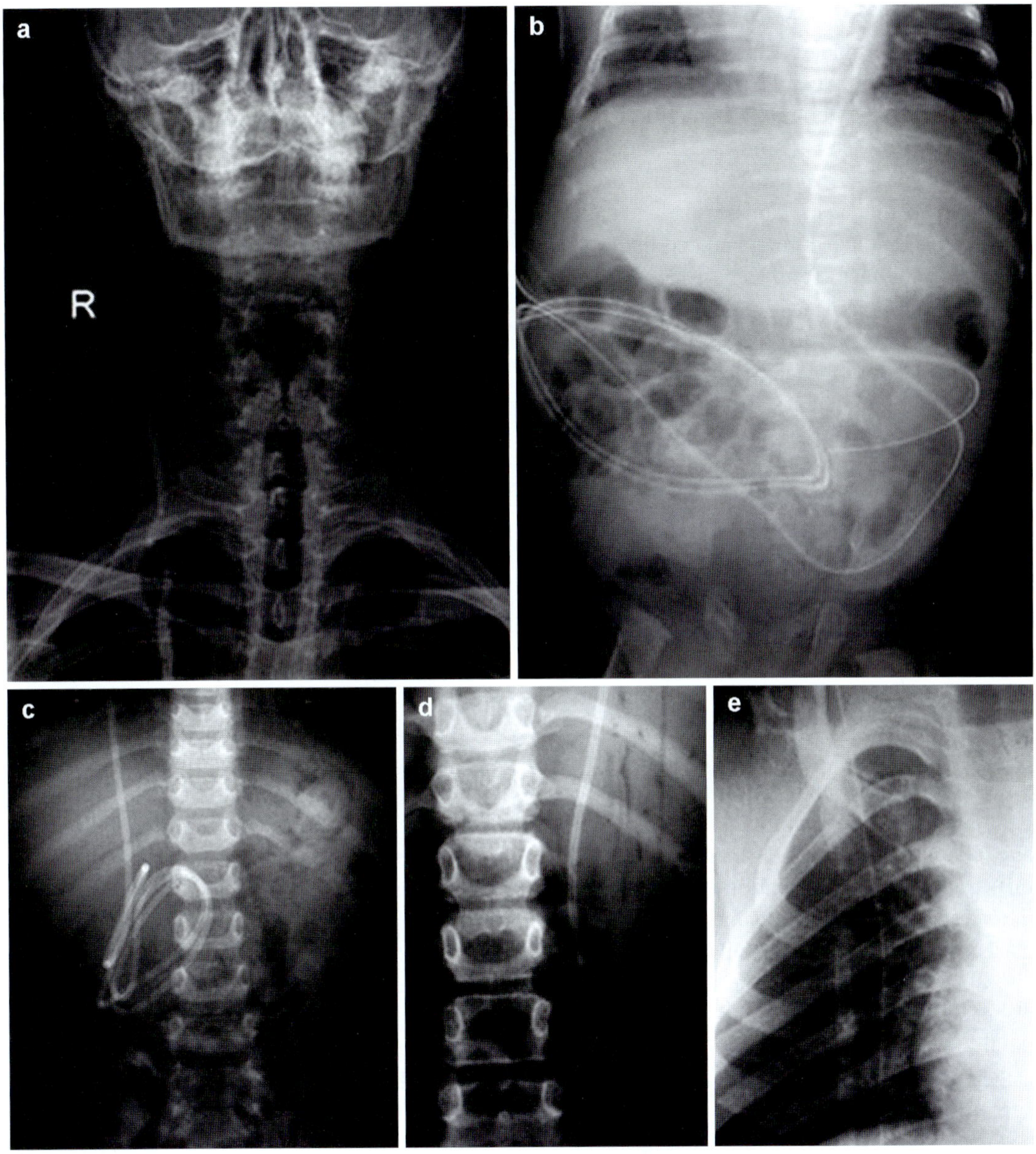

Fig. 3.16 (**a**) Thorax and neck films showing discontinuity of a heavily calcified, long-standing VP tube. (**b**) Abdominal radiograph depicting a broken and retained distal catheter. (**c**) Abdomen radiograph revealing coiling of the tube. (**d**, **e**) Chest radiographs showing short and calcified catheters

the migration of the distal fragment should it occur. The distal fragment of a VP shunt may coil completely into the peritoneal cavity [8]. Migration of the distal fragment of VA shunts is obviously more dangerous because the catheter can lodge in the right atrium causing arrhythmia or embolization to the pulmonary vessels (Fig. 3.16) [84].

3.6.3 Distal Obstruction

Pseudocyst formation is a common cause of distal catheter obstruction. Pseudocysts are loculated collections of CSF that form around the terminal end of the catheter. In patients with VP shunts, pseudocysts are caused by peritoneal adhesions or migration of the greater omentum over the shunt tip [85]. Pseudocysts can also develop around ventriculopleural shunts due to adhesions caused by chronic pleural irritation.

Conventional radiographs may show coiling of the distal catheter within an intra-abdominal soft tissue mass or a loculated pleural effusion. A definitive diagnosis can be made by CT or ultrasounds that depict the loculated fluid collection surrounding the catheter tip. Alternatively, radionuclide imaging will show localized activity around the catheter tip. Treatment entails externalization of the catheter and drainage of the pseudocyst. If the fluid is sterile, the existing shunt may be reimplanted or moved to a different site [86]. Infected pseudocysts require shunt removal, EVD placement, and antibiotics (Fig. 3.7) [3].

Other causes of distal obstruction include catheter migration or erosion into soft tissues. Children with VP shunts are at greater risk for distal catheter migration because of redundancy of the intraperitoneal catheter intentionally placed to allow for future growth of the child [5]. Erosion into a hollow viscus can present acutely with signs and symptoms of peritonitis or indolently with migration of the catheter to any location in the genitourinary or gastrointestinal tract [87]. Accumulation of CSF increases the intraperitoneal pressure that can dilate inguinal hernias and patent vaginal processes allowing catheter migration into the scrotum [81]. The catheter may also erode into solid organs, such as the liver, or into the abdominal wall. Rarely, the catheter may encircle the bowel causing mechanical intestinal obstruction [85].

Obstructions are more common at the ventricular end than at the peritoneal end of the shunt. Distal obstruction may be caused by adhesions within the peritoneum too. VP shunts with distal slit valves seem to be more prone to blockage. Another place in which obstruction may occur is the valve itself often caused by blood and debris and by substances of inflammatory origin. CSF protein concentration does not seem to play an important role on proximal or distal valve blockage. Although catheters are made of materials to avoid collapse of the tubing, kinking of the catheter (sometimes due to technical failure in placing the shunt) may also cause a functional block. Kinking may also result from bowel adhesions and displacement among visceral structures or from retraction of the tube outside the peritoneum. Most of these complications may be correctly be diagnosed by plain radiographs, ultrasounds, and CT studies.

3.6.4 Pneumothorax and Subcutaneous Emphysema

Postoperative pneumothorax with or without subcutaneous emphysema complicates 10–20 % of ventriculopleural shunt surgeries but can occur with any shunt type. Air may enter the subcutaneous tissues via the surgical incision. Other sources of air entry after ventriculopleural shunting include bronchopleural fistulas at the pleural space in the setting of positive-pressure ventilation [88]. Subcutaneous emphysema is usually clinically nonsignificant, but occasionally it may cause upper airway obstruction or tension pneumomediastinum (Fig. 3.18) [88]. There are few reports of distal ventriculopleural catheter migration, possibly because of the relative rarity of its use. Erosion of a ventriculopleural shunt into the chest wall resulting in subcutaneous edema and shunt malfunction has also been documented [89].

3.6.5 Hydrothorax (Pleural Effusion)

In 1954, Ransohoff reported the use of ventriculopleural (VPL) shunting in patients with tumoral hydrocephalus [92]. Nevertheless, VPL drainage has not gained widespread acceptance owing to fears of complications as pneumothorax or CSF pleural effusions [90, 93]. Its use has even been considered dangerous or contraindicated in children [91]. Cranially placed valves and devices with antisiphon mechanisms have decreased the incidence of symptomatic pleural effusions of CSF [91]. VPL shunting has seldom been considered as an alternative route for CSF drainage

[94]. However, some series document the feasibility and safety of VPL shunt and of subdural–pleural shunting [90, 97]. A few authors have even used VPL shunting as the first option for treating hydrocephalus [97].

Reports on complications of VPL shunting have obscured the benefits of its use in clinical practice. Symptomatic tension hydrothorax, pneumothorax, fibrothorax, pleural empyema, CSF galactorrhea, and even tumor spread through the shunt tubing have been documented following VPL anastomosis [90, 93–95, 99]. The most frequent complication of pleural shunts is symptomatic tension hydrothorax causing respiratory distress [90, 93]. Some reports argue that pleural effusion is an age-related event [98]; accordingly, the use of VPL shunting has been discouraged especially in children. In contrast, other authors have demonstrated that the diversion of CSF to the pleural cavity constitutes a valid alternative in children as young as 3 years old.

In evaluating the results of VPL shunting, we must consider that this route is often utilized in particularly problematic cases, its use being reserved for cases in which the abdominal and/or the vascular routes have already failed, especially after persistent valve infection with peritonitis [100]. These facts preclude valid comparisons with other routes for CSF shunting [97]. Jones et al. used an antisiphon device connected with the valve, with the aim of preventing the formation of clinically significant CSF pleural effusions [91]. These authors reported that only 1 of 52 children developed a symptomatic hydrothorax that required conversion to a VP shunt [91]. Nevertheless, the use of antisiphon devices in children frequently induces symptoms of underdrainage owing to the narrow margins that these devices achieve for effectively controlling raised ICP.

The presence of a pleural collection of fluid observed on the chest radiographs of patients with VPL shunting should be of no concern in the absence of respiratory symptoms [91]. In our opinion, the finding of small hydrothoraces in otherwise asymptomatic children indicates that the shunt is functioning. However, we consider that children with VPL shunts must be regularly followed up in view of the reports on tension pleural effusions that can appear at any time, as a result of changes in the valve pressure or in the absorption capability of the pleural cavity [91]. Megison and Benzel warned about the use of VPL shunting in adults with pulmonary diseases [97]. The ventilatory reserve must be considered with particular care especially in meningomyelocele patients with kyphoscoliosis and in cases of Chiari malformation [97]. In all these cases, the burden of a pleural fluid effusion in an already restricted ventilatory capacity might precipitate a frank respiratory failure [97]. Some authors use VPL shunts only as a temporary solution for CSF drainage, especially during management of VP or VA shunt infection and before definitive tumor removal [101, 102].

Small asymptomatic effusions do not necessitate treatment [91] although larger collections may produce symptoms of respiratory involvement especially if they are under tension [90]. Shunt catheter irritation or infection results in accumulation of bacteria, leukocytes, and inflammatory mediators that mix with the protein-rich CSF that, together with the shunted CSF volume, contribute to the accumulation of pleural fluid. Lung atelectasis further reduces the pleural surface also impairing fluid absorption [90]. Children, particularly infants, are more prone to hydrothorax because of the relatively smaller pleural surface available for absorption and due to enhanced immune responses from frequent viral infections and routine immunizations. Antisiphon devices and newer valves that prevent overdrainage have decreased the incidence of hydrothorax [101].

A different origin of CSF hydrothorax is the resulting from the intrathoracic migration of a VP distal catheter. This complication may be due to technical complications or to preexisting anatomical conditions [76, 77]. Symptomatic and tension hydrothorax secondary to VP shunting has also been described in the absence of transthoracic catheter migration [81, 103, 104]. Although more common in children due to suboptimal peritoneal absorption, adult cases have also been reported [105]. Diagnosis is made radiographically by injecting contrast material or

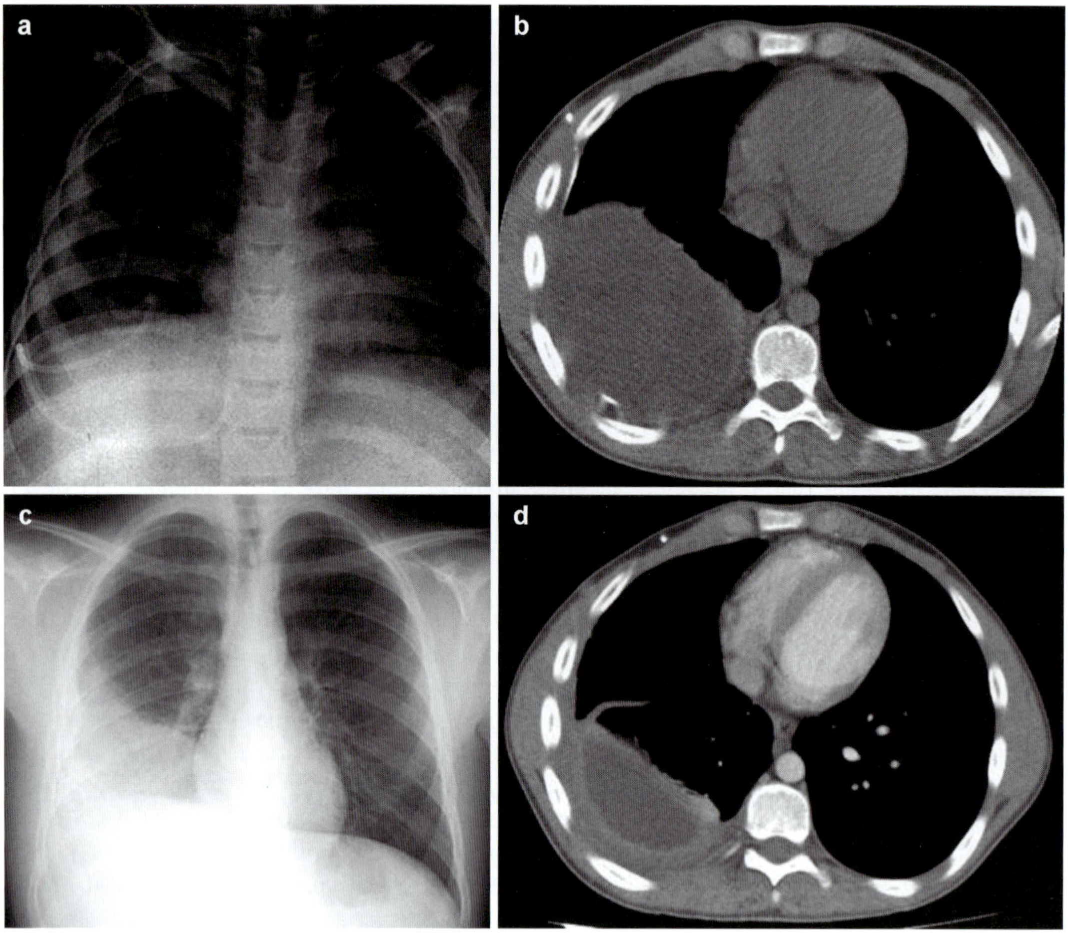

Fig. 3.17 Pleural effusion due to ventriculopleural shunt in a 30-year-old man. (**a**) Chest radiograph and (**b**) transaxial CT image show tip of ventriculopleural shunt coiled within the right pleural effusion. (**c**) Chest radiograph and (**d**) transaxial CT image after a month that shows an improvement in the right pleural collection after ventriculopleural shunt removal

radionuclide into the shunt reservoir and visualizing their accumulation in the pleural space [106]. Thoracocentesis and chemical analysis can also confirm the presence of CSF in the pleural fluid (Fig. 3.17) [103].

Hydrothoraces are usually well defined in plain chests radiographs and in thoracic CT.

3.6.6 Fibrothorax

Fibrothorax with lung entrapment is a rare complication of VPL shunts [107]. Fibrosis of the pleural cavity is believed to be caused by an inflammatory reaction to CSF proteins or chronic low-grade infection. The duration of VPL shunting required to develop fibrosis is highly variable [107]. The confirmation of fibrothorax requires radiographic studies.

3.6.7 Complications Related to Shunt Variants

Alternative types of shunts have been tried in patients who develop complications associated with standard VP shunts (e.g., CSF pseudocysts, recurrent distal obstruction). In these shunt systems, the distal shunt is placed in the right atrium, pleural space, fallopian tube, stomach, ureter, gallbladder, etc. The gallbladder may also be used for distal shunt placement when difficult shunt placement or ineffectual use of peritoneal shunts justifies the risk of potential infection of the biliary system. In the setting of acute cholecystitis and ventriculocholecystic shunt malfunction, gallbladder wall thickening, and sludge are nonspecific findings at sonography, and hepatobiliary radioisotope studies show no activity in the gallbladder.

3.6.8 Tricuspid Valve Pathology

Chronic mechanical irritation of the tricuspid valve by the distal catheter may cause fibrosis, calcification, and stenosis of the tricuspid valve [108]. The catheter may also damage the valve, directly leading to tricuspid regurgitation. Other causes of catheter-related heart damage include endocarditis and bland thrombus. This entity often requires the use of echocardiography for diagnosis together with a more thorough cardiologic evaluation.

3.6.9 Thromboembolic Disease and Pulmonary Arterial Hypertension

Ventriculovascular CSF drainage has been used when the peritoneum is no longer usable because of adhesions or to recent peritoneal infection. VA shunts have a number of severe and even fatal complications. Shunt nephritis, pulmonary emboli, shunt infection during bacteremia, and the need for periodic catheter lengthening have all led to the reduced use of vascular CSF shunting in recent years. The intravascular catheter promotes clot formation in the internal jugular vein, which may then propagate into the superior vena cava or at the tip of the catheter in the right atrium [85]. These thrombi may calcify.

Inappropriate position of the catheter tip in the superior vena cava increases the risk of venous thrombosis. Real-time 2D echocardiography is used to determine the size, site, and area of attachment for surgical planning. Catheter or CT angiography will show occlusion of the superior vena cava with concomitant collateral vessels. Coronary sinus thrombosis with acute myocardial infarction has been reported. Although rare in children, the prevalence of pulmonary arterial hypertension after VA shunting in adults may be as high as 8 % on the basis of echocardiography and lung function testing. Pulmonary hypertension may be secondary to chronic thromboembolic disease because pulmonary embolism with infarction occurs in up to 50 % of patients with VA shunts [109]. Because of the potential serious complications of pulmonary hypertension, surveillance echocardiography and pulmonary function testing are recommended every 12 months for patients with VA shunts [110].

Unlike VP shunts, the length of the distal VA catheter cannot be initially redundant to allow for growth of the child because the excess tubing would impinge on the atrial wall [85]. Consequently, as the patient grows, the catheter tip often rises into the superior vena cava, a position that is suboptimal for CSF drainage and requires shunt lengthening that can also be performed prophylactically. Failure of VA shunts may be caused by migration within the right atrium or through a patent foramen ovale to a position where drainage is impaired. Erosion of the distal catheter tip through the free wall of the right ventricle into the pericardial space has been reported, resulting in massive CSF pericardial effusion and life-threatening cardiac tamponade. Erosion through the interatrial septum creates a conduit for paradoxical emboli [111].

3.6.10 Abdominal Complications

Ventriculoperitoneal shunting is regarded as the safest route for CSF diversion, although several conditions, such as adhesions, abdominal cysts, and recent peritonitis, can produce loss of the capability of the peritoneum to absorb CSF [94].

3.6.10.1 Abdominal CSF Pseudocysts

A pseudocyst is a loculated intra-abdominal fluid collection that develops around the peritoneum. Pseudocysts are more common than ascites.

Symptoms consistent with bowel obstruction can be evident if the pseudocyst is large. Abdominal CSF pseudocysts are reported with a frequency ranging between 1 and 10 % [112, 113]. The pseudocyst formation is related to inflammatory processes affecting the peritoneal cavity, leading to mesentery wrapping around the peritoneal catheter and to loculated fluid collections. The complication may depend on both infectious and aseptic causes [3, 112]. In case of an infective etiology, a low-grade sepsis, usually due to the presence of *Staphylococcus epidermidis*, is the most frequent finding. Aseptic etiologies include inflammatory reactions to the presence of the catheter, to the CSF protein, or to tumor cells disseminated via the shunt. Previous abdominal surgical operations represent another risk factor for this complication. The observation by some authors that smaller pseudocysts are infected and larger ones are sterile was not confirmed by others (Fig. 3.7) [2, 100].

3.6.10.2 Ascites

Ascites in shunted patients results from an accumulation of CSF in the peritoneal cavity due either to a reduced absorptive capacity or to an excessive volume of CSF. A suboptimal peritoneal absorption capacity has been propounded in infants who have a smaller peritoneal surface than older children and who are more exposed to viral infections [81]. Infection is, however, the most common etiological factor by interfering with the peritoneal absorption of CSF (in case of diffuse abdominal inflammatory reactions) or by increasing the production of hyperproteic CSF (in case of ventriculitis). Hyperproteic CSF is an independent risk factor for ascites when tumoral hydrocephalus is present, as in children harboring optic gliomas or craniopharyngiomas [114, 116, 117]. Tumoral hydrocephalus can also cause ascites because of tumor cells dissemination within the peritoneal cavity thus interfering with peritoneal absorption [86, 114]. Furthermore, in case of hydrocephalus due to choroid plexus papillomas, a pure hypersecretory mechanism has been hypothesized.

The absorptive capacity of the peritoneum can also be reduced by scarring from previous peritonitis or previous surgical procedures [115]. Oncotic pressure of intraperitoneal fluid is increased by inflammation from infection, foreign body reactions to the catheter, or shunt-disseminated metastasis [86]. Ascites with abdominal distention and respiratory compromise may occur within weeks, months, or even years after shunt placement. Ascites is also a contributory factor in the production of inguinal hernia and hydrocele (Fig. 3.18) [81, 118]. Ascites is easily visualized with ultrasound or CT.

3.6.10.3 Inguinal Hernia and Hydrocele

The most common abdominal complications of VP shunts are inguinal hernia and/or hydrocele that occur in 3.8–16.8 % of the peritoneal shunt insertions [80]. The incidence of such a complication rises to 30 % of cases when a CSF shunt is placed in the first few months of life vs. nearly 10 % at 1 year of age. Insufficient peritoneal CSF absorption (in part favored by the possible seeding of glia into the peritoneal cavity) [119], raised intra-abdominal pressure, and patency of the processus vaginalis (60–70 % of cases at 3 months of life, 50–60 % at 1 year, and 40 % at 2 years) [73] are the factors that are thought that intervene in the pathogenesis of inguinal hernia/hydrocele and that also explain its increased incidence in infants. Signs and symptoms may occur either early (1 day) or after several months from surgery, and bilateral involvement has been demonstrated in up to 50 % of cases [120]. These complications are mainly diagnosed on clinical grounds but usually require radiographic or ultrasonographic studies for confirmation and surgical planning.

3.6.10.4 Visceral–Intestinal Perforation

Thanks to the introduction of soft and flexible silicone tubes, the incidence of visceral perforation, which was before a rare complication of peritoneal shunts, has even been further reduced [121]. However, it remains a severe complication of VP shunting and is associated with a mortality rate as high as 15 % [121]. The perforation may occur *early*, at the time of the insertion of the

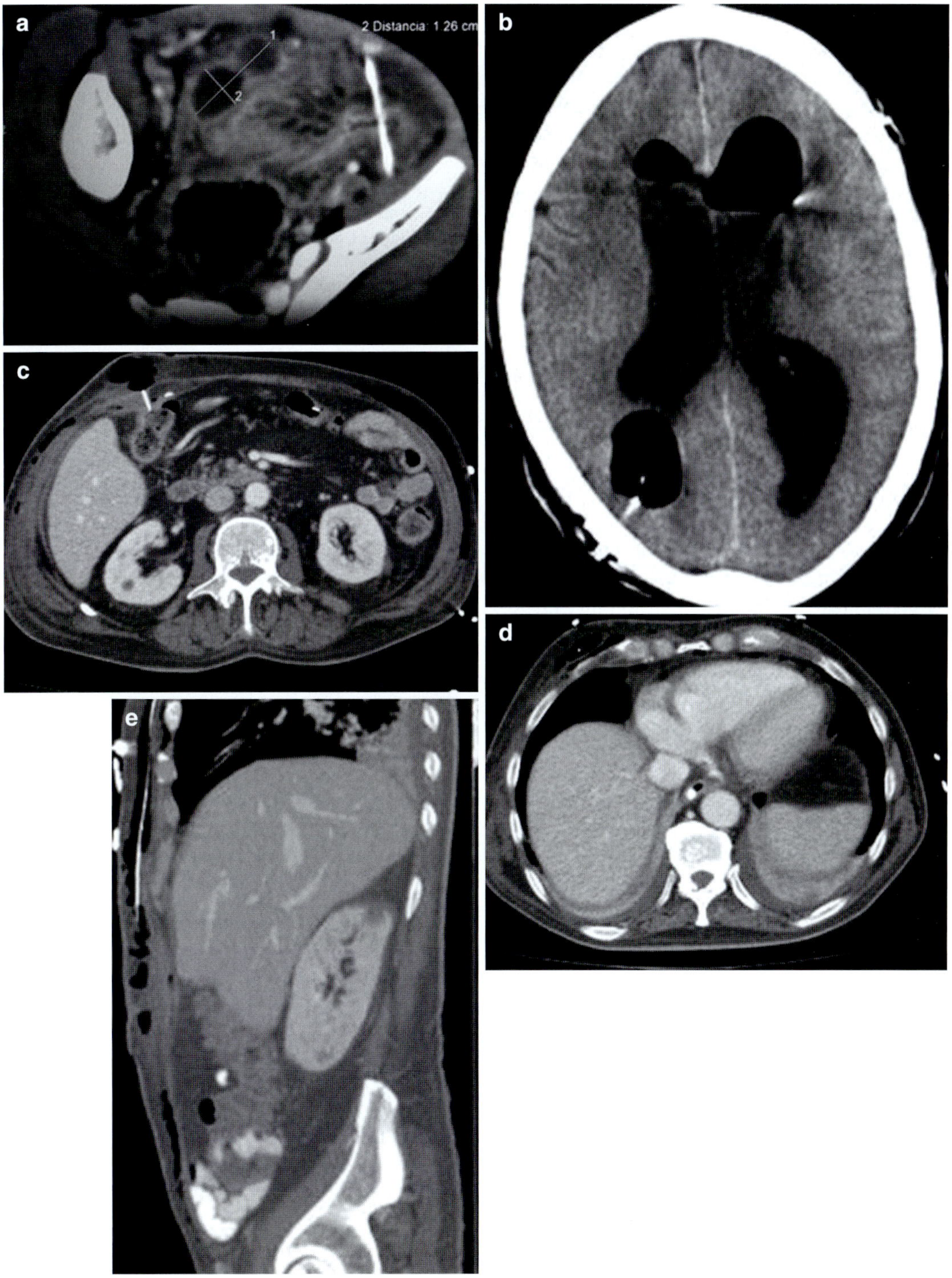

Fig. 3.18 (**a**) Transaxial CT image shows peritoneal pseudocyst and ascites around the terminal end of the catheter. (**b–e**) A 50-year-old-man with a ventriculoperitoneal shunt who presented with altered mental status, abdominal pain, nausea, and vomiting. (**b**) Transaxial CT image shows diffuse hydrocephalus and pneumoventriculus with air around the catheter. (**c**, **d**) Transaxial CT image shows pneumomediastinum and subcutaneous emphysema after colonic perforation. (**e**) Sagittal reconstruction showing subcutaneous emphysema around the catheter

CSF shunt device or later, even after several years from its implant [121, 122]. Peritoneal adhesions, improper skin incision, and inability by the surgeon to differentiate between peritoneum and viscus wall during placement of the peritoneal catheter are the most frequent causes of this complication occurring during shunt placement. Direct peritoneal puncture by trochar is thought not to increase the incidence of visceral perforation, except for infants with myelodysplasia with an overdistended bladder.

Concerning *late* perforation, local inflammation, and adhesions of the distal catheter to the viscus wall, in addition to chronic friction, have been proposed as the main risk factors for visceral perforation [121, 123]. The bowel is the site more frequently involved (0.1 % of overall CSF shunt complications), followed by the bladder, the stomach, the liver, the gallbladder, the scrotum, and the vagina (Fig. 3.18). Visceral perforation by abdominal catheters need a thorough investigation and often requires radiographic, ultrasonographic, and CT studies together with the close collaboration of the pediatric or general surgeon.

Conclusions

Shunt failure occurs in 40–50 % of patients during the first 2 years after shunt surgery. The diagnosis is initially suspected on the basis of history and physical examination, often with findings of increased ICP. However, imaging is often needed for confirming the diagnosis and for establishing the cause of the shunt failure. Therefore, radiologists should be familiar with the neuroimaging and other radiodiagnostic techniques for assessing shunt malfunction and shunt complications.

Malfunctions and complications are expected, although unwanted, risks associated with the use of CSF shunts. Correlative imaging modalities constitute essential adjuncts in the workup of patients with CSF shunt failure. Radiologists manage a variety of diagnostic tools they can use to disclose the cause of the malfunction or complication. Close communication with the treating clinicians is essential for tailoring the diagnostic imaging workup to the particular problem.

References

1. Weprin BE, Swift DM (2002) Complications of ventricular shunts. Tech Neurosurg 7(3):224–242
2. Goeser CD, McLeary MS, Young LW (1998) Diagnostic imaging of ventriculoperitoneal shunt malfunctions and complications. Radiographics 18:635–651
3. Browd SR, Gottfried ON, Ragel BT, Kestle JR (2006) Failure of cerebrospinal fluid shunts: part II: overdrainage, loculation, and abdominal complications. Pediatr Neurol 34:171–176
4. Wallace AN, McConathy J, Menias CO, Bhalla S, Wippold FJ II (2014) Imaging evaluation of CSF shunts. AJR Am J Roentgenol 202:38–53
5. Sivaganesan A, Krishnamurthy R, Sahni D, Viswanathan C (2012) Neuroimaging of ventriculoperitoneal shunt complications in children. Pediatr Radiol 42:1029–1046
6. Lehnert BE, Rahbar H, Relyea-Chew A, Lewis DH, Richardson ML, Fink JR (2011) Detection of ventricular shunt malfunction in the ED: relative utility of radiography, CT, and nuclear imaging. Emerg Radiol 18:299–305
7. Desai KR, Babb JS, Amodio JB (2007) The utility of the plain radiograph "shunt series" in the evaluation of suspected ventriculoperitoneal shunt failure in pediatric patients. Pediatr Radiol 37:452–456
8. Browd S, Ragel B, Gottfried O (2006) Failure of cerebrospinal fluid shunts. Part I: obstruction and mechanical failure. Pediatr Neurol 34:83–92
9. Dinçer A, Özek MM (2011) Radiologic evaluation of pediatric hydrocephalus. Childs Nerv Syst 27:1543–1562
10. Van Lindert EJ, Beems T, Grotenhuis JA (2006) The role of different imaging modalities: is MRI a condition sine qua non for ETV? Childs Nerv Syst 22:1529–1536
11. Martínez-Lage JF, Torres J, Campillo H, Sanchez-del-Rincón I, Bueno F, Zambudio G et al (2000) Ventriculopleural shunting with new technology valves. Childs Nerv Syst 16:867–871
12. Udayasankar UK, Braithwaite K, Arvaniti M, Tudorascu D, Small WC, Little S et al (2008) Low-dose nonenhanced head CT protocol for follow-up evaluation of children with ventriculoperitoneal shunt: reduction of radiation and effect on image quality. AJNR Am J Neuroradiol 29:802–806
13. Guillaume DJ (2010) Minimally invasive neurosurgery for cerebrospinal fluid disorders. Neurosurg Clin N Am 21:653–672
14. Inoue T, Kuzu Y, Ogasawara K, Ogawa A (2005) Effect of 3-tesla magnetic resonance imaging on various pressure programmable shunt valves. J Neurosurg 103:163–165
15. Lillis SS, Mamourian AC, Vaccaro TJ, Duhaime AC (2010) Programmable CSF shunt valves: radiographic identification and interpretation. AJNR Am J Neuroradiol 31:1343–1346

16. Dincer A, Yildiz E, Kohan S, Ozek M (2011) Analysis of endoscopic third ventriculostomy patency by MRI: value of different pulse sequences, the sequence parameters, and the imaging planes for investigation of flow void. Childs Nerv Syst 27:127–135
17. Dincer A, Kohan S, Ozek MM (2009) Is all "communicating" hydrocephalus really communicating? Prospective study on the value of 3D-constructive interference in steady state sequence at 3 T. AJNR Am J Neuroradiol 30:1898–1906
18. Kim SK, Wang KC, Cho BK (2000) Surgical outcome of pediatric hydrocephalus treated by endoscopic III ventriculostomy: prognostic factors and interpretation of postoperative neuroimaging. Childs Nerv Syst 16:161–168
19. Schroeder HW, Schweim C, Schweim KH (2000) Analysis of aqueductal cerebrospinal fluid flow after endoscopic aqueductoplasty by using cine phase contrast magnetic resonance imaging. J Neurosurg 93:237–244
20. Doll A, Christmann D, Kehrli P, Abu Eid M, Gillis C, Bogorin A et al (2000) Contribution of 3D CISS MRI for pre and post-therapeutic monitoring of obstructive hydrocephalus. J Neuroradiol 27:218–225
21. Laitt RD, Mallucci CL, Jaspan T, McConachie NS, Vloeberghs M, Punt J (1999) Constructive interference in steady-state 3D Fourier-transform MRI in the management of hydrocephalus and third ventriculostomy. Neuroradiology 41:117–123
22. Warf BC, Campbell JW, Riddle E (2011) Initial experience with combined endoscopic third ventriculostomy and choroid plexus cauterization for post-hemorrhagic hydrocephalus of prematurity: the importance of prepontine cistern status and the predictive value of FIESTA MRI imaging. Childs Nerv Syst 27:1063–1071
23. Kim DS, Choi JU, Huh R, Yun PH, Kim DI (1999) Quantitative assessment of cerebrospinal fluid hydrodynamics using a phasecontrast cine MR image in hydrocephalus. Childs Nerv Syst 15:461–467
24. Stoquart-El Sankari S, Lehmann P, Gondry-Jouet C, Fichten A, Godefroy O, Meyer ME et al (2009) Phase-contrast MR imaging support for the diagnosis of aqueductal stenosis. AJNR Am J Neuroradiol 30:209–214
25. Battal B, Kocaoglu M, Bulakbasi N, Husmen G, Tuba Sanal H, Tayfun C (2011) Cerebrospinal fluid flow imaging by using phase-contrast MR technique. Br J Radiol 84:758–765
26. Connor SE, O'Gorman R, Summers P, Simmons A, Moore EM, Chandler C et al (2001) SPAMM, cine phase contrast imaging and fast spin-echo T2-weighted imaging in the study of intracranial cerebrospinal fluid (CSF) flow. Clin Radiol 56:763–772
27. Barkovich AJ (1996) Pediatric neuroimaging, 2nd edn. Lippincott-Raven, Philadelphia, pp 439–475
28. Ellegaard L, Mogensen S, Juhler M (2007) Ultrasound-guided percutaneous placement of ventriculoatrial shunts. Childs Nerv Syst 23:857–862
29. Drake JM (1993) Ventriculostomy for treatment of hydrocephalus. Neurosurg Clin N Am 4:657–666
30. Dias MS, Li V (1998) Pediatric neurosurgical disease. Pediatr Clin North Am 45:1539–1578
31. Teo C, Jones R (1996) Management of hydrocephalus by endoscopic third ventriculostomy in patients with myelomeningocele. Pediatr Neurosurg 25:57–63
32. Teo C, Kadrian D, Hayhurst C (2013) Endoscopic management of complex hydrocephalus. World Neurosurg 79:S21.e 1–7
33. Di Rocco C, Massimi L, Tamburrini G (2006) Shunts vs endoscopic third ventriculostomy in infants: are there different types and/or rates of complications? A review. Childs Nerv Syst 22:1573–1589
34. Beems T, Grotenhuis JA (2004) Long-term complications and definition of failure of neuroendoscopic procedures. Childs Nerv Syst 20:868–877
35. Schroeder HWS, Niendorf W-R, Gaab MR (2002) Complications of endoscopic third ventriculostomy. J Neurosurg 96:1032–1040
36. Schönauer C, Bellotti A, Tessitore E, Parlato C, Moraci A (2000) Traumatic subependymal hematoma during endoscopic third ventriculostomy in a patient with a third ventricle tumor: case report. Minim Invasive Neurosurg 43:135–137
37. Fukuhara T, Vorster S, Liciano MG (2000) Risk factor for failure of endoscopic third ventriculostomy for obstructive hydrocephalus. Neurosurgery 46:1100–1111
38. Buxton N, Macarthur D, Mallucci C, Punt J, Vloeberghs M (1998) Neuroendoscopy in the premature population. Childs Nerv Syst 14:649–652
39. Koch D, Wagner W (2004) Endoscopic third ventriculostomy in infants of less than 1 year of age: which factors influence the outcome? Childs Nerv Syst 20:405–411
40. Tamburrini G, Caldarelli M, Di Rocco C (2002) Diagnosis and management of shunt complications in the treatment of childhood hydrocephalus. Rev Neurosurg 3:1–34
41. Tubbs RS, Banks JT, Soleau S, Smyth MD, Wellons JC III, Blount JP et al (2005) Complications of ventriculosubgaleal shunts in infants and children. Childs Nerv Syst 21:48–51
42. Aguiar PH, Shu EB, Freitas AB, Leme RJ, Miura FK, Marino R Jr (2000) Causes and treatment of intracranial haemorrhage complicating shunting for paediatric hydrocephalus. Childs Nerv Syst 16:218–221
43. Oi S, Shimoda M, Shibata M, Honda Y, Togo K, Shinoda M et al (2000) Pathophysiology of long-standing overt ventriculomegaly in adults. J Neurosurg 92:933–940
44. Hamada H, Hayashi N, Kurimoto M, Umemura K, Hirashima Y, Nogami K et al (2004) Tension pneumocephalus after neuroendoscopic procedure—case report. Neurol Med Chir 44:205–208
45. Saxena S, Ambesh SP, Saxena HN, Kumar R (1999) Pneumocephalus and convulsion after ventriculoscopy: a potentially catastrophic complication. J Neurosurg Anesthesiol 11:200–202
46. Schreffler RT, Schreffler AJ, Wittler RR (2002) Treatment of cerebrospinal fluid shunt infections: a decision analysis. Pediatr Infect Dis J 21:632–636

47. Whitehead WE, Kestle JRW (2001) The treatment of cerebrospinal fluid shunt infections. Pediatr Neurosurg 35:205–210
48. Schroeder HWS, Oertel J, Gaab MR (2004) Incidence of complications in neuroendoscopic surgery. Childs Nerv Syst 20:878–883
49. Hopf NJ, Grunert P, Fries G, Resch KDM, Perneczky A (1999) Endoscopic third ventriculostomy: outcome analysis of 100 consecutive procedures. Neurosurgery 44:795–806
50. Baird C, O'Connor D, Pittman T (2000) Late shunt infections. Pediatr Neurosurg 32:269–273
51. Filka J, Hutova M, Tuharsky J, Sagat T, Kralinski K, Krcmery V Jr (1999) Nosocomial meningitis in children after ventriculoperitoneal shunt insertion. Acta Paediatr 88:576–578
52. Drake JM, Kestle JR, Tuli S (2000) CSF shunts: 50 years on past, present and future. Childs Nerv Syst 16:800–804
53. Park CK, Wang KC, Seo JK, Cho BK (2000) Transoral protrusion of a peritoneal catheter: a case report and literature review. Childs Nerv Syst 16:184–189
54. Dominguez CJ, Tyagi A, Hall G, Timothy J, Chumas PD (2000) Sub-galeal coiling of the proximal and distal components of a ventriculo-peritoneal shunt. An unusual complication and proposed mechanism. Childs Nerv Syst 16:493–495
55. Martínez-Lage JF, Pérez-Espejo MA, Almagro MJ, Ros de San Pedro J, López F, Piqueras C et al (2005) Syndromes of overdrainage of ventricular shunting in childhood hydrocephalus. Neurocirugia 16:124–133
56. Martínez-Lage JF, Ruíz-Espejo AM, Almagro MJ, Alfaro R, Felipe-Murcia M, López-Guerrero A (2009) CSF overdrainage in shunted intracranial arachnoid cysts: a series and review. Childs Nerv Syst 25:1061–1069
57. Kestle J, Drake J, Milner R (2000) Long-term follow-up data from the Shunt Design Trial. Pediatr Neurosurg 33:230–236
58. Eldredge EA, Rockoff MA, Medlock MD (1997) Postoperative cerebral edema occurring in children with slit ventricles. Pediatrics 99:625–630
59. Rohde C, Weinzierl M, Mayfrank L, Gilsbach JM (2002) Postshunt insertion CSF leaks in infants treated by an adjustable valve opening pressure reduction. Childs Nerv Syst 18:702–704
60. Foltz EL (1993) Hydrocephalus: slit ventricles, shunt obstructions, and third ventricle shunts: a clinical study. Surg Neurol 40:119–124
61. Epstein F, Lapras C, Wisoff JH (1988) "Slit-ventricle syndrome": etiology and treatment. Pediatr Neurosci 14:5–10
62. Engel M, Carmel PW, Chutorian AM (1979) Increased intraventricular pressure without ventriculomegaly in children with shunts: "normal volume" hydrocephalus. Neurosurgery 5:549–552
63. Albright AL, Tyler-Kabara E (2001) Slit-ventricle syndrome secondary to shunt-induced suture ossification. Neurosurgery 48:764–769
64. Buxton N, Punt J (1999) Subtemporal decompression: the treatment of noncompliant ventricle syndrome. Neurosurgery 44:513–518
65. Di Rocco C, Tamburrini G (2003) Shunt dependency in shunted arachnoid cysts: a reason to avoid shunting. Pediatr Neurosurg 38:164–168
66. Di Rocco C, Velardi F (2003) Acquired Chiari type I malformation managed by supratentorial cranial enlargement. Childs Nerv Syst 19:800–807
67. Berger MS, Sundsten J, Lemire RJ, Silbergeld D, Newell D, Shurtleff D (1990) Pathophysiology of isolated lateral ventriculomegaly in shunted myelodysplastic children. Pediatr Neurosurg 16:301–304
68. James HE (1990) Spectrum of the syndrome of the isolated fourth ventricle in post-hemorrhagic hydrocephalus of the premature infant. Pediatr Neurosurg 16:305–308
69. Montgomery CT, Winfield JA (1993) Fourth ventricular entrapment caused by rostrocaudal herniation following shunt malfunction. Pediatr Neurosurg 19:209–214
70. Barada W, Najjar M, Beydoun A (2009) Early onset tension pneumocephalus following ventriculoperitoneal shunt insertion for normal pressure hydrocephalus: a case report. Clin Neurol Neurosurg 111:300–302
71. Drake J, Kestle J, Milner R et al (1998) Randomized trial of CSF shunt valve design in pediatric hydrocephalus. Neurosurgery 43:294–305
72. Woerdeman PA, Hanlo PW (2006) Ventriculoperitoneal shunt occlusion due to spontaneous intraabdominal knot formation in the catheter. Case report. J Neurosurg 105(3 Suppl):231–232
73. Oktem IS, Akdemir H, Koc K, Menku A, Tucer B, Selcuku A, Turan C (1998) Migration of abdominal catheter of ventriculoperitoneal shunt into the scrotum. Acta Neurochir 140:167–170
74. Hermann EJ, Zimmermann M, Marquardt G (2009) Ventriculoperitoneal shunt migration into the pulmonary artery. Acta Neurochir (Wien) 151:647–652
75. Fewel ME, Garton HJ (2004) Migration of distal ventriculoperitoneal shunt catheter into the heart: case report and review of the literature. J Neurosurg 100(2 Suppl Pediatrics):206–211
76. Martin LM, Donaldson-Hugh ME, Cameron MM (1997) Cerebrospinal fluid hydrothorax caused by transdiaphragmatic migration of a ventriculoperitoneal catheter through the foramen of Bochdalek. Childs Nerv Syst 13:282–284
77. Di Roio C, Mottolese C, Cayrel V, Artru F (2000) Respiratory distress caused by migration of ventriculoperitoneal shunt catheter into the chest cavity. (letter). Intensive Care Med 26:818
78. Doh JW, Bae HG, Lee KS, Yun IG, Byun BJ (1995) Hydrothorax from intrathoracic migration of a ventriculoperitoneal shunt catheter. Surg Neurol 43:340–343
79. Bryant M (1998) Abdominal complications of ventriculoperitoneal shunts. Am Surg 54:50–54
80. Guillén A, Costa JM, Castelló I, Claramunt E, Cardona E (2002) Unusual abdominal complication of ventriculoperitoneal shunt. Neurocirugia 4:401–404
81. Hadzikaric N, Nasser M, Mashani A, Ammar A (2002) CSF hydrothorax—VP shunt complication

without displacement of a peritoneal catheter. Childs Nerv Syst 18:179–182
82. Sainte-Rose C, Piatt JH, Renier D et al (1991) Mechanical complications in shunts. Pediatr Neurosurg 17:2–9
83. Cuka GM, Hellbusch LC (1995) Fractures of the peritoneal catheter of cerebrospinal fluid shunts. Pediatr Neurosurg 22:101–103
84. Irie W, Furukawa M, Murakami C et al (2009) A case of V-A shunt catheters migration into the pulmonary artery. Leg Med (Tokyo) 11:25–29
85. Murtagh FR, Quencer RM, Poole CA (1980) Extracranial complications of cerebrospinal fluid shunt function in childhood hydrocephalus. AJR Am J Roentgenol 135:763–766
86. Kariyattil R, Steinbok P, Singhal A, Cochrane DD (2007) Ascites and abdominal pseudocysts following ventriculoperitoneal shunt surgery: variations of the same theme. J Neurosurg 106(5 Suppl):350–353
87. Haralampopoulos F, Iliadis H, Karniadakis S, Koutentakis D (1996) Invasion of a peritoneal catheter into the inferior vena cava: report of a unique case. Surg Neurol 46:21–22
88. Haret DM, Onisei AM, Martin TW (2009) Acute-recurrent subcutaneous emphysema after ventriculopleural shunt placement. J Clin Anesth 21:352–354
89. Pearson B, Bui CJ, Tubbs RS, Wellons JC 3rd (2007) An unusual complication of a ventriculopleural shunt: case illustration. J Neurosurg 106(5 Suppl):410
90. Beach C, Manthey DE (1998) Tension hydrothorax due to ventriculopleural shunting. J Emerg Med 16:33–36
91. Jones RF, Currie BG, Kwok BC (1988) Ventriculopleural shunts for hydrocephalus: a useful alternative. Neurosurgery 23:753–755
92. Ransohoff J (1954) Ventriculopleural anastomosis in treatment of midline obstructional masses. J Neurosurg 11:295–301
93. Sanders DY, Summers R, Derouen L (1997) Symptomatic pleural collection of cerebrospinal fluid caused by a ventriculoperitoneal shunt. South Med J 90:831–832
94. Detwiler PN, Porter RW, Rekate HL (1999) Hydrocephalus – clinical features and management. In: Choux M, Di Rocco C, Hockley A, Walker M (eds) Pediatric neurosurgery. Churchill-Livingstone, London, pp 253–274
95. Iosif G, Fleischman J, Chitkara R (1991) Empyema due to ventriculopleural shunt. Chest 99:1538–1539
96. Moron MA, Barrow DL (1994) Cerebrospinal fluid galactorrhea after ventriculo-pleural shunting: case report. Surg Neurol 42:227–230
97. Piatt JH Jr (1994) How effective are ventriculopleural shunts? Pediatr Neurosurg 21:66–70
98. Willison CD, Kopitnik TA, Gustafson R, Kaufman HH (1992) Ventriculoperitoneal shunting used as a temporary diversion. Acta Neurochir 115:62–68
99. Yellin A, Findler G, Barzylay Z, Lieberman Y (1992) Fibrothorax associated with a ventriculopleural shunt in a hydrocephalic child. J Pediatr Surg 27:1525–1526
100. Roitberg BZ, Tomita T, McLone DG (1998) Abdominal cerebrospinal fluid pseudocysts: a complication of ventriculoperitoneal shunts in children. Pediatr Neurosurg 29:267–273
101. Grunberg J, Rebori A, Verocay MC, Ramela V, Alberti R, Cordoba A (2005) Hydrothorax due to ventriculopleural shunting in a child with spina bifida on chronic dialysis: third ventriculostomy as an alternative of cerebrospinal diversion. Int Urol Nephrol 37:571–574
102. Kanev PM, Park TS (1993) The treatment of hydrocephalus. Neurosurg Clin N Am 4:611–619
103. Born M, Reichling S, Schirrmeister J (2008) Pleural effusion: beta-trace protein in diagnosing ventriculoperitoneal shunt complications. J Child Neurol 23:810–812
104. Adeolu AA, Komolafe EO, Abiodun AA, Adetiloye VA (2006) Symptomatic pleural effusion without intrathoracic migration of ventriculoperitoneal shunt catheter. Childs Nerv Syst 22:186–188
105. Matushita H, Cardeal D, Pinto FC, Plese JP, de Miranda JS (2008) The ventriculoomental bursa shunt. Childs Nerv Syst 24:949–953
106. Chang CP, Liu RS, Liu CS et al (2007) Pleural effusion resulting from ventriculopleural shunt demonstrated on radionuclide shuntogram. Clin Nucl Med 32:47–48
107. Khan TA, Khalil-Marzouk JF (2008) Fibrothorax in adulthood caused by a cerebrospinal fluid shunt in the treatment of hydrocephalus. J Neurosurg 109:478–479
108. Akram Q, Saravanan D, Levy R (2011) Valvuloplasty for tricuspid stenosis caused by a ventriculoatrial shunt. Catheter Cardiovasc Interv 77:722–725
109. Milton CA, Sanders P, Steele PM (2001) Late cardiopulmonary complication of ventriculo-atrial shunt. Lancet 358:1608
110. Kluge S, Baumann HJ, Regelsberger J et al (2010) Pulmonary hypertension after ventriculoatrial shunt implantation. J Neurosurg 113:1279–1283
111. El-Eshmawi A, Onakpoya U, Khadragui I (2009) Cardiac tamponade as a sequela to ventriculoatrial shunting for congenital hydrocephalus. Tex Heart Inst J 36:58–60
112. Pathi R, Sage M, Slavotinek J, Hanieh A (2004) Abdominal cerebrospinal fluid pseudocysts. Australas Radiol 48:61–63
113. Rainov N, Schobess A, Heidecke V, Buckert W (1994) Abdominal CSF pseudocysts in patients with ventriculo-peritoneal shunts. Report of fourteen cases and review of the literature. Acta Neurochir 127:73–78
114. Kumar R, Sahay S, Gaur B, Singh V (2003) Ascites in ventriculoperitoneal shunt. Indian J Pediatr 70:859–864
115. Diluna ML, Johnson MH, Bi WL, Chiang VL, Duncan CC (2006) Sterile ascites from a ventriculoperitoneal shunt: a case report and review of the literature. Childs Nerv Syst 22:1187–1193
116. Olavarria G, Reitman AJ, Goldman S, Tomita T (2005) Post-shunt ascites in infants with optic chiasmal hypothalamic astrocytoma: role of ventricular gallbladder shunt. Childs Nerv Syst 21:382–384

117. Mobley LW 3rd, Doran SE, Hellbusch LC (2005) Abdominal pseudocyst: predisposing factors and treatment algorithm. Pediatr Neurosurg 41:77–83
118. Kimura T, Tsutsumi K, Morita A (2011) Scrotal migration of lumboperitoneal shunt catheter in an adult: case report. Neurol Med Chir (Tokyo) 51:861–862
119. Magee JF, Barker NE, Blair GK, Steinbok P (1996) Inguinal herniation with glial implants: possible complication of ventriculoperitoneal shunting. Pediatr Pathol Lab Med 16:591–596
120. Ammar A, Ibrahim AW, Nasser M, Rashid M (1993) CSF hydrocele—unusual complication of V-P shunt. Neurosurg Rev 14:141–143
121. Sathyanarayana S, Wylen EL, Baskaya MK, Nanda A (2000) Spontaneous bowel perforation after ventriculoperitoneal shunt surgery: case report and review of 45 cases. Surg Neurol 54:388–396
122. Kin S, Imamura J, Ikeyama Y, Jimi Y, Yasukura S (1997) Perforation of the intestine by a peritoneal tube 10 years after a ventriculo-peritoneal shunt. No Shinkei Geka 25:573–575
123. Shetty PG, Fatterpekar GM, Sahani DV, Shroff MM (1999) Pneumocephalus secondary to colonic perforation by ventriculoperitoneal catheter. Br J Radiol 72:704–705

Part II

Complications of Extrathecal CSF Shunts

4 Introduction: The Use of Extrathecal CSF Shunts, Optional vs Mandatory, Unavoidable Complications

Rizwan A. Khan

Contents

4.1 **Types of Extrathecal Shunts** 75

4.2 **Indications** 77

4.3 **Unavoidable Complications** 78
4.3.1 Complications Due to Material 78
4.3.2 Complications Due to Design 79
4.3.3 Complication Due to Age 79
4.3.4 Complications Due to Miscellaneous Causes 79

References 79

R.A. Khan, MD, MS, MCh
Department of Pediatric Surgery, JNMC, AMU, Aligarh, India
e-mail: drrizwanahmadkhan@yahoo.co.in

4.1 Types of Extrathecal Shunts

Since 1895 when Gartner proposed shunting the CSF into extrathecal low-pressure compartments such as the venous or lymphatic system or the abdominal cavity, the treatment of hydrocephalus has come a long way [1]. The idea was first applied by Fergusson in 1898 and later was taken up by several authors, including Cushing, but the results were mostly disappointing. The modern shunting era began with Nulsen and Spitz, creating a one-way pressure-regulated valve which they placed in the atrium via the jugular vein (Figs. 4.1 and 4.2). There are various types of extrathecal shunts, some of which are only of historical importance. Extrathecal shunts still in vogue are lumboperitoneal, ventriculovenous, ventriculoatrial, ventriculopleural, ventriculoureteric, ventriculo-gallbladder, and ventriculoperitoneal shunts [2, 3]:

1. Lumboperitoneal (LP) shunts are used in patients with communicating hydrocephalus or small slit ventricles (due to overdrainage caused by other extrathecal shunts like ventriculoperitoneal and ventriculoatrial shunts) and patients who have had multiple ventricular shunt malfunctions. These shunts have the advantage of avoiding injury by the ventricular catheter, maintaining the patency of ventricles (unlike ventricular shunts where the ventricles tend to collapse leading to shunt malfunction), and have lower risk of obstruction and infection. However, LP shunts are more prone to malfunction from mechanical

C. Di Rocco et al. (eds.), *Complications of CSF Shunting in Hydrocephalus: Prevention, Identification, and Management*, DOI 10.1007/978-3-319-09961-3_4,

failures like migration out of the spine or peritoneum and carry a definite risk of development of hindbrain herniation over a period of time especially in children. The assessment of function of a lumbar shunt is more difficult as compared to ventricular shunt [4].

2. Ventriculoatrial (VA) shunts are provided to divert cerebrospinal fluid from the cerebral ventricle into the right atrium. These are not chosen as the first-line method to redirect the CSF rather when there have been multiple failure of the VP shunt (Table 4.1). The intraoperative appropriate vein selection and exact shunt placement are important to reduce complications such as obstruction [5].
3. Ventriculopleural shunts were introduced as a management option for hydrocephalus by Ransohoff in 1954. Ventriculopleural shunts have been used infrequently in the management of hydrocephalus and have become the "next preferred procedure" in case if the ventriculoperitoneal shunt fails. It has low complication rates and is easy to perform, but involvement and collaboration of the thoracic surgery team is required. The risk of pleural effusion is highest among the infants which seemed to be reduced with the introduction of antisiphon device [6].
4. Ventriculoureteric shunt (VUS) is rarely used nowadays in neurosurgical practice owing to much better techniques that are available. It is technically demanding – exposure of the renal pelvis and ureter requires the help of an urologist. As previously thought, it no more requires nephrectomy and reimplantation of the ureter, but to prevent expulsion, flanged at the distal catheter must be used. Hyponatremia is a known metabolic complication immediately following the VUS [7].
5. Ventriculo-gallbladder shunts (VGS) are used because of the ability of the biliary tree to adequately control intracranial pressure, low risk of infection due to the sterility of bile, and also the prospect for electrolyte reabsorption from the small intestine (Table 4.1). But it is not the first line of treatment. Indications described are multiple shunt revisions, abdominal pseudocysts, and ascites secondary to shunts in optic chiasmal hypothalamic astrocytomas. Bile calculus causing a distal

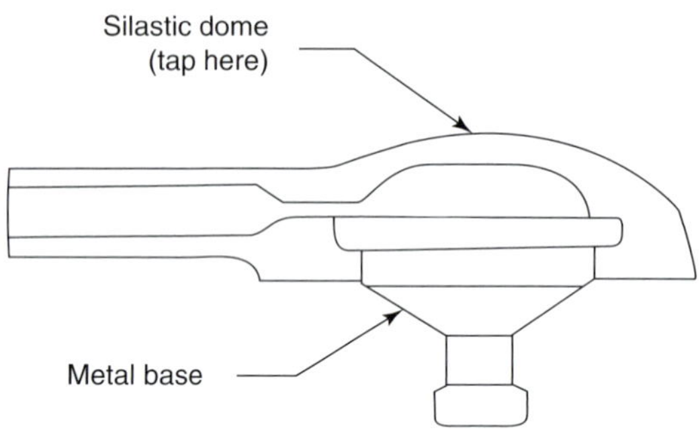

Fig. 4.1 Conventional ventriculoperitoneal shunt

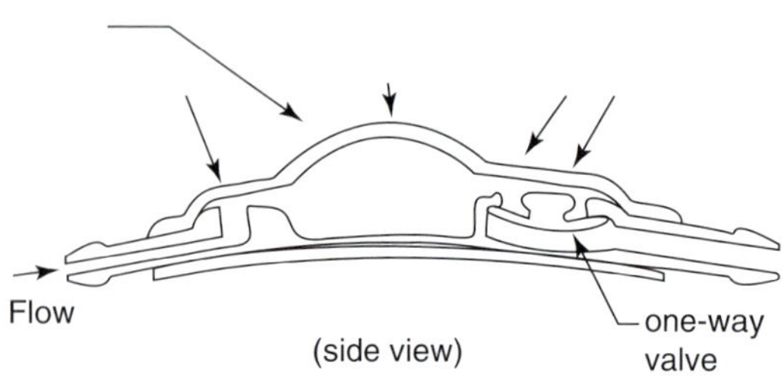

Fig. 4.2 Ventriculoperitoneal shunt with antisiphon device

Table 4.1 Showing features of the extrathecal shunts

Type of extrathecal shunt	Drainage into	Practicality	Common complication
Ventriculoperitoneal	Peritoneal cavity	Most commonly performed	Mechanical, fracture, infection
Ventriculopleural	Pleural cavity	Second most commonly performed procedure	Pleural effusion
Ventriculoatrial	Right atrium	Multiple failure of VP shunt	Obstruction, embolic episodes
Ventriculoureteric	Ureter/renal pelvis	Rarely used	Hyponatremia
Ventriculo-gallbladder	Gallbladder	Multiple failures	Bile calculus with distal obstruction
Lumboperitoneal	Lumbar space to peritoneum	Overdrainage syndrome due to other extrathecal shunts	Mechanical complications, hindbrain herniation

obstruction in the VG shunt catheter is a frequently reported complication. There are also chances of cholecystitis causing retrograde and descending shunt infections [8].

6. It is widely accepted that ventriculoperitoneal shunts represent the most common extracranial CSF diversion choice, given that the peritoneal cavity is the most efficient and reliable location for CSF absorption. The peritoneal cavity is the preferred drainage site in children because it enables the implantation of drainage catheter of sufficient length to allow for the growth and predisposes to less severe complications than does the right atrium and ease of shunt revision. The first ventriculoperitoneal shunt is probably attributed to Kaush. In 1908 he reported a patient in whom he connected a lateral ventricle to the peritoneum using a rubber tube, but the patient died because of overdrainage.

4.2 Indications

It is easy to identify patients who would benefit from CSF diversion if the presentation includes clear evidence of increased intracranial pressure (ICP), manifested as severe headaches with projectile vomiting, diplopia, upward gaze paresis, and a dilated ventricular system on radiologic imaging [2, 9] (Table 4.1).

1. In adults with occlusive hydrocephalus with raised ICP, CSF diversion is indicated to prevent permanent neurologic deficits or neurologic deficits progress. To supplement clinical findings, radiological evidence of ventricular enlargement may be assessed with Evan's index which is a ratio of greatest width of the frontal horns of the lateral ventricles to the maximal internal diameter of the skull. An index exceeding 0.3 is indicative of a hydrocephalus. T2-weighted MR images can show transependymal flow of CSF and subependymal white matter damage.
2. Assessing patients of NPH for CSF diversion is difficult. Contrary to its name, there are periodical fluctuations of intracranial pressure in the early stages of the disease. Presence of this intermittent elevation of ICP provides a justification for treatment by shunting, which cuts off the peaks of increased ICP damaging the brain. On radiology widened temporal horns and flattened cortical sulci at the top of the brain are also found in NPH. A twenty-four-h ICP monitoring showing B-waves is regarded to be a good indicator of NPH likely to benefit from shunting. Patients with NPH who are considered for shunting should have gait disturbances and at least one of the two other elements of the triad: disturbances of urination and cognition. Patterns of concentration of biomarkers like NFL (neurofilament protein light) may also help in reaching the diagnosis [10].
3. The most important point to be considered in decision making in premature infants is the rapid head growth with bulging and tense anterior fontanelle. There may be prominent scalp vein and episodes of apnea and bradycardia. Term infants may also show irritability, vomiting, drowsiness, axial hypotonia, and setting-sun sign. Retinal hemorrhages may be present, but papilledema is uncommon. Older children may show headaches, projectile vomiting, diplopia (abducens nerve palsy), blurred vision, loss of visual acuity, and papilledema. Transfontanellar craniosonography may help in showing the progress of ventricular enlargement, and CT and MRI can be used to assess the severity by measuring Evan's ratio or by the presence of transependymal CSF absorption [11]. The most difficult is the evaluation of a child with macrocephaly and normal development. Computed tomography scanning shows increased extra-axial collections, with a normal or mildly enlarged ventricle. This entity, sometimes referred to as benign extra-axial collections of infancy, may be a stage of transient communicating hydrocephalus that may resolve in a period of 12–18 months with a normal outcome. It is a clinical and not an imaging diagnosis, and it must be distinguished from true communicating hydrocephalus. If the child is

developing normally, close observation with neurodevelopmental examination and head circumference measurements are adequate. If the child is neurologically abnormal, then a radionuclide cisternogram plays a role in evaluating the contribution of abnormal fluid dynamics. It has been used to identify patients with communicating hydrocephalus. A high lumbar pressure, poor 4-h urinary excretion (normal 50 %, borderline 30–40 %, definitely abnormal <30 %), persistence of ventricular filling at 24 h, and poor flow over convexity are highly suggestive of communicating hydrocephalus and an indication for CSF diversion [12].

4.3 Unavoidable Complications

Shunt system is a foreign body placed for relieving the intracranial pressure and will have some complications inherent to its very presence inside the body. There are many complications associated with the shunt like infection, obstruction, overdrainage, underdrainage, loculation, etc. These complications can be avoided or best minimized with proper precautions and use of appropriate shunting device. But there are certain complications that are going to be present, and the neurosurgeon has no control over these complications.

4.3.1 Complications Due to Material

Holter developed the first shunt to employ silicone with multiple slit valve design. Medical grade silicone (dimethyl polysiloxane), the indispensible material for the shunt systems of current generation, meets all the criteria of biocompatibility, nonimmunogenic, noncarcinogenic, fatigue-free (which could withstand the severe, long-term mechanical stress they were subject to particularly in the right atrium), thermally resistant (ideal for heat sterilization), and electrical stability. Although chemically inert, silicones are not necessarily biologically inert, and there are several evidences of silicone allergy in some patients with silicone shunts. At the time of insertion of a ventricular catheter, the blood–brain barrier is not healed for 2–3 weeks. This leads to adherence of the platelets and serum proteins including immunoglobulins, albumin, fibronectin, and fibrinogen which in turn potentiate the inflammatory response and also adhere to silicone rubber and alter the function of more distal shunt components (e.g., the valve mechanism). In the peritoneal cavity, shunt catheters can be obstructed by ingrowth of mesothelial cells and fibroblasts, and adsorption of protein is associated with greater adhesion of inflammatory cells.

The body's reaction to silicone can be classified into three types: local reaction and granuloma formation, silicone migration, and autoimmune disease. In all cases following the implantation of silicone, there is the development of a chronic type of reaction to the implant, which includes the formation of a fibrous tissue pseudocapsule with minimal inflammatory reaction. This is best represented by the very familiar shunt tract. Another form of reaction that has been recognized is the formation of granulomas, focal collections of macrophages, histiocytes, epithelioid cells, giant cells, lymphocytes, and plasma cells often termed "siliconomas." These are seen along the tract in patient with multiple revisions. Silicone allergy is known to affect an implant in a patient by the phenomenon of migration. This spread can occur by lymphatic, hematogenous, and local route. This is seen more commonly in patients with breast implants and cardiac valve prosthesis, in those undergoing cardiopulmonary bypass, and in patients on frequent hemodialysis. Autoimmune disease can occur following implantation of silicone polymers. This is also seen more commonly in women who have undergone injection or implantation of silicone for breast augmentation. Symptoms include arthritis, arthralgia, and local and regional lymphadenopathy.

In patients with suspected or documented silicone allergy, the use of polyurethane or CO2-extracted silicone catheters has been postulated but not proven to offer some advantage in reducing the risk of recurrent malfunctions [13, 14].

4.3.2 Complications Due to Design

A physical design modification, i.e., addition of soft radial flanges to push the catheter away from the brain tissue and protect the catheter lumen from the problem of tissue ingrowth, has not been successful. It has since become clear that the simple addition of flanges does not prevent tissue ingrowth, and in fact some neurosurgeons report that tissue ingrowths on flanged catheters are even more tenacious than those associated with standard design catheters.

The technological advancements made to valve systems (like the staircase mechanism of the Codman Medos valve) have provided additional CSF pathways that are turbulent and susceptible to areas of buildup of debris that may be a reason for the higher failure rate. Diaphragm-based antisiphon devices are prone to obstruction from encapsulation. There is no evidence that using an open system has any advantage over using a closed system, but theoretically any malfunction in an open system would result only in loss of antisiphon function, without obstruction to CSF flow as against the closed system, in which the flow stops once the pressure reaches zero. In flow control devices, patients develop nighttime or early morning headaches. This is because these patients have limited pressure volume compensatory reserve and there can be an excessive increase in ICP during cardiovascular fluctuations, especially at night [15]. Silicone rubber components of CSF shunts, especially in the subcutaneous compartment, degrade with time, becoming fragile and likely to fracture. This occurs because of deposition of calcium phosphate and aluminum in the external layers of shunt tubing. Evidence suggests that the barium used in the silicone catheters is probably not an important factor in promoting calcification and degradation. But using barium-free catheters makes it difficult to assess a shunt system on radiologic imaging [16].

4.3.3 Complication Due to Age

Age at which the shunt is performed is also a predictor of shunt survival. Patients older than 2 years have a longer shunt survival period than those who were younger. It has been suggested that this observation is related to both immunological deficiency and particular bacterial flora in infants. Prematurity at first shunt insertion also predisposes to subsequent shunt revisions. This point to some fundamental tissue reaction occurs in response to shunt insertion [17].

4.3.4 Complications Due to Miscellaneous Causes

Concurrent surgical procedure is noted to increase the risk of shunt failure. Shunt surgery is generally performed as a single procedure but, sometimes, like in patients with tumors requiring a biopsy, it is done as simultaneous procedure. But in such a setting the procedure becomes long and the risk of infection and malfunction increases [18].

It has been seen that whites have significantly longer shunt survival times than nonwhites. Multiple factors especially increased incidence of prematurity and general immunocompromised state among nonwhites may be responsible for this [19].

As a matter of fact there is no ideal or flawless shunt up to this time. An ideal shunt still needs to be the goal in the future of treating hydrocephalus. The ideal shunt would allow for a flow-regulated control to drain a specific amount of fluid, which could be tailored to an individual patient's needs. All the CSF shunt systems that are currently available show a given failure rate, and therefore search for the perfect shunt continues.

References

1. Greenberg MS (1997) Handbook of neurosurgery, 4th edn. Greenberg Graphics, Lakeland
2. Milhorat TH (1995) Hydrocephalus: pathophysiology and clinical features. In: Wilkins RH, Rengachary SS (eds) Neurosurgery, vol 3, 2nd edn. McGraw Hill, New York, pp 3625–3632
3. Nulsen FE, Spitz EB (1952) Treatment of hydrocephalus by direct shunt from ventricle to jugular vein. Surg Forum 2:399–403

4. Aoki N (1990) Lumboperitoneal shunt: clinical applications, complications, and comparison with ventriculoperitoneal shunt. Neurosurgery 26:998–1003
5. Nash DL, Schmidt K (2010) Complications and management of ventriculoatrial (VA) shunts, a case report. Cerebrospinal Fluid Res 7(Suppl 1):S42
6. Piatt JH Jr (1994) How effective are ventriculopleural shunts? Pediatr Neurosurg 21:66–70
7. Pittman T, Steinhardt G, Weber T (1992) Ventriculo-ureteral shunt without nephrectomy. Br J Neurosurg 6:261–263
8. Aldana PR, James HE, Postlethwait RA (2008) Ventriculogallbladder shunts in pediatric patients. J Neurosurg Pediatr 1:284–287
9. Kausch W (1908) Die Behandlung des Hydrocephalus der Kleinen Kinder. Arch Klin Chir 87:709–796
10. Gallia GL, Rigamonti D, Williams MA (2006) The diagnosis and treatment of normal pressure hydrocephalus. Nat Clin Pract Neurol 2:375–381
11. Robinson S, Kaufman BA, Park TS (2002) Outcome analysis of initial neonatal shunts: does the valves make the difference? Pediatr Neurosurg 37:287–294
12. Fouyas IP, Casey AH, Thompson D, Harkness WF, Hayward RD, Rutka JT et al (1996) Use of intracranial pressure monitoring in the management of childhood hydrocephalus and shunt-related problems. Neurosurgery 38(4):726–732
13. Jimenez DF, Keating R, Goodrich JT (1994) Silicone allergy in ventriculoperitoneal shunts. Childs Nerv Syst 10(1):59–63
14. Snow RB, Kossovsky N (1989) Hypersensitivity reaction associated with sterile ventriculoperitoneal shunt malfunction. Surg Neurol 31:209–214
15. Drake JM, Kestle J, Milner R et al (1998) Randomized trial of CSF shunt value design in paediatric hydrocephalus. Neurosurgery 43:294–305
16. Echizenya K, Satoh M, Murai H et al (1987) Mineralization and biodegradation of CSF shunting systems. J Neurosurg 67:584–619
17. Serlo W, Fernell E, Heikkinen E et al (1990) Functions and complications of shunts in different etiologies of childhood hydrocephalus. Childs Nerv Syst 6:92–94
18. Shurtleff DB, Stuntz JT, Hayden PW (1985/1986) Experience with 1201 cerebrospinal fluid shunt procedures. Pediatr Neurosci 12:49–57
19. Vinchon M, Dhellemmes P (2006) Cerebrospinal fluid shunt infection: risk factors and long-term follow-up. Childs Nerv Syst 22:692–697

Iatrogenic Complications of CSF Shunting

5

Juan F. Martínez-Lage, Miguel Angel Pérez-Espejo, and Ahmet Tuncay Turgut

Contents

5.1 **Introduction** 82
5.1.1 What Is Iatrogenesis? 82

5.2 **Wrong Indications** 82
5.2.1 Neonatal and Infantile Hydrocephalus 82
5.2.2 Pediatric Normal Pressure Hydrocephalus 83
5.2.3 Asymptomatic Pediatric Ventriculomegaly 83
5.2.4 Adult Normal Pressure Hydrocephalus 84
5.2.5 Posttraumatic Hydrocephalus Versus Posttraumatic Brain Atrophy 84
5.2.6 Unrecognized Shunt Malfunction 84
5.2.7 Apparent Clinically Arrested Hydrocephalus 85
5.2.8 Extracerebral Fluid Collections 86

5.3 **Iatrogenesis in Diagnostic Procedures** 88
5.3.1 Reservoir Pumping 88
5.3.2 Shunt Tap 88
5.3.3 ICP Measurement 88
5.3.4 Iatrogenesis Related to Neuroimaging Studies 89
5.3.5 Miscellaneous Tests 89

5.4 **Technical Problems** 90
5.4.1 Preparations for Surgery 90
5.4.2 Patient Position, Local Anesthetics, and Skin Preparation 91
5.4.3 Skin Incision, Burr Hole, and Dural Opening 92
5.4.4 Ventricular Catheter Insertion-Related Pitfalls 92
5.4.5 Peritoneal Access 95
5.4.6 Tunneling and Subcutaneous Passage of the Distal Catheter 95
5.4.7 Rupture, Disconnection, and Migration 96
5.4.8 Reservoirs, Valves, and Antisiphon Devices 96
5.4.9 Connection of the Shunt Parts, Closure, and Wound Dressing 97

5.5 **"Friendly Fire" from Other Specialties** 97

5.6 **Iatrogenesis in Diverse Indications and Distal Draining Locations** 98
5.6.1 Ventriculoatrial Shunting 98
5.6.2 Ventriculopleural Shunting 99
5.6.3 Lumboperitoneal Shunting 99
5.6.4 Ventriculogallbladder Shunting 99
5.6.5 Ventriculoureteral Shunting 99
5.6.6 Ventriculosubgaleal Shunting 99
5.6.7 Subduroperitoneal Shunting 100
5.6.8 Arachnoid-Cyst Shunting 100
5.6.9 Multiloculated Hydrocephalus and Fourth Ventricle Cysts 100

5.7 **Programmable Valves** 101

5.8 **Shunt Infection** 102

5.9 **Follow-Up, Education, and Continuity of Care** 102

Conclusions 102

References 102

J.F. Martínez-Lage, MD (✉) • M.A. Pérez-Espejo, MD
Pediatric Neurosurgery Section and Regional Service of Neurosurgery, Virgen de la Arrixaca University Hospital, El Palmar, Murcia 30120, Spain
e-mail: juanf.martinezlage@gmail.com; miguelangelperezespejomartinez@gmail.com

A.T. Turgut, MD
Department of Radiology, Ankara Training and Research Hospital, Ankara TR-06590, Turkey
e-mail: ahmettuncayturgut@yahoo.com

C. Di Rocco et al. (eds.), *Complications of CSF Shunting in Hydrocephalus: Prevention, Identification, and Management*, DOI 10.1007/978-3-319-09961-3_5,

5.1 Introduction

5.1.1 What Is Iatrogenesis?

The word iatrogenesis refers to the effects (good or bad) related to illnesses caused by medical examinations or treatments. This term is currently employed to designate an untoward consequence of any kind of therapy or medical act that is, as a rule, preventable. In a broad sense, iatrogenesis may result from drug administration, surgical procedures, chance, error, or negligence. Iatrogenic effects are specifically identifiable and easily recognizable in complications arising after a surgical procedure. Thus, the term is commonly utilized referring to a preventable harm resulting from a surgical (or medical) treatment. However, some overlapping exists between expressions such as untoward effect, side effect, ill effect, complication, and iatrogenic harm without a clear-cut border that differentiates them. Iatrogenic failure has also been referred to as "friendly fire." The surgical scars produced for placing a shunt are an example of iatrogenesis, although their production is inevitable. Infection of an external ventricular drainage (EVD) is another example of an iatrogenic damage but it does occur in spite of the strictest preventive measures. Consequently, in this chapter we will deal with a variety of iatrogenic effects of hydrocephalus treatments bearing in mind that they are, at least in part, potentially preventable. However, we must remember that there is not a single medical act that can be regarded as completely free of doing harm and this includes even the physicians' words.

A recent survey of medical-device-associated complications in the USA during the 2-year period of 2004 and 2005, consisting of 144,799 reported events, yielded an estimate rate of 5,205 VP shunting adverse events of which 3,340 required hospitalization [63]. This high number of VP-shunt-related complications contributed to the largest rate of hospitalization across all pediatric age groups (63 %) [63]. A study on hospital utilization, charges, comorbidities, and deaths related to CSF shunting showed that hydrocephalus is a chronic illness, and that its management uses a disproportionate share of hospital days and healthcare charges in the USA [127]. Several studies also showed that patients with hydrocephalus have increased in age and comorbidities and that hydrocephalus-related conditions require an increase in research efforts and funding [127, 156].

Given the large number of reported complications of CSF shunts, some reflections are necessary before undertaking CSF shunting. Some general principles include the following:

(a) Shunt implantation is necessary.
(b) There is not a better option.
(c) Preoperative planning and surgical technique are undertaken in detail.
(d) Trainees are appropriately taught and supervised.
(e) Patients are in their best physical condition.
(f) CSF infections and coagulation disorders have been previously corrected.
(g) The appropriate equipment, including a reserve valve, has been checked and at hand.

5.2 Wrong Indications

A sound indication for CSF shunting is the first measure for avoiding iatrogenic complications. The goal of diagnosis and management of hydrocephalus is to determine (a) the need for treatment, (b) the nature of treatment, (c) its probable outcome, and (d) the introduction of treatment modifications [156]. In the presence of well-known clinical manifestations (headaches, vomiting, and impaired consciousness), the indication for CSF shunting is straightforward. Ventricular size alone cannot direct the diagnosis or the decision to treat [156]. Anatomical imaging is usually insufficient as a sole diagnostic tool for hydrocephalus. The authors analyze in the following sections some difficulties and uncertainties on the indications for CSF shunting in several common conditions with impaired CSF dynamics, aimed at preventing the occurrence of iatrogenic problems.

5.2.1 Neonatal and Infantile Hydrocephalus

Hydrocephalus in neonates and infants usually presents with macrocephaly, a tense fontanel, split sutures, irritability, and poor feeding [160].

Serial routine measurements of head circumference (HC) constitute a key sign for diagnosing hydrocephalus in children below 1 year of age [160]. A bulging fontanel and suture diastasis are highly reliable indicators of hydrocephalus in this age group [49, 153]. In the newborn with posthemorrhagic hydrocephalus, cranial growth measurements should be recorded in HC charts. Obviously, these signs (bulging fontanel and suture diastasis) cannot be elicited when the skull has already fused. Excessive head enlargement usually parallels ventricular increase in serial ultrasound (US) studies. Before placing a definitive CSF valve in this patient population, several management options must have been tried for controlling raised intracranial pressure (ICP), namely serial lumbar punctures, EVD, reservoir taps, or ventriculosubgaleal shunting according to institutional customs and guidelines [11]. These procedures try to avoid needless shunt operations, although some authors favor early valve insertion for prevention of brain damage due to prolonged conservative measures [119]. There is much debate regarding the most appropriate valve and the optimal timing for shunt insertion in this group of patients [11, 119]. A recent study comprising 5,416 infants (younger than 1 year of age) comparing ETV and CSF shunting has demonstrated a higher rate of surgical failures in patients treated with ETV, especially in those under 90 days of life [63]. A higher failure rate of ETV was associated with prematurity, intraventricular hemorrhage, and spina bifida [63]. In infants, we customarily use a programmable valve that allows matching the valve pressure setting to the changing needs of the infants' developing brain. With these valves, we aim at preventing not only early manifestations of over- or undershunting, but also the late appearance of overdrainage especially those of slit-ventricle syndrome (SVS) and craniocerebral disproportion [82]. Criteria for delaying shunting in newborn posthemorrhagic hydrocephalus include (a) the presence of a bloody CSF, (b) CSF infection, and (c) a high CSF protein content. Standards for placing a definitive CSF valve comprise: (a) HC increases greater than 1.5 cm per week, (b) maximum transverse atrial diameter of 10 mm, and (c) decrease of Doppler diastolic velocity and increase of pulsatility index. Bradycardia and apneic spells in these children indicate the need for an urgent CSF decompression procedure.

In myelomeningocele patients, some authors tried to reduce the rate of shunt insertion [19]. Taking into account that the normal rate of hydrocephalus in myelomeningocele is approximately 80 %, these authors reported that, with their policy, the incidence of valve insertion was reduced to only 52 %. Their established criteria for valve placement include (a) symptoms of raised ICP, bulging fontanels, bradycardia, sun-setting eyes, and progressive head growth; and (b) increasing ventriculomegaly in serial US or computerized tomography (CT) [19]. On the contrary, they do not consider pseudomeningocele or wound CSF leak as indicators of the need for shunting [19].

5.2.2 Pediatric Normal Pressure Hydrocephalus

There is also a group of children with so-called *occult hydrocephalus* [36] whose clinical picture does not suggest intracranial hypertension. This group is regarded as the pediatric counterpart (or precursor) of chronic adult hydrocephalus or normal pressure hydrocephalus (NPH). The children show up with nonspecific signs and symptoms such as slight macrocrania, failing vision, mild psychomotor retardation, unsteady gait, increased tone and deep reflexes in the lower limbs, impaired ocular movements, epilepsy, and endocrine dysfunction [36]. In some patients, the history suggested a probable etiology as perinatal hemorrhage or meningitis, but in most instances no cause could be elicited. All children underwent CSF shunting that led to total recovery in 30 instances [36]. The decision to operate on these children is not so obvious and indicates the need for complementary diagnostic tools for establishing an accurate diagnosis.

5.2.3 Asymptomatic Pediatric Ventriculomegaly

Asymptomatic children with ventriculomegaly *detected on neuroimaging studies* as CT or magnetic resonance imaging (MRI) constitutes a more problematic situation. Some authors believe that children below the age of 3 years with moderate or greater ventriculomegaly should be operated on based on the fact that we cannot guarantee that they will not undergo a future brain damage and that it is preferable to err on the side of implanting a valve [86]. Children beyond 5 years of age with stable ventriculomegaly might be watched if their intellectual achievements are in the normal range and remain stable. These children probably constitute the precursor of the condition denominated LOVA (long-standing overt ventriculomegaly of adults) [100, 115]. The distinction between ventriculomegaly and brain atrophy often requires complementary investigations as intracranial pressure (ICP) monitoring or dynamic CSF tests [122]. However, patients with unclear diagnosis of hydrocephalus usually also offer equivocal results on these tests. When the decision of not to operate a child is made, close observation based on objective data, such as serial ophthalmological and psychometric testing, is crucial. A survey performed among pediatric neurosurgeons to know their attitudes toward shunting asymptomatic children with ventriculomegaly showed that there exists a general conservative attitude for recommending surgery [34]. In conclusion, ventriculomegaly alone in the absence of clinical support must not be treated, as a wrong indication may lead only to iatrogenic complications.

5.2.4 Adult Normal Pressure Hydrocephalus

In adults, the association of dementia, urinary incontinence and ataxic gait together with enlarged ventricles and a normal CSF opening pressure, with no apparent cause, point toward the diagnosis of idiopathic NPH. However, many doubts may arise regarding the correct diagnosis of NPH, especially for distinguishing it from brain atrophy given that both hydrocephalus and atrophy may occur in the elderly and may coexist with arterial hypertension, diabetes mellitus, and vascular conditions related to aging. To avoid iatrogenic failures in these patients, the diagnosis needs to be confirmed by one or more of the following tests: serial high-volume lumbar punctures, psychometric tests, intracranial pressure measurements, and/or infusion tests. Screening tests reported to date for diagnosing NPH, excepting serial lumbar punctures and external lumbar drainage, do not have enough sensitivity and specificity to offer better results than those obtained with automatic shunt placement [15]. Patients must be selected for avoiding an expensive, potentially hazardous, and ineffective shunt procedure in those unlikely to benefit from it [15, 147]. The costs, invasiveness, and potential complications of external lumbar drainage (e.g., meningitis) limit the utility of this test for predicting the success of shunting in presumed NPH patients [147]. For treatment, most authors recommend placing a low-pressure valve. However, a low-pressure valve may trigger the iatrogenic appearance of subdural hematomas and hygromas. On the other hand, medium-pressure valves or antisiphon devices may induce underdrainage. Programmable valves and antigravitational devices are being investigated that might decrease the incidence of iatrogenic failure in patients with NPH.

5.2.5 Posttraumatic Hydrocephalus Versus Posttraumatic Brain Atrophy

To assess what survivors of a severe head injury would benefit from shunt placement, ICP recording, bolus injection, pressure/volume index, and resistance for CSF absorption are used. These tests may help in differentiating posttraumatic hydrocephalus from posttraumatic brain atrophy.

5.2.6 Unrecognized Shunt Malfunction

Shunt revision for shunt malfunction is one of the most common operations performed by pediatric neurosurgeons. Shunt revision surgery is seldom elective and seems to occur always at inopportune hours, shunt revision being often more urgent than the initial procedure [114]. Failure in detecting shunt dysfunction constitutes a potential source of iatrogenic complications. In the first place, the differential diagnosis of shunt failure in children must be established against other common childhood diseases as viral diseases or even appendicitis. Shunt series, CT or MRI studies, and shunt taps are often performed to avoid harm due to "failure to diagnose," that is, performing defensive medicine [156]. The value of comparing the ventricular size on neuroimaging at the time of shunt dysfunction with that seen on baseline studies is of utmost importance.

However, ventricular dilatation is a frequent, but not constant, finding of CSF shunt failure. Some patients with protracted symptoms consistent with CSF shunt malfunction and normal ventricular size will be finally found to have a malfunctioning shunt at surgical revision [158]. Even a shunt tap can give equivocal results in the presence of an incomplete block of the proximal catheter. A slow CSF flow from the valve reservoir can indicate partial catheter block, CSF hypotension, or ventricular collapse. Continuous intraventricular pressure recording may clarify the diagnosis in doubtful cases of shunt dysfunction [35, 122]. In a study of children with shunt failure that presented with subtle deterioration, dynamic CSF studies showed abnormally compliant pressure-volume curves in the absence of acute episodic pressure waves [41]. Physicians usually trust neuroimaging studies, but approximately 10 % of shunted patients do not develop ventricular dilatation at the time of shunt failure. Undue delay in the identification and treatment in this setting leads to iatrogenic neurological or intellectual damage, blindness, or even to the patients' death [146]. Some clinical guidelines have been suggested for the evaluation of suspected shunt dysfunction in the emergency setting [102].

5.2.7 Apparent Clinically Arrested Hydrocephalus

In compensated hydrocephalus, as occurs in patients known to harbor a long-standing nonfunctional shunt, the situation may not be necessarily permanent due to the uncertain nature of the equilibrium between CSF production and absorption. Late decompensation of hydrocephalus might occur either spontaneously, after inflammatory conditions, or after a minor head injury [107]. Some adolescents and young adults, especially those with spina bifida, those with intraventricular hemorrhage hydrocephalus, and some with tumoral hydrocephalus may evolve with apparent clinically arrested hydrocephalus. Spina bifida patients with presumed compensated hydrocephalus often experience long periods of silent and subtle deterioration or refer vague symptoms such as tiredness, mental dulling, and so on. They may even experience clinical manifestations of spinal cord involvement due to hydromyelia that develops over many years. These individuals must be followed-up and searched for minimal neurological or cognitive changes. Diagnosis is based on periodic neuropsychological testing and on ICP monitoring in selected patients. Patients with arrested hydrocephalus are often found during a routine outpatient clinic visit to have a broken shunt and deny having any symptom. In the same way, their neurological examination, including funduscopy, is normal. The explanation for this fact is that there may exist some flow through the fibrous pericatheter tract that allows some intermittent drainage of CSF [25]. Another explanation is the maturation of CSF absorptive mechanisms. Successful removal of CSF shunts could be performed in 27 out of 850 children (3.2 %), this being the most reliable prognostic factor initial shunt insertion below 1 year of age [56]. As the patients remain asymptomatic for long periods, shunt revision or replacement is not advised, in the hope that they have become shunt-independent. However, these patients must undergo close observation during a period whose duration has not yet been well defined. The patients are also instructed to attend hospital urgently should they note the appearance of symptoms of raised ICP. Neglecting these simple precautionary measures might lead to iatrogenic neurological damage and even to the patient's death.

5.2.8 Extracerebral Fluid Collections

Several conditions may be associated with neuroimaging findings of extra-axial fluid collections. The pitfalls for the categorization of these fluid accumulations have been amply discussed [6, 55, 88, 97, 116]. These collections are presented in the following text.

5.2.8.1 Benign Pericerebral Collections of Fluid

Benign external hydrocephalus refers to enlarged subarachnoid spaces, mainly in the frontoparietal convexity of the cerebral hemispheres, which manifest with macrocrania and a large anterior fontanel. Benign pericerebral collections of fluid are generally asymptomatic but may cause doubtful or minimal developmental delay. The condition is often of familial presentation and is more prevalent in boys. The collections might be considered abnormal in the presence of clinical signs of raised ICP and of associated ventriculomegaly [99]. These fluid accumulations are of benign nature and decrease during the first year of life and usually disappear by the age of 3 years without surgery (Fig. 5.1) [6, 54, 88]. Benign subarachnoid accumulations of fluid require only periodic clinical observation and serial neuroimaging [88]. Their origin has been attributed to a defective capacity of the *arachnoid villi* for fluid absorption, or represents a mismatch in the development of the skull and the brain, their main significance being that they place affected infants at a higher risk for developing a subdural hematoma [97]. Mistaking these collections of fluid with chronic subdural hematomas may lead to unnecessary placement of a subduroperitoneal shunt with the potential for developing CSF leaks through the surgical wound in the short term [6] or iatrogenic overdrainage in the long term [81].

5.2.8.2 Posttraumatic and Postinfectious Subdural Collections

Posttraumatic and postinfectious collections of fluid, with bloody or xanthochromic fluid (subdural effusions), may produce brain compression. They also evolve with macrocephaly and are accompanied by neurological symptoms and require surgical treatment as subdural taps, burr-hole drainage, temporary external derivation, or they may even necessitate a subduroperitoneal shunt. On MRI, the fluid appears more intense than normal CSF. The most often used treatment is subduroperitoneal shunting.

5.2.8.3 Initial Stages of Communicating Hydrocephalus

Initial communicating hydrocephalus may show up with dilatation of the subarachnoid spaces, the cerebral fissures and cisterns, and with slightly enlarged ventricles [55, 16]. In this context, serial neuroimaging studies, preferably MRI, are mandatory to not delay surgery of true hydrocephalus. Diagnostic methods for differentiating subdural hygroma from communicating hydrocephalus include neuroimaging studies and also measurements of the subdural pressure with a manometer during trephine drainage [55].

5.2.8.4 Brain Atrophy

Similarly, dilated arachnoid spaces at the convexities, cerebral fissures, and cisterns do occur in conditions associated with brain atrophy. Logically, shunting these ex vacuo fluid spaces triggers a number of iatrogenic complications and does not afford any clinical benefit.

5.2.8.5 Leptomeningeal Seeding of Tumors

Exceptionally, external hydrocephalus may result from occult leptomeningeal seeding of a benign or malignant brain tumor [134]. In this case, subdural postcontrast enhancement will reveal the true nature of the condition.

5.2.8.6 Arachnoid Cysts

Correct management of intracranial arachnoid cysts represents a difficult issue due to the lack of guidelines and to the many possible surgical options. Certain complications related to the treatment of intracranial arachnoid cysts are of iatrogenic nature and are due to overzealous surgical management based on wrong indications. Some arachnoid cysts merely represent a form of localized hydrocephalus associated with a certain degree of focal atrophy.

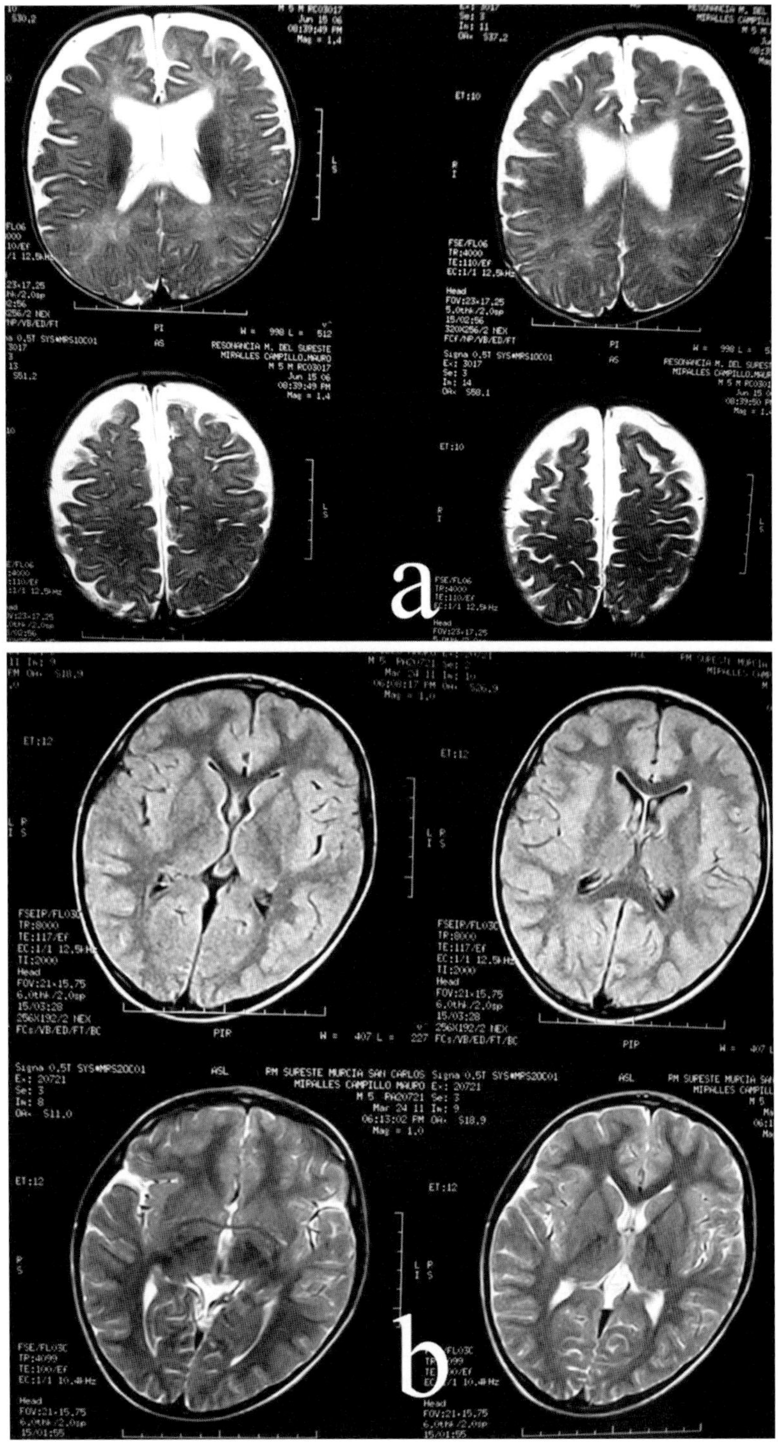

Fig. 5.1 (**a**) MRI showing benign external hydrocephalus in a 6-month-old boy. (**b**) Spontaneous resolution of the pericerebral collection and ventriculomegaly at age 3 years

Indications for arachnoid cyst shunting must be established on *clinical criteria* as most diagnostic methods are unable to discriminate which cysts benefit from surgery [83]. Arachnoid pouches may produce clinical symptoms depending on the patient's age, cyst size, focal cerebral compression, and brain shifts apart from symptoms of raised ICP. An arachnoid cyst discovered on neuroimaging studies in an otherwise asymptomatic patient needs only periodic observation [83]. Options for arachnoid cyst treatment include endoscopic fenestration, cyst excision or fenestration by craniotomy, and cyst shunting. Until recently, the preferred method of treatment was cystoperitoneal shunting, a procedure that is fraught with a multitude of complications as happens with VP shunts. Current trends favor the use of neuroendoscopic or open surgical fenestration for obviating shunt-related complications. In a recent paper from our institution we insisted on two facts [84]. First, many arachnoid cysts merely constitute incidental discoveries and need only clinical observation. Second, undue shunt placement usually leads to iatrogenic overdrainage manifestations such as orthostatic headaches in the short term, and to more serious complications such as shunt dependency, slit- ventricle syndrome, pseudotumor syndrome, posterior fossa overcrowding, or even to tonsillar herniation (acquired Chiari malformation) in the long term [7, 17, 50, 76, 83].

5.3 Iatrogenesis in Diagnostic Procedures

5.3.1 Reservoir Pumping

The neurosurgeon often assesses shunt patency by pumping the valve reservoir. This method is of limited utility but it can give an estimate of valve functioning in the appropriate clinical setting [106]. A reservoir that does not refill after a few flushing maneuvers probably indicates ventricular catheter block, but a slow replenishment of the flushing device may also indicate low ICP, partial catheter block, or ventricular collapse. The diagnosis of shunt block is more dependable if the reservoir remains umbilicated. On the contrary, a reservoir that is felt hard upon pumping represents valve or distal catheter block. Parents should be discouraged from pumping the valve as repeated flushing of the reservoir may precipitate an iatrogenic shunt block [13].

5.3.2 Shunt Tap

Puncture of the valve reservoir is also performed to test shunt function and to obtain CSF for biochemical and bacteriological examination [91, 96, 117, 129]. The technique includes meticulous skin preparation and disinfection and the use of a thin 23G or 25G needle (often a butterfly system) that can be connected to a manometer [96]. In normal conditions, the recorded pressure must be equal or slightly higher than the opening pressure of the valve and fluid must drip spontaneously. Slight aspiration with a small syringe can be applied if there is scanty spontaneous CSF flow. When no fluid comes out with these maneuvers, there likely exists a proximal obstruction. A higher recorded pressure than that of the opening pressure of the valve indicates distal obstruction. Equivocal readings may occur in the presence of a shunt block later demonstrated at surgery [150]. The technique is quite safe but it may cause several iatrogenic complications: (a) shunt infection; (b) breakage of the reservoir; and (c) superficial or cerebral hemorrhage when aspiration is applied [91].

5.3.3 ICP Measurement

Several methods are usually employed to assess ICP before first shunt implantation and also for evaluation of presumed shunt failure [35, 49, 122, 155]. Lumbar puncture manometry has significant inaccuracies. Continuous pressure recording via the valve reservoir is difficult to be maintained for a significant time and is almost impossible to perform in small children due to poor collaboration. Transfontanelar ICP recording represents a safe noninvasive method that provides useful information on ICP in patients with doubtful signs of progressive hydrocephalus or of shunt malfunction [49]. Intraventricular pressure recording has long been considered as the gold standard for ICP measurements but its use is limited due to: (a) the possibility of infection, (b) limited length of utilization, and (c) the difficulties for cannulating a compressed ventricle.

Subdural monitoring is another method for ICP recording but has not gained widespread acceptance. Epidural sensors give less exact readings than those of intraventricular devices and present measurement drifts over time. However, in daily practice, epidural monitoring represents a good method for ICP recording. Epidural sensors can be kept in place for a prolonged period and possess less risks due to the barrier that the dura mater offers against infection. The most frequently used monitoring systems at present are the intraparenchymal sensors. Their use in hydrocephalus has two main indications: hydrocephalus of chronic evolution and suspicion of gradual shunt failure. This method constitutes a minimally invasive procedure, although it may be fraught by brain damage, hemorrhage, or infection [155].

5.3.4 Iatrogenesis Related to Neuroimaging Studies

Three main aspects of neuroimaging studies deserve consideration: (a) the risk of misinterpretation of the tests [48, 59]; (b) the dangers associated with the repeated use of ionizing radiation, especially in children; and (c) the diagnostic yield of the study. At present, physicians other than neurosurgeons are often called on to evaluate complex cases of suspected shunt malfunction and they rely on neuroimaging reports that do not mention or diagnose shunt malfunction [59]. Of reported methods currently utilized for checking shunt function, *ultrasonography* doubtless constitutes the most innocuous one. US studies are dependable, cheap, noninvasive, can be repeated as needed, can be performed at the bedside and require no sedation. Drawbacks of US include the lack of definition of the convexities and the posterior fossa, and its impracticability in children with a closed skull.

The so-called *shunt series* are often performed as a routine procedure at emergency departments in suspected shunt failure. X-ray studies are necessary for assessment of shunt integrity, for example, when breakage or disconnection is suspected and for depicting the catheter position. Generally speaking, the diagnostic yield of the shunt series is low [31, 143]. Shunt tube integrity in children and thin individuals can also be explored by simple palpation of the subcutaneous trajectory of the shunt from its cranial to its abdominal ends. As many shunted patients ("difficult shunt patients") repeatedly attend the emergency services, shunt series should be performed only when this study is strictly necessary and never for defensive medicine [31, 143, 141].

CT and MRI are more dependable than shunt series in the evaluation of shunt malfunction (Fig. 5.2) [71]. *CT head scan* constitutes the *gold standard* for emergency assessment of shunt malfunction. CT scans are also requested very often, accounting for a cumulative exposure to ionizing radiation. CT scanning usually takes a short time; in most cases it does not require sedation or general anesthesia; and CT machines are usually available 24 h a day. In addition, some radiology departments use a rapid-sequence, low-dose CT scanning technique that does not reduce image quality [93, 141]. Plain radiographs and CT scanning have low sensitivity for identifying shunt failure, indicating that neurosurgical consultation should be sought in cases of suspected shunt failure [59, 85].

The best method for imaging the cerebral ventricles is *MRI*, but this technique is not always accessible in many hospitals during the whole day, and it requires sedation or even anesthesia in children and in uncooperative patients. Data acquisition involves a longer time, which makes it impractical in the emergency setting. A rapid-sequence MRI protocol for evaluation of hydrocephalus in children has also been developed [8].

To determine shunt patency, a *shuntogram* can be obtained by injecting a contrast medium (or an isotope) in the valve reservoir obtaining skull and abdominal images. Isotopic shuntogram is now rarely used with the same indication and is of no use in emergent situations.

5.3.5 Miscellaneous Tests

Biomarkers of infection such as C-reactive protein and routine blood analyses are of utmost

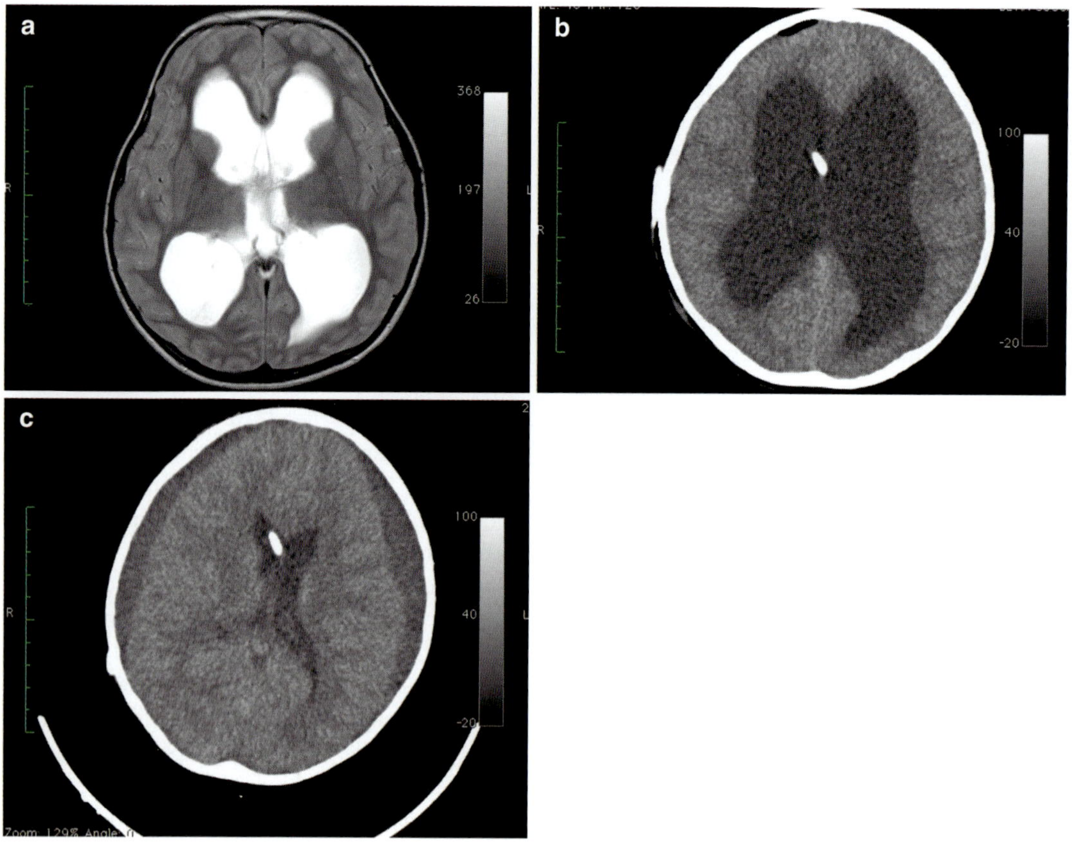

Fig. 5.2 MR (**a**) and serial CT (**b**, **c**) scans depicting the development of subdural hygroma in a 52-year-old female patient having undergone ventriculoperitoneal shunting due to hydrocephalus (Courtesy of Recep Brohi MD, Ankara, Turkey)

value for the diagnosis of shunt infection, although the most reliable test in suspected infection is culture of CSF obtained from the valve reservoir. Several other tests are also utilized for establishing the diagnosis, for indicating surgical treatment, and for assessing shunt function, for example, EEG, evoked potentials, and so on. Most of them are noninvasive and lack significant complications, but they are impractical in the acute setting although useful in the evaluation of chronic failure.

5.4 Technical Problems

Many technical problems related to shunt treatment derive from the lack of established criteria for selecting the most appropriate treatment as are (a) choosing between ETV or shunting, (b) deciding the technique for shunt insertion, and (c) choosing the type of valve. If iatrogenic complications are to be avoided, the philosophy underlying shunt insertion must no more be considered as a sophisticated "plumbing work." Cerebral pulsatility, bulk CSF volume flow, and hydrodynamic properties of the whole craniospinal axis have also to be taken into account in the design and performance of novel devices and in the search of new biomaterials. Table 5.1 summarizes the steps for shunt surgery.

5.4.1 Preparations for Surgery

In this section, a standard VP shunt insertion is described (especially as performed in our

Table 5.1 Steps for shunt surgery

Summary of steps for shunt surgery	
1	Surgery is necessary
2	Better treatment not indicated
3	Shunt placement is not contraindicated
4	General and skin conditions are adequate
5	Choose the type of surgery/ shunting
6	Careful planning
7	Meticulous surgical technique

Table 5.2 Common iatrogenic causes of VP shunt failures

Part of shunt insertion	Complication/cause
Ventricular catheter	Wrong length
	Malposition of catheter tip
	Ventricular migration
	Bleeding at catheter replacement
Reservoir	Inadequate contour/size
Valve	Inadequate valve
Subcutaneous tunneling	Skin breakdown from superficial passage
	Intrathoracic penetration
	Liver, gallbladder, lung penetration
	Lung apex perforation
Abdominal catheter	Preperitoneal placement
	Viscus perforation
	Vascular perforation
	Urinary bladder perforation
Connections	Disconnections: avoid connectors in growing patients

institution). The shunt we currently use consists of: (a) ventricular catheter, (b) a burr-hole-type reservoir, and (c) a programmable (Sophysa-Polaris®) valve with a unitized peritoneal catheter. Table 5.2 gives an account of common iatrogenic failures in VP shunting.

(a) The patients must be in their best general status. Infections, sepsis, and coagulation disorders should have been previously corrected. Prior medications are usually continued. Preoperative anesthetic assessment is highly desirable. In premature newborns, temporary measures to delay surgery till they achieve a satisfactory weight are also advisable (in our institution this limit is 1,300 g). If necessary, a latex-free operating room and latex-free accessory materials are prepared.

(b) The medical records (including the signed informed consent form) and the neuroimaging studies are taken to the operating room with the patient.

(c) The necessary equipment (including two sets of valves) must also be ready. Pressure settings of programmable valves are adjusted beforehand while the valve is still in the sterile package.

(d) Prophylactic antibiotics are given preoperatively and repeated at 8–12 h intervals for 1 or 2 days.

(e) The hair is washed with an antiseptic shampoo. Hair shaving is performed immediately before surgery to avoid contamination of small scalp erosions [12].

5.4.2 Patient Position, Local Anesthetics, and Skin Preparation

5.4.2.1 Position

The patient is usually positioned supine, the head rotated to the side opposite to that of the planned skin incision, placing the head, neck, thorax, and abdomen in a flat horizontal plane to facilitate the passage of the tunneling device.

5.4.2.2 Skin

The skin is disinfected with an iodine solution (or clorhexidine if the patient is allergic to iodine) applied for 10 min and dried with sterile towels. Surgical drapes are placed around the planned surgical field and covered with adhesive plastic transparent films. Importantly, in shunt revisions, all the skin overlying the shunt trajectory is prepared as described to have the opportunity of revising both proximal and distal ends of the shunt.

5.4.2.3 Local Anesthetic

A local anesthetic is injected in the planned surgical incision for analgesia, prevention of bleeding, and for separation of the skin layers.

5.4.3 Skin Incision, Burr Hole, and Dural Opening

5.4.3.1 Skin Incisions

The cranial incision is usually made curved or as a small skin flap. Lineal incisions are not recommended as they would contact with the shunt hardware in case of wound infection. Incisions should not be performed in the proximity of tracheostomy or gastrostomy wounds. Dissection of the galea aponeurotica and the pericranium are of great importance, especially in infants, to achieve a watertight closure at the end of the operation.

5.4.3.2 Burr Hole

A burr hole of sufficient size, placed on the desired point of catheter insertion (frontal, posterior parietal, or occipital), is performed. At present, there is no scientific evidence on the superiority between frontal and posterior catheter placements [3, 14]. When a burr-hole-type reservoir is used, the bone opening must be large enough to accommodate it, avoiding a too large orifice that would favor the intracranial migration of the reservoir (or valve).

5.4.3.3 Dural Opening

The dura mater and brain are coagulated with monopolar cautery to make an opening of the same size as the proximal catheter. A too large dural orifice will facilitate the escape of fluid around the tube. At the same time, any dural or cortical bleeding points are coagulated.

5.4.4 Ventricular Catheter Insertion-Related Pitfalls

5.4.4.1 Choice of the Ventricular Catheter

Ventricular catheter length is calculated from preoperative CT or MRI scans. The catheter tip is placed in front of the foramen of Monro to avoid the choroid plexus [3]. Placement is not problematic in patients with large ventricles but in instances with smaller ventricles, US, stereotaxy, or navigation may be used [157].

5.4.4.2 Ventricular Cannulation

The catheter with its stylet is then gently introduced. Entry within the ventricle is felt by the surgeon's hands and confirmed by the spontaneous flow of CSF. A sample of CSF is sent for analysis and bacteriological study. Excessive escape of CSF is avoided to prevent pneumocephalus and early overdrainage. The ventricular catheter can be irrigated or replaced if fluid does not flow properly. Proximal shunt block is the most frequent cause of shunt malfunction; accordingly, emphasis must be placed in confirming a good flow of CSF. Several ventricular catheter models with different holes and diameters have been designed for avoiding (or retarding) obstruction [43]. Nonstraight catheters, and those with flanged tips, are not recommended because they do not prevent blockage and, on the contrary, they increase the risk for hemorrhage during revision surgery. During reoperations, the ventricular catheter is placed without the stylet using the previous tract.

5.4.4.3 Misplacement of Ventricular Catheters

The ventricular catheter tip may be involuntarily positioned within the ventricular wall, embedded in the brain parenchyma, within the septum, in the temporal horn, or even in the cisterns (Fig. 5.3). Planning of the length and trajectory prevents this complication. Catheter impaction within the brain parenchyma usually results in its block. Treatment consists of shunt revision and catheter replacement. Sudden death has been reported by brain stem impaction of a fourth ventricle catheter [75].

5.4.4.4 Intracranial Migration and Retention of Ventricular Catheters

Proximal catheters may disconnect from the attached reservoir (or valve) due to a too-loose ligature, use of absorbable sutures ties, or by suction into the ventricle during catheter replacement. BioGlide proximal catheters seem to be more prone to disconnections making retrieval difficult or impossible [20]. One-piece shunts

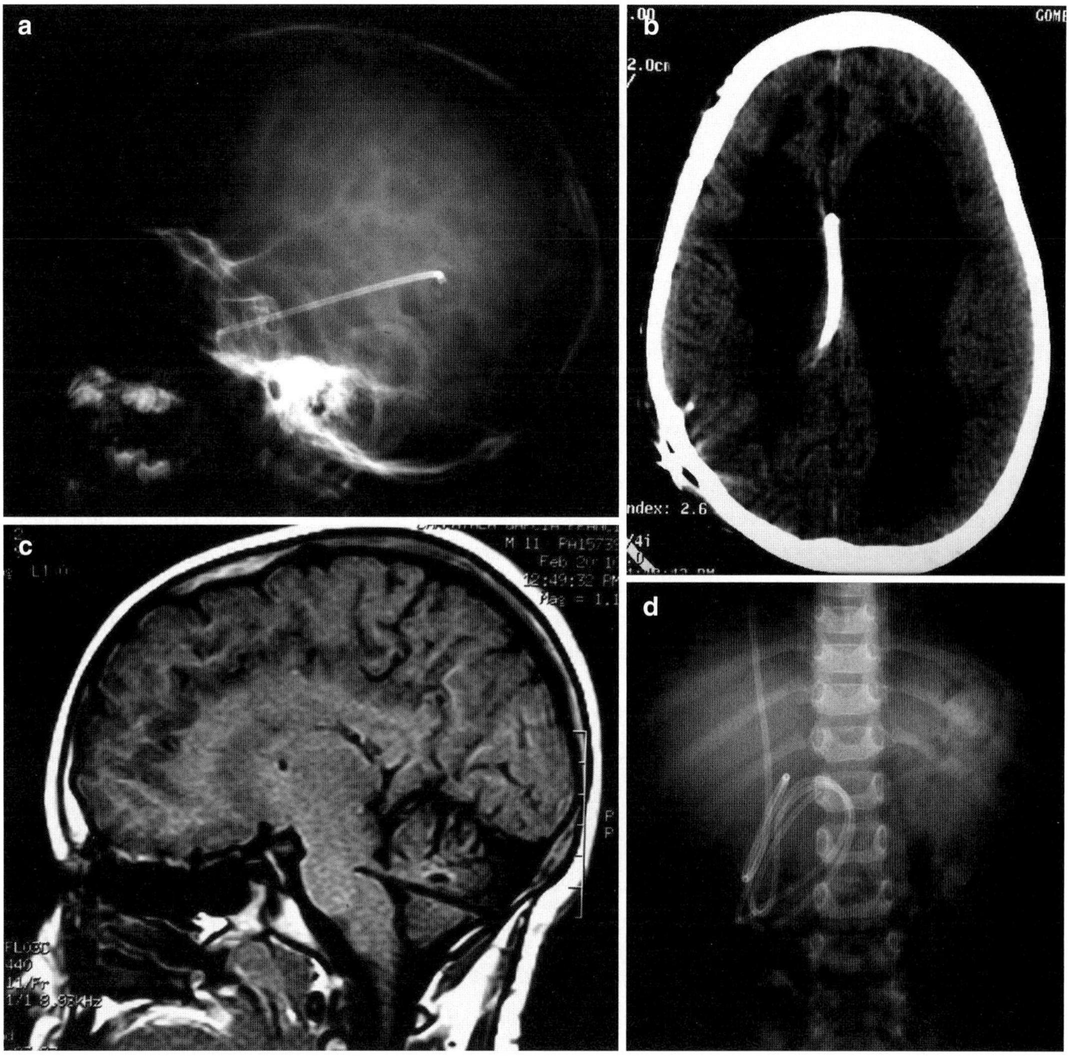

Fig. 5.3 Examples of iatrogenic malposition: (**a**) skull radiograph of a tightly adhered ventricular catheter that was initially placed in the temporal horn; (**b**) CT in shunt malfunction due to a misplaced proximal catheter within the septum; (**c**) MRI showing impaction of fourth ventricular catheter in the brain stem, (**d**) radiograph showing a peritoneal catheter placed in the preperitoneal space

have also been reported to migrate within the ventricles due to their uniform diameter and to a faulty fixation to the pericranium. In the same manner, catheters may also be pulled out of the skull during the patients' growth.

5.4.4.5 Intraventricular Hemorrhage in Shunt Revision

Problematic intraventricular hemorrhage happens more often in proximal catheter revision than in new insertions [67]. The reported incidence of ventricular hemorrhage during shunt revisions is approximately 30 % [14]. On removing the catheter, it will often come out easily, but not infrequently it is firmly attached to the choroid plexus, septum, or ventricular wall. Attempts at removal have to be made with great care. If the catheter still continues to be adhered, it is better to leave it in situ. Forceful maneuvers for removing the proximal catheter often are the cause of iatrogenic hemorrhages. Proposed maneuvers for safe catheter removal include gentle traction, delicate rotation of the tube, irrigation with saline, and intraluminal coagulation with the stylet or with a flexible neuroendoscopy electrode, or laser coagulation through a separate burr hole [14, 80, 130]. Unfortunately, none of these methods completely avoids bleeding. Intraventricular urokinase has been used for reducing the duration of the external drainage and to prevent a new catheter block [83]. Delayed hemorrhage from an iatrogenic aneurysm has been documented after removal of a long-standing VP shunt [62, 139].

5.4.4.6 Intraparenchymal Hemorrhage

Intracerebral bleeding from ventricular catheter insertion is quite rare, but some asymptomatic instances may escape detection if CT scans are not routinely performed after shunt placement or revision [89]. The origin of these hemorrhages may be at the cortical vessels (arteries or veins) or along the proximal catheter tract. Bleeding is more frequent in older patients and in individuals with cerebrovascular conditions, brain edema, unrecognized coagulopathies, and bleeding disorders. They may also occur after repeated maneuvers for ventricular cannulation. Intracerebral bleeding may happen early after shunt placement or in a delayed form. Many of these hemorrhages may give no clinical manifestations and require no surgery. However, instances with neurological involvement may necessitate revision for hemostasis or even craniotomy. Prevention consists of careful coagulation of dural and cortical vessels and of avoiding multiple attempts for ventricular cannulation. Hemorrhages may also occur at sites distant from the ventricular catheter (extradural or subdural spaces) and are usually related to sudden CSF depletion (Fig. 5.4) [2, 109].

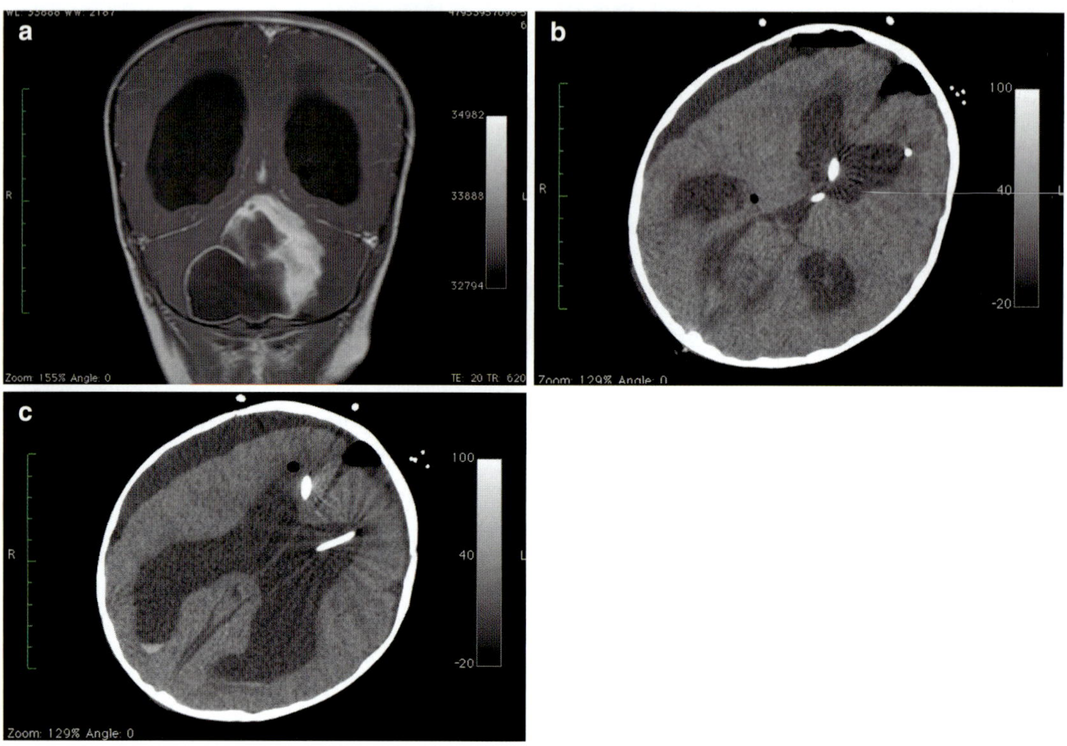

Fig. 5.4 (**a**) Preoperative cranial CT scan of a 15-month-old boy who was operated because of a tumoral lesion in the posterior fossa with the histopathological diagnosis of grade 2 pilomyxoid astrocytoma. (**b**, **c**) CT scans showing the development of subdural hematoma in the same patient having undergone ventriculoperitoneal shunting because of a persistent hydrocephalus due to a malfunctioning ventriculocisternal (Torkildsen's) shunt (Courtesy of Recep Brohi MD, Ankara, Turkey)

5.4.5 Peritoneal Access

The habitual abdominal skin incision is a transverse paraumbilical one. Skin incision should be away from gastrostomy or colostomy wounds. The peritoneum can be entered by one of the following three methods:

5.4.5.1 Open Surgery

The open technique we routinely perform is a mini-laparotomy. After skin incision, the subcutaneous layer is dissected, the fascia is opened horizontally, and the muscles split vertically to expose the peritoneum. This layer is pulled up, away from the bowel, with straight mosquito forceps, and opened with dural scissors. In this way, the neurosurgeon can inspect under direct vision the intestinal loops and prevent the inadvertent placement of the distal catheter in the preperitoneal space (one of the most common preventable causes of iatrogenic shunt failure at the abdominal end). A thin brain spatula may be used for introducing the distal tube within the peritoneum.

5.4.5.2 Trocar Insertion

A trocar may also be utilized to access the peritoneum. Although extremely rare, the aorta and the iliac arteries [29], the cava, the bladder, the stomach, or the bowel can be perforated accidentally by the trocar, a method that we have abandoned after having experienced some unfortunate accidents. The risk of perforation is higher in infants and undernourished patients and in those who have peritoneal adhesions from previous abdominal surgeries. Before trocar insertion, it is mandatory to empty the bladder (especially in spina bifida patients) and to stop muscle relaxants. In our view, trocar use does not offer substantial advantages and, on the contrary, it may cause extremely severe injuries. The collaboration of a general surgeon should be sought when technical abdominal problems are anticipated. Bowel perforation occurring *early* after shunt surgery is undoubtedly an iatrogenic complication. *Late* bowel perforation is unrelated to the technique. It was earlier reported with the use of spring-reinforced shunts [105, 126]. Intestinal perforation can give rise to severe complications caused by Gram negative or anaerobic organisms, for instance peritonitis, ventriculitis, septic pneumocephalus, and brain abscess [105, 126].

5.4.5.3 Endoscopic Laparoscopy

This technique is increasingly being used for new shunt insertions and for revisions. Indications include prior abdominal surgery, obesity, previous peritoneal infections, retained fragments of broken devices, and pseudocysts [77]. However, it has the inconvenience of requiring the collaboration of an endoscopic surgeon with the appropriate equipment. Laparoscopic surgery is not devoid of risks of visceral or vascular perforation [29].

Intraperitoneal parts of broken or disconnected distal catheters can be retrieved both by open surgery and by laparoscopy. Nevertheless, retained abdominal catheters that cannot be removed during shunt revision can be safely left within the peritoneal cavity, as they produce no harm. Detailed accounts of shunt-related abdominal complications have been published [30, 46] and will be also discussed in another chapter of this book.

5.4.6 Tunneling and Subcutaneous Passage of the Distal Catheter

Placing the patient in a flat position is essential for making shunt passage easier. The shunt-passer can be introduced from scalp to abdominal incision or in the opposite way (the one we prefer). Saline can be injected in the subcutaneous tissue of the planned shunt course to facilitate the tunneller passage especially in infants and children. Then, the shunt-passer is advanced carefully, controlling the displacement of its tip under the subcutaneous trajectory by digital palpation.

Three sites call for special attention during tunneling [123], the passage above the lower ribs (to not damage the liver, gallbladder, or lungs), the pleural apex (to not produce a pneumothorax), and the junction of the cranial and cervical aponeurosis to avoid intracranial penetration in children with open sutures [108, 135]. During tunneling, passing beneath the breast in female patients is avoided to prevent late complications should breast surgery be performed as mastectomy, breast implants, etc. [121]. Care should also be taken to not perforate the thin skin of infants all along the passage of the tunneling device. Most shunt-passers are malleable and permit molding to adapt best to the patient's anatomy. In adults, one or more intermediate skin incisions may be required for passing the shunt.

In shunt revisions, the previous tract can be used to pass subcutaneously the new catheter by suturing with a 4/0 silk suture, the end of the new tube to the end of the catheter that is being removed and pulling from it slowly. This maneuver is usually successful in cases of malfunctions occurring early after initial shunt placement and in patients with spring-reinforced shunts, but not when the tubing has become hardened over time. The tubing may break into pieces at removal, making difficult the extraction of fragments that will have to be left in place to avoid multiple unsightly cutaneous incisions.

When the shunt has to be taken out of the abdomen because of peritoneal infection, the tube must be removed from the abdominal incision and not from the cranial one because pulling it out through the scalp incision would contaminate the whole subcutaneous tract of the shunt producing severe cellulitis.

Connectors should not be employed in children at the level of the chest or abdomen in cases of shunt rupture or disconnection because the tubing will become detached again. In this case, replacing the whole distal catheter at the cranial end seems to be preferable.

5.4.7 Rupture, Disconnection, and Migration

Innumerable adverse events related to biodegradation, rupture, disconnections, and migration with or without protrusion (or extrusion) of the distal catheter have been reported that are mainly unrelated to the surgical technique and that cannot be regarded as iatrogenic [10, 68]. These complications include hydrothorax, migration of the distal catheter into the chest [27, 135], bronchus, heart [64], subscalp coiling [53], retrograde subcutaneous migration [79], migration and/or extrusion in the subdural space, ventricles [125], stomach or bowel, bladder, vagina [103], scrotum [111], umbilicus [1], mouth [45], nose, anus, skin incisions [32, 154], etc. Most of them are noniatrogenic in nature and their appearance is unpredictable and, hence, unpreventable [10, 42, 68, 79]. Intraventricular migration has been reported with valveless and cylindrical or unitized shunts, which suggests the possible prevention by a tighter fixation of the tubes to the pericranium and by avoiding these types of shunts [53, 125].

5.4.8 Reservoirs, Valves, and Antisiphon Devices

5.4.8.1 Reservoirs

Most neurosurgeons consider essential using a reservoir for testing shunt patency and for CSF sampling [96, 106, 117, 129]. Reservoirs may be of burr-hole type or placed in-line with the valve. Fortunately, reservoirs and flushing devices cause few iatrogenic problems, skin necrosis and occlusion being the most frequent [78].

5.4.8.2 Valves

Most valves drain CSF when there is a gradient of pressure between the ventricles and the end of the distal catheter. There are basically two main types: differential pressure and flow-regulated valves. There are three basic models of standard valves: low, medium, and high pressure, which refer to their closing pressure. Flow-controlled valves as the Orbis Sigma I and II provide a more physiological drainage but due to their increased resistance to flow they may not work in NPH and in infants with open sutures. So-called programmable valves permit the transcutaneous adjustment of pressure settings by using a magnet. Closed-ended and distal slit valves are not recommended because they are more prone to distal obstruction [28]. Presently, new devices that include an antisiphon or an antigravitational mechanism are also employed. No notable differences have been reported to exist with the use of one of these shunting devices [37, 107, 140].

Table 5.3 Patient-specific treatments at our institution

Type of hydrocephalus	Procedure/valve
Standard size ventricles	Programmable or medium-pressure valve
Premature and newborn infants	Programmable set at low pressure, low-pressure valve, small-contoured valve
Large ventricles, chronic hydrocephalus, adult NPH	Programmable, flow-regulated (OS-II), gravity valve/antisiphon devices
Slitlike ventricles Overdrainage	Programmable flow-regulated gravity valve antisiphon devices
Obstructive hydrocephalus	Endoscopic third ventriculostomy
	CSF shunt
Multiloculated hydrocephalus, arachnoid cysts, trapped fourth ventricle	Neuroendoscopy DVP with one or two catheters connected in Y

The valve may be implanted on the burr hole or on the adjacent skull. In Table 5.3, we summarize the currently accepted indications for each type of surgery and valve according to the patient's characteristics and the etiology of hydrocephalus. Under- and overdrainage may occur in most types of shunts and will be dealt with in the corresponding chapters. For avoiding skin necrosis over the valve (or reservoir dome) one can: (a) place the burr hole away from the parietal zone; (b) make a subcutaneous pocket for the valve; (c) use low-profile devices and small reservoirs; (d) avoid laying the patient's head on the side of the valve; and (e) in premature and newborn children, choose a low-pressure or a programmable valve adjusted at low-pressure setting to facilitate CSF drainage that would counteract the tension produced by the reservoir on a distended scalp. These measures are especially advised for small babies and for debilitated patients.

Electing the most adequate shunt requires expertise and scientific knowledge. Nevertheless, we agree with the general recommendation of implanting the valve to which one is accustomed to and is more confident with.

5.4.8.3 Antisiphon Devices

Antisiphon devices may be added to most valves. Their main value consists of decreasing the siphoning effect of differential-pressure shunts. Antisiphon valves are not recommended in infants given that they lead to underdrainage. Some antisiphon models fail to function owing to the fibrosis that forms on the antisiphon mechanism.

5.4.8.4 In-Line Filters

In-line filters were formerly used for preventing tumor cell seeding through the shunt although they are now rarely utilized given that they become blocked easily.

5.4.9 Connection of the Shunt Parts, Closure, and Wound Dressing

The components of the shunt are assembled together with a 2/0 silk ligature (thinner threads cut the silastic tubes as do nylon sutures). Reabsorbable sutures are not advised as they give rise to disconnections. The ligature knots are placed facing the skull to avoid skin necrosis from knot pressure. The reservoir is then fixed to the pericranium with 4/0 silk sutures. Before closure, the correct functioning of the valve is checked by observing the drip of CSF through the distal tube after placing the distal catheter tip below the level of the patient's body, by pumping the reservoir, or by aspirating with a small syringe. Only then, the peritoneal catheter is introduced within the peritoneum and the abdominal and cranial incisions are closed in layers. The wound is again disinfected and a slightly compressive wound dressing is placed on the incisions.

5.5 "Friendly Fire" from Other Specialties

Ignoring the presence of a VP shunt may initiate diverse iatrogenic complications. Colleagues pertaining to other specialties must look at the patient's past history so as not to overlook the presence of the shunt. For example, unwary anesthetists when dealing with shunted patients may puncture the distal catheter during catheterization of the jugular vein [21]. Subcutaneous drug-delivery ports (Port-a-cath type) are best inserted on the side opposite to that of the valve. A lumbar puncture or spinal anesthesia in a shunted patient may also trigger a shunt malfunction [33]. Some general surgeons fail to note the presence of the shunt and may inadvertently cut the tube on performing abdominal operations. For instance, we have seen shunt damage during a hiatus hernia repair, a cholecystectomy, and an appendicitis operation; and also the inadvertent opening of the stomach during a VP shunt revision due to confusion of the viscus wall with peritoneal adhesions. Laparoscopic procedures in the presence of VP shunt are reported to be safe [77]. A case of pneumocephalus has been documented in this context [113]. In addition, the induced pneumoperitoneum can increase the intraabdominal pressure and hinder CSF drainage through the peritoneal catheter [142].

The possibility of a nonshunt-related cause of symptoms in hydrocephalic children, for example, abdominal pain due to appendicitis, must also be taken into account. In the presence of appendicitis (or other clean-contaminated abdominal surgeries), a prudent attitude is to leave the distal catheter in place, but when there is peritoneal infection it is advisable to externalize the shunt [38, 72, 110]. Although infrequently, percutaneous and laparoscopic gastrostomy procedures may also interfere with VP shunt function [9]. Peritoneal dialysis may also produce peritonitis but contamination of the CSF shunt is exceptional in this context [47]. Shunt perforation can also be produced by neurosurgeons during skull fixation with head-holder pins. All the aforementioned iatrogenic complications do occur very rarely but close collaboration of the neurosurgeon with these specialists seems to be highly advisable.

5.6 Iatrogenesis in Diverse Indications and Distal Draining Locations

Complications related to the diverse distal places for CSF drainage will be discussed extensively in the diverse chapters of this book. Table 5.4 summarizes some current iatrogenic complications in shunts other than VP shunts.

Table 5.4 Common iatrogenic complications in non-VP shunts

Type of drainage system	Complication/causes
Ventriculoatrial	Inappropriate length of atrial catheter
	Delay in recognizing complications
	Forceful atrial catheter insertion
	Forceful atrial catheter removal
Ventriculopleural	Lung puncture
	Pneumothorax
Lumboperitoneal	Valveless shunts
	Failure in recognizing complications
	Overdrainage (tonsillar descent, etc.)
Ventriculogallbladder	Biliary tract infection
Ventriculoureteral	Hypertonic bladder
	Urinary infection
Subduroperitoneal	Wrong diagnosis/indication
	Malposition
	Cortical damage at shunt removal
Cystoperitoneal shunt (in arachnoid cysts)	Wrong indication
	Use of valveless shunts
Loculated hydrocephalus	Wrong position
Posterior fossa drainages	Use of multiple shunts

5.6.1 Ventriculoatrial Shunting

At present, ventriculoatrial (VA) valves are implanted in many centers as a second-line shunting procedure. Cor pulmonale, chronic pulmonary thromboembolism, pericardial tamponade, shunt nephritis, inferior vena cava and hepatic vein thrombosis, septicemia, bronchopulmonary fistula, pleural effusion, and catheter malposition and shortening have been reported after VA shunt implantation [39, 74, 161]. The main drawbacks of VA shunting depend on the need for prophylactic lengthening, the higher severity of complications, and its higher mortality rate. Malposition of the atrial catheter is an iatrogenic complication that can be obviated by using anatomical surface marks, intraoperative radiograph, ECG, or echocardiography when inserting the shunt. Vascular and cardiac rupture is a preventable complication that may be obviated by avoiding forceful insertion and strong pulling of the atrial catheter at shunt revision [40, 137].

5.6.2 Ventriculopleural Shunting

Ventriculopleural (VPL) shunting has not gained widespread acceptance owing to feared thoracic complications as hydrothorax, tension pneumothorax, fibrothorax, pleural empyema, and tumor seeding to the pleura through the shunt. At our institution, VPL shunting constitutes the second-line procedure for CSF derivation even in children [136]. Pleural insertion of the distal tube can be performed by open surgery or by endoscopy. Iatrogenic complications of VPL shunting include lung puncture and pneumothorax, which need to be appropriately prevented and managed. Hydrothoraces can be treated, at least temporarily, with diamox and repeated pleural punctures.

5.6.3 Lumboperitoneal Shunting

Lumboperitoneal (LP) shunting is used in communicating hydrocephalus, idiopathic intracranial hypertension, NPH, pseudomeningocele, and CSF leaks. LP shunts can be placed in patients with collapsed ventricles. These shunts obviate a transcerebral access, thus preventing brain injury and hemorrhage. They also decrease infection and epilepsy rates. The main drawbacks of LP shunting consist of the difficulties for checking its patency. In addition, this type of shunt does not avoid overdrainage. Complications related with its use comprise back pain, sciatica, scoliosis, posterior fossa crowding, acquired Chiari malformation, syringomyelia, and even death [23, 24, 152, 149]. Most complications occur after placement of percutaneous valveless LP shunts, but they are infrequent with "T" type shunts and other valved LP systems. Treatment of these complications consists of LP shunt conversion to a VP shunt and of foramen magnum decompression for cases with posterior fossa crowding, acquired Chiari, and syringomyelia [23, 24, 148].

5.6.4 Ventriculogallbladder Shunting

Ventriculogallbladder shunt is rarely utilized today although its reported complication rate is similar to that of other shunts [44, 132]. Ventriculogallbladder shunt is usually performed after failure of VP, VA, and VPL shunting, and is contraindicated in biliary tract diseases. Specific complications include gallbladder atony and gallstones. There was a reported fatality with this type of shunt due to bile reflux ventriculitis [44, 132].

5.6.5 Ventriculoureteral Shunting

This type of CSF derivation is presently practically abandoned. Complications specific to this technique include ascending urinary infection, shunt migration out of the ureter, distal migration into the bladder, and electrolyte imbalance due to volume depletion [58]. Complications may be prevented by avoiding placing this type of shunt especially in patients with a hypertonic bladder or with urinary infections [58].

5.6.6 Ventriculosubgaleal Shunting

Ventriculosubgaleal shunt placement is a temporary method for CSF derivation and is utilized in premature infants with hydrocephalus, shunt infections, tumors, etc. The large surface of the pericranial pocket permits collecting fluid from the ventricles (or subdural space), via a low-pressure valve, into the subgaleal pouch. Complications consist of obstruction, infection, fluid leaks, skin ulceration, intracranial bleeding from CSF hypotension, and skull deformation from pressure by the fluid collection [138]. Iatrogenic skin disruption and fluid leaks can be prevented by a watertight two-layered closure and treated by oversewing the skin even at the bedside.

5.6.7 Subduroperitoneal Shunting

Neurosurgical treatments of chronic subdural hematomas in children include transcutaneous taps, external drainage, subdurogaleal shunts and subduroperitoneal shunts [87]. A 26 % complication rate has been reported in subduroperitoneal shunts that comprise obstruction, migration, skin necrosis, infection, subdural empyema, bowel perforation, and ileus. Migration was seen with unitized-shunts and skin necrosis in children with reservoirs. Proximal tube adhesions to the dura or cortex at the time of shunt removal have also been reported. Migrations (upward or downward) can be prevented by tight fixation of the tube to the pericranium or by placing a reservoir. Proximal tube obstruction may even cause the patient's death [112]. Shunt removal must be performed as soon as the collection is no longer necessary to avoid iatrogenic cortical injury and also to prevent overshunting [81].

5.6.8 Arachnoid-Cyst Shunting

The availability of modern neuroimaging tools and concerns about the large size of some arachnoid cysts has led to overtreatment of patients who perhaps should have never been shunted [84]. Criteria for success of arachnoid-cyst shunting consist of achieving alleviation of the patient's symptoms and not of the total resolution of the cyst on imaging. We do not recommend placing valveless shunts as they cause severe manifestations of CSF hypotension and dangerous brain shifts. One of the main indications of programmable valves is precisely its use in arachnoid-cyst management that permits to adjust the shunt pressure to the patient's needs. In cases of arachnoid cyst associated with hydrocephalus, treatment with a combined cysto-VP shunt is preferable for avoiding dangerous intercompartment differences of pressure. Complications in arachnoid-cyst shunting comprise orthostatic headaches, CSF leaks from the cranial wound, and subdural hygromas and hematomas. However, the most severe complications in this type of shunting are those related to late effects of overshunting, as slit-ventricle syndrome, craniosynostosis, craniocerebral disproportion, posterior fossa overcrowding, and acquired tonsillar herniation [7, 17, 50, 76, 84].

5.6.9 Multiloculated Hydrocephalus and Fourth Ventricle Cysts

5.6.9.1 Multiloculated Hydrocephalus

Multiloculated hydrocephalus is a severe condition in which no single treatment has shown to be superior [162]. It may originate from congenital or from acquired conditions (infection, hemorrhage, and overdrainage). Symptoms and signs derive from gradients of pressure between the isolated compartments. The objectives of treatment are threefold and consist of improving the patient's symptoms, reducing the number of operations, and of decreasing surgical-related complications. Failure to achieve these goals may lead to innumerable shunt revisions, progressive deterioration, or even cause the patient's death. Placement of multiple catheters or multiple shunts [65] is to be avoided, as they will merely contribute to multiply the number of shunt failures. At present, one should consider communicating the isolated compartment with the ventricles by neuroendoscopic techniques such as septum pellucidum fenestration and communication of isolated cavities, with or without associated shunt placement [101, 162]. Microsurgical communication of supratentorial and infratentorial isolated ventricles has also been advocated, although these procedures carry a higher morbidity and mortality rate [4, 95, 120].

5.6.9.2 Posterior Fossa Cysts, Trapped Fourth Ventricle, and Dandy-Walker Cyst

Fourth-ventricular shunting is commonly used for treating symptomatic isolated fourth ventricle, posterior fossa cysts, and Dandy-Walker malformation [69]. Several iatrogenic complications have been reported with these shunts such as appearance of new cranial nerve deficits, intracystic hemorrhage, and impaction of the catheter into the brain stem [69, 75]. Placing the catheter in the brain stem is avoided by using a more lateral route for catheter insertion (Fig. 5.3c) [69, 75]. Some authors propound a microsurgical approach for communicating the fourth ventricle with the cisterns or using neuroendoscopic procedures in trapped fourth ventricle and in Dandy-Walker malformation [4, 92, 145]. Upward transtentorial herniation as an iatrogenic complication of supratentorial shunting in Dandy-Walker malformation has also been described [94]. For treatment of these cystic lesions we usually place a combined "Y" shunt with a single valve that communicates the supra- and infratentorial cavities, thus avoiding a gradient of pressure between compartments that often causes cranial nerve deficits. We also utilize a suboccipital craniotomy followed by a microsurgical approach in selected cases as a second-line treatment.

5.7 Programmable Valves

Externally adjustable valves are preferred by some neurosurgeons who argue that these devices (a) reduce costs by decreasing the number of shunt revisions, (b) may prevent overdrainage syndromes, and (c) contribute to programmed shunt removal [82, 133]. However, there is not a generalized opinion to support these views [51, 151]. Patients and their relatives have to be instructed on the need of checking the valve pressure setting (and eventually of readjustment) after performing an MRI study. Medical devices such as MRI machines, cochlear implants, transcranial magnetic stimulation, and vagus nerve stimulator are reported to interfere with the function of these valves [18, 61, 70]. Several magnetic objects such as cell phones, toy magnets, tablet computer, portable game machines, iPad2 and 3, television sets, other home appliances, and the Japanese magnetic suspension railway have all been reported to induce changes in the valve pressure adjustments [5, 90, 98, 124, 131]. Increasing concerns on the interaction of new technological devices when they are implanted in the same individual, especially in children, have been the subject of recent analyses [104, 124, 148]. In spite of these drawbacks, programmable shunts (which were formerly used in special cases of hydrocephalus in our institution) have become the standard shunt we use in the majority of CSF drainage procedures (Fig. 5.5). A new generation of MRI-stable valves (Polaris, Sophysa) have been developed that overcome problems related with accidental reprogramming of the valve pressure settings by magnets, by using a self-locking system [57, 73].

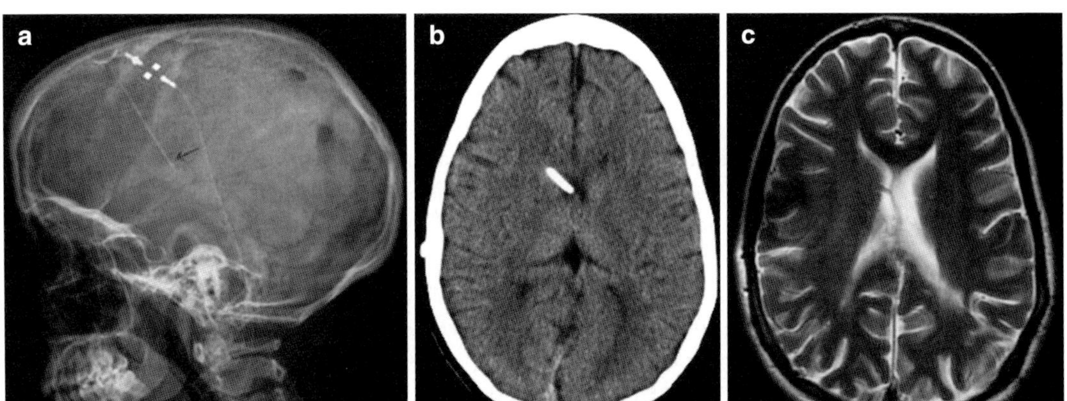

Fig. 5.5 Correction of mildly symptomatic slit ventricle by readjustment of an externally programmable valve: (**a**) radiograph showing a programmable valve adjusted at 150 mm H_2O; (**b**) CT scan corresponding to the same patient; (**c**) MRI showing slight increase in ventricular size following upgrading of the valve pressure setting

5.8 Shunt Infection

Issues corresponding to shunt infection are dealt with in a separate chapter. However, a few comments appear to be opportune regarding iatrogenic factors concerning shunt-related infection. First, knowledge of predictors of CSF shunt infection should be made available to physicians and emergency departments for avoiding delay in diagnosis and management of shunt infection [118]. Second, adopting protocols and guidelines for infection prevention and using a meticulous surgical technique seem to be crucial for avoiding shunt contamination [22, 144, 159]. Third, standardization and hospital-based infection control registries may help to recognize factors contributing to CSF shunt infection and to improve preventive measures [128, 159].

5.9 Follow-Up, Education, and Continuity of Care

Most shunt failures occur during the first year after shunt insertion and shunt infection mainly presents during the first 3 months after surgery. Accordingly, close follow-up visits are usually advised especially during the first year after initial valve placement. The evolution of ventricular changes after shunting in infants are best monitored by serial US. The convenience of obtaining a baseline CT scan is widely accepted. Initially, we perform a visit at 3 months after shunt insertion, then at 6 and 12 months, and then annually up to the age of 5 years. Subsequent visits are scheduled at 2-year intervals or more frequently as dictated by the patient's special needs. After the age of 18 years, follow-up visits are scheduled every 5 years. US and MRI studies to avoid radiation risks are gradually replacing ventricular size assessment by CT scans. In addition, we follow an "open door" policy and patients may be revised either at the emergency department or at the outpatient clinic according to the patients' perceived necessities.

Our service, which is the only one existing in our autonomous community, gathers the vast majority of shunted individuals, making follow-up easier. In the same way, shunted children and adults are followed-up by the same neurosurgical team, ensuring a satisfactory continuity of care. However, we noted that some patients fail to attend the scheduled follow-up visits during adolescence and adulthood and come back only when they present symptoms of suspected shunt dysfunction. Several authors have signaled that hydrocephalus is a chronic disease that needs continued medical surveillance, either by pediatricians and family doctors or by neurosurgeons, and have stressed the importance of educating patients (and their relatives) on the manifestations that indicate the suspicion of shunt malfunction [26, 52, 66, 127]. Preventive measures are also disseminated by lectures delivered to the spina bifida and hydrocephalus patients' associations and to pediatricians of our geographic region too. Some authors have stressed the negative consequences that may arise from failure in carrying out an adequate follow-up, which might result in severe neurological deterioration or even in death [16, 60].

Conclusions

The high incidence and severity of CSF shunt failure indicates the need of rapid detection and treatment. Many shunt failures are preventable. Analyses of their causative factors and improvements in shunt technology and materials will undoubtedly contribute to decreasing their occurrence and to diminishing their devastating consequences. Hydrocephalus is a chronic condition and, as such, it deserves improvement in promoting research and technological progress. Attention to transition and continuity of care also seem to be crucial for decreasing morbidity and mortality related to shunt placement and surgical revisions and for improving these patients' quality of life.

References

1. Adeloye A (1973) Spontaneous extrusion of the abdominal tube through the umbilicus complicating peritoneal shunt for hydrocephalus. J Neurosurg 38:758–759
2. Aguiar PH, Shu EBS, Freiras ABR et al (2000) Causes and treatment of intracranial haemorrhage

complicating shunting for pediatric hydrocephalus. Childs Nerv Syst 16:218–221
3. Albright LA, Haines SJJ, Taylor FH (1988) Function of parietal and frontal shunts in childhood hydrocephalus. J Neurosurg 69:883–886
4. Ambruster L, Kunz M, Ertl-Wagner B et al (2012) Microsurgical outlet restoration in isolated fourth ventricular hydrocephalus: a single-institutional experience. Childs Nerv Syst 28:2101–2107
5. Anderson RCE, Walker ML, Viner JM, Kestle JRW (2004) Adjustment and malfunction of a programmable valve after exposure of toy magnets. J Neurosurg 101(Suppl 2):222–225
6. Anderson H, Elfverson J, Svendsen P (1984) External hydrocephalus in infants. Childs Brain 11: 398–402
7. Aoki N, Sakai T, Umezawa Y (1990) Slit ventricle syndrome after cyst-peritoneal shunting for the treatment of intracranial arachnoid cysts. Childs Nerv Syst 6:41–43
8. Ashley WW Jr, McKinstry RC, Leonard JR et al (2005) Use of rapid-sequence magnetic resonance imaging for evaluation of hydrocephalus in children. J Neurosurg Pediatr 103(Suppl 2):124–130
9. Backman T, Berglund Y, Sjövie H, Arnbjörnsson E (2007) Complications in video-assisted gastrostomy in children with or without a ventriculoperitoneal shunt. Pediatr Surg Int 23:665–668
10. Boch AL, Hermelin E, Sainte-Rose C, Sgouros S (1998) Mechanical dysfunction of ventriculoperitoneal shunts caused by calcification of the silicone rubber catheter. J Neurosurg 88:975–982
11. Bravo C, Cano P, Conde R et al (2011) Posthemorrhagic hydrocephalus in the preterm infant: current evidence in diagnosis and treatment. Neurocirugia (Astur) 22:381–400
12. Broekman MLD, Van Beijnum J, Peul WC, Regli L (2011) Neurosurgery and shaving: what's the evidence? J Neurosurg 11:670–678
13. Bromby A, Czosnyka Z, Allin D et al (2007) Laboratory study on 'intracranial hypotension' created by pumping the chamber of the hydrocephalus shunt. Cerebrospinal Fluid Res 4:2
14. Brownlee RD, Dold ONR, Myles ST (1995) Intraventricular hemorrhage complicating ventricular catheter revision: incidence and effect on shunt survival. Pediatr Neurosurg 22:315–320
15. Burnett MG, Sonnad SS, Stein SC (2006) Screening tests for normal-pressure hydrocephalus; sensitivity, specificity and cost. J Neurosurg 105:823–829
16. Buxton N, Punt J (1998) Failure to follow patients with hydrocephalus shunts can lead to death. Br J Neurosurg 12:399–401
17. Caldarelli M, Novegno F, Di Rocco C (2009) A late complication of CSF shunting: acquired Chiari I malformation. Childs Nerv Syst 25:443–452
18. Chadwick KA, Moore J, Tye GW, Coelho H (2013) Management of patients with cochlear implants and ventriculoperitoneal shunts. Cochlear Implants Int 15:185–190
19. Chakraborty A, Crimmins D, Hayward R, Thompson D (2008) Toward reducing shunt placement rates in patients with myelomeningocele. J Neurosurg Pediatr 1:361–365
20. Chen HH, Riva-Cambrin J, Brockmeyer DL et al (2011) Shunt failure due to intracranial migration of BioGlide ventricular catheters. J Neurosurg Pediatr 7:408–412
21. Cho KH, Yoon SH, Kim SH et al (2004) Neck mass after catheterization of a neck vein in a child with a ventriculoperitoneal shunt. Pediatr Neurosurg 40:182–186
22. Choux M, Genitori L, Lang D, Lena G (1992) Shunt implantation: reducing the incidence of shunt infection. J Neurosurg 77:875–880
23. Chumas PD, Armstrong DC, Drake JM et al (1993) Tonsillar herniation: the rule more than the exception after lumboperitoneal shunting in the pediatric population. J Neurosurg 78:568–573
24. Chumas PD, Kulkarni AV, Drake JM et al (1993) Lumboperitoneal shunting: a retrospective study in the pediatric population. Neurosurgery 32:376–383
25. Clyde BL, Albright AL (1995) Evidence for a patent fibrous tract in fractured, outgrown, or disconnected ventriculoperitoneal shunts. Pediatr Neurosurg 23:20–25
26. Çolak A, Albright AL, Pollack IF (1997) Follow-up of children with shunted hydrocephalus. Pediatr Neurosurg 27:208–210
27. Cooper JR (1978) Migration of the ventriculoperitoneal shunt into the chest. Case report. J Neurosurg 48:146–147
28. Cozzens JW, Chandler JP (1997) Increased risk of distal ventriculoperitoneal shunt obstruction associated with slit valves or distal slits in the peritoneal catheter. J Neurosurg 87:682–686
29. Danan D, Winfree CJ, McKhann GM II (2008) Intra-abdominal vascular injury during trocar-assisted ventriculoperitoneal shunting: case report. Neurosurgery 63:E613
30. Davidson RI (1976) Peritoneal bypass in the treatment of hydrocephalus: historical review and abdominal complications. J Neurol Neurosurg Psychiatry 39:640–646
31. Desai KP, Babb JS, Amodio JB (2007) The utility of plain radiograph "shunt series" in the evaluation of suspected ventriculoperitoneal shunt failure in pediatric patients. Pediatr Radiol 37:452–456
32. DeSousa AL, Worth RM (1979) Extrusion of peritoneal catheters through abdominal incision: report of a rare complication of ventriculoperitoneal shunt. Neurosurgery 5:504–506
33. Dias MS, Li V, Pollina J (1999) Low-pressure shunt 'malfunction' following lumbar puncture in children with shunted obstructive hydrocephalus. Pediatr Neurosurg 30:146–150
34. Dias MS, Shaffer ML, Iantosca MR, Hill KL Jr (2011) Variability among pediatric neurosurgeons in the threshold for ventricular shunting in asymptomatic children with hydrocephalus. J Neurosurg Pediatr 7:134–142
35. Di Rocco C, McLone DG, Shimoji T, Raimondi AJ (1975) Continuous intraventricular cerebrospinal fluid

pressure recording in hydrocephalus children during wakefulness and sleep. J Neurosurg 42:683–689
36. Di Rocco C, Caldarelli M, Ceddia A (1989) 'Occult' hydrocephalus in children. Childs Nerv Syst 5:71–75
37. Drake JD (2008) The surgical management of pediatric hydrocephalus. Neurosurgery 62(SCH Suppl 2):SCH633–SCH642
38. Ein SH, Miller S, Rutka JT (2006) Appendicitis in the child with a ventriculo-peritoneal shunt: a 30-year experience. J Pediatr Surg 41:1255–1258
39. Forrest DM, Cooper DGW (1968) Complications of ventriculo-atrial shunts. A review of 455 cases. J Neurosurg 29:506–512
40. Foy PM, Shaw MD, Mercer JL (1980) Shunt catheter impacted in the vena cava. Case report. J Neurosurg 52:109–110
41. Fried A, Shapiro K (1986) Subtle deterioration in shunted childhood hydrocephalus. A biomechanical and clinical profile. J Neurosurg 65:211–216
42. Fukamachi A, Wada H, Toyoda O et al (1982) Migration or extrusion of shun catheters. Acta Neurochir (Wien) 64:159–166
43. Galarza M, Gimenez A, Valero J et al (2014) Computational fluid dynamics of ventricular catheters used for the treatment of hydrocephalus: a 3D analysis. Childs Nerv Syst 30:105–116
44. Girotti ME, Singh RR, Rodgers BM (2009) The ventriculo-gallbladder shunt in he treatment of refractory hydrocephalus: a review of the current literature. Am Surg 75:734–737
45. Griffith JA, De Feo D (1987) Peroral extrusion of a ventriculoperitoneal shunt catheter. Neurosurgery 21:259–261
46. Grosfeld JL, Cooney DR, Smith J et al (1976) Intraabdominal complications following ventriculoperitoneal shunt procedures. Pediatrics 54:791–796
47. Grunberg J, Rebori A, Verocay MC (2003) Peritoneal dialysis in children with spina bifida and ventriculoperitoneal shunt: one center's experience and review of the literature. Perit Dial Int 23:481–486
48. Guimaraes CVA, Leach JL, Jones BV (2011) Trainee misinterpretations on pediatric neuroimaging studies: classification, imaging analysis, and outcome assessment. AJNR Am J Neuroradiol 32: 1591–1599
49. Hanlo PW, Gooskens RHJM, Faber JAI et al (1996) Relationship between anterior fontanelle pressure measurements and clinical signs in infantile hydrocephalus. Childs Nerv Syst 12:200–209
50. Hassounah MI, Rahm BE (1994) Hindbrain herniation: an unusual occurrence after shunting of intracranial arachnoid cyst. J Neurosurg 81:126–129
51. Hatlen TH, Schurtleff DB, Loeser JD et al (2012) Nonprogrammable and programmable cerebrospinal fluid shunt valves: a 5-year study. J Neurosurg Pediatr 9:462–467
52. Hayward RD (2004) What should we be doing for the 'teenage shunt'. Acta Neurochir (Wien) 146:1175–1176
53. Heim RC, Kaufman BA, Park TS (1994) Complete migration of peritoneal shunt tubing to the scalp. Childs Nerv Syst 10:399–400
54. Hellbrusch LC (2007) Benign extracerebral fluid collections in infancy: clinical presentation and long-term follow-up. J Neurosurg Pediatr 107(Suppl 2):119–125
55. Huh PW, Yoo DS, Cho KS et al (2006) Diagnostic method for differentiating external hydrocephalus from simple subdural hygroma. J Neurosurg 105:65–70
56. Ianelli A, Rea G, Di Rocco C (2005) CSF shunt removal in children with hydrocephalus. Acta Neurochir (Wien) 147:503–507
57. Inoue T, Kuzu Y, Ogasawara K, Ogawa A (2005) Effect of 3-tesla magnetic resonance imaging on various pressure programmable shunt valves. J Neurosurg 103(Suppl 2):163–165
58. Irby PB 3rd, Wolf JS Jr, Schaeffer CS, Stoller ML (1993) Long-term follow-up of ventriculoureteral shunts for treatment of hydrocephalus. Urology 42:193–197
59. Iskandar BJ, McLaughlin C, Mapstone TB et al (1998) Pitfalls in the diagnosis of ventricular shunt dysfunction: radiology reports and ventricular size. Pediatrics 101:1031–1036
60. Iskandar BJ, Tubbs RS, Mapstone TB et al (1998) Death in shunted hydrocephalic children in the 1990s. Pediatr Neurosurg 28:173–176
61. Jandial R, Aryan H, Hughes S, Levy ML (2004) Effect of vagus nerve stimulator magnet on programmable shunt settings. Neurosurgery 55:627–630
62. Jenkinson MD, Basu S, Broome JC et al (2006) Traumatic cerebral aneurysm formation following ventriculoperitoneal shunt insertion. Childs Nerv Syst 22:193–196
63. Jernigan SC, Berry JG, Graham DA, Goumnerova L (2014) The comparative effectiveness of ventricular shunt placement versus endoscopic third ventriculostomy for initial treatment of hydrocephalus in infants. J Neurosurg Pediatr 13:295–300
64. Kang JK, Jeun SS, Chung DS et al (1996) Unusual proximal migration of ventriculoperitoneal shunt into the heart. Childs Nerv Syst 12:176–179
65. Kaiser G (1986) The value of multiple shunt systems in the treatment of nontumoral infantile hydrocephalus. Childs Nerv Syst 2:200–205
66. Kimmings E, Kleinlugtebeld A, Casey ATH, Hayward RD (1996) Does the child with shunted hydrocephalus require long-term neurosurgical follow-up? Br J Neurosurg 10:77–81
67. Kuwamura K, Kokunai T (1982) Intraventricular hematoma secondary to a ventriculoperitoneal shunt. Neurosurgery 10:384–386
68. Langmoen IA, Lundar T, Vatne K, Hovind KH (1992) Occurrence and management of fractured peripheral catheters in CSF shunts. Childs Nerv Syst 8:222–225
69. Lee M, Leahu D, Weiner HL et al (1995) Complications of fourth-ventricular shunts. Pediatr Neurosurg 22:309–314
70. Lefranc M, Ko JY, Peltier J et al (2010) Effects of transcranial magnetic stimulation on four types of pressure-programmable valves. Acta Neurochir (Wien) 152:689–697

71. Lehnert BE, Rahbar H, Relyea-Chew A et al (2011) Detection of ventricular shunt malfunction in the ED: relative utility of radiography, CT, and nuclear imaging. Emerg Radiol 18:299–305
72. Li G, Dutta S (2008) Perioperative management of ventriculoperitoneal shunts during abdominal surgery. Surg Neurol 70:492–497
73. Lüdermann W, Rosahl SK, Kaminsky J, Samii M (2005) Reliability of a new adjustable shunt device without the need for readjustment following 3-Tesla MRI. Childs Nerv Syst 21:227–229
74. Lundar T, Langmoen IA, Hovind KH (1997) Fatal cardiopulmonary complications in children treated with ventriculoatrial shunts. Childs Nerv Syst 7:215–217
75. MacGee EE (1980) Shunt position within the brain stem: a preventable complication. Neurosurgery 6:99–100
76. Maixner VJ, Besser M, Johnston IH (1992) Pseudotumor syndrome in treated arachnoid cysts. Pediatr Neurosurg 37:178–185
77. Martin K, Baird R, Farmer JP et al (2011) The use of laparoscopy in ventriculoperitoneal shunt revisions. J Pediatr Surg 46:2146–2150
78. Martínez-Lage JF, Poza M, Esteban JA (1992) Mechanical complications of the reservoirs and flushing devices in ventricular shunt systems. Br J Neurosurg 6:321–326
79. Martínez-Lage JF, Poza M, Izura V (1993) Retrograde migration of the abdominal catheter as a complication of ventriculoperitoneal shunts: the fishhook sign. Childs Nerv Syst 9:425–427
80. Martínez-Lage JF, López F, Poza M, Hernández M (1998) Prevention of intraventricular hemorrhage during CSF shunt revisions by means of a flexible coagulating electrode: a preliminary report. Childs Nerv Syst 14:203–206
81. Martínez-Lage JF, Ruiz-Espejo Vilar A, Pérez-Espejo MA et al (2006) Shunt-related craniocerebral disproportion: treatment with cranial vault expanding procedures. Neurosurg Rev 29:229–235
82. Martínez-Lage JF, Almagro MJ, Sanchez del Rincón I et al (2008) Management of neonatal hydrocephalus: feasibility of use and safety of two programmable (Sophy and Polaris) valves. Childs Nerv Syst 24:546–556
83. Martínez-Lage JF, Almagro MJ, Ruíz-Espejo A et al (2009) Keeping CSF valve function with urokinase in children with intraventricular hemorrhage and CSF shunts. Childs Nerv Syst 25:981–986
84. Martínez-Lage JF, Ruíz-Espejo AM, Almagro MJ et al (2009) CSF overdrainage in shunted intracranial arachnoid cysts: a series and review. Childs Nerv Syst 25:1061–1069
85. Mater A, Shroff M, Al-Farsi S et al (2008) Test characteristics of neuroimaging in the emergency department evaluation of children for cerebrospinal fluid shunt malfunction. CJEM 10:131–135
86. McLone DG, Partington MD (1993) Arrest and compensation of hydrocephalus. Neurosurg Clin N Am 4:621–624
87. Melo JRT, Di Rocco F, Bourgeois M et al (2014) Surgical options for treatment of traumatic subdural hematomas in children younger than 2 years of age. J Neurosurg Pediatr. doi:10.3171/2014.1.PEDS13393
88. Ment LR, Duncan OC, Geehr R (1981) Benign enlargement of the subarachnoid spaces in the infant. J Neurosurg 54:504–508
89. Misaki K, Uchiyama N, Hayashi Y, Hamada JI (2010) Intracerebral hemorrhage secondary to ventriculoperitoneal shunt insertion. Neurol Med Chir (Tokyo) 50:76–79
90. Miwa K, Kondo H, Sakai N (2001) Pressure changes observed in Codman-Medos programmable valves following magnetic exposure and filliping. Childs Nerv Syst 17:150–153
91. Moghal NE, Quinn MW, Levene MI, Puntis JWL (1991) Intraventricular haemorrhage after aspiration of ventricular reservoirs. Arch Dis Child 67:448–449
92. Mohanty A, Biswas A, Satish S et al (2006) Treatment for Dandy-Walker malformation. J Neurosurg 105(Suppl 5):348–356
93. Morton RP, Reynols RM, Ramakrishna R et al (2013) Low-dose head computed tomography in children: a single institutional experience in pediatric radiation risk reduction. J Neurosurg Pediatr 12:406–410
94. Naidich TP, Radkowski MA, McLone DG, Leetsma J (1996) Chronic cerebral herniation in shunted Dandy-Walker malformation. Radiology 158:431–434
95. Nida TY, Haines SJ (1993) Multiloculated hydrocephalus: craniotomy and fenestration of intraventricular septations. J Neurosurg 78:70–76
96. Noetzl MJ, Baker RP (1984) Shunt fluid examination: risks and benefits in the evaluation of shunt malfunction and infection. J Neurosurg 61:328–332
97. Nogueira GJ, Zaglul HF (1991) Hypodense extracerebral images on computed tomography in children. 'External hydrocephalus': a misnomer. Childs Nerv Syst 7:336–341
98. Nomura S, Fujisawa H, Suzuki M (2005) Effect of cell-phone magnetic fields on adjustable cerebrospinal fluid shunt valves. Surg Neurol 63:467–468
99. Odita JC (1992) The widened frontal subarachnoid space. A CT comparative study between macrocephalic, microcephalic and normocephalic infants and children. Childs Nerv Syst 8:36–39
100. Oi S, Shimoda M, Shibata M et al (2000) Pathophysiology of long-standing overt ventriculomegaly in adults. J Neurosurg 92:933–940
101. Oi S, Abbot R (2004) Loculated ventricles and isolated compartments in hydrocephalus: their pathophysiology and the efficacy of neuroendoscopic surgery. Neurosurg Clin N Am 15:77–87
102. Park JK, Frim DM, Schwartz MS et al (1997) The use of clinical practice guidelines (CPGs) to evaluate practice and control costs in ventriculoperitoneal shunt management. Surg Neurol 48:536–541
103. Patel CD, Matloub H (1973) Vaginal perforation as a complication of ventriculoperitoneal shunt. Case report. J Neurosurg 38:761–762
104. Peña C, Browsher K, Samuels-Reid J (2004) FDA-approved neurologic devices intended for use in infants, children, and adolescents. Neurology 63:1163–1167

105. Peirce KR, Loeser JD (1975) Perforation of the intestine by a Raimondi peritoneal catheter. Case report. J Neurosurg 43:112–113
106. Piatt JH Jr (1992) Physical examination of patients with cerebrospinal fluid shunts: is there any useful information in pumping the shunt? Pediatrics 89:470–473
107. Pople IF (2002) Hydrocephalus and shunts: what the neurologist should know. J Neurol Neurosurg Psychiatry 73(Suppl 1):i17–i22
108. Portnoy HD, Croissan PD (1973) Two unusual complications of a ventriculoperitoneal shunt. J Neurosurg 39:775–776
109. Power D, Ali-Khan F, Drage M (1999) Contralateral extradural haematoma after insertion of a programmable-valve ventriculoperitoneal shunt. J R Soc Med 92:360–361
110. Pumberg W, Löbl M, Geissler W (1998) Appendicitis in children with a ventriculoperitoneal shunt. Pediatr Neurosurg 28:21–26
111. Ramani PS (1974) Extrusion of abdominal catheter of ventriculoperitoneal shunt into the scrotum. J Neurosurg 40:772–773
112. Ransohoff J (1975) Chronic subdural hematoma treated by subduro-pleural shunt. Pediatrics 20:561–564
113. Raskin J, Guillaume DJ, Ragel BT (2010) Laparoscopic-induced pneumocephalus in a patient with a ventriculoperitoneal shunt. Pediatr Neurosurg 46:390–391
114. Rekate HL (1991–1992) Shunt revision: complications and their prevention. Pediatr Neurosurg 17:155–162
115. Rekate HL (2007) Longstanding overt ventriculomegaly in adults: pitfalls in treatment with endoscopic third ventriculostomy. Neurosurg Focus 22(4):E6
116. Robertson WC Jr, Gomez MR (1978) External hydrocephalus. Early finding in congenital communicating hydrocephalus. Arch Neurol 35:541–544
117. Rocque BG, Lapsiwala S, Iskandar BJ (2008) Ventricular shunt tap as a predictor of proximal shunt malfunction in children: a prospective study. J Neurosurg Pediatr 1:439–443
118. Rogers EA, Kimia A, Madsen JR et al (2012) Predictors of ventricular shunt infection among children presenting to a pediatric emergency department. Pediatr Emerg Care 28:405–409
119. Romero L, Ros B, Rius F et al (2014) Ventriculoperitoneal shunt as a primary neurosurgical procedure in newborn posthemorrhagic hydrocephalus: report of a series of 47 shunted patients. Childs Nerv Syst 30:91–95
120. Sandberg D, McComb JG, Krieger MD (2005) Craniotomy and fenestration of multiloculated hydrocephalus in pediatric patients. Neurosurgery 57(ONS Suppl 1):ONS-100–ONS106
121. Schrot RJ, Ramos-Boudreau C, Boggan JE (2012) Breast-related CSF shunt complications: literature review with illustrative case. Breast J 18:479–483
122. Schuhmann MU, Sood S, McAllister JP et al (2008) Value of overnight monitoring of intracranial pressure in hydrocephalic children. Pediatr Neurosurg 44:269–279
123. Schul DB, Wolf S, Lumenta CB (2010) Iatrogenic tension pneumothorax resulting in pneumocephalus after insertion of a ventriculoperitoneal shunt: an unusual complication. Act Neurochir (Wien) 152:143–144
124. Schneider T, Knauff U, Nitsch J, Firsching R (2002) Electromagnetic hazards involving adjustable shunt valves in hydrocephalus. J Neurosurg 96:331–334
125. Scott M, Wycis HT, Murtagh F, Reyes V (1955) Observations on ventricular and subarachnoid peritoneal shunts in hydrocephalic children. J Neurosurg 12:165–175
126. Shetty PG, Fatterpekar GM, Sahani DV, Shiroff MM (1999) Pneumocephalus secondary to colonic perforation by ventriculoperitoneal shunt catheter. Br J Radiol 72:704–705
127. Simon TD, Riva-Cambrin J, Srivastava R et al (2008) Hospital care for children with hydrocephalus in the United States: utilization, charges, comorbidities, and deaths. J Neurosurg Pediatr 1:131–137
128. Simon TD, Hall M, Riva-Cambrin J et al (2009) Infection rates following initial cerebrospinal fluid placement across pediatric hospitals in the United States. J Neurosurg Pediatr 4:156–165
129. Sood S, Kim S, Ham SD et al (1993) Useful components of the shunt tap for evaluation of shunt function. Childs Nerv Syst 9:157–162
130. Steinbok P, Cochrane DD (1998) Removal of adherent ventricular catheter. Technical note. Pediatr Neurosurg 18:167–168
131. Strahle J, Selzer BJ, Muraszko KM et al (2012) Programmable shunt valve affected by exposure to a tablet computer. J Neurosurg Pediatr 10:118–120
132. Stringel G, Turner M, Crase T (1993) Ventriculo-gallbladder shunts in children. Childs Nerv Syst 9:331–333
133. Takahashi I (2001) Withdrawal of shunt systems – clinical use of the programmable shunt system and its effect on hydrocephalus in children. Childs Nerv Syst 17:472–477
134. Tarnakis A, Edwards RJ, Lowis SP, Pople IK (2005) Atypical external hydrocephalus with visual failure due to occult leptomeningeal dissemination of a pontine glioma. J Neurosurg 102(Suppl 2):224–227
135. Taub E, Lavyne MM (1994) Thoracic complications of ventriculoperitoneal shunts: case report and review of the literature. Neurosurgery 34:181–184
136. Torres Lanzas J, Ríos Zambudio A, Martínez-Lage JF et al (2002) Tratamiento de la hidrocefalia mediante la derivación ventrículopleural. Arch Bronconeumol 38:511–514
137. Tsingoglou S, Eksteins HB (1981) Pericardial tamponade by Holter ventriculoatrial shunts. J Neurosurg 35:695–699
138. Tubbs RS, Banks JT, Soleau S et al (2005) Complications of ventriculosubgaleal shunts. Childs Nerv Syst 21:48–51
139. Tubbs RS, Acakpo-Satchivi L, Blount JP et al (2006) Pericallosal artery pseudoaneurysm secondary to endoscopic-assisted ventriculoperitoneal shunt placement. J Neurosurg Pediatr 105(Suppl 2):140–142
140. Turner MS (1995) The treatment of hydrocephalus: a brief guide to shunt selection. Surg Neurol 43:314–319

141. Udayasankar UK, Braithwaite K, Arvaniti M et al (2008) Low-dose non-enhancement head CT protocol for follow-up evaluation of children with ventriculoperitoneal shunt: reduction of radiation and effect on image quality. AJNR Am J Neuroradiol 29:802–806
142. Uzzo RG, Bilsky M, Mininberg DT, Poppas DP (1997) Laparoscopic surgery in children with ventriculoperitoneal shunts: effect of pneumoperitoneum. Urology 49:735–737
143. Vassilyadi M, Tataryn ZL, Alkherayf F et al (2010) The necessity of shunt series. J Neurosurg Pediatr 6:468–473
144. Venes JL (1976) Control of shun infection: report of 150 consecutive cases. J Neurosurg 45:311–314
145. Villavicencio AT, Wellons JC III, George TM (1998) Avoiding complicated shunt systems by open fenestration of symptomatic fourth ventricular cysts associated with hydrocephalus. Pediatr Neurosurg 29:314–319
146. Vinchon M, Fichten A, Delestret I, Dhellemmes P (2003) Shunt revision for asymptomatic failure: surgical and clinical results. Neurosurgery 52:347–356
147. Walchenbach R, Geiger E, Thomeer RTWM, Vanneste JAL (2002) The value of temporary external lumbar CSF drainage in predicting the outcome of shunting on normal pressure hydrocephalus. J Neurol Neurosurg Psychiatry 72:503–506
148. Wang C, Hefflin B, Cope JU et al (2010) Emergency department visits for medical device-associated adverse events among children. Pediatrics 126:247–259
149. Wang VY, Barbaro NM, Lawton MT et al (2007) Complications of lumboperitoneal shunts. Neurosurgery 60:1045–1049
150. Watkins L, Hayward R, Andar U, Harkness W (1994) The diagnosis of blocked cerebrospinal fluid shunts: a prospective study of referral to a pediatric neurosurgical unit. Childs Nerv Syst 10:87–90
151. Weinzierl MR, Rohde V, Gilsbach JM, Korinth M (2008) Management of hydrocephalus in infants by using shunts with adjustable valves. J Neurosurg Pediatr 2:1–18
152. Welch K, Shillito J, Strand R et al (1981) Chiari I malformation- an acquired disorder? J Neurosurg 55:604–609
153. Wellons JC III, Holubkov R, Browd R et al (2013) The assessment of bulging fontanel and splitting of sutures in premature infants: an interrater reliability study by the Hydrocephalus Clinical Research Network. J Neurosurg Pediatr 11:12–14
154. Whittle IR, Johnston IH (1983) Extrusion of peritoneal catheter through neck incision: a rare complication of ventriculoperitoneal shunting. Aust N Z J Surg 53:177–178
155. Wiegand C, Richards P (2007) Measurement of intracranial pressure in children: a critical review of current methods. Dev Med Child Neurol 49: 935–941
156. Williams MA, McAllister JP, Walker ML et al (2007) Priorities for hydrocephalus research: report from a National Institutes of Health-sponsored workshop. J Neurosurg 107(Suppl 5):345–357
157. Wilson TJ, Stetler WR Jr, Al-Holou WN, Sullivan SE (2013) Comparison of the accuracy of ventricular catheter placement using freehand placement, ultrasonic guidance, and stereotactic navigation. J Neurosurg 119:66–70
158. Winston KR, Lopez JA, Freeman J (2006) CSF shunt failure with stable normal ventricular size. Pediatr Neurosurg 42:151–155
159. Winston KR, Dolan SA (2011) Multidisciplinary approach to cerebrospinal fluid shunt infection with an appeal for attention to details in assessment and standardization in reporting. J Neurosurg Pediatr 7:452–461
160. Zahl SM, Wester K (2008) Routine measurement of head circumference as a tool for detecting intracranial expansion in infants. What is the gain? A national survey. Pediatrics 121:e416–e420
161. Zamora I, Lurbe A, Alvarez-Garijo A et al (1984) Shunt nephritis: a report of five children. Childs Brain 11:183–187
162. Zuccaro G, Ramos JG (2011) Multiloculated hydrocephalus. Childs Nerv Syst 27:1609–1619

Complications Related to the Choice of the CSF Shunt Device

6

Kevin Tsang, William Singleton, and Ian Pople

Contents

6.1 **Introduction** ... 109

6.2 **Basic Hydrodynamics** ... 110

6.3 **Types of Valves** ... 110
6.3.1 Flow-Regulated Valves ... 110
6.3.2 Differential Pressure Valves ... 111
6.3.3 Gravitational Valves ... 111
6.3.4 Adjustable or 'Programmable' Valves ... 112

6.4 **Catheter Characteristics** ... 112
6.4.1 Material Properties ... 112
6.4.2 Physical Properties and Interplay with the Valve Complex ... 114

6.5 **Patient Factors** ... 115

Conclusions ... 116

References ... 116

K. Tsang, MD • W. Singleton, MD
I. Pople, MD (✉)
Department of Neurosurgery,
North Bristol NHS Trust, Bristol, UK
e-mail: ikpople@hotmail.com

6.1 Introduction

Specific complications of CSF shunting are sometimes associated with certain aspects of shunt design and manufacture. Complications may arise that are specific to the type of catheter and valve selected and may reflect peculiarities to the component itself, or be related to the aetiology of the hydrocephalus being treated.

Although many surgeons prefer to use only one or two types of valves for most of their patients, there are some situations where careful decision-making regarding valve selection is paramount. A good understanding of both valve hydrodynamics and the underlying CSF dynamic disorder in the patient being treated is vital to avoid complications that may arise from poor valve selection. The use of shunt adjuncts, such as anti-siphon devices, adds another level of complexity and potential for complication if improperly selected.

In this chapter, we will first describe the different types of shunt valves available on the market currently, and the principles of pressure and flow regulation, as well as reasons for choosing adjustable systems. We then go onto describe the possible complications associated with each type of system and the specific problems that may arise in neonates, children, adults and the elderly in turn. Complications have arisen from specific catheter designs, which will also be discussed here.

C. Di Rocco et al. (eds.), *Complications of CSF Shunting in Hydrocephalus: Prevention, Identification, and Management*, DOI 10.1007/978-3-319-09961-3_6,

6.2 Basic Hydrodynamics

Familiarity with the relationship between pressure, flow and resistance greatly assists in the understanding of hydrocephalus and shunt mechanisms, which is obviously an integral part of choosing the most appropriate device [19]. The factors affecting CSF flow through a shunt is dependent on various factors. These include the intraventricular pressure (IVP), the hydrostatic pressure (p), the valve's opening pressure (OPV) and the pressure within the cavity in which the shunt is placed (e.g. intra-abdominal pressure, IAP). From principles of physics, one can derive that the pressure gradient between the two ends of a shunt system $(\Delta P) = \text{IVP} + p - \text{OPV} - \text{IAP}$. From hydrostatic studies, the hydrostatic pressure is known to be the product of the height of the column (h), density of CSF (ρ) and gravitational force (g).

In any given patient, the OPV is a constant for the particular system chosen, whereas IVP and IAP may fluctuate within a small range given a particular posture. However, the main variable would be the height of the column influencing the hydrostatic pressure.

These are important as the flow, F, through a tube is equivalent to the differential pressure, ΔP, divided by the resistance in the tube and valve, that is, $F = \Delta P/(R_T + R_V)$. The resistance of the tube can be calculated using Poiseuille's law and is a constant for the particular system chosen. Therefore, the determinants of CSF flow, and hence the choice of a device, will be mainly regulated by the following: (1) patient's underlying condition and IVP; (2) patient's position (and hence the possible need for an anti-siphon device); and (3) the resistance provided by the shunt system.

6.3 Types of Valves

There are four main groups of valves: flow-regulated, differential pressure, gravitational or adjustable ('programmable'). Most of the data on efficacy of various valves are reported by proponents of the device and no randomised controlled trials are available to compare these devices. It is therefore important for the treating physician to understand the properties of these shunts and choose the most appropriate system on an individual basis.

6.3.1 Flow-Regulated Valves

This type of valve utilises variable resistance (i.e. R_V) to control the flow of CSF. One example would be the Integra OSV II® system, which allows flow rates of either 18–30 or 8–17 ml/h. These valves consist of a synthetic ruby pin within a moveable ring. They will work as a differential pressure valve until the ICP is high enough to displace the ruby pin downwards, reducing the outflow aperture and thus increasing resistance to flow. This allows a relatively constant flow rate at a range of ICP (normally up to 25 mmHg). With further increases in ICP, the moveable ring becomes displaced downwards, opening the aperture and reducing the resistance to flow.

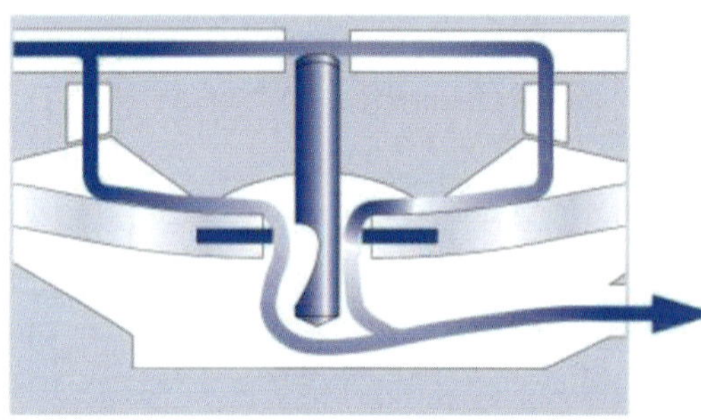

Displaced pin - maintaining constant flow

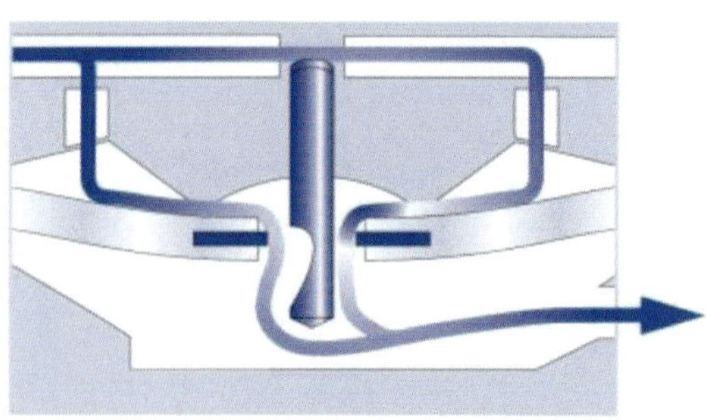

High ICP - displaced ring to increase flow

This type of valve may be of benefit in patients with siphoning and over-drainage problems or in those with a high risk of developing slit-ventricle syndrome. Current data have shown a benefit in improving symptoms of low ICP but no difference in their revision rates compared to other types of valves. In fact, these valves tend to have a smaller orifice, which may act as a site for obstruction.

6.3.2 Differential Pressure Valves

This type of valve utilises a very simple concept – opening and closing pressures. When the ICP is above the valve's opening pressure, CSF will flow, and vice versa. However, due to the valve's mechanisms, the closing pressure may be lower than the quoted opening pressure and symptoms of over-drainage may occur without siphoning. A large variety of these valves exist in the market, examples include the Codman® Precision Valve and the Sophysa Pulsar® Valve, and each one is subdivided according to their pressure range (high, medium and low). They can be roughly placed into four groups according to their mechanism of actions: diaphragm valve, ball-in-cone valve, mitre valve and slit valve.

Diaphragm valves are the most common type and include the Sophysa Pulsar® Valve. They consist of a silicon membrane which deflects in response to ICP changes, thus controlling the flow rate. These devices differ from one another in terms of the position of the membrane (proximal or distal to reservoir) and therefore would affect one's ability to utilise the valve for examination and intrathecal drug delivery.

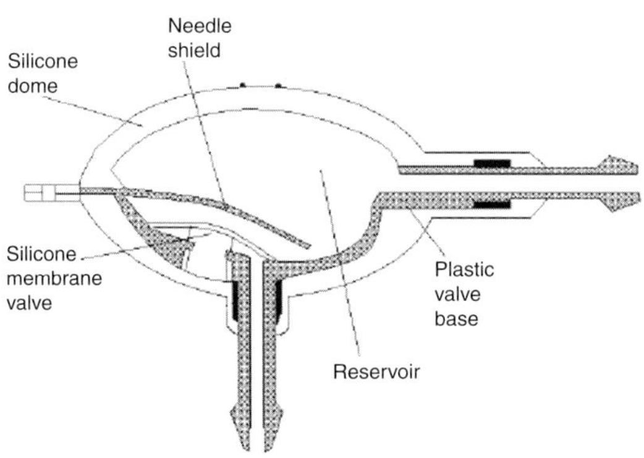

Ball-in-cone valves include the Codman® Hakim system where a ball sits in the middle of a cone or a spring. The opening pressure is determined by the properties of the spring whilst the flow rate is then determined by the diameter of the outflow aperture, the diameter of the ball and the cone angle. As ICP increases, the ball is displaced away from the cone and therefore flow increases. These valves seem to be less prone to the ageing effects of materials compared to the mitre and slit valves but may be more prone to obstruction (e.g. in post-intraventricular haemorrhage neonates).

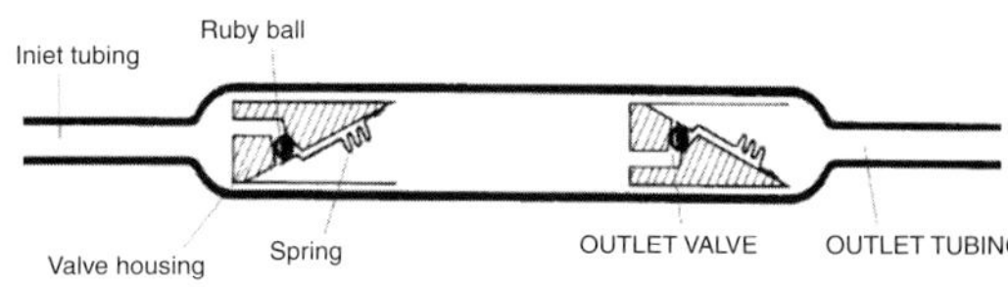

The mitre valves include the Integra™ Mischler Valve which is essentially a system with a direct flow path to resist occlusion and may therefore be useful in those with high CSF protein levels. The main determinants for their control of CSF flow include the size, shape, length and thickness of the silicone leaflets.

Slit valves are made of silicone rubber material with cuts or slits within them [27]. These slits are malleable and will open in response to rising ICP. The number of slits and the stiffness of the membrane will determine the opening pressure and flow rate. An example would be the Sophysa Phoenix system. They can be placed either proximally (e.g. Holter-Hausner® valve) or distally (e.g. Codman® Unishunt) – the more distal the placement, the lower the resistance to flow.

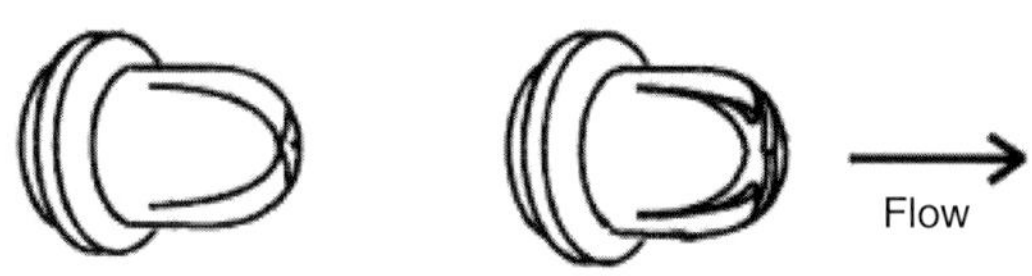

6.3.3 Gravitational Valves

This type of valve has been designed to reduce the siphoning effects of change in patient's posture by altering the opening pressure, using gravity. They are basically ball-in-cone differential pressure valves but with an additional gravitational unit. This is composed of a ball which would displace into the cone when the patient is upright, thus increasing resistance and reducing flow. This results in the valve having two different opening pressures depending on the patient's posture [21]. As with any differential pressure valve, they come in a range of different opening pressures and given that this is dependent on the height of the column (see hydrodynamics above), the choice should be based on the height of the patient. Examples of gravitational valves include the Integra™ H-V valve and the Miethke DualSwitch™ valve.

6.3.4 Adjustable or 'Programmable' Valves

These are differential pressure valves which have a mechanism that allows adjustment of the opening pressure by the user externally, but otherwise the design is similar to a normal differential pressure valve as described above. The obvious benefit is the ability to alter the opening pressure according to the patient's symptoms and hence negating the need for revision surgery. They may therefore be useful in normal pressure hydrocephalus patients to allow a gradual reduction in ventricular size without causing subdural haematomas [15]. However, there are no class I data to compare their efficacy to other types of valves. In addition, due to the magnetic design of these valves, a strong magnetic field such as an MRI may alter the shunt setting. This has been attempted to be overcome, such as in the Polaris and proGav valves [2, 1]

A number of adjustable valves are available in the market, including Codman® Medos valve, Strata® adjustable pressure valve and Miethke proSA™ valve [9, 31]. These are, in the main, indicated in the management of idiopathic Normal Pressure Hydrocephalus and have been shown to reduce post-operative over-drainage and subdural formation in these patients [10] However, a surgeon may choose to use these more expensive valves in younger adults with very large ventricles or perhaps in children primarily, as a way of allowing gradual upgrading of valve pressure as the child grows taller [5, 38]. Whether this lowers the risk of long-term over-drainage complications or blockage in the individual child is not yet clear from longitudinal studies [6].

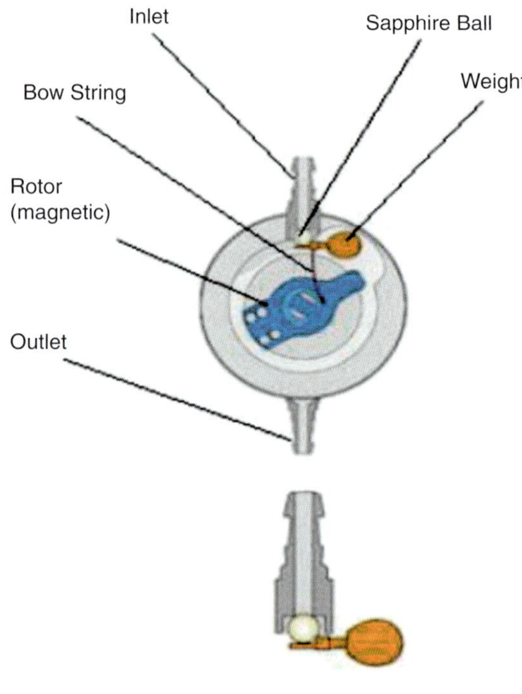

6.4 Catheter Characteristics

It is now well recognised that delayed shunt complications (defined here as greater than 5 years) are often a consequence of catheter failure [45]. The entity of catheter occlusion by in-growing choroid plexus, ependyma and glia is covered elsewhere in this book. Here we are interested in the details of catheter design and material that may dispose it to degrade, calcify and become brittle over time [12]. This may lead to catheter fracture, migration and cause subsequent shunt dysfunction as well as possible visceral injury, depending on the site of the distal catheter [3, 4, 11, 18, 23]. Catheter technology has developed with greater understanding of the resistance associated with the tube itself and how this affects CSF drainage. Tissue response to the catheter itself has changed the materials used in shunt manufacture [13, 14].

6.4.1 Material Properties

Modern shunt catheter tubing is made of plain silicone, and initial concerns about silicone allergy in shunted patients have largely been clinically unfounded [30]. Initial shunt catheters sometimes contained a spiral wire re-enforcement in order to reduce the chance of kinking but were associated with a high rate of abdominal complications. There are many reports of catheter migration and visceral perforation (usually of the rectum or vagina) associated with the Raimondi wired shunt in the literature, so they are not used in modern neurosurgical practice for these reasons [36, 39, 40, 42, 43, 46, 49].

Catheter material tends to degrade and calcify over time. This makes the catheter more brittle and likely to fracture during patient movement. Calcified or degraded catheter tubing can become fixed to subcutaneous tissue. If this fixation takes place before the patient stops growing, there is an increased risk of fracture or migration. It also makes removal of a catheter at revision surgery much more difficult and it is far more likely that shunt products are retained within the patient. This is associated with developing later abdominal complications such as intestinal obstruction and perforation (Fig. 6.1) [48].

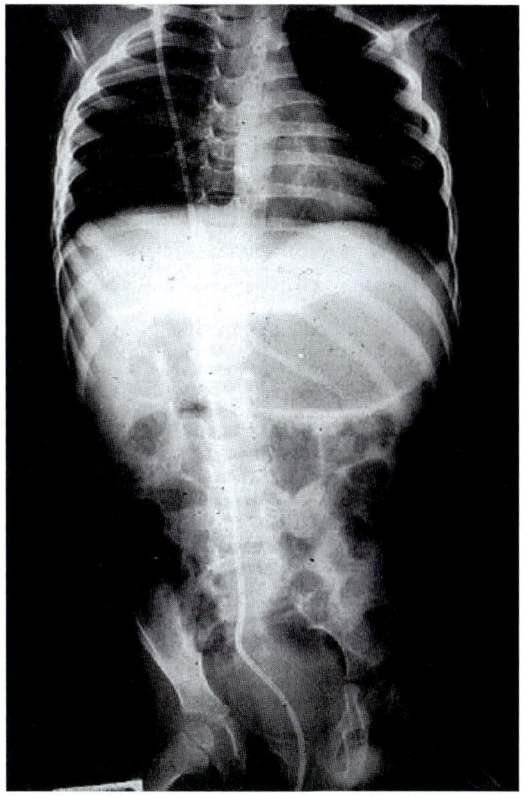

Fig. 6.1 Delayed rectal extrusion of a distal shunt catheter in an infant shown on plain radiography caused by colonic erosion without clinical evidence of peritonism or bowel perforation

Calcification in shunt catheters occurs in vivo by dystrophic calcification, which is characterised by a normal concentration of serum calcium but altered cellular metabolism caused by cell death or damage. This type of calcification seen in silicone implants is thought to occur due to the cellular debris that accumulates next to the implant. This could be the result of direct trauma or tissue reaction to the catheter itself. Dystrophic calcification is augmented by the presence of surface irregularities on the catheter caused by catheter degradation and by barium.

Biopolymers deteriorate in four ways: (1) the structure is altered by hydration; (2) covalent bonds of the chains are weakened; (3) these bonds are broken, which reduces the molecular weight of the polymer; and (4) certain soluble fragments are digested by macrophages, which causes host-cell-mediated inflammation, and can accelerate calcification. In the human body, silicones have to resist chemical and mechanical insults for a number of years.

Interestingly, the cerebral parenchyma and peritoneal cavity do not degrade silicone catheters, suggesting that it is the subcutaneous environment that promotes polymer breakdown. However, this cannot be completely the case as ventriculoatrial catheters have also been shown to degrade with time. Mechanical forces applied during movement can facilitate the breaking down of non-covalent bonds in a silicone polymer, which may explain the differential degradation of catheters along its length. Catheter fracture is often observed at the level of the neck; this is the part of the catheter that is under most dynamic stress during the lifetime of the shunt system and several reports have indicated that the most common site of shunt fracture was 2–4 cm above the clavicle.

The presence of barium coating of shunt catheters is associated with an increased rate of catheter calcification. Both platinum- and barium-coated silicon catheters have been reported to have an early calcification and fracture rate. For these reasons, it is generally recommended that they are no longer used in clinical practice. One may hypothesise that the coating is more likely to form microscopic cracks with time that may cause local micro-cellular damage and hence activate local host inflammation and accelerate dystrophic calcification as described above. The development of plain silicon-coated shunt catheters has increased the longevity of shunt catheters, but they are still susceptible to calcification and subsequent fracture in the long term. Improvements in shunt longevity will be dictated by research in biomaterials that do not interact with the host environment and do not calcify or degrade over time.

The impregnation of catheters with antibiotics (e.g. Bactiseal), or coating with substances that reduce bacterial adhesion (Silverline, or Bioglide), has been developed to reduce the rate of shunt failure from infection and have variable amounts of evidence to support their efficacy. Some surgeons with historically high shunt infection rates have chosen to use these catheters routinely for all patients at considerably increased expense to their department, whereas others with low infection rates may only use them selectively on those patients with specific risk factors (e.g. infants under the age of 6 months, patients with poor skin condition, previously infected patients). These anti-microbial catheters do not completely eliminate the risk of infection in such patients, but provide some defence against the more common pathogens causing shunt infections. A UK multicentre randomised trial (BASICS) is underway to assess the efficacy of these different products [7].

6.4.2 Physical Properties and Interplay with the Valve Complex

As previously described, a variety of valves are commercially available, which differ not only in the way they regulate CSF dynamics but also in the way they are manufactured. The profile of the valve and the mechanism by which it connects to the catheter is of relevance to late mechanical

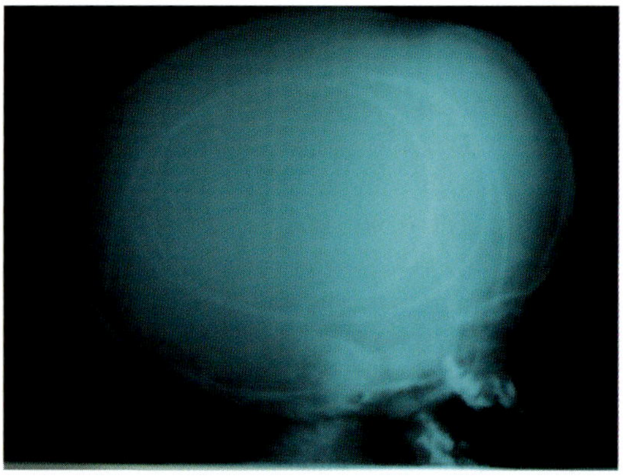

Fig. 6.2 Migration of whole of a low-profile shunt system upwards into grossly enlarged cerebral ventricles. Most migrations of low-profile systems occur distally into the peritoneal cavity

complications. A low-profile tubular valve in the catheter line, such as the Hakim valve (Codman) is often chosen in paediatric practice to minimise tension in the overlying thin skin, but has a tendency to migrate downwards because it becomes pulled by a fixed subcutaneous calcified distal catheter as the child grows older. By comparison, the round-bodied valves (Orbis-Sigma), or a flushing burr-hole valve cannot migrate distally with traction caused by growth. In these systems, disconnection or fracture of the distal catheter is more likely to result from the traction applied to the aging degraded material. Rarely, a low-profile tubular valve system can migrate proximally and sometimes fully including the valve (Fig. 6.2).

Physical design of shunt systems will determine how frequently catheters become disconnected and displaced. Unitised systems were introduced in an attempt to lower the risk of disconnections by avoiding the need to attach the tubing to connectors and fix it with a silk or nylon ligature. However, they are more difficult to revise than systems with separate components and overall the longevity of the shunt has not been shown to be any better for these systems. Some type of valves have connectors that need considerable effort and manipulation to attach a catheter securely ('fiddly') and would seem more likely to be associated with complications such as disconnections or leakage from iatrogenic holes in the catheter. A surgeon should become familiar with the valve shape and characteristic of the connectors to lower the risk of these types of mechanical complications.

The outflow mechanism from a distal catheter influences shunt function. The presence of drainage slits (not valves) at the end of the distal catheters is associated with a higher incidence of distal shunt failure, and in our practice these are always removed prior to shunting into the peritoneum or pleura [17]. Catheter length has an impact on shunt function [16]. As described above the flow is dependant on resistance – as defined by Poiseuille's law. The resistance will increase as the length of the catheter increases. Shorter catheters will have a higher flow rate and will, therefore, more likely over-drain. Conversely, very long distal catheters occasionally under-drain in premature babies. This has an obvious implication when shunting very small children. This will be discussed further below.

6.5 Patient Factors

The choice of the most appropriate shunt components for an individual patient can become a complicated science and a full understanding of the aforementioned mechanical characteristics is important in order to minimise complications. Obviously, the various patient characteristics including the underlying reason for the need for shunting are vital in the decision-making process too. These are covered in more detail in the separate chapters in this book and a brief description will be given here.

The underlying diagnosis often determines an individual's CSF dynamics, as does the patient's age. It is well documented that CSF production declines with age whilst the resistance to CSF outflow increases with age [20]. This means that older patients are more likely to suffer from low-pressure symptoms secondary to shunt overdrainage [32, 37]. This effect is further amplified by the increased siphoning effect of a long distal catheter, compared to a shorter catheter in a child or baby. Therefore, the treating physician may consider avoiding low-pressure valves in older patients (e.g. those with normal-pressure hydrocephalus, NPH), or in the case of a programmable shunt, to start at a higher setting and gradually reduce it according to symptoms [51]. This approach will also allow for the increased risk of subdural haematoma secondary to overdrainage in the setting of an atrophic brain with reduced compliance [24, 34, 44]. The treating physician may also consider the use of an antisiphon adjunct which may either be built into the valve (as in the case of a gravitational valve) or as an addition (e.g. Delta chamber, 'shunt assistant' or SiphonGuard) [25, 29, 35, 41, 50].

In infants, especially pre-term babies suffering from intraventricular haemorrhage, a low-pressure valve may occasionally be more suitable as the relatively low ICP, shorter distal catheter and higher intra-abdominal pressure, compared to adults, mean there is reduced siphoning and a medium- or high-pressure valve may sometimes result in inadequate CSF diversion. Conversely, in choosing some valves in these babies, particularly differential low-pressure systems, there is the risk of development of subdural collections and slit-ventricle syndrome (SVS), so the surgeon may consider upgrading the valve pressure as the child grows, or employing a flanged catheter to help maintain ventricular patency (Fig. 6.3) [26, 33, 47]. There is some evidence that the use of a flow-controlled valve (e.g. OSV II), or gravitational valve may reduce the development of SVS but conflicting evidence exist in the literature and there is no class I publication available [8, 22, 28].

In some children who have suffered severe meningitis complicated by post-meningitic hydrocephalus, the CSF compliance can be abnormally high and their ventricles continue to expand radiologically and symptomatically under relatively low intracranial pressure. A low pressure or preferably an adjustable valve is an appropriate choice in this situation and a degree of siphoning is often required initially to bring the ventricles down and improve the clinical condition of the child.

In other children who have developed low CSF compliance ('brittle ventricles') from chronic shunt over-drainage, the choice of valve design and opening pressure in situations of shunt

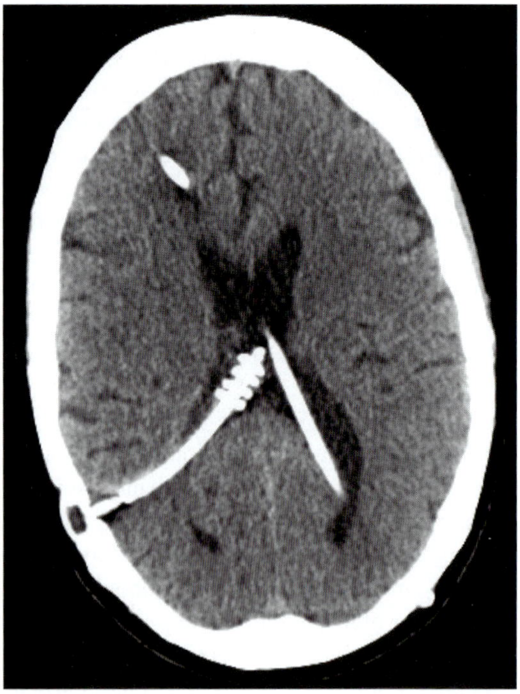

Fig. 6.3 Cranial CT showing a right-sided flanged proximal catheter. These are not commonly used nowadays, but were designed to reduce the rate of proximal blockage due to obstructing choroid plexus or ependyma. They are not popular due to the potential difficulties associated with removal when revising a dysfunctional system

revision or complete renewal is critical as these children will deteriorate quickly and dramatically without the correct (usually pre-existing) valve pressure and degree of siphoning.

Patient factors such as CSF red cell count or protein levels may affect the surgeon's choice of valve in that some ball valves may not tolerate sustained increased levels of red cells and protein as effectively as valves with simpler diaphragm designs, leading to earlier shunt blockage. In some patients with extremely high levels of CSF protein, as may occur in children with tumours, it may become necessary to omit the valve component altogether.

Conclusions

The choice of shunt components on the current market can often seem overwhelming. This probably reflects the fact that no one system is perfect and all have their specific limitations. The neurosurgeon needs to be aware of the principles of shunt design and their subtle differences. Most importantly, an understanding of how shunt components will interact with the patient and influence CSF dynamics is paramount before deciding on the appropriate shunt components to be used. A poorly judged selection will influence the risk of early post-operative complications and may leave a patient either chronically under- or over-shunted.

References

1. Allin DM, Czosnyka M, Richards HK, Pickard JD, Czosnyka ZH (2008) Investigation of the hydrodynamic properties of a new MRI-resistant programmable hydrocephalus shunt. Cerebrospinal Fluid Res 5:8
2. Allin DM, Czosnyka ZH, Czosnyka M, Richards HK, Pickard JD (2006) In vitro hydrodynamic properties of the Miethke ProGAV hydrocephalus shunt. Cerebrospinal Fluid Res 3:9
3. Alonso-Vanegas M, Alvarez JL, Delgado L, Mendizabal R, Jiménez JL, Sanchez-Cabrera JM (1994) Gastric perforation due to ventriculo-peritoneal shunt. Pediatr Neurosurg 21(3):192–194
4. Aras M, Altaş M, Serarslan Y, Akçora B, Yılmaz A (2013) Protrusion of a peritoneal catheter via abdominal wall and operated myelomeningocele area: a rare complication of ventriculoperitoneal shunt. Childs Nerv Syst [Epub ahead of print]
5. Arnell K, Eriksson E, Olsen L (2006) The programmable adult Codman Hakim valve is useful even in very small children with hydrocephalus. A 7-year retrospective study with special focus on cost/benefit analysis. Eur J Pediatr Surg 16(1):1–7
6. Aschoff A, Krämer P, Benesch C, Klank A (1991) Shunt-technology and overdrainage–a critical review of hydrostatic, programmable and variable-resistance-valves and flow-reducing devices. Eur J Pediatr Surg 1(Suppl 1):49–50
7. BASICS trial. (http://www.nets.nihr.ac.uk/projects/hta/1010430)
8. Beez T, Sarikaya-Seiwert S, Bellstädt L, Mühmer M, Steiger HJ (2014) Role of ventriculoperitoneal shunt valve design in the treatment of pediatric hydrocephalus-a single center study of valve performance in the clinical setting. Childs Nerv Syst 30:293–297
9. Belliard H, Roux FX, Turak B, Nataf F, Devaux B, Cioloca C (1996) The Codman Medos programmable shunt valve. Evaluation of 53 implantations in 50 patients. Neurochirurgie 42(3):139–145; discussion 145–6
10. Bergsneider M, Black PM, Klinge P, Marmarou A, Relkin N (2005) Surgical management of idiopathic

normal-pressure hydrocephalus. Neurosurgery 57(3 Suppl):S29–S39; discussion ii–v
11. Berhouma M, Messerer M, Houissa S, Khaldi M (2008) Transoral protrusion of a peritoneal catheter: a rare complication of ventriculoperitoneal shunt. Pediatr Neurosurg 44(2):169–171
12. Boch AL, Hermelin E, Sainte-Rose C, Sgouros S (1998) Mechanical dysfunction of ventriculoperitoneal shunts caused by calcification of the silicone rubber catheter. J Neurosurg 88(6):975–982
13. Browd SR, Gottfried ON, Ragel BT, Kestle JR (2006) Failure of cerebrospinal fluid shunts: part II: overdrainage, loculation, and abdominal complications. Pediatr Neurol 34(3):171–176
14. Browd SR, Ragel BT, Gottfried ON, Kestle JR (2006) Failure of cerebrospinal fluid shunts: part I: obstruction and mechanical failure. Pediatr Neurol 34(2):83–92
15. Carmel PW, Albright AL, Adelson PD, Canady A, Black P, Boydston W, Kneirim D, Kaufman B, Walker M, Luciano M, Pollack IF, Manwaring K, Heilbrun MP, Abbott IR, Rekate H (1999) Incidence and management of subdural hematoma/hygroma with variable- and fixed-pressure differential valves: a randomized, controlled study of programmable compared with conventional valves. Neurosurg Focus 7(4):e7
16. Couldwell WT, LeMay DR, McComb JG (1996) Experience with use of extended length peritoneal shunt catheters. J Neurosurg 85(3):425–427
17. Cozzens JW, Chandler JP (1997) Increased risk of distal ventriculoperitoneal shunt obstruction associated with slit valves or distal slits in the peritoneal catheter. J Neurosurg 87(5):682–686
18. Cuka GM, Hellbusch LC (1995) Fractures of the peritoneal catheter of cerebrospinal fluid shunts. Pediatr Neurosurg 22:101–103
19. Czosnyka Z, Czosnyka M, Richards HK, Pickard JD (2002) Laboratory testing of hydrocephalus shunts – conclusion of the U.K. Shunt evaluation programme. Acta Neurochir (Wien) 144(6):525–538; discussion 538
20. Czosnyka M, Czosnyka Z, Whitfield P, Donovan T, Pickard J (2001) Age dependence of cerebrospinal pressure-volume compensation in patients with hydrocephalus. J Neurosurg 94:482–486
21. Deininger MH, Weyerbrock A (2009) Gravitational valves in supine patients with ventriculo-peritoneal shunts. Acta Neurochir (Wien) 151(6):705–709; discussion 709
22. Drake JM, Kestle JR, Milner R, Cinalli G, Boop F, Piatt J Jr, Haines S, Schiff SJ, Cochrane DD, Steinbok P, MacNeil N (1998) Randomized trial of cerebrospinal fluid shunt valve design in pediatric hydrocephalus. Neurosurgery 43(2):294–303; discussion 303–5
23. Ghritlaharey RK, Budhwani KS, Shrivastava DK, Gupta G, Kushwaha AS, Chanchlani R, Nanda M (2007) Trans-anal protrusion of ventriculo-peritoneal shunt catheter with silent bowel perforation: report of ten cases in children. Pediatr Surg Int 23(6):575–580
24. Gölz L, Lemcke J, Meier U (2013) Indications for valve-pressure adjustments of gravitational assisted valves in patients with idiopathic normal pressure hydrocephalus. Surg Neurol Int 4:140
25. Gruber R, Jenny P, Herzog B (1984) Experiences with the anti-siphon device (ASD) in shunt therapy of pediatric hydrocephalus. J Neurosurg 61(1):156–162
26. Gruber RW, Roehrig B (2010) Prevention of ventricular catheter obstruction and slit ventricle syndrome by the prophylactic use of the Integra antisiphon device in shunt therapy for pediatric hypertensive hydrocephalus: a 25-year follow-up study. J Neurosurg Pediatr 5(1):4–16
27. Hahn YS (1994) Use of the distal double-slit valve system in children with hydrocephalus. Childs Nerv Syst 10(2):99–103
28. Hanlo PW, Cinalli G, Vandertop WP, Faber JA, Bøgeskov L, Børgesen SE, Boschert J, Chumas P, Eder H, Pople IK, Serlo W, Vitzthum E (2003) Treatment of hydrocephalus determined by the European Orbis Sigma Valve II survey: a multicenter prospective 5-year shunt survival study in children and adults in whom a flow-regulating shunt was used. J Neurosurg 99(1):52–57
29. Hassan M, Higashi S, Yamashita J (1996) Risks in using siphon-reducing devices in adult patients with normal-pressure hydrocephalus: bench test investigations with Delta valves. J Neurosurg 84(4):634–641
30. Jimenez DF, Keating R, Goodrich JT (1994) Silicone allergy in ventriculoperitoneal shunts. Childs Nerv Syst 10(1):59–63
31. Katano H, Karasawa K, Sugiyama N, Yamashita N, Ohkura A, Kamiya K (2003) Clinical evaluation of shunt implantations using Sophy programmable pressure valves: comparison with Codman-Hakim programmable valves. J Clin Neurosci 10(5):557–561
32. Khan QU, Wharen RE, Grewal SS, Thomas CS, Deen HG Jr, Reimer R, Van Gerpen JA, Crook JE, Graff-Radford NR (2013) Overdrainage shunt complications in idiopathic normal-pressure hydrocephalus and lumbar puncture opening pressure. J Neurosurg 119(6):1498–1502
33. Kiekens R, Mortier W, Pothmann R, Bock WJ, Seibert H (1982) The slit-ventricle syndrome after shunting in hydrocephalic children. Neuropediatrics 13(4):190–194
34. Lemcke J, Meier U, Müller C, Fritsch MJ, Kehler U, Langer N, Kiefer M, Eymann R, Schuhmann MU, Speil A, Weber F, Remenez V, Rohde V, Ludwig HC, Stengel D (2013) Safety and efficacy of gravitational shunt valves in patients with idiopathic normal pressure hydrocephalus: a pragmatic, randomised, open label, multicentre trial (SVASONA). J Neurol Neurosurg Psychiatry 84(8):850–857
35. Lemcke J, Meier U (2010) Improved outcome in shunted iNPH with a combination of a Codman Hakim programmable valve and an Aesculap-Miethke ShuntAssistant. Cent Eur Neurosurg 71(3):113–116
36. Lucantoni D, Magliani V, Galzio R, Zenobii M, Cristuib L (1985) Cranial intraventricular migration of Raimondi uni-shunt system. J Neurosurg Sci 29(2):157–158
37. McCullough DC, Fox JL (1974) Negative intracranial pressure hydrocephalus in adults with shunts and its

relationship to the production of subdural hematoma. J Neurosurg 40(3):372–375

38. McGirt MJ, Buck DW 2nd, Sciubba D, Woodworth GF, Carson B, Weingart J, Jallo G (2007) Adjustable vs set-pressure valves decrease the risk of proximal shunt obstruction in the treatment of pediatric hydrocephalus. Childs Nerv Syst 23(3):289–295
39. Miserocchi G, Sironi VA, Ravagnati L (1984) Anal protrusion as a complication of ventriculo-peritoneal shunt. Case report and review of the literature. J Neurosurg Sci 28(1):43–46
40. Peirce KR, Loeser JD (1975) Perforation of the intestine by a Raimondi peritoneal catheter. Case report. J Neurosurg 43(1):112–113
41. Portnoy HD, Schulte RR, Fox JL, Croissant PD, Tripp L (1973) Anti-siphon and reversible occlusion valves for shunting in hydrocephalus and preventing post-shunt subdural hematomas. J Neurosurg 38(6):729–738
42. Raimondi AJ, Matsumoto S (1967) A simplified technique for performing the ventriculo-peritoneal shunt. Technical note. J Neurosurg 26(3):357–360
43. Raimondi AJ, Robinson JS, Kuwawura K (1977) Complications of ventriculo-peritoneal shunting and a critical comparison of the three-piece and one-piece systems. Childs Brain 3(6):321–342
44. Ringel F, Schramm J, Meyer B (2005) Comparison of programmable shunt valves vs standard valves for communicating hydrocephalus of adults: a retrospective analysis of 407 patients. Surg Neurol 63(1):36–41; discussion 41
45. Sainte-Rose C, Piatt JH, Renier D (1991/1992) Mechanical complications in shunts. Pediatr Neurosurg 17:2–9
46. Sakamoto T, Kojima H, Futawatari K, Kowada M (1986) Spontaneous transection of a Raimondi peritoneal catheter–a case report with scanning electron microscopic study of the transected tube. No Shinkei Geka 14(8):1039–1042
47. Salmon JH (1978) The collapsed ventricle: management and prevention. Surg Neurol 9(6):349–352
48. Sekhar LN, Moossy J, Guthkelch AN (1982) Malfunctioning ventriculoperitoneal shunts. Clinical and pathological features. J Neurosurg 56(3):411–416
49. Turner MS, Goodman J (1989) Extrusion of a Raimondi peritoneal catheter from the thigh. Neurosurgery 25(5):833–834; discussion 835
50. Zachenhofer I, Donat M, Roessler K (2012) The combination of a programmable valve and a subclavicular anti-gravity device in hydrocephalus patients at high risk for hygromas. Neurol Res 34(3):219–222
51. Zemack G, Romner B (2000) Seven years of clinical experience with the programmable Codman Hakim valve: a retrospective study of 583 patients. J Neurosurg 92(6):941–948

Functional Complications: Hyperdrainage

7

Erdal Kalkan, Bülent Kaya, Fatih Erdi, and Ahmet Tuncay Turgut

Contents

7.1 **Introduction** 119
7.2 **Historical Review** 119
7.3 **Incidence** 120
7.4 **The Siphoning Effect** 120
7.5 **Complications of Overdrainage** 120
7.5.1 Extra-axial Fluid or Blood Collections ... 120
7.5.2 Management of Extra-axial Fluid or Blood Collections 122
7.5.3 The Slit Ventricle Syndrome 123
7.5.4 Management of Slit Ventricle Syndrome 124
7.5.5 Premature Closure of Cranial Sutures or Iatrogenic Craniosynostosis 125
References 126

E. Kalkan, MD (✉) • B. Kaya, MD • F. Erdi, MD
Department of Neurosurgery,
Necmettin Erbakan University,
Meram Faculty of Medicine, Konya,
Akyokus/Meram 42080, Turkey
e-mail: erdalkalkan62@yahoo.com;
drbulentkaya1977@gmail.com;
mferdinrs@gmail.com

A.T. Turgut, MD
Department of Radiology,
Ankara Training and Research Hospital,
Ankara TR-06590, Turkey
e-mail: ahmettuncayturgut@yahoo.com

7.1 Introduction

Functional complications including cerebrospinal fluid (CSF) overdrainage represent one of the most frequent complications in both pediatric and adult hydrocephalic shunt-treated patients [1]. The term overdrainage has been previously defined as the excessive evacuation of CSF from the ventricular system [2]. More recently Browd et al. referred overdrainage to several scenarios in which a shunt is functioning properly but is removing more fluid than is necessary for that particular patient [3].

In this chapter, we aimed to identify the functional complication of "overdrainage" in shunted patients and to present strategies for its management.

7.2 Historical Review

Dandy was the first observer of overdrainage in 1932 as immediate and rapid postoperative conduction of CSF which caused intracranial hypotension and collapse of ventricular system, leading to subdural hematomas [4]. Nevertheless, the term 'overdrainage' was first used in the literature by Becker and Nulsen in 1968 in a report on the complications of valvular arterio-venous shunts [5]. In another study, Faulhauer and Schmitz reported 84 patients with symptoms or signs of overdrainage in a series of 400 patients [2]. Later, Pudenz and Foltz published a summary

C. Di Rocco et al. (eds.), *Complications of CSF Shunting in Hydrocephalus: Prevention, Identification, and Management*, DOI 10.1007/978-3-319-09961-3_7,

of the current understanding of overdrainage in 1991 [6]. The relation between overdrainage and siphoning was investigated in this study where intracranial and CSF hydrodynamics during postural changes were examined. In 1995, Aschoff et al. critically compared the different valve types and flow-reducing devices for overcoming overdrainage and concluded that the problem of shunt overdrainage remains unsolved [7].

7.3 Incidence

The reported incidence of symptomatic overdrainage ranges widely from 3 to 71 % in different studies [1]. Long ago, it was concluded that the effects of overdrainage occur at different age groups, but the average incidence is 10–12 % and time of occurrence after first shunting is approximately 6.5 years [6]. Tschan et al. reported an average incidence of 20 % in this context and noted that shunt failures in pediatric population have been attributed to overdrainage in 40 % of patients [1]. Recently, Cheok et al. emphasized the straightforward correlation between overdrainage along with its complications and ventricular shunting [4].

7.4 The Siphoning Effect

Siphoning is a complication of shunting and has been stated as the primary cause of overdrainage [4, 8]. It has been shown that negative intracranial pressure (ICP) values are generated by gravity-dependent drainage [9]. In physiological conditions, CSF circulates within the craniospinal compartment where it is being produced and absorbed. Within this compartment CSF and blood are at the same hydrostatic level at any site of absorption independent from body's position. When the body is horizontal after shunting, the absorbing cavity (pleural, peritoneal, right atrium, etc.) has approximately the same hydrostatic level. However when the body is in vertical position, the absorbing cavity has a lower hydrostatic level and due to this hydrostatic pressure difference, CSF is siphoned down [10].

Hydrostatic pressure difference is related not only with the vertical level of CSF in the craniospinal compartment but also with the fluid level in the absorbing cavity. As a result, the changes in body height and weight affect vertical hydrostatic difference. In addition, the changes in the compliance of either the craniospinal compartment or the absorbing cavity will lead to some changes in the vertical hydrostatic difference. For example, an infant with a large open anterior fontanel or an adult with cranial decompression shows increased craniospinal compliance whereas spinal stenosis, a Chiari type-I malformation, pseudotumor cerebri, or a large intracranial mass lesion could result in a decrease of the craniospinal compliance. Weight loss or extreme constipation is reported to be among factors affecting the intraperitoneal compliance [10].

CSF and blood are transferred from the cranial compartment to the spinal compartment in a balanced fashion when the body is in erect position. The degree of this transition is variable in hydrocephalic patients depending on the localization and the degree of CSF flow obstruction. This variety makes the balanced cotransfer of CSF and blood more complicated and harder to predict.

These interactions may also explain why the effects of overdrainage occur sequentially at different age groups and have different time of occurrence after first shunting [6]. Due to significant variety of these interactions, we cannot easily predict who will develop overdrainage after shunting and which shunting system is entirely favorable.

7.5 Complications of Overdrainage

7.5.1 Extra-axial Fluid or Blood Collections

As the ventricles decrease in size after shunting, the brain/CSF volume decreases in the cranial vault, allowing a space to develop in the subdural space. This space leads to accumulation of fluid or blood around the brain. Most commonly

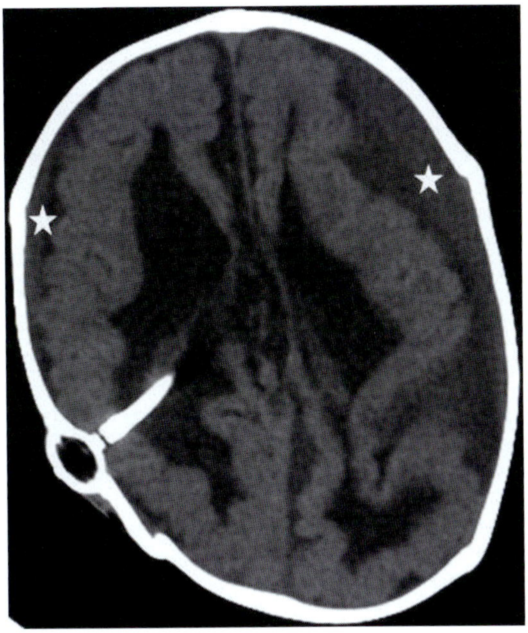

Fig. 7.1 Axial noncontrast computed tomography depicting an example of shunt overdrainage with subsequent development of bilateral extra-axial fluid collection (*asterisks*)

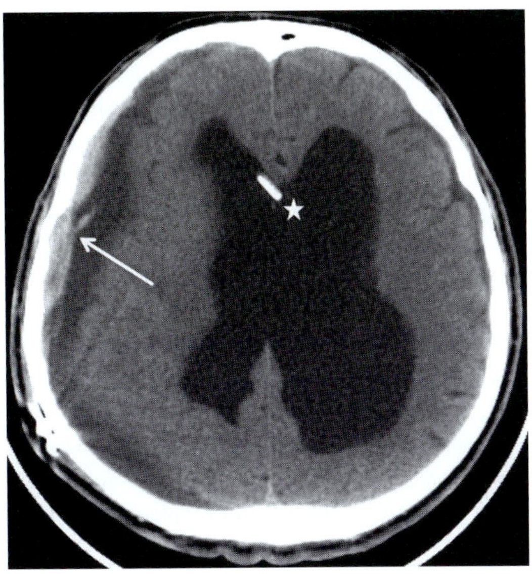

Fig. 7.2 Right frontoparietal hyperdense extra-axial fluid collection (*arrow*) consistent with acute subdural hematoma. *Asterisk* denotes ventricular catheter

benign CSF collections (effusions) are observed (Fig. 7.1); however, the development of subdural hematomas is also possible (Fig. 7.2) [3].

The incidence of subdural hematoma following shunting and effusion varies considerably in the literature. Indeed, asymptomatic postoperative subdural hematomas and effusions have been noted more frequently with wider availability of imaging tools as well as technical advances in neuroradiology [6].

Despite being uncommon, most practitioners have dealt with this complication in the past. Earlier, Faulhauer and Schmitz reported 17 subdural hematomas (4 %) in a series of 400 shunted patients [2]. Only five of these patients required surgical evacuation, which was combined with occlusion of the shunt to promote relative increase in ICP to "occlude" subdural spaces. On the other hand, Drake et al. reported 12 (3.5 %) extra-axial fluid accumulation in a series of 344 shunted patients [11].

The formation of subdural effusions is considered to be a precursor to and/or risk factor for subdural hematoma formation. Clearly, most stable small subdural effusions do not transition into subdural hematomas. However, expanding and/or large (>8 mm) subdural effusions are at higher risk of hemorrhagic condition. Therefore, it is logical to correlate the risk of subdural hematoma formation with the incidence of subdural effusions after shunt procedures [12].

Siphoning has been previously noted to be the major factor for the cause of subdural collections. Multiple valve designs and antisiphon devices have been developed over the years to prevent the effects of siphoning [12]. Nevertheless, the opening pressure of the existing valve seems to be another significant factor having a role in the pathophysiology of subdural collections. A subdural effusion incidence of 70 % was reported in "The Dutch Normal Pressure Hydrocephalus Study" whereas the same incidence was reported to be 30 % with low- and medium-pressure differential pressure valves, respectively, in the aforementioned study [13]. Later, Bergsneider et al. encountered a 4 % incidence among iatrogenic normal pressure hydrocephalus (iNPH) patients with an initial valve setting of 200 mmH_2O and concluded that siphoning played a lesser role in the generation of overdrainage complications with iNPH [12].

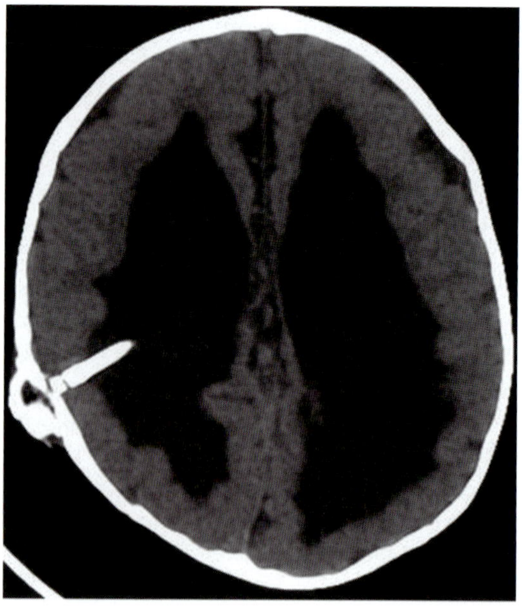

Fig. 7.3 Resolution of extra-axial fluid collection after substituting the initial valve with an adjustable one and setting a higher resistance

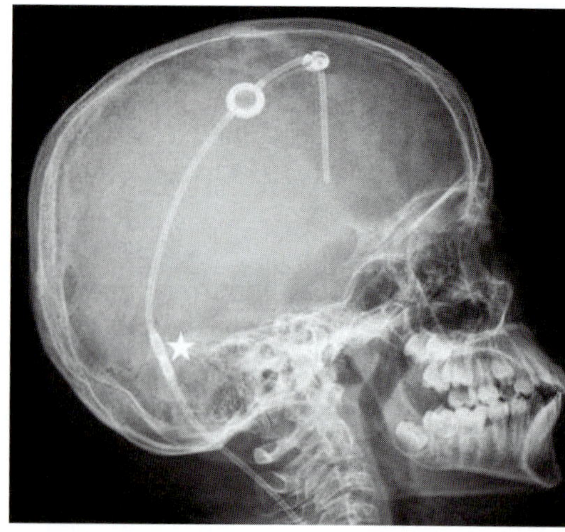

Fig. 7.4 *Asterisk* denotes an antisiphon device which was inserted for preventing overdrainage

7.5.2 Management of Extra-axial Fluid or Blood Collections

Treatment options vary depending on the symptoms, type, and extent of the collection. Mainly three options have been proposed for this purpose. First, it may be possible to manage these collections conservatively if they are small (≤8 mm) with no accompanying brain compression or herniation. Second option is to treat the overdrainage by raising the opening pressure of the shunt's valve. This can be achieved by substituting the valve with a higher resistance one or raise the opening pressure if the valve is adjustable (Fig. 7.3). Alternatively, inserting an antisiphon device can be considered (Fig. 7.4). Finally, the drainage of the extra-axial fluid collection either alone or in combination with second option can be applied as the third alternative [3].

Bergsneider et al. reported their clinical experience in shunted iNPH patients with adjustable valves in some different scenarios [12]. Briefly, they performed the follow-up of the asymptomatic and relatively small effusions (≤8 mm), conservatively. In the presence of moderate effusions (8–15 mm) in asymptomatic patients, it was recommended to raise the initial opening pressure and perform the follow-up with computed tomography (CT). If the patient is symptomatic (headache or focal neurological deficit), it was recommended to act depending on the degree of morbidity. In this regard, it was recommended to raise the initial opening pressure and perform the follow-up with CT in cases with minimal morbidity. If morbidity is moderate/severe, on the other hand, it was recommended to raise the initial opening pressure for smaller subdural effusions. Finally, the placement of a temporary subdural drain or a subdural-peritoneal shunt is reserved for large (>15 mm) or moderate/severe symptomatic collections.

Drainage may be accomplished by a burr hole and a temporary drain or via a subdural catheter that is spliced into the existing shunt system below the valve. This latter system (i.e., combination intraventricular catheter and spliced subdural catheter) commonly results in reexpansion of the brain with resolution of the extra-axial fluid collections. Reexpansion occurs due to relative pressure gradient from the ventricular system to the extra-axial fluid space resulting in brain expansion and obliteration of the subdural space [3].

In the case of a subdural hematoma whether it is primary or associated with the hemorrhagic conversion of subdural effusion, patients should be treated urgently. Accordingly, previous anticoagulation should be reversed and/or antiplatelet medication interrupted. Besides, the application of prophylactic anticonvulsants should be considered. Smaller, asymptomatic subdural hematoma collections can often be resolved after increasing the valve pressure. On the other hand, larger and/or symptomatic subdural hematoma collections typically require surgical evacuation in addition to valve pressure adjustments [12].

This complication is best prevented by avoiding overdrainage through selection of appropriate valve systems. Albeit previous studies showed a reduction of overdrainage by using high-pressure valves or flow-controlled shunts, clinical outcomes were disappointing due to insufficient CSF drainage in the horizontal position [3].

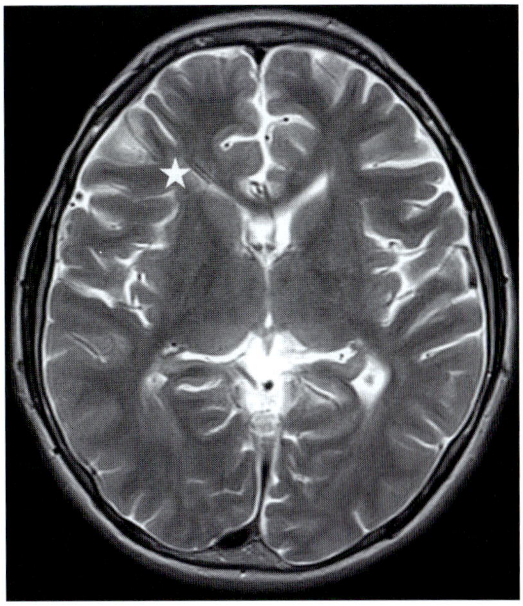

Fig. 7.5 Axial T2-weighted MRI scan demonstrating the collapse of the lateral ventricles in a patient with slit ventricle syndrome. A portion of the shunt ventricular catheter is seen (*asterisk*). The patient presented with signs of shunt failure despite the presence of small, slit-like ventricular system

7.5.3 The Slit Ventricle Syndrome

Although the exact definition of the slit ventricle syndrome (SVS) is unclear in the pediatric neurosurgery literature, the characteristic finding of the syndrome is symptomatic small ventricles. SVS is a condition in which the clinical picture is one of acute or semiacute headache, nausea, vomiting, and/or lethargy. The headache could be episodic, typically presenting as pressure waves, often terminating in vomiting or hyperventilation, and is sometimes associated with bradycardia and systemic hypertension [14]. Browd et al. defined this condition as shunt malfunction in spite of the presence of a patent shunt system [3]. SVS can be seen in both pediatric and adult patients. Clinically, symptomatic, shunted patient with "slit" or collapsed ventricles or intracranial hypertension syndrome without any neuroradiological findings can be seen during the course [3, 12, 14].

Patients with SVS often have a patent shunt system which was inserted several years ago and radiographic studies (CT or MRI) revealed small in size ventricles (Fig. 7.5). Recently, Larysz et al. indicated the importance of appreciating the existence of small ventricles after placement of a ventriculoperitoneal shunt with proper positioning of ventricular catheter for exclusion of intracranial hypertension [14]. Although the incidence of slit ventricle syndrome is low, it accounts for a disproportionate number of shunt revisions and is a common problem in the pediatric neurosurgery literature. Di Rocco et al. reported excessive drainage in less than 1 % of all newly shunted patients [15].

The common complaints of the patients are body position-dependent symptoms such as headaches, nausea, and/or vomiting in the vertical position. These symptoms generally improve quickly by lying down. Orthostatic headaches, dizziness, and/or lack of concentration in school children can be also encountered. This group also showed clinically unclassifiable symptoms such as orthostatic whole body pain or a feeling of heaviness in the legs immediately after standing up [1].

Intermittent proximal catheter obstruction during the course of SVS can lead to intermittent headaches due to fluctuated ICP. An acute presentation with loss of appetite and lethargy can be rarely seen. Augmented fatigue, restlessness, and/or constant weeping in patients younger than 5 years are reported as other symptoms [1].

The patients with SVS has been classified by Rekate into five subgroups: those with (1) extreme low pressure headaches, probably from siphoning of CSF from the brain by the shunt, (2) intermittent obstruction of the proximal shunt catheter, (3) normal volume hydrocephalus with diminished buffering capacity of the CSF, (4) intracranial hypertension associated with working shunts, and (5) headaches (in shunted children) unrelated to intracranial pressure or shunt function [16, 17].

The underlying pathophysiological events leading to SVS have been proposed as overdrainage caused by siphoning at the distal catheter, either by gravity alone or, in the case of atrial or pleural shunts, by negative pressure at the distal end of the catheter tubing [3].

If overdrainage occurs during the period of brain growth, the brain fills the intracranial space completely and the ventricles remain collapsed consequently. This leads to an impairment in brain compliance and intermittent obstruction of the ventricular catheter by the collapsed ventricular system. Obstruction may be symptomatic without a measurable change in ventricle size because of poor compensatory mechanisms. Occasionally this obstruction leads to severe life-threatening complications [3].

The incidence of the SVS is variable among different studies. The Shunt Design Trial demonstrated SVS in only one case out of the 344 patients included to the study (follow-up 1.0–5.5 years, median 3 years) [18]. In a series of 120 patients with ventriculoatrial shunts with a long-term follow-up (average 11 years) an incidence of 1.8 % was reported [19]. It is a well-known phenomenon that SVS occurs generally several years after shunt insertion [20]. Thus, the lower incidence documented in some studies may be related to insufficient follow-up period [3]. Long ago, Sgouros et al. reported a SVS incidence of 10 % among 70 patients with 16-year follow-up [21]. On the contrary, Serlo et al. noted that slit ventricles occurred in 75 of 141 (53 %) patients in their series [22].

Although relatively few shunted patients develop SVS, Browd et al. made a point of the disproportionate number of shunt-related consultations and procedures among these patients [3].

7.5.4 Management of Slit Ventricle Syndrome

7.5.4.1 Medical Treatment

Supine rest during the day in a scheduled period may be beneficial in some patients with mild symptoms. Although it is unclear whether therapeutic success is a reflection of misdiagnosis or of efficacious therapy, antimigraine therapy has offered an alternative first step treatment. The therapeutic effects of antimigraine therapy depend on its stabilizing or reducing effects on cerebral blood flow. By means of these effects the intracranial volume decreases and symptomatic relief occurs [3]. Acetazolamide and in some cases short-term dexamethasone administration has also been used in the setting of SVS [14, 23]. However, it should be remembered that conservative approaches are more appropriate in the setting of infrequent symptoms without limitations of daily activities and can serve as a prompt way of lowering the intracranial pressure as a temporary measure until a decision regarding the surgical procedure.

7.5.4.2 Surgical Treatment

Various surgical options including subtemporal craniectomy, cranial expansion, shunt revision with higher pressure valves, adjustable valves, adding an antisiphon device, third ventriculostomy either endoscopic or not have been proposed in the management of SVS previously [1, 3, 6, 24].

Historically some original techniques have been proposed. Yelin and Ehni suggested that surrounding the ventricular catheter with a perforated red rubber tube prevents obstruction from coaptation of the ventricular walls [25]. Subtemporal craniectomy for the treatment of SVS was introduced by Epstein et al. in 1974 [26]. The authors noted that this procedure makes three important contributions to the management of shunt-dependent children with SVS: First venting of increased ICP, second enlargement of the ipsilateral ventricle, and the last ability of the surgeon to evaluate ICP by observation and palpation of the craniectomy area [26]. Papadakis and Epstein mentioned that the effectiveness of subtemporal craniectomy in venting the ICP reduction is also dependent on the size of the craniectomy and expansibility of the dura mater [27]. Incising the outer layer of dura especially in adults have been advocated for increasing expansibility [26]. More recently Roth et al. used a modified bilateral subtemporal decompression technique with dura and arachnoid opening and found this strategy very curative for severe and resistant SVS [28]. The authors concluded that further cranial expansion may be reserved for children with recurrent SVS symptoms who do not respond to subtemporal decompression and remain with very small ventricles [28].

For the treatment of resistant SVS despite prior treatment with antisiphon devices, addition of shunt valves operating at higher pressures, and subtemporal craniectomy, Reddy et al. recommended third ventriculostomy with cisternal and lamina terminalis opening by a subfrontal approach [29]. This technique was used previously by Cohen with a 15-year patency in 1949 [30].

While the original antisiphon valves (ASV) were reported by Portnoy et al. in 1973 [8], they have become the method of choice in management of SVS with time [6]. Gruber et al. started to use ASV routinely in 1977 in the management of pediatric hydrocephalus patients and achieved effective prevention from siphoning and significant reduction in postoperative ventricular catheter obstruction [31]. They reported four time less annual complication rate after ASV [31].

McLaurin and Olivi mentioned the amendatory effects of implantation of an ASV with upgrading valve resistance in their review of 15 SVS cases [32]. More recently, Browd et al. concluded that shunt revision should be the preferred initial treatment of SVS, based on past experiences [3]. But this option have some special difficulties. First of all, intraventricular catheter revisions in these patients can be difficult due to ventricular collapse. Several technical options have been proposed to cope with this difficulty including dilating the ventricular system under close observation and intracranial pressure monitoring, followed by performing a third ventriculostomy and using endoscopy, fluoroscopy, or stereotaxis during the revision [3].

Endoscopic third ventriculostomy (ETV) is increasingly used for the treatment of shunt-related complications in hydrocephalic patients, particularly if the etiology of the underlying hydrocephalus is of obstructive nature [33].

7.5.5 Premature Closure of Cranial Sutures or Iatrogenic Craniosynostosis

A group of hydrocephalic patients shunted at an early age will develop craniocerebral disproportion, an iatrogenic mismatch between the fixed intracranial volume and the growing brain implying an iatrogenic craniosynostosis [34]. Premature fusion of the sutures was first reported by Strenger in 1963, and since then, ventricular shunting has been a widely recognized cause of secondary craniosynostosis [35, 36]. Faulhauer and Schmitz calculated an overall microcephaly incidence of 6 % in their series of 400 shunted hydrocephalic patients. They noted that the most common skull deformity encountered after shunting was dolichocephaly (sagittal suture synostosis) [2]. Doorenbosch et al. noted an incidence of 1.0–12.4 % in their review and found the dolicocephaly as the most common type of iatrogenic craniosynostosis consistent with previous reports [36]. Different strategies including conservative treatment with close clinico-radiological follow-up, inserting an adjustable valve and raising the opening pressure, strip craniectomies and osteotomies, and other calvarial remodeling techniques have been recommended in previous reports for the management of iatrogenic craniosynostosis [36]. For the surgical treatment an exact radiological, especially CT-proven craniosynostosis diagnosis should be made. It is also recommended to use an adjustable valve and raising the opening pressure for dilating the ventricles postoperatively to prevent the development of a subdural fluid collection [36].

References

1. Tschan CA, Antes S, Huthmann A, Vulcu S, Oertel J, Wagner W (2014) Overcoming CSF overdrainage with the adjustable gravitational valve proSA. Acta Neurochir (Wien) 156(4):767–776
2. Faulhauer K, Schmitz P (1978) Overdrainage phenomena in shunt treated hydrocephalus. Acta Neurochir (Wien) 45(1–2):89–101
3. Browd SR, Gottfried ON, Ragel BT, Kestle JR (2006) Failure of cerebrospinal fluid shunts: part II: overdrainage, loculation, and abdominal complications. Pediatr Neurol 34(3):171–176
4. Cheok S, Chen J, Lazareff J (2014) The truth and coherence behind the concept of overdrainage of cerebrospinal fluid in hydrocephalic patients. Childs Nerv Syst 30(4):599–606
5. Becker DP, Nulsen FE (1968) Control of hydrocephalus by valve-regulated venous shunt: avoidance of complications in prolonged shunt maintenance. J Neurosurg 28(3):215–226
6. Pudenz RH, Foltz EL (1991) Hydrocephalus: overdrainage by ventricular shunts. A review and recommendations. Surg Neurol 35(3):200–212
7. Aschoff A, Kremer P, Benesch C, Fruh K, Klank A, Kunze S (1995) Overdrainage and shunt technology. A critical comparison of programmable, hydrostatic and variable-resistance valves and flow-reducing devices. Childs Nerv Syst 11(4):193–202
8. Portnoy HD, Schulte RR, Fox JL, Croissant PD, Tripp L (1973) Anti-siphon and reversible occlusion valves for shunting in hydrocephalus and preventing post-shunt subdural hematomas. J Neurosurg 38(6):729–738
9. Chapman PH, Cosman ER, Arnold MA (1990) The relationship between ventricular fluid pressure and body position in normal subjects and subjects with shunts: a telemetric study. Neurosurgery 26(2):181–189
10. Kurtom KH, Magram G (2007) Siphon regulatory devices: their role in the treatment of hydrocephalus. Neurosurg Focus 22(4):E5
11. Drake JM, Kestle JR, Milner R, Cinalli G, Boop F, Piatt J Jr, Haines S, Schiff SJ, Cochrane DD, Steinbok P, MacNeil N (1998) Randomized trial of cerebrospinal fluid shunt valve design in pediatric hydrocephalus. Neurosurgery 43(2):294–303
12. Bergsneider M, Miller C, Vespa PM, Hu X (2008) Surgical management of adult hydrocephalus. Neurosurgery 62(Suppl 2):643–659
13. Boon AJ, Tans JT, Delwel EJ, Egeler-Peerdeman SM, Hanlo PW, Wurzer HA, Avezaat CJ, de Jong DA, Gooskens RH, Hermans J (1998) Dutch Normal-Pressure Hydrocephalus Study: randomized comparison of low- and medium-pressure shunts. J Neurosurg 88(3):490–495
14. Larysz D, Larysz P, Klimczak A, Mandera M (2010) Is neuroradiological imaging sufficient for exclusion of intracranial hypertension in children? Intracranial hypertension syndrome without evident radiological symptoms. Acta Neurochir Suppl 106:203–208
15. Di Rocco C, Marchese E, Velardi F (1994) A survey of the first complication of newly implanted CSF shunt devices for the treatment of nontumoral hydrocephalus. Cooperative survey of the 1991–1992 Education Committee of the ISPN. Childs Nerv Syst 10(5):321–327
16. Rekate HL (1993) Classification of slit-ventricle syndromes using intracranial pressure monitoring. Pediatr Neurosurg 19(1):15–20
17. Rekate HL (2008) Shunt-related headaches: the slit ventricle syndromes. Childs Nerv Syst 24(4):423–430
18. Kestle J, Drake J, Milner R, Sainte-Rose C, Cinalli G, Boop F, Piatt J, Haines S, Schiff S, Cochrane D, Steinbok P, MacNeil N (2000) Long-term follow-up data from the Shunt Design Trial. Pediatr Neurosurg 33(5):230–236
19. Vernet O, Campiche R, de Tribolet N (1995) Long-term results after ventriculo-atrial shunting in children. Childs Nerv Syst 11(3):176–179
20. Major O, Fedorcsák I, Sipos L, Hantos P, Kónya E, Dobronyi I, Paraicz E (1994) Slit-ventricle syndrome in shunt operated children. Acta Neurochir (Wien) 127(1–2):69–72
21. Sgouros S, Malluci C, Walsh AR, Hockley AD (1995) Long-term complications of hydrocephalus. Pediatr Neurosurg 23(3):127–132
22. Serlo W, Saukkonen AL, Heikkinen E, von Wendt L (1989) The incidence and management of the slit ventricle syndrome. Acta Neurochir (Wien) 99(3–4): 113–116
23. Fattal-Valevski A, Beni-Adani L, Constantini S (2005) Short-term dexamethasone treatment for symptomatic slit ventricle syndrome. Childs Nerv Syst 21(11):981–984
24. Chernov MF, Kamikawa S, Yamane F, Ishihara S, Hori T (2005) Neurofiberscope-guided management of slit-ventricle syndrome due to shunt placement. J Neurosurg 102(3 Suppl):260–267
25. Yelin FS, Ehni G (1969) Percallosal sump ventriculostomy for shunt-dependent hydrocephalic patient with small ventricles. Case report. J Neurosurg 31(5): 570–573
26. Epstein FJ, Fleischer AS, Hochwald GM, Ransohoff J (1974) Subtemporal craniectomy for recurrent shunt obstruction secondary to small ventricles. J Neurosurg 41(1):29–31
27. Papadakis N, Epstein F (1975) Letter: subtemporal craniectomy for recurrent shunt obstruction. J Neurosurg 42(1):115–117
28. Roth J, Biyani N, Udayakumaran S, Xiao X, Friedman O, Beni-Adani L, Constantini S (2011) Modified bilateral subtemporal decompression for resistant slit ventricle syndrome. Childs Nerv Syst 27(1):101–110
29. Reddy K, Fewer HD, West M, Hill NC (1988) Slit ventricle syndrome with aqueduct stenosis: third ventriculostomy as definitive treatment. Neurosurgery 23(6):756–759
30. Cohen I (1949) Third ventriculostomy proven patent after 15 years. J Neurosurg 6(1):89–94

31. Gruber R, Jenny P, Herzog B (1984) Experiences with the anti-siphon device (ASD) in shunt therapy of pediatric hydrocephalus. J Neurosurg 61(1):156–162
32. McLaurin RL, Olivi A (1987) Slit-ventricle syndrome: review of 15 cases. Pediatr Neurosci 13(3): 118–124
33. Boschert JM, Krauss JK (2006) Endoscopic third ventriculostomy in the treatment of shunt-related overdrainage: Preliminary experience with a new approach how to render ventricles navigable. Clin Neurol Neurosurg 108(2):143–149
34. Weinzweig J, Bartlett SP, Chen JC, Losee J, Sutton L, Duhaime AC, Whitaker LA (2008) Cranial vault expansion in the management of postshunt craniosynostosis and slit ventricle syndrome. Plast Reconstr Surg 122(4):1171–1180
35. Strenger L (1963) Complications of ventriculovenous shunts. J Neurosurg 20:219–224
36. Doorenbosch X, Molloy CJ, David DJ, Santoreneos S, Anderson PJ (2009) Management of cranial deformity following ventricular shunting. Childs Nerv Syst 25(7):871–874

8 Mechanical Complications of Shunts

Vasilios Tsitouras and Spyros Sgouros

Contents

8.1 **Fracture** 129
8.1.1 Epidemiology 129
8.1.2 The Implanted Material 130
8.1.3 Material Selection and Importance of the Hardware 132
8.1.4 Surgical Technique 133

8.2 **Dislocation** 134
8.2.1 Proximal Catheter 134
8.2.2 Distal Catheter 135
8.2.3 Presentation 137
8.2.4 Management 137

References 138

V. Tsitouras, MD
Department of Neurosurgery,
"Mitera" Childrens Hospital, Athens, Greece

S. Sgouros, MD (✉)
Department of Neurosurgery,
"Mitera" Childrens Hospital, Athens, Greece

Department of Neurosurgery,
University of Athens, Athens, Greece
e-mail: sgouros@med.uoa.gr

8.1 Fracture

8.1.1 Epidemiology

Fractures or ruptures of the shunt catheters are the causative events of 4.5–13.6 % of shunt revision surgeries [46, 63]. Besides the contribution to patients' morbidity, there is an increased impact to health care costs, considering the large numbers of patients with CSF shunts and the cumulative long time that these shunts are implanted for. An accurate conclusion regarding the exact impact of mechanical complications to shunt malfunction is difficult to draw because these problems usually present a few years after the implantation and many patients are lost to follow-up. In addition, in a group of patients with such fractures or disconnections the clinical impact is minimal or unnoticed because either the patient has become shunt-independent or the CSF diversion is still patent through a fibrous reactive sleeve over the damaged catheter [75]. Furthermore, although a great amount of research focuses on shunt infection issues, mechanical dysfunction has not gained proportionate attention in the literature over the years.

A large series of 1,719 patients shunted for hydrocephalus and followed for 10 years showed that the overall risk for shunt malfunction at the end of the study was 70 % [63]. The most frequent cause was obstruction (56 %), followed by fracture, disconnection, and late migration which accounted for 19 % of mechanical complications

C. Di Rocco et al. (eds.), *Complications of CSF Shunting in Hydrocephalus: Prevention, Identification, and Management*, DOI 10.1007/978-3-319-09961-3_8,

occurring in 13 % of the children. It was similarly noticed that such complications occurred mostly in children, treated in their early age for hydrocephalus and these catheters were placed for longer periods (>5 years) [9].

8.1.2 The Implanted Material

Materials have a wide spectrum of properties that are used to describe and quantify their features. These properties can be thermal, electrical, chemical, mechanical, etc. For materials that are used in medicine and more specifically for implantable human purposes, all these properties are important and this section will focus on the mechanical characteristics of silicone rubbers and their correlation with the host's reaction (humans) in their presence.

Polysiloxanes are mixed inorganic and organic polymers mostly known as *silicon rubber* [49]. These are based on a silicon and oxygen skeleton, instead of an organic carbon chain skeleton. Silicon as an element was first discovered in 1824 by J.J. Berzelius, but it was in the 1940s that F.S. Kipping (the father of silicon science) achieved extensive synthesis of silicone compounds and allowed the industrial production of the new material. The high resistance to heat made it superior for medical use because its physical properties were not affected by thermal sterilization. Its high flexibility and biocompatibility made silicon well suited for in vivo implantation use [23]. In the early 1950s, the silicon rubber marketed for medical use was Silastic® (Dow Corning, Midland, MI). In neurosurgery, it was introduced as the tubing material of the newly presented CSF diversion systems for the treatment of hydrocephalus, at the end of the same decade. Since then, silicon rubber has been the material that was used almost exclusively by the manufacturers of CSF shunt systems.

Calcification

It is the first step of the process that leads to: (1) degradation and weakness of the catheter and (2) cell aggregation and tethering of the tube to the surrounding tissue. The phenomenon was well studied after the first malfunctions of several silicon-made implants appeared (cardiac prostheses, breast implants) [17, 32, 34]. When the local concentration of an insoluble compound into a solution exceeds the limit of solubility, then *precipitation* of the compound from the solution occurs [9, 65, 67]. The following stages are the formation of a small *nucleus* of precipitate and then the growth of it by continuous precipitation (Fig. 8.1). This nucleation process is enhanced by the presence of solid interfaces and, especially for the precipitation of *calcium phosphate,* is accelerated in an alkaline environment [33]. Two mechanisms of calcification are known [65, 84]: *Metastatic calcification* is associated with increased calcium and phosphorus blood concentrations and is described in renal insufficiency; and *dystrophic calcification* has normal calcium and phosphorus blood concentrations but altered cellular metabolism and is the one encountered in silicone implants. An accelerated formation of nuclei from the cellular debris that accumulate in proximity to the implant has been demonstrated [9, 32]. Further formation of initial nuclei results from cracks and surface irregularities of the material which allow element extrusion and interaction with the surrounding cells.

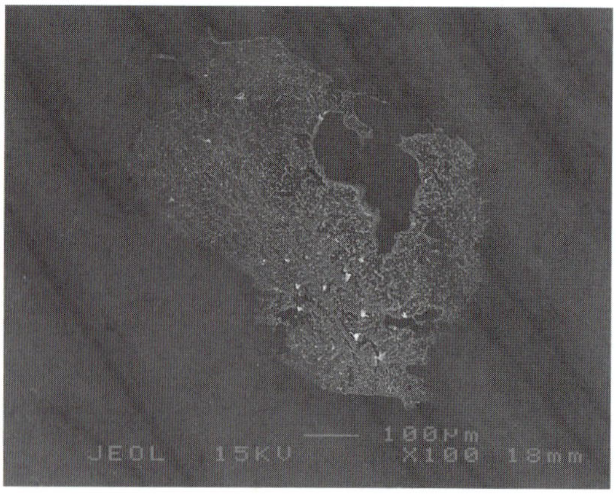

Fig. 8.1 Scanning Electron Microscopy of a shunt valve of diaphragm type, removed from a patient due to shunt malfunction. There is precipitation of crystals on the diaphragm, which with time deteriorates and interferes with the physical properties of the membrane and can block the gap between diaphragm and case (magnification ×100)

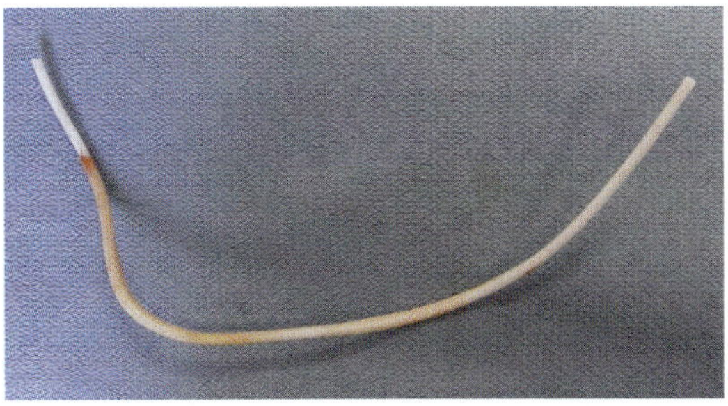

Fig. 8.2 Distal catheter removed during shunt revision. There is obvious calcification on its outer surface at the area corresponding to the neck region, where the shunt was implanted

Immune Response

Investigation of previously implanted shunts revealed eosinophils and giant cells as parts of the fibrous sleeve, indicating that a hypersensitivity reaction occurs [74]. Most of these studies applied plain radiographs, scanning electron microscopy (SEM), spectral analysis, and simple histology. The cell-mediated immunity was supported from the presence of T-cell granulomas. Others have found immunoglobulin G antibodies specifically directed against silicon, as a part of humoral immunity involvement [30]. On the other hand, some investigators only found dense hyalinized connective tissue with fibroblasts and calcific deposits [85]. Heggers et al. supported a chronic inflammatory reaction – predominantly a foreign body giant cell granuloma type – that was initiated from the release of silicon particles from the aging material [34, 38]. Some authors support that different kind of particles are responsible for the foreign body reaction such as cotton fibers, talc granules, and hair that inadvertently enter the host during surgery [66]. The most profound tissue reaction over the ventriculoperitoneal (VP) shunt tubing was noticed at the subcutaneous course of the catheter and especially at the neck area [9, 75] (Fig. 8.2). Calcification was present only in catheters placed in subcutaneous or vascular areas [46]. It is supported that the cerebral parenchyma and the peritoneal cavity are far less reactive for the silicon catheters [42]. This suits well with the "cellular reaction" theory since the subcutaneous tissue and the intravascular space are areas where migration of immunocompetent cells can occur but it does not explain the lack of calcification in the peritoneal cavity. Furthermore, some case reports of distal catheter insertion into abdominal hollow viscera suggest that a key point for that is the anchoring of the catheter to the organ serosa, which appears to be initiated by a local inflammatory reaction around the distal tip that facilitates erosion and perforation [41, 53, 64]. The clear mechanism is not yet fully understood. Regarding the most proximal compartment of the host involved, there is no cellular immunity in the cerebral parenchyma (similar to the one described for the rest of the body) and ventricular catheters do not induce a gliotic reaction inside the brain tissue as noticed by the absence of adherent cells on the silicone [9, 19].

Degradation and Altered Physical Properties

The interaction of the silicone catheter with the surrounding tissue leads to the calcification of tube. The implant becomes rigid and fragile. Besides the calcified covering sheet, the degradation process evolves. It has been shown that the dynamic properties of the silicon rubber begin to deteriorate about 6 months after the implantation; the ultimate tensile strength and extensibility gradually decreases over the first 3 years and becomes remarkably altered after 5 years [23, 76]. Different studies have found reticulation damage as an important factor [9, 23]. The four ways that biopolymers deteriorate were described by Kronenthal [43]: (a) the structure is altered by hydration; (b) some covalent bonds of the chain are weakened; (c) these bonds are broken; and (c) soluble fragments are digested by the macrophages. In the human body, the silicones are not subjected to extreme temperatures or irradiation, which are known to contribute to degradation, but the subsequent chemical and mechanical insults (especially in prolonged time periods) can have the same result. This is more evident in prosthetic heart valves that are exposed to strong biological activity (blood cells) and intense mechanical stress (heart beats and blood flow) [65, 78]. In VP (and ventriculoatrial – VA) shunts, the more mobile segment is in the neck [23, 46]. Repeatable head movements – especially extension and contralateral rotation – increase the tension of the mobile neck segment over the fixed parts. The three more vulnerable zones were found to be: (a) the connection between the distal catheter and the reservoir or the valve, (b) the point of traversing the galea, and (c) the crossing of the clavicle [24]. Shunts that are inserted in young children and remain for long time periods are exposed to additional mechanical stress due to the increasing height of the child. The vulnerable part is this case is from the occiput to the peritoneal insertion [24] (Fig. 8.3). There are reports that even a minimal-to-moderate external tension over the tethered and weakened catheter led to fracture as it was the case in two boys where the shunt was fractured over the occipital area after a haircut with clippers [45]. In addition, children have a greater tendency for shunt calcification from a physiological point of view and this maybe related to the increased serum phosphorus levels, compared to adults [9, 18]. A reduction in catheter tubing tensile strength and extensibility was demonstrated when the apparatus had been implanted for more than 6 years [23]. These changes were related to mineralization of the catheter, which resulted in a 30–40 % reduction in tubing thickness. Similar findings were reported from Tomes et al. who showed that catheters become weaker the longer they are implanted and that tubing with a greater cross-sectional area requires greater force to fracture [79].

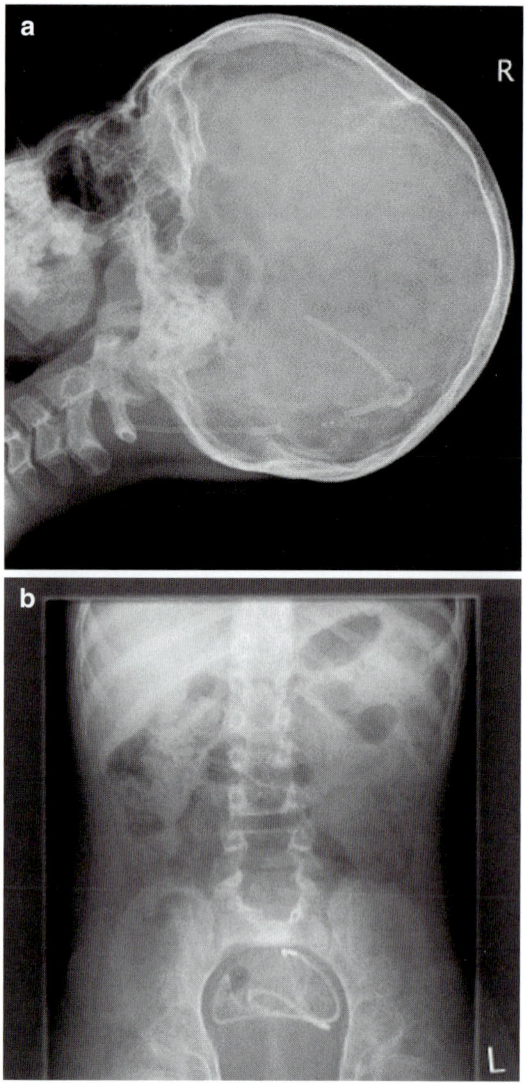

Fig. 8.3 Distal catheter fracture in the region of the neck. Plain radiographs of a 10-year-old boy, who had a shunt inserted when he was 6 months old, and he presented on this occasion with symptoms of raised intracranial pressure. (**a**) Lateral skull radiograph. The distal shunt tube is abruptly discontinued in the neck region, a few centimeters below the valve. (**b**) Abdominal plain radiograph. The remaining distal tube has "fallen" in the peritoneal cavity and coiled up at the region of Douglas pouch

8.1.3 Material Selection and Importance of the Hardware

As previously mentioned, there are reports of allergy to the implanted silicone catheters [35, 36]. In these cases, the presentation was similar to shunt infection or obstruction, but the importance is that the authors used as an alternative catheters that were made from *polyurethane*. Until recently, such choice was not available. Polyurethane is a polymer composed of a chain of organic units joined by carbamate (urethane) links. It shares many properties with silicone such as heat resistance, which allows it to be thermally sterilized, high biocompatibility, low toxicity, and high tensile strength. On the other hand, it is more rigid, making such systems less easy to manufacture than silicone-based ones [35]. Polyurethane breast implants tended to produce thicker and longer-lasting surrounding capsules compared to the silicon-based ones [70].

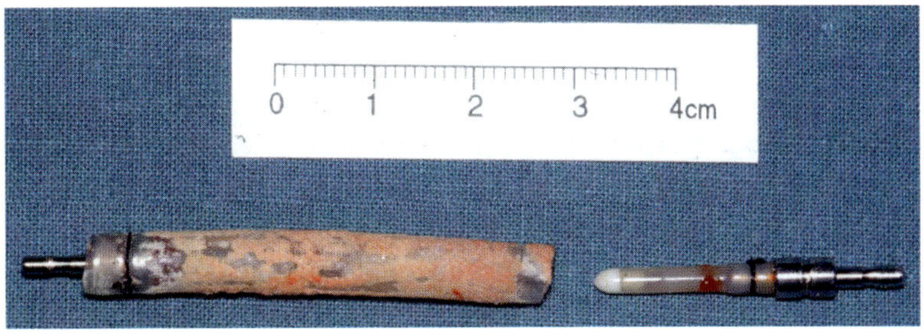

Fig. 8.4 Shunt valve of Holter type, removed during shunt revision, 20 years after implantation. The valve case has completely disintegrated due to material distruction. Extensive calcification is seen on the outer surface

On the field of CSF diversion shunt systems, the two materials have not yet been properly compared on a clinical basis.

In order to be radiographically visualized after implantation, shunt catheters must be either homogeneously *impregnated with barium* or only have a stripe of it. It has been demonstrated that barium precipitates locally as barium salts, enhancing the local immune response and increasing the focal tethering effect and subsequently the risk for catheter fracture [9]. Furthermore, catheters with barium that were tested for their tensile strength without being previously implanted, showed significantly lower values in terms of both ultimate strain and ultimate stress [79]. Similar reports were not found regarding *antibiotic-impregnated* shunt catheters. It is not mentioned if their physical properties are altered in vitro due to the presence of the antibiotics. Aryan et al. did not find significant local reaction in such externalized catheters [6]. It is unknown if their long-term fracture rates are different from the conventional type of catheters.

The valve type may influence the mechanical features and durability of the shunt system. The valve *profile* has a major impact [9]. A tubular valve in the catheter line may have a tendency to migrate especially in a growing child as it is pulled by a fixed calcified catheter. Round-bodied valves are more resistant to migration distally. If such valves are placed in the hypochondriac region (to prevent cranial MRI artifacts and skin erosion issues), there is a tendency to fracture at the side of the outlet connector as this is the point of maximal stress force due to the continuous abdominal movements over the fixed valve [2]. Shunt failure caused by valve collapse has been reported in the past [50] (Fig. 8.4) and regarded 11 patients with the Mini-Holter valve where intussusception of the valve ends into the valve tubing was noticed, possibly due to the siphoning effect. The same type of valve was mechanically disrupted in a case report in which the proximal metallic portion was "dislocated" out of its silicone sheath, possibly due to the growth-related traction applied to the fixed valve [86]. In a recent retrospective study, the fixed pressure–gravity-assisted valve paediGAV (Aesculap AG & Co. KG, Tuttligen, Germany) and the programmable differential pressure Codman Hakim (Codman &Shurtlef, Inc., Raynham, USA) were compared and there was no significant difference regarding shunt failure of mechanical etiology [7].

A critical point in mechanical complications of shunts is *the number of shunt components*. The more the pieces connected to each other, the higher the failure rates [3]. A typical shunt includes one proximal catheter, connected to a reservoir or a burr-hole-type valve and a distal catheter connected to the valve. This means two components with one connection at best, but frequently three components with two connections. In a review of 275 shunt revisions, disconnection of the system accounted for 15 % of the malfunctions [3]. It was also found that the more distal the connection was from the ventricle, the higher the likelihood of disconnection. One-piece shunt systems are described to decrease early fractures and disconnections by avoiding distal connectors [31, 59].

8.1.4 Surgical Technique

Although significant amount of data have highlighted the contribution of the surgical technique in the prevention of shunt infection and obstruction, too little evidence exists regarding the correlation of mechanical complications and surgical choices or maneuvers [22]. When shunts other than one piece are utilized, an important determinant is the competence of the connection between two parts. Most times this requires reinforcement with surgical knots. The knots have to be strong enough to secure the connection but not too tight to prevent rupture of the catheter or the suture. The choice of the suture material may have an impact. Multifilament nonabsorbable sutures are mostly preferred (Silk). They are better manipulated with minimal memory effect. Monofilament sutures are regarded safer for the prevention of infection (bacteria are attached less easily compared to multifilament material) but may tear the silicon tube. For the same reason, the size of the suture is also important. Sizes 2-0 or 3-0 are preferred. The knot has to be efficient but not too big and preferably should face downward so that it is hidden in cases of thin-skinned patients [37, 72].

Several studies and reviews highlight the significance of handling the shunt components only with instruments, avoiding any contact with gloved hands, to reduce the infection rates [10, 11, 71, 81]. If these instruments are sharp and improperly used, they may tear the shunt catheters leading to shunt malfunction if the damage is not noticed. Similarly, when passing the catheter through the tunneler, an acute angle of insertion should be avoided in order to prevent abrasions to the tube caused by the sharp end of the tunneler. Lubrication of the catheter with sterile saline is a useful maneuver. When performing a shunt revision (i.e., for proximal obstruction) many surgeons use a scalpel blade to cut the knot and disconnect the shunt components. This is hazardous for the catheter's integrity and should be performed with great caution if there is no option for insertion of new hardware. The surgeon must target the knot – not the thread – and the direction of the movement should be away from the catheter. After that, the tube is inspected for unnoticed tears. If such exist, a small piece of the catheter – containing the tear – is cut away and the rest is reconnected as usual.

The choice of the burr-hole site may influence the mechanical complications rate. As previously explained, a shunt with a frontal burr hole usually needs an additional connection and this adds to the failure likelihood. On the other hand, Aldrich et al. found that occipitally placed shunts have a significantly higher rate of dislocation than frontally placed shunts [3]. Langmoen et al. studied the differences between ventriculoperitoneal and ventriculoatrial shunts with respect to the problem of mechanical failures and they found that the fracture rates of the distal catheter were almost the same (2.9–3 %) [46].

8.2 Dislocation

Dislocation of a shunt component refers to the migration of a previously correctly placed catheter or valve. The component could be disconnected from the shunt system or not. There is a lack of uniformly applied definitions regarding mechanical complications of shunts. In addition, there is paucity in the recent literature about this specific type of shunt malfunction. Most authors focus on the rheological properties of these systems.

The prevalence of pediatric shunt malfunction was reported to be 39 % at the first year and 53 % at 2 years [21]. The rate of shunt discontinuity (fracture or disconnection) is up to 10 % and refers to either ventriculoperitoneal or subduroperitoneal shunts [48]. Migrations of proximal or distal catheters have been reported on case reports and accurate frequencies extracted from efficient series or reviews are missing.

8.2.1 Proximal Catheter

The dislocated proximal catheter could enter deeper into the cranial cavity or retract distally from the previously desired location. Most systems include an angled port where the distal part of the ventricular catheter is secured in a 90° position before the connection to the distal part. Others prefer to use burr-hole reservoirs or burr-hole-type valves which are connected to the ventricular catheter. The connection should be secured with a suture properly knotted. This connection is not always straightforward, especially in cases of slitlike ventricles where even minimal manipulation of the proximal catheter can lead to improper placement. A loose connection of the ventricular catheter may result in spontaneous proximal migration. This can also happen iatrogenically in future shunt revisions when one tries to lift the burr-hole reservoir or valve and misses the disconnected catheter. Besides the surgical aspect, recently the material of the catheter was found to be responsible for the disconnection and intracranial migration [15]. The Bioglide® catheter (Medtronic, Minneapolis, US-MN) designed to potentially decrease cell adhesion and thereby reduce shunt obstruction or infection by becoming hydrophilic and lubricious when hydrated, was prone to disconnection because of this slippery surface. It was eventually recalled by Medtronic in 2009.

8.2.2 Distal Catheter

The most case reports in the literature concerning catheter migration are about the distal ventriculoperitoneal components. The distal catheter in the majority of VP shunts starts from the distal end of the valve – usually located occipitally or frontally – and ends into the peritoneal cavity in a variety of lengths, related to the manufacturer's guidelines and the surgeon's preferences. The length varies from 15 to 120 cm. Some surgeons prefer to cut short the catheter especially in newborns. The long tube and the intestinal peristaltic movements were considered responsible in rare cases of spontaneous knot formation [14, 41]. On the other hand, short catheters may add to overdrainage as explained by the Poisseuille law. A intra-abdominal length of 30–40 cm is sufficient.

The distal catheter can migrate either distally from its previous position or proximally in a retrograde direction. As already mentioned, it can be disconnected from the shunt system or not. Usually it remains coiled into the peritoneal cavity (if disconnected) or a herniated loop protrudes

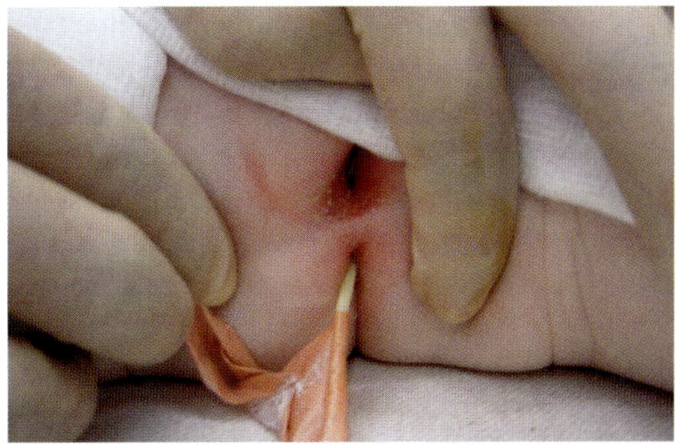

Fig. 8.5 Extrusion of distal shunt catheter through the anus, on a 28-month-old girl. The shunt was inserted in the peritoneal cavity 12 months before, through open mini-laparotomy (not with trocar)

through the peritoneal incision and part of it is fixed subcutaneously. There are case reports of distal catheter dislocation in almost every compartment of the human body. In the peritoneal cavity, the catheter can entry a hollow [40] or (much more rarely) a solid viscus [80]. The large intestine is the more probable entry site [28] and from there it protrudes through the anus. In cases of stomach perforation, transoral protrusions have been reported [8]. Additional reports include urinary bladder perforation and transurethreal protrusion [13], dislocation through the vagina [55], into the gallbladder [58], the scrotum [60], and extrusion through the abdominal wall [82], the umbilicus [1] and the lumbar region [39].

Several theories have been presented in order to explain the "transperitoneal" dislocations of the distal catheters. One is the iatrogenic perforation of the intestine during the insertion of the shunt. Some surgeons use the trocar technique, which may predispose to this complication in inexperienced hands [29]. Studies that compared mini-laparotomy and laparoscopic-assisted insertion techniques, failed to show an advantage of one against the other [44]. In obese patients and in multiple peritoneal reoperations, the laparoscopic-assisted technique should be strongly considered [29]. In general, anal protrusion of the catheter can have an early (a few weeks) or delayed presentation (from months to years) (Fig. 8.5). The "iatrogenic" theory applies mostly in the early presentation cases. For delayed presentations different explanations are given. Spring-coiled catheters had a higher tendency to relate with bowel perforation. The plain silicone catheters can initiate an allergic reaction and become adherent to the intestinal serosa with subsequent erosion into the lumen [12]. Local infective adhesions were also mentioned [53]. Some authors recommend the hydration of the silicon tube prior to insertion based on the tendency of the silicon rubber to become sticky when it remains in a dry state [41]. Another theory focuses on children with myelomeningoceles (MMC), which are reported to be more susceptible to bowel perforation due to their weaker intestinal musculature [25]. Glatstein et al. in 2011 reviewed the reported pediatric cases with catheter protrusions through the anus and showed 23 patients with ages ranging from 0.9 to 72 months (6 years) [29]. Sathyanarayana et al. in 2000 reviewed 45 adult patients and reported a bowel perforation rate of less than 0.1 % in VP shunt insertions [64].

A retrograde migration of the peritoneal catheter is also well described. In these cases, the tube can end at the thoracoabdominal subcutaneous tissue (Fig. 8.6), the breast [69], the heart [57, 61], the lateral ventricle [4, 52], the subdural space [77], or extruded through the neck incision [83]. The mechanism here is more complex and multifactorial. The migration may be the result of abdominal wall contractions that can expel the shunt catheter into the fibrous tract surrounding the catheter [69]. Increased intraabdominal pressure due to obesity, constipation, or pseudocyst formation may contribute. Anchoring of the shunt tube to a more proximal calcified point may act like a "windlass" resulting in traction of the tube. The retained memory effect of the catheters that are coiled into the manufacturer's package could be another possible explanation [20]. Forceful rotation or flexion–extension movements of the head and neck can pull out the distal catheter from the peritoneal cavity [69]. In girls the distal tube that is tunneled closely to the breast may become adherent to it and eventually, when the breast grows, can – theoretically – facilitate the upward migration of the catheter. Similar result can have the deterioration of severe scoliosis in the calcified shunt.

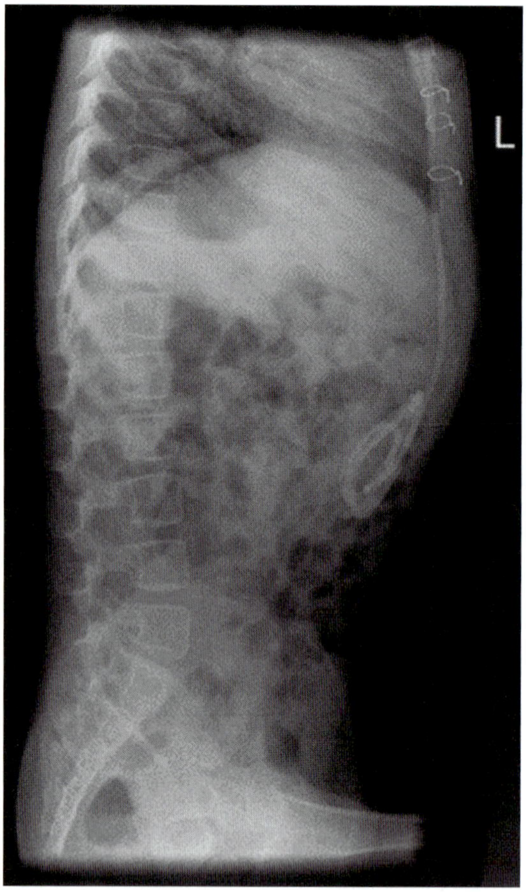

Fig. 8.6 Lateral abdominal radiograph of a 5-year-old girl who presented a few months after shunt insertion with symptoms of raised intracranial pressure. The distal catheter has coiled up in the region of the abdominal wound, outside the peritoneal cavity

The migration of the distal tube into the heart or more distally in the pulmonary vasculature is also described. Until 2011, there were 13 reported cases [57]. One mechanism proposed transvenous placement of the catheter, followed by proximal migration into the pulmonary artery. The transvenous placement must have occurred during the initial subcutaneous tunneling and further migration due to negative intrathoracic pressure and venous flow [26]. A different mechanism involved chronic erosion of a neck vein by the adherent shunt tube with subsequent proximal migration into the pulmonary artery [54].

The migration of a lumboperitoneal shunt catheter intracranially has also been described.

In this case report [5], it occurred 10 months after the insertion and the tip of it was found in the deep parenchymal structures. Possibly it was caused by spinocerebral CSF flow.

8.2.3 Presentation

Fractures, disconnections, and dislocations of shunt components usually present as shunt malfunctions. But they do not always become clinically evident. In a retrospective study it was found that from the 25 cases of disconnections in 22 patients, only 9 (40.9 %) had nonfunctioning shunts and these shunts were removed in 8 patients [48]. In the above mentioned study, only 3 out of 9 patients with nonfunctioning shunts had no symptoms [48]. It should be kept in mind that shunt failure is a neurosurgical emergency until proven otherwise and that a high index of suspicion must be maintained when receiving a shunted patient with symptoms [56]. A patient shunted in his early childhood for posthemorrhagic hydrocephalus or after MMC closure and presents after a few years with evidence of shunt disconnection is extremely likely to have signs and symptoms of increased intracranial pressure. All these patients should have proper clinical evaluation, including fundoscopy. On the other hand, many disconnections are found incidentally, usually in scheduled follow-up. The typical finding is the discontinuation of the radiolucent catheter strip, between the retroauricular area and the clavicle, in a formal shunt series (plain X-ray films). Less frequently, the ventricular catheter is found disconnected from its burr-hole attachment.

In specific cases of migration, the clinical findings are related to the organ or body compartment that is involved. External protrusion or extrusion is evident by the caregivers and often has minimal clinical sequelae. Worsening respiratory distress and "butterflies in the chest" were findings in patients with migration to the pulmonary vasculature [57]. Recurrent pneumonia was the result of a dislocated distal catheter into the lung [62] and several authors have reported CSF galactorrhea because of a distal catheter that migrated into the breast [47, 51].

8.2.4 Management

As already mentioned, a patient with a disconnected shunt should be treated with great caution, even if he/she remains asymptomatic. Besides the shunt series, Computed Tomography (CT) or Magnetic Resonance Imaging (MRI) are crucial in order to compare the findings with previous scan and appreciate any changes in the ventricular size and the subarachnoid spaces. The imaging features of the third ventricle morphology should be reviewed, in case an endoscopic third ventriculostomy (ETV) becomes an alternative option. Radionuclide shuntograms are reported to provide additional information, but are rarely performed in practice. Shunt taps are used so that the functional status of the system is assessed. Attempts to use ultrasound to verify shunt function have not been established in routine clinical practice [68]. The most reliable technique to diagnose shunt malfunction is the intraoperative exploration. A disconnected system can be replaced as a whole or in parts. Additional connections should be avoided. In all the cases, the patient is prepared and draped as if a revision of the whole system is planned.

The finding of a disconnected shunt can be a chance for the patient to become shunt free. Of course, this should be attempted with caution in selected cases. Iannelli et al. [36] showed that in 17 out of 27 children (63 %), they detected CSF shunt independency at the time of a scheduled catheter lengthening procedure. The spectrum of candidates for an ETV is becoming wider and should always be kept in mind as an alternative. Neuroendoscopy can be applied in cases of intraventricular migration of proximal catheters. Usually, the burr hole is enlarged so that the endoscope can be inserted and with a grasping forceps the catheter can be grabbed and retrieved. If that becomes difficult it should be left behind and followed.

In the specific cases of externally protruded catheters, the decision making is more straightforward. CSF samples are sent for analysis, microbiology, and cultures. If there is clinical or laboratory evidence of infection the whole system is removed, an external drain is inserted, and antibiotics are administrated intravenously and possibly intrathecally, based on the local Infectious Diseases (ID) team guidelines. If the CSF is clear, then only the distal part can be removed *outward* in a fashion that prevents spread of the infection closely to the remaining shunt. If there is no clinical or radiological evidence of recent bowel perforation, then a new catheter can be inserted into the peritoneal cavity. A general surgeon can provide his assistance in such cases or – more importantly – if there are signs of intraperitoneal perforation and infection. General surgeons are also helpful in cases of laparoscopic retrieval of disconnected catheters, even as a day-case procedures [73].

Retrieval of migrated catheters into the heart or the pulmonary artery has several options. Some authors reported a smooth removal through a retroauricular incision without any complications [61]. Others utilized fluoroscopic guidance successfully [26] or requested assistance from cardiothoracic surgeons due to potential hazards threatening the cardiac valves or chambers [27]. Endovascular methods are another vital option [16] and nevertheless, whenever the surgeon feels unfamiliar with less-known territories, asking for help from specialized expertise is always wise.

References

1. Adeloye A (1973) Spontaneous extrusion of the abdominal tube through the umbilicus complicating peritoneal shunt for hydrocephalus. Case report. J Neurosurg 38(6):758–760
2. Aihara N, Takagi T, Hashimoto N et al (1997) Breakage of shunt devices (Sophy programmable pressure valve) following implantation in the hypochondriac region. Childs Nerv Syst 13(11–12): 636–638
3. Aldrich EF, Harmann P (1990) Disconnection as a cause of ventriculoperitoneal shunt malfunction in multicomponent shunt systems. Pediatr Neurosurg 16(6):309–311; discussion 312
4. Ammar A, Nasser M (1995) Intraventricular migration of VP shunt. Neurosurg Rev 18(4):293–295
5. Anthogalidis EI, Sure U, Hellwig D, Bertalanffy H (1999) Intracranial dislocation of a lumbo-peritoneal shunt-catheter: case report and review of the literature. Clin Neurol Neurosurg 101(3):203–206
6. Aryan HE, Meltzer HS, Park MS et al (2005) Initial experience with antibiotic-impregnated silicone catheters for shunting of cerebrospinal fluid in children. Childs Nerv Syst 21(1):56–61
7. Beez T, Sarikaya-Seiwert S, Bellstadt L, Muhmer M, Steiger HJ (2014) Role of ventriculoperitoneal shunt valve design in the treatment of pediatric hydrocephalus-a single center study of valve performance in the clinical setting. Childs Nerv Syst 30(2):293–297
8. Berhouma M, Messerer M, Houissa S, Khaldi M (2008) Transoral protrusion of a peritoneal catheter: a rare complication of ventriculoperitoneal shunt. Pediatr Neurosurg 44(2):169–171
9. Boch AL, Hermelin E, Sainte-Rose C, Sgouros S (1998) Mechanical dysfunction of ventriculoperitoneal shunts caused by calcification of the silicone rubber catheter. J Neurosurg 88(6):975–982
10. Browd SR, Gottfried ON, Ragel BT, Kestle JR (2006) Failure of cerebrospinal fluid shunts: part II: overdrainage, loculation, and abdominal complications. Pediatr Neurol 34(3):171–176
11. Browd SR, Ragel BT, Gottfried ON, Kestle JR (2006) Failure of cerebrospinal fluid shunts: part I: obstruction and mechanical failure. Pediatr Neurol 34(2): 83–92
12. Brownlee JD, Brodkey JS, Schaefer IK (1998) Colonic perforation by ventriculoperitoneal shunt tubing: a case of suspected silicone allergy. Surg Neurol 49(1): 21–24
13. Burnette DG Jr (1982) Bladder perforation and urethral catheter extrusion: an unusual complication of cerebrospinal fluid-peritoneal shunting. J Urol 127(3): 543–544
14. Charalambides C, Sgouros S (2012) Spontaneous knot formation in the peritoneal catheter: a rare cause of ventriculoperitoneal shunt malfunction. Pediatr Neurosurg 48:310–312
15. Chen HH, Riva-Cambrin J, Brockmeyer DL, Walker ML, Kestle JR (2011) Shunt failure due to intracranial migration of BioGlide ventricular catheters. J Neurosurg Pediatr 7(4):408–412
16. Chong JY, Kim JM, Cho DC, Kim CH (2008) Upward migration of distal ventriculoperitoneal shunt catheter into the heart: case report. J Korean Neurosurg Soc 44(3):170–173
17. Coleman DL, Lim D, Kessler T, Andrade JD (1981) Calcification of nontextured implantable blood pumps. Trans Am Soc Artif Intern Organs 27:97–104
18. Decq P, Barat JL, Duplessis E et al (1995) Shunt failure in adult hydrocephalus: flow-controlled shunt versus differential pressure shunts–a cooperative study in 289 patients. Surg Neurol 43(4):333–339
19. Del Bigio MR, Fedoroff S (1992) Short-term response of brain tissue to cerebrospinal fluid shunts in vivo and in vitro. J Biomed Mater Res 26(8):979–987
20. Dominguez CJ, Tyagi A, Hall G, Timothy J, Chumas PD (2000) Sub-galeal coiling of the proximal and distal components of a ventriculo-peritoneal shunt. An unusual complication and proposed mechanism. Childs Nerv Syst 16(8):493–495
21. Drake JM, Kestle JR, Milner R et al (1998) Randomized trial of cerebrospinal fluid shunt valve

design in pediatric hydrocephalus. Neurosurgery 43(2):294–303; discussion 303-295
22. Drake JM, Kestle JR, Tuli S (2000) CSF shunts 50 years on–past, present and future. Childs Nerv Syst 16(10–11):800–804
23. Echizenya K, Satoh M, Murai H et al (1987) Mineralization and biodegradation of CSF shunting systems. J Neurosurg 67(4):584–591
24. Elisevich K, Mattar AG, Cheeseman F (1994) Biodegradation of distal shunt catheters. Pediatr Neurosurg 21(1):71–76
25. Etus V (2011) Ventriculoperitoneal shunt catheter protrusion through the anus: case report of an uncommon complication and literature review. Commentary. Childs Nerv Syst 27(11):2015
26. Fewel ME, Garton HJ (2004) Migration of distal ventriculoperitoneal shunt catheter into the heart. Case report and review of the literature. J Neurosurg 100(2 Suppl Pediatrics):206–211
27. Frazier JL, Wang PP, Patel SH et al (2002) Unusual migration of the distal catheter of a ventriculoperitoneal shunt into the heart: case report. Neurosurgery 51(3): 819–822; discussion 822
28. Ghritlaharey RK, Budhwani KS, Shrivastava DK et al (2007) Trans-anal protrusion of ventriculo-peritoneal shunt catheter with silent bowel perforation: report of ten cases in children. Pediatr Surg Int 23(6): 575–580
29. Glatstein M, Constantini S, Scolnik D, Shimoni N, Roth J (2011) Ventriculoperitoneal shunt catheter protrusion through the anus: case report of an uncommon complication and literature review. Childs Nerv Syst 27(11):2011–2014
30. Goldblum RM, Pelley RP, O'Donell AA, Pyron D, Heggers JP (1992) Antibodies to silicone elastomers and reactions to ventriculoperitoneal shunts. Lancet 340(8818):510–513
31. Griebel R, Khan M, Tan L (1985) CSF shunt complications: an analysis of contributory factors. Childs Nerv Syst 1(2):77–80
32. Harasaki H, McMahon J, Richards T et al (1985) Calcification in cardiovascular implants: degraded cell related phenomena. Trans Am Soc Artif Intern Organs 31:489–494
33. Harasaki H, Moritz A, Uchida N et al (1987) Initiation and growth of calcification in a polyurethane-coated blood pump. ASAIO Trans 33(3):643–649
34. Heggers JP, Kossovsky N, Parsons RW et al (1983) Biocompatibility of silicone implants. Ann Plast Surg 11(1):38–45
35. Hussain NS, Wang PP, James C, Carson BS, Avellino AM (2005) Distal ventriculoperitoneal shunt failure caused by silicone allergy. Case report. J Neurosurg 102(3):536–539
36. Iannelli A, Rea G, Di Rocco C (2005) CSF shunt removal in children with hydrocephalus. Acta Neurochir (Wien) 147(5):503–507; discussion 507
37. Israelsson LA, Jonsson T (1994) Physical properties of self locking and conventional surgical knots. Eur J Surg 160(6–7):323–327
38. Jimenez DF, Keating R, Goodrich JT (1994) Silicone allergy in ventriculoperitoneal shunts. Childs Nerv Syst 10(1):59–63
39. Joubert MJ, Stephanov S (1983) Extrusion of peritoneal catheter through the mid-lumbar region. An unusual complication of ventriculo-peritoneal shunt. Surg Neurol 19(2):120–121
40. Kang JK, Lee IW (1999) Long-term follow-up of shunting therapy. Childs Nerv Syst 15(11–12):711–717
41. Kataria R, Sinha VD, Chopra S, Gupta A, Vyas N (2013) Urinary bladder perforation, intra-corporeal knotting, and per-urethral extrusion of ventriculoperitoneal shunt in a single patient: case report and review of literature. Childs Nerv Syst 29(4):693–697
42. Koga H, Mukawa J, Nakata M, Sakuta O, Higa Y (1992) Analysis of retained ventricular shunt catheters. Neurol Med Chir (Tokyo) 32(11):824–828
43. Kronenthal RL (1975) Biodegradable polymers in medicine and surgery. In: Kronenthal RL, Oser Z, Martin E (eds) Polymers in medicine and surgery. Plenum Press, New York, pp 119–137
44. Kumar R, Singh V, Kumar MV (2005) Shunt revision in hydrocephalus. Indian J Pediatr 72(10):843–847
45. Kuo MF, Wang HS, Yang SH (2009) Ventriculoperitoneal shunt dislodgement after a haircut with hair clippers in two shunted boys. Childs Nerv Syst 25(11):1491–1493
46. Langmoen IA, Lundar T, Vatne K, Hovind KH (1992) Occurrence and management of fractured peripheral catheters in CSF shunts. Childs Nerv Syst 8(4):222–225
47. Lee SC, Chen JF, Tu PH, Lee ST (2008) Cerebrospinal fluid galactorrhea: a rare complication of ventriculoperitoneal shunting. J Clin Neurosci 15(6):698–700
48. Lee YH, Park EK, Kim DS, Choi JU, Shim KW (2010) What should we do with a discontinued shunt? Childs Nerv Syst 26(6):791–796
49. Lewis FM (1969) Elastomers by condensation polymerization. In: Kennedy JP, Tronqvist E (eds) Polymer chemistry of synthetic elastomers, part 2. Wiley, New York, pp 767–804
50. Lundar T, Langmoen IA, Hovind KH (1991) Shunt failure caused by valve collapse. J Neurol Neurosurg Psychiatry 54(6):559–560
51. Maknojia A, Caron JL (2014) Proximal subcutaneous migration of the distal end of a ventriculoperitoneal shunt presenting with recurrent cerebrospinal fluid galactorrhea. J Neurosurg 120(1):164–166
52. Mazza CA, Bricolo A (1975) Upward dislocation of peritoneal catheter into the ventricular cavity. A rare complication of the ventriculo-peritoneal shunt. Report of a case. Neuropadiatrie 6(3):313–316
53. Miserocchi G, Sironi VA, Ravagnati L (1984) Anal protrusion as a complication of ventriculo-peritoneal shunt. Case report and review of the literature. J Neurosurg Sci 28(1):43–46
54. Morell RC, Bell WO, Hertz GE, D'Souza V (1994) Migration of a ventriculoperitoneal shunt into the pulmonary artery. J Neurosurg Anesthesiol 6(2):132–134
55. Nagulic M, Djordjevic M, Samardzic M (1996) Peritoneo-vulvar catheter extrusion after shunt operation. Childs Nerv Syst 12(4):222–223

56. Neuren A, Ellison PH (1979) Acute hydrocephalus and death following V-P shunt disconnection. Pediatrics 64(1):90–93
57. Nguyen HS, Turner M, Butty SD, Cohen-Gadol AA (2010) Migration of a distal shunt catheter into the heart and pulmonary artery: report of a case and review of the literature. Childs Nerv Syst 26(8):1113–1116
58. Portnoy HD, Croissant PD (1973) Two unusual complications of a ventriculoperitoneal shunt. Case report. J Neurosurg 39(6):775–776
59. Raimondi AJ, Robinson JS, Kuwawura K (1977) Complications of ventriculo-peritoneal shunting and a critical comparison of the three-piece and one-piece systems. Childs Brain 3(6):321–342
60. Ramani PS (1974) Extrusion of abdominal catheter of ventriculoperitoneal shunt into the scrotum. Case report. J Neurosurg 40(6):772–773
61. Rizk E, Dias MS, Verbrugge J, Boop FA (2009) Intracardiac migration of a distal shunt catheter: an unusual complication of ventricular shunts. Report of 2 cases. J Neurosurg Pediatr 3(6):525–528
62. Sahin S, Shaaban AF, Iskandar BJ (2007) Recurrent pneumonia caused by transdiaphragmatic erosion of a ventriculoperitoneal shunt into the lung. Case report. J Neurosurg 107(2 Suppl):156–158
63. Sainte-Rose C, Piatt JH, Renier D et al (1991) Mechanical complications in shunts. Pediatr Neurosurg 17(1):2–9
64. Sathyanarayana S, Wylen EL, Baskaya MK, Nanda A (2000) Spontaneous bowel perforation after ventriculoperitoneal shunt surgery: case report and a review of 45 cases. Surg Neurol 54(5):388–396
65. Schoen FJ, Harasaki H, Kim KM, Anderson HC, Levy RJ (1988) Biomaterial-associated calcification: pathology, mechanisms, and strategies for prevention. J Biomed Mater Res 22(A1 Suppl):11–36
66. Sekhar LN, Moossy J, Guthkelch AN (1982) Malfunctioning ventriculoperitoneal shunts. Clinical and pathological features. J Neurosurg 56(3):411–416
67. Sgouros S, Dipple SJ (2004) An investigation of structural degradation of cerebrospinal fluid shunt valves performed using scanning electron microscopy and energy-dispersive x-ray microanalysis. J Neurosurg 100:534–540
68. Sgouros S, John P, Walsh AR, Hockley AD (1996) The value of Colour Doppler Imaging in assessing flow through ventricular shunts. Childs Nerv Syst 12:454–459
69. Shafiee S, Nejat F, Raouf SM, Mehdizadeh M, El Khashab M (2011) Coiling and migration of peritoneal catheter into the breast: a very rare complication of ventriculoperitoneal shunt. Childs Nerv Syst 27(9): 1499–1501
70. Shanklin DR, Smalley DL (1999) Dynamics of wound healing after silicone device implantation. Exp Mol Pathol 67(1):26–39
71. Shannon CN, Acakpo-Satchivi L, Kirby RS, Franklin FA, Wellons JC (2012) Ventriculoperitoneal shunt failure: an institutional review of 2-year survival rates. Childs Nerv Syst 28(12):2093–2099
72. Shaw AD, Duthie GS (1995) A simple assessment of surgical sutures and knots. J R Coll Surg Edinb 40(6):388–391
73. Short M, Solanki G, Jawaheer G (2010) Laparoscopic retrieval of disconnected shunt catheters from the peritoneal cavity as a day-case procedure in children–early feasibility report. Childs Nerv Syst 26(6):797–800
74. Snow RB, Kossovsky N (1989) Hypersensitivity reaction associated with sterile ventriculoperitoneal shunt malfunction. Surg Neurol 31(3):209–214
75. Stannard MW, Rollins NK (1995) Subcutaneous catheter calcification in ventriculoperitoneal shunts. AJNR Am J Neuroradiol 16(6):1276–1278
76. Swanson JW, Lebeau JE (1974) The effect of implantation on the physical properties of silicone rubber. J Biomed Mater Res 8(6):357–367
77. Thauvoy C (1989) Unusual complication of peritoneal drainage: migration of a shunt in the subdural space. Childs Nerv Syst 5(5):279
78. Thubrikar MJ, Deck JD, Aouad J, Nolan SP (1983) Role of mechanical stress in calcification of aortic bioprosthetic valves. J Thorac Cardiovasc Surg 86(1): 115–125
79. Tomes DJ, Hellbusch LC, Alberts LR (2003) Stretching and breaking characteristics of cerebrospinal fluid shunt tubing. J Neurosurg 98(3):578–583
80. Touho H, Nakauchi M, Tasawa T, Nakagawa J, Karasawa J (1987) Intrahepatic migration of a peritoneal shunt catheter: case report. Neurosurgery 21(2): 258–259
81. Vinchon M, Rekate H, Kulkarni AV (2012) Pediatric hydrocephalus outcomes: a review. Fluids Barriers CNS 9(1):18
82. Wakai S (1982) Extrusion of a peritoneal catheter through the abdominal wall in an infant. Case report. J Neurosurg 57(1):148–149
83. Whittle IR, Johnston IH (1983) Extrusion of peritoneal catheter through neck incision: a rare complication of ventriculoperitoneal shunting. Aust N Z J Surg 53(2):177–178
84. Woodward SC (1981) Mineralization of connective tissue surrounding implanted devices. Trans Am Soc Artif Intern Organs 27:697–702
85. Yamamoto S, Ohno K, Aoyagi M, Ichinose S, Hirakawa K (2002) Calcific deposits on degraded shunt catheters: long-term follow-up of V-P shunts and late complications in three cases. Childs Nerv Syst 18(1–2):19–25
86. Yoshida M, Ohtsuru K, Kuramoto S (1991) External dislocation of the metallic device of a shunt valve, an unusual long-term complication of the Holter valve–case report. Kurume Med J 38(2):109–112

9 Infective Complications

Ali Akhaddar

Contents

9.1 **Introduction** 141
9.2 **Epidemiology and Risk Factors** 142
9.3 **Pathogens** 142
9.4 **Clinical Presentation** 143
9.5 **Diagnostic Studies** 144
9.6 **Treatment and Outcome** 145
9.7 **Prevention** 146
Conclusion 146
References 146

A. Akhaddar, MD
Department of Neurosurgery,
Avicenne Military Hospital of Marrakech,
University of Mohammed V Souissi,
Rabat 10100, Morocco
e-mail: akhaddar@hotmail.fr

Abbreviations

CNS	Central nervous system
CSF	Cerebrospinal fluid
CT-scan	Computed tomography scan
MRI	Magnetic resonance imaging

9.1 Introduction

Cerebrospinal fluid shunting devices are foreign bodies internally or externally placed in a patient with the aim of monitoring and treatment of intracranial hypertension related to a variety of underlying pathologies. Among CSF shunt complications, infection continues to be a serious cause of shunt failure and is the major source of morbidity and mortality. Additionally, shunt infection is an important contributor to the cost of care (long hospital stays and costly interventions) and a true frustrating problem for clinicians [2].

The term “shunt infection” was defined when the CSF or the shunt tip was contaminated with bacteria and the patient shows clinical signs of acute bacterial meningitis and symptoms of shunt malfunction or obstruction [27]. Infection can occur in any part of the shunt system or the structures through which it travels resulting in meningitis, infected shunt device, infected body cavity (peritoneum, right atrium, or pleural space), and/or wound infection.

C. Di Rocco et al. (eds.), *Complications of CSF Shunting in Hydrocephalus: Prevention, Identification, and Management*, DOI 10.1007/978-3-319-09961-3_9,

9.2 Epidemiology and Risk Factors

The reported incidence of shunt infection varies with the study design, definition of infection, and duration of surveillance. The infection rate may be reported as the number of infections per population or the number on infections per procedure, inclusive of revisions. Overall, the incidence of shunt-related infection is reported to be between 0.33 and 41 % with most recent reporting rates of approximately 7–12 % of patients and 3–8 % per procedure [5, 15, 26, 28, 30, 32]. Additionally, the incidence of infection related to external ventricular drainage (ventriculostomy) is higher than the infection rate secondary to ventriculoperitoneal shunt [17]. Although all shunt implant procedures are associated with a high risk of infection, the rate of infection does not appear to differ greatly between ventriculoatrial, ventriculopleural, and ventriculoperitoneal shunts [6].

Most infections in shunt systems are diagnosed within 6 months of placement (90 %) with the high incidence observed during the first 2 months [24, 26]. The majority of early infections originated from bacterial contamination introduced at the time of surgery, often from the skin flora. On the contrary, delayed infections can occur many years after shunt surgery and are likely caused by sending off of infection from remote sites such as the urinary tract or lungs [4].

Several risk factors have been reported to be associated with increased risk of infection. However, many of these factors are controversial and have not been confirmed or have been contradicted by subsequent studies [10, 22, 30]. Several authors accepted some high-risk factors like young age, the different types of hydrocephalus, and the presence of a previous external ventricular drainage or shunt system [10, 15, 17–19, 26–28, 33, 37] (Table 9.1).

Table 9.1 Risk factors for CSF shunt infection

High risks	Young age (especially children younger than 1 year)
	Premature birth
	Immunosuppressive states
	Etiology of hydrocephalus (myelomeningocele, intraventricular hemorrhage)
	CSF leak
	Previous or concomitant systemic infection
	Shunt revision
Low or controversial risks	Long hospital stays
	Prior exposure to antibiotics or steroid treatment
	Poor skin conditions
	Gender (male patient?)
	Disturbance of consciousness
	Former radiotherapy or chemotherapy
	Neurosurgeon experience
	Long duration of shunt surgery
	Use of a single glove
	Intraoperative hypothermia
	Increased CSF protein level
	Location of the ventricular catheter (frontal or occipital)
	Number of people present in the operating room

9.3 Pathogens

The bacteria most often responsible for shunt infection are coagulase-negative staphylococci, with *Staphylococcus epidermidis* the most often reported causative organism (60–70 %) followed by *Staphylococcus aureus* (20–30 %), particularly in patients with concomitant skin infections [11, 19, 22]. After adhesion to the inner surfaces of the shunt tubing, the coagulase-negative staphylococci produce an extracellular mucoid biofilm (slime) embedding the bacteria and protecting them from the immune system and antibiotics [24, 27].

Anaerobic organisms such as *Propionibacterium acnes* and *Corynebacterium diphtheriae* account for less than 10 % of infections [19, 35]. The other causative microorganisms that may be found are Gram-negative bacteria (especially *Escherichia coli, Pseudomonas*, and *Enterobacter*) and are usually associated with corresponding abdominal and bladder pathology. Less frequently, other Gram-positive cocci (*Streptococcus*, *Micrococcus*, and *Enterococcus*) were isolated. In some cases, no pathogen could be identified. On the contrary,

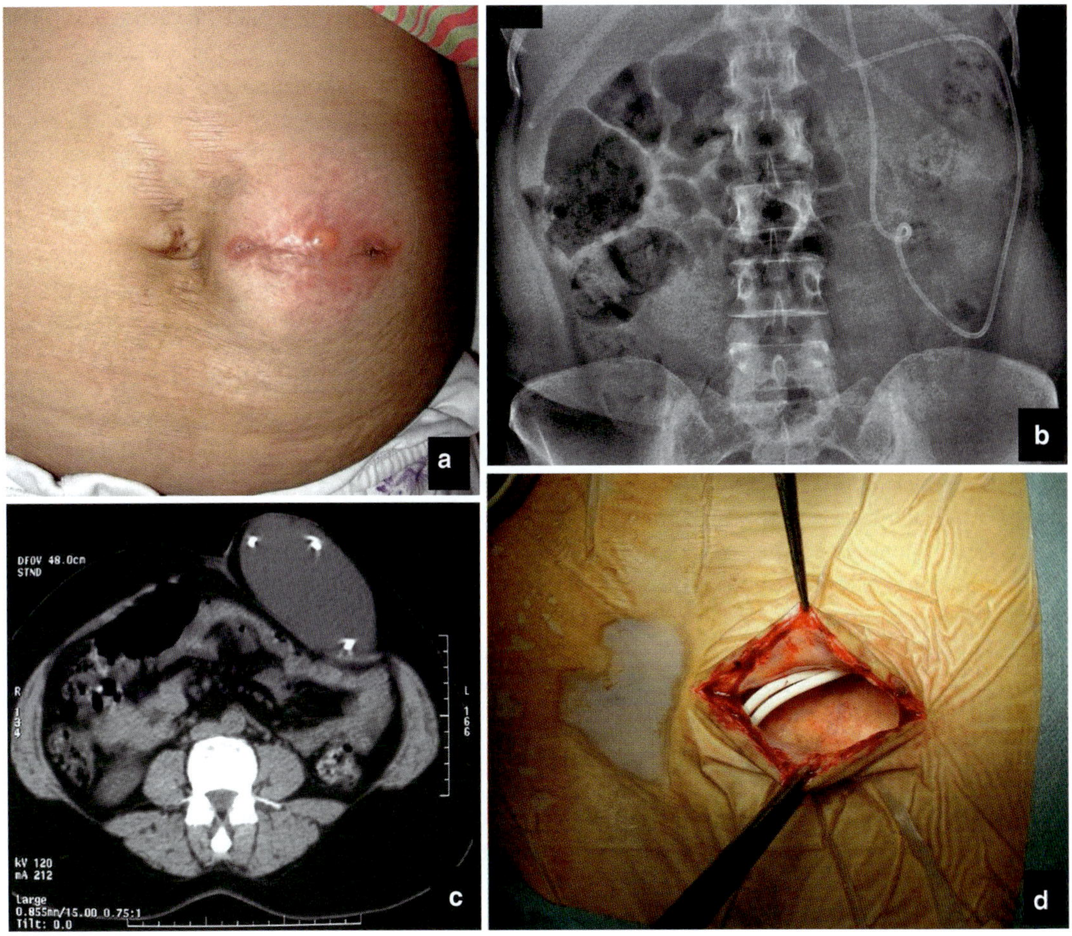

Fig. 9.1 Erythematous paraumbilical abdominal wound with swelling (**a**). Plain abdominal plain radiography without particular abnormalities (**b**). Axial abdominal CT-scan showing an extraperitoneal subcutaneous pseudocyst with the distal shunt catheter in the middle of a fluid collection (**c**). Operative findings showing the subcutaneous enrolled distal catheter (**d**)

polymicrobial infections account for up to 20 % of infections and are often associated with an abdominal origin, a contaminated head wound, or a systemic coinfection [33]. Non-bacterial shunt infections are rare and most commonly fungal infections (*Candida albicans*), usually in premature infants or immunocompromised patients [3, 24].

9.4 Clinical Presentation

The clinical presentation can vary greatly depending on the site of infection, the age of the patient, and the timing of infection (acute or chronic).

Early infection occurs days to weeks after the placement of the shunt. A high index of suspicion and proximity to a recent shunt manipulation makes this infective complication more likely. The patient is usually febrile (>38.5 °C). *Staphylococcus aureus* infections often present with erythema along the shunt track and may have a purulent drainage from the wound or visible shunt components (Fig. 9.1a) [21]. On the contrary, chronic shunt infections occur weeks to months after the shunt has been placed. In those cases, the most common presentation is that of repeated malfunctions (headache, irritability, nausea, vomiting, and lethargy) with or without fever [19, 22]. It is clear that the absence of fever does not rule out an infection.

Neonates may manifest apneic episodes, anemia, hepatosplenomegaly, and stiff neck [11]. Less commonly, patients may present with signs of meningeal irritation or seizures. Infected ventriculoatrial shunts may present with subacute bacterial endocarditis and "shunt nephritis"—an immune complex disorder that resembles acute glomerulonephritis (hepatosplenomegaly, hematuria, proteinuria and hypertension)—this rare condition is secondary to persistent stimulation of the immune system due to chronic infection, especially by *Staphylococcus epidermidis* [13]. Abdominal pain, gastrointestinal symptoms, and signs of intra-abdominal infection were seen with ventriculoperitoneal shunt infection. Ventriculopleural shunt infections may present with respiratory symptoms such as shortness of breath or a pleuritic chest pain.

9.5 Diagnostic Studies

CSF cultures are the most definitive method of diagnosis, although other laboratory values and imaging studies may point to an infection. Administration of antibiotics to a patient with suspected shunt infection before obtaining CSF culture reduces the likelihood of obtaining a positive culture.

In cases with high suspicion of shunt infection, a shunt tap should be performed and CSF sent for laboratory analysis. Studies should include CSF glucose, protein, cell counts, culture (bacterial and fungal), and sensitivities. Some advocate sending both aerobic and anaerobic cultures with the initial CSF tap [4]. Although a lumbar puncture is also possible (caution in obstructive hydrocephalus with a nonfunctioning shunt), CSF obtained this way is often sterile, even in patients who are later proven to have a ventricular shunt infection [11, 34].

Classically, CSF often shows a mild to moderate white blood cell count elevation (with predominantly polymorphonuclear cells), pleocytosis, low glucose level (a glucose ratio (CSF glucose/serum glucose) of <0.4), and elevated protein. For McClinton and colleagues, the combination of fever history and ventricular fluid neutrophils >10 % had a 99 % specificity for shunt infection and 93 positive predictive value [20]. Recurrent shunt malfunctions in a short time period can be indicative of infection, even with sterile CSF cultures, so the surgeon should have a high index of suspicion. In some doubtful situations, it is often helpful to re-tap the shunt to differentiate between a contaminant and true indolent infection [4]. A recent study showed that CSF vascular endothelial growth factor (VEGF) levels were associated with the subsequent development of shunt infection [18].

Routine blood tests often show a peripheral leukocytosis (75 %) and erythrocyte sedimentation rate is rarely normal. Blood cultures are positive in less than one-third of cases [11]. Elevated C-reactive protein (CRP) levels may also be observed in nearly three-fourths of cases [36]. In addition, any apparent sites of infection (especially open wounds) should be cultured.

Imaging studies of the patient with a suspected shunt infection include plain radiographies of the shunt system to establish continuity of the shunt hardware. Brain CT-scan and/or MRI were used to evaluate shunt configuration and location as well as the size of the ventricles and possible etiology. After contrast or gadolinium administration, patients may exhibit signs of infection: meningeal enhancement, ventriculitis (ependymal enhancement), and brain abscess. When a distal infection is suspected or there is evidence of distal malfunction, an abdominal ultrasound or CT-scan should be performed to detect a pseudocyst, the exact localization of the distal shunt catheter (Fig. 9.1), or possible pathological abdominal complications. For Kariyattil and colleagues, it is important to distinguish between CSF pseudocyst and CSF ascites (failure to absorb CSF) [14]. However, the presence of an abdominal pseudocyst is usually suggestive of infection until proven otherwise [11]. In patients with a ventriculoatrial shunt, an echocardiography must be used to look for vegetations if shunt infection is suspected.

9.6 Treatment and Outcome

Multiples studies have been performed to find the best strategy to manage CSF shunt infections [1, 11, 16, 19, 30, 33, 37]. The following are some gold questions:

(a) Should the shunt be removed? If removed, should it be replaced immediately or secondary after a temporal EVD?

Four options are commonly discussed: *First*, the infection may be treated by antibiotic therapy alone, either systematically or intrathecally; *second*, removal of the shunt with re-implantation of a new shunt immediately at the same time of the surgery; *third*, externalization of the shunt system followed by placement of a new shunt system later after the CSF becomes sterile, and *fourth*, removal of the shunt with placement of an EVD followed by shunt re-implantation at a later time when the infection has cleared (consecutive negative CSF cultures, CSF white blood cell count <30, glucose ratio (*CSF glucose/serum glucose*) of <0.4,and CSF protein <0.5 g/L).

The highest treatment success rate was reported with shunt removal/EVD placement and the highest failure rate reported was treatment with antibiotics only [15]. Treatment with antibiotics without shunt removal is therefore recommended only in cases where the patient is terminally ill, has a poor anesthetic risk, or has slit ventricles that might be difficult to catheterize [11]. In cases of abdominal pseudocyst, the new shunt must be placed in a different abdominal site or at another different site such as the atrium or pleural cavity.

(b) What is the optimal duration of antibiotic therapy?

The optimal duration has not been yet defined but it seems that a shorter duration of antibiotic treatment is correlated with a higher risk of reinfection. Generally, the treatment duration is 10–14 days after the culture becomes negative. But the treatment for virulent or highly resistant organisms may be longer [11].

(c) How long should the patient remain externalized before shunt re-implantation?

Most authors agree that the shunt should be reinserted after CSF sterilization.

(d) What is the most efficacious antibiotic regime?

There are many antibiotic protocols. The choice of antibiotic therapy is generally guided by the susceptibility patterns of the infecting organism, degree of antibiotic penetrance into the CSF, previous personal experience, and local practice patterns [1]. The initial antibiotic choice should cover a broad spectrum of microbial flora with substantial coverage of the most common Gram-positive organisms that are overwhelmingly predominant in shunt infections (see Sect. 9.3 *about pathogens*). Intraventricular injection of antibiotics may be used in addition to intravenous therapy (EVD should then be clamped for 30 min after injection) [11, 35].

The prognosis of a CSF shunt infection is dependent primarily on the health and the underlying neurological pathology. A patient with relatively normal brain organization has a better outcome than a patient with abnormal morphology especially in the pediatric population.

In general, Gram-positive organisms correlate with a better prognosis than Gram-negative ones. However, since the last decade, the increasing occurrence of nosocomial infections especially due to methicillin-resistant *Staphylococcus aureus* (MRSA) has been a particular concern [8, 19, 31]. Inadequate or inappropriate treatment can cause recurrent shunt infections (reinfection) in about 20–30 % of patients [37].

If treated promptly and vigorously, shunt infections usually resolve without sequelae. Complications, however, can include cerebritis with cortical damage, polycystic ventricles, seizure, brain abscess, peritoneal CSF malabsorption, decreased intellectual performance, psychomotor retardation, increased risk of seizures, and death [4].

9.7 Prevention

There are only a few centers in the world in which the shunt infection rate has remained below 1 %. Those centers employ precautions that are difficult to duplicate in most hospitals especially in developing countries and teaching hospitals with trainees [27]. Furthermore, prevention of infection is essential, and many simple techniques have been promoted to minimize the risk factors (Table 9.1). These techniques include control of the operative theater with limited traffic, performing surgery early in the day, washing hands preoperatively, double gloving, limited handing of implants, no-touch technique (the surgical team manipulates the shunt equipment with sterile instruments as much as possible rather than with their gloved hands), handling the shunt with Silastic-tipped forceps, affixing antibiotic or iodine-impregnated sponges or adhesive drapes to the skin edges during the operation, bathing the shunt in antibiotic solution prior to insertion, close attention to surgical wound closure to prevent CSF leakage, use of antibiotic-impregnated sutures for wound closure, shorter operation times, and use of experienced staff and surgeons whenever possible [4, 10, 15, 17]. Some recent studies have suggested that antibiotic-impregnated catheters may reduce the rates of infection [9, 12, 27]. While these catheters are more expensive to implant, one could argue that there is cost saving realized in terms of the reported decreased incidence of shunt infection and subsequent hospitalizations.

Perioperative antibiotics for preventing shunt infection are widely used. Cefazolin is effective against staphylococci, streptococci, *Escherichia coli, Proteus mirabilis, and Klebsiella pneumoniae*. Since cefazolin covers the most likely surgical site pathogens, it is considered by many clinicians worldwide to be the drug of choice for neurosurgical prophylaxis [7], but vancomycin has been shown to be more effective than cephalosporins. Vancomycin is bactericidal against staphylococci but it is not active against Gram-negative pathogens. It does not usually cross the blood-brain barrier but may do so if the meninges are inflamed [23]. Recent studies proved that vancomycin was useful in reducing postsurgical infections in patients with ventricular shunts [31]. The use of intraventricular antibiotics (gentamicin and vancomycin) at the time of shunt placement has also been advocated as a method to decrease the shunt infection rate from 6.5 to 0.4 % [25].

On the other hand, it was suggested that patients with an existing shunt should receive an antibiotic prophylaxis when dental, gastrointestinal, intra-abdominal, or urological procedures are planned [29].

Conclusion

Shunt infection remains a true frustrating problem for clinicians despite a number of acceptable management options for both prevention and treatment. The most important method of diagnosis is a high level of clinical suspicion at the time of presentation, supported by CSF studies and imaging. Treatment of infection requires hospital admission, surgical removal of the shunt, placement of a temporary external ventricular drainage, intravenous antibiotic therapy for a variable period of time, and implantation of a new shunt system when the infection has been eradicated. It should not be forgotten that the timely usage of appropriate antibiotics according to the antimicrobial susceptibility testing is essential for successful treatment and outcome. Neurosurgeons must consider prevention of infection to be a problem of such seriousness that it warrants meticulous techniques that minimize the risk of infection.

References

1. Ackerman LL (2008) Controversies in the treatment of shunt infections. In: Iskander BJ (ed) Pediatric neurosurgery. Pan Arab Neurosurgical Journal, MSD Printing Press, Kingdom of Saudi Arabia, pp 13–25
2. Arthur AS, Whitehead WE, Kestle JRW (2002) Duration of antibiotic therapy for the treatment of shunt infection: a surgeon and patient survey. Pediatr Neurosurg 36:256–259
3. Baallal H, El Asri AC, Eljebbouri B, Akhaddar A, Gazzaz M, El Mostarchid B, Boucetta M (2013)

Cryptococcal meningitis in a patient with a ventriculoperitoneal shunt and monitoring for pulmonary sarcoidosis (in French). Neurochirurgie 59:47–49
4. Campbell JW (2008) Shunt infections. In: Albright AL, Pollack IF, Adelson PD (eds) Principles and practice of pediatric neurosurgery. Thieme, New York, pp 1141–1147
5. Choux M, Genitori L, Lang D, Lena G (1992) Shunt implantation: reducing the incidence of shunt infection. J Neurosurg 77:875–880
6. Crnich CJ, Safdar N, Maki DG (2003) Infections associated with implanted medical devices. In: Finch RG, Greenwood D, Norrby SR, Whitley RJ (eds) Antibiotic and chemotherapy: anti-infective agents and their use in therapy, 8th edn. Churchill Livingstone, Edinburgh, pp 575–618
7. Dempsey R, Rapp RP, Young B, Johnston S, Tibbs P (1988) Prophylactic parenteral antibiotics in clean neurosurgical procedures: a review. J Neurosurg 69: 52–57
8. Fluit AC, Wielders CL, Verhoef J, Schmitz FJ (2001) Epidemiology and susceptibility of 3,051 Staphylococcus aureus isolates from 25 university hospitals participating in the European SENTRY study. J Clin Microbiol 39: 3727–3732
9. Govender ST, Nathoo N, van Dellen JR (2003) Evaluation of an antibiotic- impregnated shunt system for the treatment of hydrocephalus. J Neurosurg 99: 831–839
10. Grandhi R, Harrison G, Tyler-Kabara EC (2013) Implanted devices and central nervous system infection. In: Hall WA, Kim PD (eds) Neurosurgical infectious disease: surgical and nonsurgical management. Thieme, New York, pp 280–296
11. Greenberg MS (2006) Shunt infection. In: Greenberg MS (ed) Handbook of neurosurgery. Thieme, New York, pp 214–216
12. Gutiérrez-González R, Boto GR (2010) Do antibiotic-impregnated catheters prevent infection in CSF diversion procedures? Review of the literature. J Infect 61:9–20
13. Haffner D, Schindera F, Aschoff A et al (1997) The clinical spectrum of shunt nephritis. Nephrol Dial Transplant 12:1143–1148
14. Kariyattil R, Steinbok P, Singhal A, Cochrane DD (2007) Ascites and abdominal pseudocysts following ventriculoperitoneal shunt surgery: variations of the same theme. J Neurosurg 106:350–353
15. Kestle JR, Garton HJ, Whitehead WE et al (2006) Management of shunt infections: a multicenter pilot study. J Neurosurg 105:177–181
16. Kestle JR, Riva-Cambrin J, Wellons JC 3rd et al (2011) A standardized protocol to reduce cerebrospinal fluid shunt infection: the Hydrocephalus Clinical Research Network Quality Improvement Initiative. J Neurosurg Pediatr 8:22–29
17. Kim JH, Desai NS, Ricci J et al (2012) Factors contributing to ventriculostomy infection. World Neurosurg 77:135–140
18. Lee JH, Back DB, Park DH et al (2012) Increased vascular endothelial growth factor in the ventricular cerebrospinal fluid as a predictive marker for subsequent ventriculoperitoneal shunt infection: a comparison study among hydrocephalic patients. J Korean Neurosurg Soc 51:328–333
19. Lee JK, Seok JY, Lee JH et al (2012) Incidence and risk factors of ventriculoperitoneal shunt infections in children: a study of 333 consecutive shunts in 6 years. J Korean Med Sci 27:1563–1568
20. McClinton D, Carraccio C, Englander R (2001) Predictors of ventriculoperitoneal shunt pathology. Pediatr Infect Dis J 20:593–597
21. Meftah M, Boumdim H, Akhaddar A et al (2003) Migration du cathéter de dérivation ventriculo-péritonéale par voie anale. A propos d'un cas (In French). Med Maghreb 106:29–31
22. Moores LE, Ellenbogen RG (2000) Cerebrospinal fluid shunt infections. In: Hall WA, McCutcheon IE (eds) Infections in neurosurgery. The American Association of Neurological Surgeons, Park Ridge, pp 141–154
23. Pons VG, Denlinger SL, Guglielmo BJ et al (1993) Ceftizoxime versus vancomycin and gentamicin in neurosurgical prophylaxis: a randomized, prospective, blinded clinical study. Neurosurgery 33:416–423
24. Prusseit J, Simon M, von der Brelie C et al (2009) Epidemiology, prevention and management of ventriculoperitoneal shunt infections in children. Pediatr Neurosurg 45:325–336
25. Ragel BT, Browd SR, Schmidt RH (2006) Surgical shunt infection Significant reduction when using intraventricular and systemic antibiotic agents. J Neurosurg 105:242–247
26. Reddy GK, Bollam P, Caldito G (2012) Ventriculoperitoneal shunt surgery and the risk of shunt infection in patients with hydrocephalus: long-term single institution experience. World Neurosurg 78:155–163
27. Ritz R, Roser F, Morgalla M et al (2007) Do antibiotic-impregnated shunts in hydrocephalus therapy reduce the risk of infection? An observational study in 258 patients. BMC Infect Dis 7:38
28. Sacar S, Turgut H, Toprak S et al (2006) A retrospective study of central nervous system shunt infections diagnosed in a university hospital during a 4-year period. BMC Infect Dis 6:43
29. Sandford JP, Gilbert DN, Sande MA (1996) Guide to antimicrobial therapy 1996. Antimicrobial therapy, Dallas
30. Simon TD, Hall M, Riva-Cambrin J, Hydrocephalus Clinical Research Network et al (2009) Infection rates following initial cerebrospinal fluid shunt placement across pediatric hospitals in the United States. J Neurosurg Pediatr 4:156–165
31. Tacconelli E, Cataldo MA, Albanese A, Tumbarello M, Arduini E, Spanu T, Fadda G, Anile C, Maira G, Federico G, Cauda R et al (2008) Vancomycin versus cefazolin prophylaxis for cerebrospinal shunt placement in a hospital with a high prevalence of methicillin-resistant Staphylococcus aureus. J Hosp Infect 69: 337–344

32. Talbot TR, Kaiser AB (2005) Postoperative infections and antimicrobial prophylaxis. In: Mandell GL, Bennett JE, Dolin R (eds) Principle and practice of infectious diseases, 6th edn. Elsevier/Churchill Livingstone, Edinburgh, pp 3533–3567
33. Tuan TJ, Thorell EA, Hamblett NM, Kestle JR, Rosenfeld M, Simon TD et al (2011) Treatment and microbiology of repeated cerebrospinal fluid shunt infections in children. Pediatr Infect Dis J 30: 731–735
34. Tunkel AR, Drake JM (2010) Cerebrospinal fluid shunt infections. In: Mandell GL, Bennett JE, Dolin R (eds) Mandell, Douglas, and Bennett's principles and practice of infectious diseases, 7th edn. Churchill Livingstone/Elsevier, Philadelphia, pp 1231–1236
35. Wilkie MD, Hanson MF, Statham PF, Brennan PM (2013) Infections of cerebrospinal fluid diversion devices in adults: the role of intraventricular antimicrobial therapy. J Infect 66:239–246
36. Wong GKC, Wong SM, Poon WS (2011) Ventriculoperitoneal shunt infection: intravenous antibiotics, shunt removal and more aggressive treatment? ANZ J Surg 81:307
37. Yilmaz A, Musluman AM, Dalgic N et al (2012) Risk factors for recurrent shunt infections in children. J Clin Neurosci 19:844–848

Posthemorrhagic and Postinflammatory Complications

10

Joanna Y. Wang and Edward S. Ahn

Contents

10.1	**Posthemorrhagic Hydrocephalus**	149
10.1.1	Introduction	149
10.1.2	Pathophysiology of PHH	150
10.1.3	Shunting in PHH and Complications	150
10.1.4	Alternatives to Shunting and Adjunctive Therapies	153
10.1.5	Long-Term Outcomes of PHH and Shunting	153
10.2	**Postinflammatory Hydrocephalus**	153
10.2.1	Introduction	153
10.2.2	Pathophysiology of PIH	154
10.2.3	Management of PIH and Complications	154
10.2.4	Long-Term Outcomes of PIH	155
References		155

J.Y. Wang • E.S. Ahn, MD (✉)
Division of Pediatric Neurosurgery,
The Johns Hopkins Hospital,
600 N. Wolfe St., Phipps 560,
Baltimore, MD 21287, USA
e-mail: eahn4@jhmi.edu

10.1 Posthemorrhagic Hydrocephalus

10.1.1 Introduction

Although the incidence of intraventricular hemorrhage (IVH) and posthemorrhagic hydrocephalus (PHH) in preterm infants is decreasing, these conditions are still associated with poor neurodevelopmental and functional outcomes [1]. Additionally, with the growing viability of infants born at younger estimated gestational ages (EGAs), these conditions remain significant burdens as IVH severity increases with prematurity. Despite improvements in neonatal care, there still lacks a uniform paradigm for the treatment and management of PHH. Patients with PHH typically are initially treated with a temporizing device that allows for these infants to develop more favorable immunologic and nutritional statuses; a permanent ventriculoperitoneal (VP) shunt is later inserted in cases of persistent ventricular dilation and symptomatic hydrocephalus. This patient population is at high risk for temporizing device and shunt complications, especially shunt obstruction and infection, slit-ventricle syndrome, and the development of loculated hydrocephalus. The impact of these complications on long-term neurodevelopmental outcomes is unclear; however, there are few alternative methods to avoid prolonged shunt dependence in these patients.

C. Di Rocco et al. (eds.), *Complications of CSF Shunting in Hydrocephalus: Prevention, Identification, and Management*, DOI 10.1007/978-3-319-09961-3_10,

10.1.2 Pathophysiology of PHH

Preterm infants are at risk for an extensive array of neurologic complications, the most commonly observed of which is IVH. The susceptibility of these patients to cerebrovascular injury is not fully understood, but is thought to be in part due to a combination of several factors, including dysregulation of cerebral vasculature with systemic hemodynamic instability, the immaturity of several structures including the highly vascular germinal matrix, and underdeveloped cardiac and respiratory systems [2–4]. IVH typically results from rupture of vessels in the germinal matrix, a critical area of cellular proliferation in the developing brain. This area is extremely vulnerable to hemorrhage due to the fragility of its vascular network, but typically disappears around 33–35 weeks gestation.

Reports of the rate of PHH following IVH vary from 25 to 74 % [5]. The likelihood of IVH progressing to PHH depends in part on the severity of the initial hemorrhagic event, which can be assessed by the Papile grading scale [6, 7]. A grade I IVH involves less than 10 % of the ventricle, while a grade II IVH extends to less than 50 % of the ventricle. Grade III indicates involvement of more than 50 % of the ventricle with ventricular dilation, and a grade IV hemorrhage indicates ventricular dilation with periventricular white matter involvement. It has been theorized that PHH develops from IVH due to insufficient fibrinolysis of microthrombi which cause obstruction of arachnoid villi, impairing CSF resorption. Larger blood clots may also obstruct flow within regions of the ventricular system. Additionally, the breakdown of blood products is thought to result in the recruitment of pro-inflammatory factors and the deposition of extracellular matrix, leading to meningeal fibrosis and subependymal gliosis. These processes can obstruct CSF outflow from the aqueduct of Sylvius and the foramina of the fourth ventricle [5, 8].

10.1.3 Shunting in PHH and Complications

Clinical findings consistent with hydrocephalus, including vomiting, poor feeding, lethargy, and apnea, with increasing head circumference and fontanelle fullness along with corresponding findings of ventriculomegaly on imaging are indications for treatment. Though temporizing, nonsurgical methods such as serial lumbar punctures or ventricular taps may be attempted in some patients, many patients display persistently dilated ventricles or elevated intracranial pressures (ICP) and require surgical intervention. Previous studies of patients managed by serial tapping did not find an effect of treatment on neurodevelopmental outcomes or shunt dependence, and recurrent tapping was associated with high rates of central nervous system (CNS) infection [9]. For patients with rapidly progressive hydrocephalus, temporary external ventricular drainage (EVD) has been employed and offers the advantages of ICP monitoring and control. A catheter is inserted into the lateral ventricle and is tunneled subcutaneously under the scalp to connect to an external drainage system. However, these devices are associated with several complications, including device infection, dislocation, and occlusion, as well as overdrainage and the development of subdural hygromas. Infection rates vary from 5.4 to 7.1 % in prior reports, and infection of EVD systems have been associated with poor long-term outcomes [9–12]. Moreover, the rates of these patients who eventually need permanent shunting are high, ranging from 64 to 68 % [11, 13].

Typically, one of two temporizing devices, the ventricular reservoir or the ventriculosubgaleal shunt (VSGS), is initially placed upon diagnosis of PHH to delay placement of a permanent VP shunt. A retrospective study found that early VP shunt insertion is associated with higher rates of shunt infection and mechanical obstruction [14]. In comparing shunt outcomes between patients who initially received VP shunts and those who initially had ventricular reservoirs inserted, it was found that despite the fact that directly shunted patients were at higher weights and EGAs, they experienced higher rates of shunt revision [15]. Therefore, initial treatment with a reservoir prior to shunt insertion seems to be beneficial. The risks associated with early VP shunt insertion have been theorized to be related in part to the presence of blood breakdown products in the

CSF; however, a study which examined the relationship between shunt outcomes and CSF parameters including cell count, protein level, and glucose levels did not find an association between alterations in CSF content and shunt complications [16]. Other proposed benefits of initial insertion of a temporary device include allowing time for optimization of patient factors, including nutritional and immunologic statuses, and the potential for avoiding permanent shunting; however, timing and choice of the initial intervention relies heavily on clinical judgment.

The ventricular reservoir was first introduced in the 1980s and requires CSF to be manually removed by serial reservoir taps. One of the primary complications of reservoir insertion is device infection, thought to be related to the requirement for repeated reservoir access. Early reports found infection rates ranging from 8 to 10 %, but subsequent series have reported that infection rates have decreased over time to approximately 5 % [17–21]. A proposed advantage of ventricular tapping is the removal of CSF and clearance of blood breakdown products and cellular debris; however, this theorized benefit has not been borne out in studies [22]. An important practical consideration with reservoirs is the frequency of taps and the volume of CSF removed with each tap. Depending on the rate of fluid reaccumulation and patient symptomatology, patients may require daily CSF removal. However, there is significant variability in tapping practices with respect to regularity of tapping, the amount of fluid removed, and the use of clinical features and imaging to guide tapping. A study of patients treated with reservoirs found that only taps that achieved ICPs of less than 7 cm H_2O were able to achieve appreciable differences in cerebral blood flow velocity [23]. Removal of a consistent volume of CSF at regular intervals is also not ideal and results in rapid fluctuations in ICP [24]. Ultimately, most patients initially managed with reservoirs ultimately require permanent shunting, with studies reporting rates of VP shunting at 75–88 % [2].

An alternative temporizing device, the VSGS, consists of a ventricular reservoir, from which CSF is redirected to a subgaleal scalp pocket for reabsorption (Fig. 10.1). Because the device does not necessitate repeated manual CSF removal, the risk for device infection is theoretically lower. However, studies have not demonstrated a significant difference in device infection rates between patients treated with the reservoir and VSGS, with rates in VSGS patients ranging from 0 to 14 % (Table 10.1) [25, 26]. It has been proposed that the comparable risk of

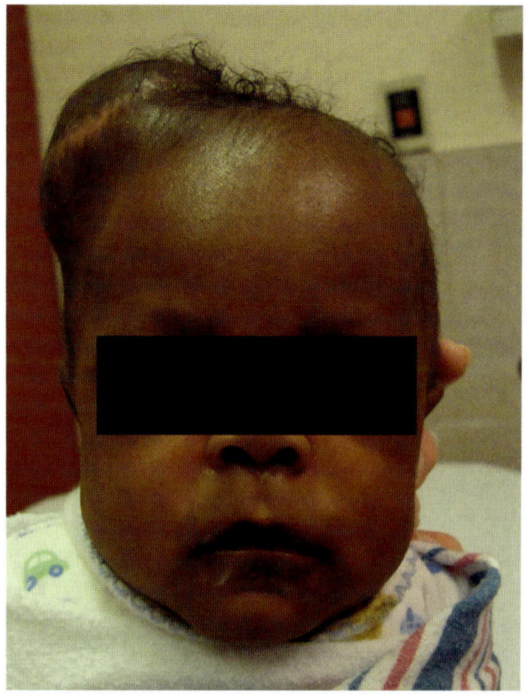

Fig. 10.1 An ex-premature infant who developed grade 4 IVH and PHH and was treated with a VSGS

Table 10.1 Rates of infection and permanent shunting in VSGS patients as reported in the literature

Series	Number of patients with PHH treated with VSGS	Rate of device infection (%)	Rate of shunting (%)
Fulmer et al. (2000) [26]	20	0	100
Tubbs et al. (2005) [25]	71	5.9	NR
Wellons et al. (2009) [27]	36	14	86
Lam et al. (2009) [29]	16	6.3	71.4
Limbrick et al. (2010) [28]	30	3.3	66.7

infection may be a result of CSF stasis within the subgaleal pocket. The rates of permanent shunt insertion in this population have also been comparable to those treated with the reservoir, at approximately 60–100 % [2, 26]. A multicenter retrospective study found that reservoir patients experienced lower rates of VP shunt insertion compared to VSGS patients [27]. However, other studies which have directly compared the two temporizing devices have found comparable rates of shunt infection and revision, permanent shunt placement, and mortality (Table 10.1) [28, 29]. In previous studies, reported VSGS revision rates ranged from 25 to 28 %; in most of these cases, revisions occurred due to the development of adhesions within the subgaleal pocket rather than shunt dysfunction [30]. Reports of mortality rates varied from 9 to 20 %; however, the causes of death were not reported, and the severity of the preceding IVH was not accounted for [30, 31]. Other less common complications seen with the VSGS include CSF leakage from the incision site, catheter migration, and intraparenchymal hemorrhage. The rates of CSF leakage vary from 4.7 to 32 % in studies; much of this variation appears to be due to surgical technique [25, 26, 32]. Intraparenchymal hemorrhage appears rare and has been reported in two studies, with three cases total in the literature [25, 26, 30]. The impact of treatment with the VSGS on long-term neurodevelopmental outcomes has yet to be fully investigated.

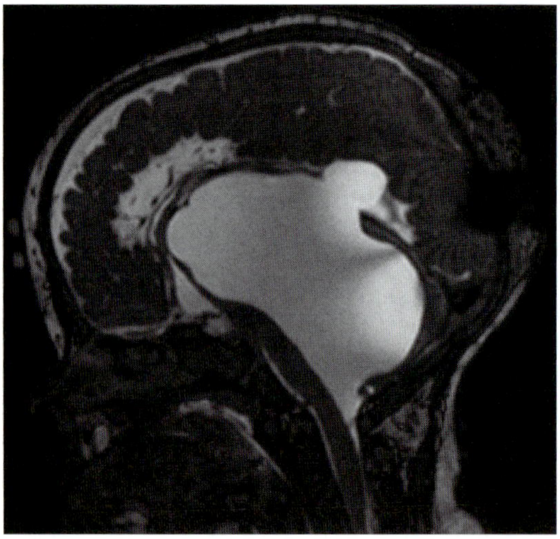

Fig. 10.2 T2-weighted MRI of a 16-month-old patient with a history of prematurity and PHH and multiple CSF infections. There is a loculated fourth ventricle with outlet obstruction with considerable mass effect on the brainstem and cerebellum. There is also supratentorial extension

Although efforts are made to avoid permanent shunting in infants with PHH to prevent long-term shunt dependence, the overall rate of permanent shunt insertion ranges from 0 to 20 % in patients with IVH [15, 28, 33, 34]. The majority of patients initially treated with temporizing devices ultimately undergo permanent shunt placement. The most commonly inserted device is the VP shunt, although selected individuals require CSF diversion to other locations. Even after a temporizing device has been initially inserted, timing of permanent shunting is controversial and relies on clinical judgment of a patient's surgical candidacy and evaluation of factors including infant weight, medical stability, and CSF profile [9]. Several studies have found that compared to infants with hydrocephalus of other etiologies, those with PHH are at increased risk of complications including shunt infection and occlusion requiring revision, slit-ventricle syndrome, and loculated hydrocephalus (Fig. 10.2) [35]. Rates of VP shunt infection in PHH patients have been reported at approximately 13 %, compared to 4–8.5 % overall in shunted populations [2, 5, 36–39]. The high rates of shunt infection seen in this population have been hypothesized to be in part due to an immature and dysregulated immune system. The use of antibiotic-impregnated shunt catheters has been proposed, and a prospective study of these devices reported an infection rate of 6.8 % [40]. IVH and PHH are also associated with a need for multiple shunt revisions, for which the most common indication is shunt failure secondary to obstruction [41]. A recent retrospective study reported a revision rate of 71.6 % and a multiple revision rate of 55 % for complications including obstruction and overdrainage; lower birth weight and EGA were found to be risk factors for multiple revisions [42].

10.1.4 Alternatives to Shunting and Adjunctive Therapies

VP shunting is currently the mainstay of treatment in PHH, but several alternative medical and surgical treatment methods have been proposed. Trials of diuretic therapy with acetazolamide or furosemide have found that drug treatment with CSF tapping is associated with higher rates of eventual permanent shunt insertion and increased risk for motor impairment and nephrocalcinosis compared to management with CSF removal alone [43, 44]. Currently, there is no evidence to support the use of diuretic therapy in PHH. The use of fibrinolytics in preventing the development of hydrocephalus in IVH has also been suggested, but two randomized trials investigating the effects of intraventricular streptokinase in PHVD have not shown any benefit with respect to rates of permanent shunting or neurodevelopmental outcomes [45]. A multicenter randomized trial on PHH prevention with intraventricular tissue plasminogen activator (tPA) with a procedure involving drainage, irrigation, and fibrinolytic therapy (DRIFT) also did not find an effect of this management protocol on the rates of permanent shunting. However, although DRIFT was found to be associated with an increased risk for secondary hemorrhage, patients in the treatment group experienced better neurodevelopmental outcomes compared to the control group, with lower rates of mortality and cognitive disability [46, 47].

A promising surgical approach for PHH is endoscopic third ventriculostomy (ETV). Though outcomes of cases managed with ETV alone are inconsistent, recent studies of ETV with choroid plexus coagulation (CPC) are encouraging. In selected PHH patients, ETV with CPC may offer a means of continued CSF diversion without long-term shunt dependence [2, 48].

10.1.5 Long-Term Outcomes of PHH and Shunting

Improvement in neurodevelopmental outcomes after IVH and PHH has been largely attributed to improvements in neonatal care. Early studies from 1970 to 1980 reported significant cognitive disability and mortality associated with grade IV IVH [49]. Later reports detailed high rates of neurodevelopmental problems including sensory and motor deficits, visual impairment, hearing loss, seizures, and cognitive and behavioral disturbances in patients with severe IVH [50–52]. As these patients typically also suffer from an extensive array of medical comorbidities, poor outcomes are unlikely to be due to IVH and PHH alone. However, the effect of permanent shunting on long-term outcomes is incompletely understood. Although some studies have found that shunt insertion and complications are risk factors for poor outcomes, a study of functional outcomes in PHH patients did not find differences in the rates of functional independence in shunted and non-shunted patients [53–55]. The most critical determinant of neurologic outcome appears to be IVH severity, with patients who develop periventricular hemorrhagic infarction are at highest risk for the development of complications including cerebral palsy [33].

10.2 Postinflammatory Hydrocephalus

10.2.1 Introduction

Hydrocephalus which results from CNS infection poses a unique set of challenges with respect to treatment. The pathophysiologic mechanisms of hydrocephalus development are incompletely understood, but obstruction of CSF flow is thought to result from the inflammatory debris within the subarachnoid space and meningeal scarring. Patients with persistent hydrocephalus despite infection resolution are typically treated with permanent shunt insertion. Studies have demonstrated that patients with postinflammatory hydrocephalus (PIH) are at increased risk for shunt complications, including shunt infection and obstruction requiring surgical revision, compared to patients with hydrocephalus of other etiologies. Although there have been few reports on long-term outcomes of shunting in this population, avoidance of shunt dependence remains an important goal of management. Alternative interventions including ETV have demonstrated promise in selected patients with favorable ventricular anatomy.

10.2.2 Pathophysiology of PIH

The mechanism of PIH is believed to be secondary to obstruction of the basal cisterns and blockage of CSF outflow secondary to inflammation and meningeal fibrosis and scarring [56]. Neonatal meningitis is also considered a risk factor for the development of multiloculated hydrocephalus [56–59]. However, the mechanism of hydrocephalus often varies by pathogen. With *Toxoplasmosis gondii*, the parasites are thought to cause obstruction of the ventricular system via damage to the ependymal linings of the lateral ventricles. Other studies have suggested that hydrocephalus develops as a result of leptomeningeal inflammation in reaction to the parasite. Acquisition of CMV during the in utero period is associated with the development of hydrocephalus *ex vacuo* secondary to cortical atrophy as well as obstructive hydrocephalus from periventricular inflammation [5].

In the postnatal period, the most common cause of PIH is bacterial infection. Studies performed in the 1980s of children afflicted with bacterial meningitis have reported PIH rates at approximately 30 % [5, 57, 60]. However, the incidence of post-meningitic hydrocephalus in the pediatric population has not been well established since advancements in neonatal care. Brain abscesses can also result in obstructive hydrocephalus from mass effect and ventricular compression. Additionally, abscesses can lead to the development of loculated hydrocephalus, thought to be due to subependymal inflammation and infarction resulting in cyst formation. The pathogenesis of hydrocephalus from viral infections varies by virus; viruses often have specific tropisms for ependymal or meningeal cells.

Special consideration should be given to hydrocephalus in patients with tuberculosis with CNS involvement. Tuberculous meningitis typically favors the base of the brain, where infection results in exudate that obstructs the basal cisterns, preventing CSF outflow from the foramina of the fourth ventricle. Less commonly, intracerebral tuberculomas can cause hydrocephalus by compression of the ventricular system. Fungal pathogens including *Cryptococcus neoformans* and *Coccidioides immitis* can cause post-meningitic hydrocephalus; however, the pathogenesis of hydrocephalus in these cases is less well understood [5].

10.2.3 Management of PIH and Complications

An active infection and progressive hydrocephalus presents a therapeutic challenge, as insertion of a foreign device to divert CSF may exacerbate the infection. In the acute setting, repeated lumbar or ventricular taps may be required for management. Studies from the 1960s and 1970s of post-meningitic hydrocephalus reported high mortality rates with placement of a ventricular reservoir or with EVD [61]. Persistent hydrocephalus is typically managed by VP shunt insertion, though there is considerable variability in practice depending on patient and pathogen. Depending on the pathogen, CNS infection can result in a wide range of other sequelae and complications not causally related to the development of hydrocephalus. Regardless, studies have shown that patients with PIH are at increased risk for shunt complications including shunt infection, occlusion, and multiple shunt failures and are also at risk for development of loculated hydrocephalus (Fig. 10.3) [41, 62]. Preexisting multiloculated hydrocephalus appears to increase the risk for shunt complications, especially device infection, and for poor outcomes overall. Management options include placement of multiple shunts and fenestration of intraventricular septations, but there are no evidence-based guidelines regarding treatment choice [57].

There is a dearth of literature on methods for reducing shunt complications and alternatives to shunting for PIH. A study of the use of VSGS in PIH found that compared to patients with PHH,

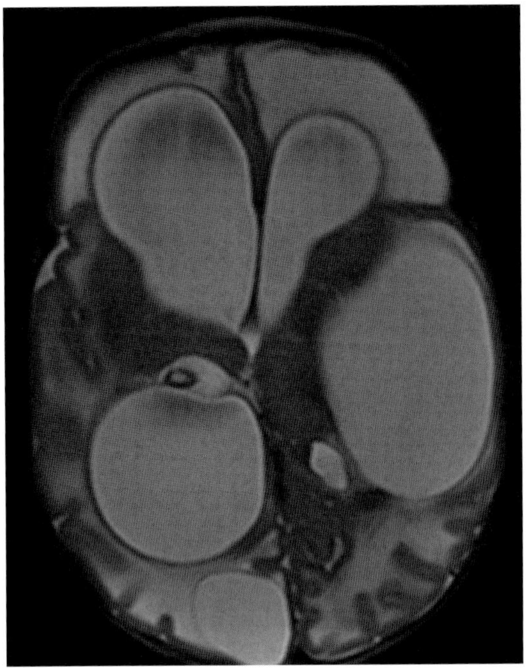

Fig. 10.3 MRI of a 4-month-old patient with a history of multiple intracranial abscesses secondary to S. aureus meningitis who developed loculated hydrocephalus requiring multiple shunt placements with endoscopic fenestrations

VSGS complication rates are comparable between the two groups except with device infection, for which PIH patients experienced higher rates [63]. ETV has had encouraging results in patients with PIH, though patients need to be carefully selected based on ventricular system anatomy. In a study of non-shunted and shunt-dependent patients with PHH or PIH, the success rate of ETV in causing durable resolution of hydrocephalus was 60 % in PIH patients [64].

Recently, ETV has received attention for its promise as a cost-effective therapy for PIH in the developing world. A study of long-term outcomes in 149 Ugandan infants with PIH compared treatment with ETV with or without CPC and those treated with permanent shunt insertion and found no significant differences in survival between the two groups. Though ETV patients experienced a lower incidence of functional dependence and disability, this was attributed mostly to treatment selection and shunting of infants with the most severe cases of PIH. The authors cited that ETV success was dependent on the absence of scarring within the prepontine cistern [65].

10.2.4 Long-Term Outcomes of PIH

The neurodevelopmental outcomes of patients with PIH vary widely, but studies have found that these patients experience higher rates of epilepsy and cognitive and functional impairment and experience lower quality of life compared to pediatric patients with hydrocephalus of other etiologies [38, 66–71]. Most of these studies only include a small number of PIH patients; in a 2007 questionnaire-based study with four PIH patients, one patient attended normal primary school, two patients were without motor disability, and one patient eventually developed epilepsy. Outcomes were assessed with the Hydrocephalus Outcomes Questionnaire; overall, there were no significant differences between PIH patients and other hydrocephalus patients in the cognitive, physical, and social-emotional health domains [66, 72]. A study of hydrocephalus outcomes in adulthood found that patients with childhood post-meningitic hydrocephalus were at higher risk for developing cognitive impairment compared to those patients who developed hydrocephalus at older ages or as a result of a focal brain lesion. Though many studies support the idea that PIH itself is associated with poor functional outcomes, few studies have examined the impact of PIH on long-term shunt outcomes and the effects of shunting and shunt complications on neurodevelopment.

References

1. Mathews TJ, Minino AM, Osterman MJ, Strobino DM, Guyer B (2011) Annual summary of vital statistics: 2008. Pediatrics 127(1):146–157. doi:10.1542/peds.2010-3175
2. Robinson S (2012) Neonatal posthemorrhagic hydrocephalus from prematurity: pathophysiology and current treatment concepts. J Neurosurg Pediatr 9(3): 242–258. doi:10.3171/2011.12.PEDS11136
3. du Plessis AJ (2008) Cerebrovascular injury in premature infants: current understanding and challenges

for future prevention. Clin Perinatol 35(4):609–641. doi:10.1016/j.clp.2008.07.010
4. du Plessis AJ (2009) The role of systemic hemodynamic disturbances in prematurity-related brain injury. J Child Neurol24(9):1127–1140.doi:10.1177/0883073809339361
5. Cinalli G, Maixner WJ, Sainte-Rose C (2004) Pediatric hydrocephalus. Springer, Milan
6. Papile LA, Burstein J, Burstein R, Koffler H (1978) Incidence and evolution of subependymal and intraventricular hemorrhage: a study of infants with birth weights less than 1,500 gm. J Pediatr 92(4):529–534
7. Volpe JJ (2008) Neurology of the newborn. Elsevier Health Sciences, Philadelphia
8. Cherian S, Whitelaw A, Thoresen M, Love S (2004) The pathogenesis of neonatal post-hemorrhagic hydrocephalus. Brain Pathol 14(3):305–311
9. Shooman D, Portess H, Sparrow O (2009) A review of the current treatment methods for posthaemorrhagic hydrocephalus of infants. Cerebrospinal Fluid Res 6:1. doi:10.1186/1743-8454-6-1
10. Weninger M, Salzer HR, Pollak A, Rosenkranz M, Vorkapic P, Korn A, Lesigang C (1992) External ventricular drainage for treatment of rapidly progressive posthemorrhagic hydrocephalus. Neurosurgery 31(1):52–57; discussion 57–58
11. Rhodes TT, Edwards WH, Saunders RL, Harbaugh RE, Little CL, Morgan LJ, Sargent SK (1987) External ventricular drainage for initial treatment of neonatal posthemorrhagic hydrocephalus: surgical and neurodevelopmental outcome. Pediatr Neurosci 13(5): 255–262
12. Berger A, Weninger M, Reinprecht A, Haschke N, Kohlhauser C, Pollak A (2000) Long-term experience with subcutaneously tunneled external ventricular drainage in preterm infants. Childs Nerv Syst 16(2): 103–109; discussion 110
13. Cornips E, Van Calenbergh F, Plets C, Devlieger H, Casaer P (1997) Use of external drainage for posthemorrhagic hydrocephalus in very low birth weight premature infants. Childs Nerv Syst 13(7):369–374
14. Taylor AG, Peter JC (2001) Advantages of delayed VP shunting in post-haemorrhagic hydrocephalus seen in low-birth-weight infants. Childs Nerv Syst 17(6):328–333
15. Willis B, Javalkar V, Vannemreddy P, Caldito G, Matsuyama J, Guthikonda B, Bollam P, Nanda A (2009) Ventricular reservoirs and ventriculoperitoneal shunts for premature infants with posthemorrhagic hydrocephalus: an institutional experience. J Neurosurg Pediatr 3(2):94–100. doi:10.3171/2008.11.PEDS0827
16. Fulkerson DH, Vachhrajani S, Bohnstedt BN, Patel NB, Patel AJ, Fox BD, Jea A, Boaz JC (2011) Analysis of the risk of shunt failure or infection related to cerebrospinal fluid cell count, protein level, and glucose levels in low-birth-weight premature infants with posthemorrhagic hydrocephalus. J Neurosurg Pediatr 7(2):147–151. doi:10.3171/2010.11.PEDS10244
17. Brouwer AJ, Groenendaal F, van den Hoogen A, Verboon-Maciolek M, Hanlo P, Rademaker KJ, de Vries LS (2007) Incidence of infections of ventricular reservoirs in the treatment of post-haemorrhagic ventricular dilatation: a retrospective study (1992-2003). Arch Dis Child Fetal Neonatal Ed 92(1):F41–F43. doi:10.1136/adc.2006.096339
18. Hudgins RJ, Boydston WR, Gilreath CL (1998) Treatment of posthemorrhagic hydrocephalus in the preterm infant with a ventricular access device. Pediatr Neurosurg 29(6):309–313, doi:28744
19. Brockmeyer DL, Wright LC, Walker ML, Ward RM (1989) Management of posthemorrhagic hydrocephalus in the low-birth-weight preterm neonate. Pediatr Neurosci 15(6):302–307; discussion 308
20. Benzel EC, Reeves JP, Nguyen PK, Hadden TA (1993) The treatment of hydrocephalus in preterm infants with intraventricular haemorrhage. Acta Neurochir 122(3–4):200–203
21. Gurtner P, Bass T, Gudeman SK, Penix JO, Philput CB, Schinco FP (1992) Surgical management of posthemorrhagic hydrocephalus in 22 low-birth-weight infants. Childs Nerv Syst 8(4):198–202
22. Whitelaw A (2001) Repeated lumbar or ventricular punctures in newborns with intraventricular hemorrhage. Cochrane Database Syst Rev (1):CD000216. doi: 10.1002/14651858.CD000216
23. Maertzdorf WJ, Vles JS, Beuls E, Mulder AL, Blanco CE (2002) Intracranial pressure and cerebral blood flow velocity in preterm infants with posthaemorrhagic ventricular dilatation. Arch Dis Child Fetal Neonatal Ed 87(3):F185–F188
24. Bass JK, Bass WT, Green GA, Gurtner P, White LE (2003) Intracranial pressure changes during intermittent CSF drainage. Pediatr Neurol 28(3):173–177
25. Tubbs RS, Banks JT, Soleau S, Smyth MD, Wellons JC 3rd, Blount JP, Grabb PA, Oakes WJ (2005) Complications of ventriculosubgaleal shunts in infants and children. Childs Nerv Syst 21(1):48–51. doi:10.1007/s00381-004-0967-6
26. Fulmer BB, Grabb PA, Oakes WJ, Mapstone TB (2000) Neonatal ventriculosubgaleal shunts. Neurosurgery 47(1):80–83; discussion 83–84
27. Wellons JC, Shannon CN, Kulkarni AV, Simon TD, Riva-Cambrin J, Whitehead WE, Oakes WJ, Drake JM, Luerssen TG, Walker ML, Kestle JR (2009) A multicenter retrospective comparison of conversion from temporary to permanent cerebrospinal fluid diversion in very low birth weight infants with posthemorrhagic hydrocephalus. J Neurosurg Pediatr 4(1):50–55. doi:10.3171/2009.2.PEDS08400
28. Limbrick DD Jr, Mathur A, Johnston JM, Munro R, Sagar J, Inder T, Park TS, Leonard JL, Smyth MD (2010) Neurosurgical treatment of progressive post-hemorrhagic ventricular dilation in preterm infants: a 10-year single-institution study. J Neurosurg Pediatr 6(3):224–230. doi:10.3171/2010.5.PEDS1010
29. Lam HP, Heilman CB (2009) Ventricular access device versus ventriculosubgaleal shunt in post hemorrhagic hydrocephalus associated with prematurity. J Matern Fetal Neonatal Med 22(11):1097–1101. doi:10.3109/14767050903029576

30. Koksal V, Oktem S (2010) Ventriculosubgaleal shunt procedure and its long-term outcomes in premature infants with post-hemorrhagic hydrocephalus. Childs Nerv Syst 26(11):1505–1515. doi:10.1007/s00381-010-1118-x
31. Acakpo-Satchivi L, Shannon CN, Tubbs RS, Wellons JC 3rd, Blount JP, Iskandar BJ, Oakes WJ (2008) Death in shunted hydrocephalic children: a follow-up study. Childs Nerv Syst 24(2):197–201. doi:10.1007/s00381-007-0408-4
32. Sklar F, Adegbite A, Shapiro K, Miller K (1992) Ventriculosubgaleal shunts: management of posthemorrhagic hydrocephalus in premature infants. Pediatr Neurosurg 18(5–6):263–265
33. Brouwer A, Groenendaal F, van Haastert IL, Rademaker K, Hanlo P, de Vries L (2008) Neurodevelopmental outcome of preterm infants with severe intraventricular hemorrhage and therapy for post-hemorrhagic ventricular dilatation. J Pediatr 152(5):648–654. doi:10.1016/j.jpeds.2007.10.005
34. Lee IC, Lee HS, Su PH, Liao WJ, Hu JM, Chen JY (2009) Posthemorrhagic hydrocephalus in newborns: clinical characteristics and role of ventriculoperitoneal shunts. Pediatr Neonatol 50(1):26–32. doi:10.1016/S1875-9572(09)60026-7
35. Vinchon M, Rekate H, Kulkarni AV (2012) Pediatric hydrocephalus outcomes: a review. Fluids Barriers CNS 9(1):18. doi:10.1186/2045-8118-9-18
36. Kulkarni AV, Drake JM, Lamberti-Pasculli M (2001) Cerebrospinal fluid shunt infection: a prospective study of risk factors. J Neurosurg 94(2):195–201. doi:10.3171/jns.2001.94.2.0195
37. Odio C, McCracken GH Jr, Nelson JD (1984) CSF shunt infections in pediatrics. A seven-year experience. Am J Dis Child 138(12):1103–1108
38. Bourgeois M, Sainte-Rose C, Cinalli G, Maixner W, Malucci C, Zerah M, Pierre-Kahn A, Renier D, Hoppe-Hirsch E, Aicardi J (1999) Epilepsy in children with shunted hydrocephalus. J Neurosurg 90(2):274–281. doi:10.3171/jns.1999.90.2.0274
39. Renier D, Lacombe J, Pierre-Kahn A, Sainte-Rose C, Hirsch JF (1984) Factors causing acute shunt infection. Computer analysis of 1174 operations. J Neurosurg 61(6):1072–1078. doi:10.3171/jns.1984.61.6.1072
40. Sciubba DM, Noggle JC, Carson BS, Jallo GI (2008) Antibiotic-impregnated shunt catheters for the treatment of infantile hydrocephalus. Pediatr Neurosurg 44(2):91–96. doi:10.1159/000113109
41. Lazareff JA, Peacock W, Holly L, Ver Halen J, Wong A, Olmstead C (1998) Multiple shunt failures: an analysis of relevant factors. Childs Nerv Syst 14(6):271–275
42. Chittiboina P, Pasieka H, Sonig A, Bollam P, Notarianni C, Willis BK, Nanda A (2013) Posthemorrhagic hydrocephalus and shunts: what are the predictors of multiple revision surgeries? J Neurosurg Pediatr 11(1):37–42. doi:10.3171/2012.8.PEDS11296
43. Whitelaw A, Kennedy CR, Brion LP (2001) Diuretic therapy for newborn infants with posthemorrhagic ventricular dilatation. Cochrane Database Syst Rev (2):CD002270. doi: 10.1002/14651858.CD002270
44. International randomised controlled trial of acetazolamide and furosemide in posthaemorrhagic ventricular dilatation in infancy. International PHVD Drug Trial Group (1998). Lancet 352 (9126):433–440
45. Yapicioglu H, Narli N, Satar M, Soyupak S, Altunbasak S (2003) Intraventricular streptokinase for the treatment of posthaemorrhagic hydrocephalus of preterm. J Clin Neurosci 10(3):297–299
46. Whitelaw A, Jary S, Kmita G, Wroblewska J, Musialik-Swietlinska E, Mandera M, Hunt L, Carter M, Pople I (2010) Randomized trial of drainage, irrigation and fibrinolytic therapy for premature infants with posthemorrhagic ventricular dilatation: developmental outcome at 2 years. Pediatrics 125(4):e852–e858. doi:10.1542/peds.2009-1960
47. Whitelaw A, Aquilina K (2012) Management of posthaemorrhagic ventricular dilatation. Arch Dis Child Fetal Neonatal Ed 97(3):F229-3. doi:10.1136/adc.2010.190173
48. Warf BC, Campbell JW, Riddle E (2011) Initial experience with combined endoscopic third ventriculostomy and choroid plexus cauterization for post-hemorrhagic hydrocephalus of prematurity: the importance of prepontine cistern status and the predictive value of FIESTA MRI imaging. Childs Nerv Syst 27(7):1063–1071. doi:10.1007/s00381-011-1475-0
49. Pikus HJ, Levy ML, Gans W, Mendel E, McComb JG (1997) Outcome, cost analysis, and long-term follow-up in preterm infants with massive grade IV germinal matrix hemorrhage and progressive hydrocephalus. Neurosurgery 40(5):983–988; discussion 988–989
50. Boynton BR, Boynton CA, Merritt TA, Vaucher YE, James HE, Bejar RF (1986) Ventriculoperitoneal shunts in low birth weight infants with intracranial hemorrhage: neurodevelopmental outcome. Neurosurgery 18(2):141–145
51. Adams-Chapman I, Hansen NI, Stoll BJ, Higgins R (2008) Neurodevelopmental outcome of extremely low birth weight infants with posthemorrhagic hydrocephalus requiring shunt insertion. Pediatrics 121(5):e1167–e1177. doi:10.1542/peds.2007-0423
52. Gupta N, Park J, Solomon C, Kranz DA, Wrensch M, Wu YW (2007) Long-term outcomes in patients with treated childhood hydrocephalus. J Neurosurg 106(5 Suppl):334–339. doi:10.3171/ped.2007.106.5.334
53. Vassilyadi M, Tataryn Z, Shamji MF, Ventureyra EC (2009) Functional outcomes among premature infants with intraventricular hemorrhage. Pediatr Neurosurg 45(4):247–255. doi:10.1159/000228982
54. Maitre NL, Marshall DD, Price WA, Slaughter JC, O'Shea TM, Maxfield C, Goldstein RF (2009) Neurodevelopmental outcome of infants with unilateral or bilateral periventricular hemorrhagic infarction. Pediatrics 124(6):e1153–e1160. doi:10.1542/peds.2009-0953
55. Resch B, Gedermann A, Maurer U, Ritschl E, Muller W (1996) Neurodevelopmental outcome of hydrocephalus following intra-/periventricular hemorrhage in preterm infants: short- and long-term results. Childs Nerv Syst 12(1):27–33

56. Handler L, Wright M (1978) Postmeningitic hydrocephalus in infancy. Neuroradiology 16(1):31–35
57. Nida TY, Haines SJ (1993) Multiloculated hydrocephalus: craniotomy and fenestration of intraventricular septations. J Neurosurg 78(1):70–76. doi:10.3171/jns.1993.78.1.0070
58. Albanese V, Tomasello F, Sampaolo S (1981) Multiloculated hydrocephalus in infants. Neurosurgery 8(6):641–646
59. Kalsbeck JE, DeSousa AL, Kleiman MB, Goodman JM, Franken EA (1980) Compartmentalization of the cerebral ventricles as a sequela of neonatal meningitis. J Neurosurg 52(4):547–552. doi:10.3171/jns.1980.52.4.0547
60. Lorber J, Pickering D (1966) Incidence and treatment of post-meningitic hydrocephalus in the newborn. Arch Dis Child 41(215):44–50
61. De Villiers J, Clüver PV, Handler L (1978) Complications following shunt operations for post-meningitic hydrocephalus. In: Treatment of hydrocephalus computer tomography. Springer, Berlin, pp 23–27
62. Tuli S, Drake J, Lawless J, Wigg M, Lamberti-Pasculli M (2000) Risk factors for repeated cerebrospinal shunt failures in pediatric patients with hydrocephalus. J Neurosurg 92(1):31–38. doi:10.3171/jns.2000.92.1.0031
63. Nagy A, Bognar L, Pataki I, Barta Z, Novak L (2013) Ventriculosubgaleal shunt in the treatment of post-hemorrhagic and postinfectious hydrocephalus of premature infants. Childs Nerv Syst 29(3):413–418. doi:10.1007/s00381-012-1968-5
64. Smyth MD, Tubbs RS, Wellons JC 3rd, Oakes WJ, Blount JP, Grabb PA (2003) Endoscopic third ventriculostomy for hydrocephalus secondary to central nervous system infection or intraventricular hemorrhage in children. Pediatr Neurosurg 39(5):258–263, doi:72871
65. Warf BC, Dagi AR, Kaaya BN, Schiff SJ (2011) Five-year survival and outcome of treatment for postinfectious hydrocephalus in Ugandan infants. J Neurosurg Pediatr 8(5):502–508. doi:10.3171/2011.8.PEDS11221
66. Platenkamp M, Hanlo PW, Fischer K, Gooskens RH (2007) Outcome in pediatric hydrocephalus: a comparison between previously used outcome measures and the hydrocephalus outcome questionnaire. J Neurosurg 107(1 Suppl):26–31. doi:10.3171/PED-07/07/026
67. Kao CL, Yang TF, Wong TT, Cheng LY, Huang SY, Chen HS, Chan RC (2001) The outcome of shunted hydrocephalic children. Zhonghua Yi Xue Za Zhi (Taipei) 64(1):47–53
68. Vinchon M, Baroncini M, Delestret I (2012) Adult outcome of pediatric hydrocephalus. Childs Nerv Syst 28(6):847–854. doi:10.1007/s00381-012-1723-y
69. Sgouros S, Malluci C, Walsh AR, Hockley AD (1995) Long-term complications of hydrocephalus. Pediatr Neurosurg 23(3):127–132
70. Vinchon M, Dhellemmes P (2006) Cerebrospinal fluid shunt infection: risk factors and long-term follow-up. Childs Nerv Syst 22(7):692–697. doi:10.1007/s00381-005-0037-8
71. Casey AT, Kimmings EJ, Kleinlugtebeld AD, Taylor WA, Harkness WF, Hayward RD (1997) The long-term outlook for hydrocephalus in childhood. A ten-year cohort study of 155 patients. Pediatr Neurosurg 27(2):63–70
72. Kulkarni AV, Rabin D, Drake JM (2004) An instrument to measure the health status in children with hydrocephalus: the hydrocephalus outcome questionnaire. J Neurosurg 101(2 Suppl):134–140. doi:10.3171/ped.2004.101.2.0134

11 Complications Related to the Type of Hydrocephalus: Normal Pressure Hydrocephalus

María Antonia Poca and Juan Sahuquillo

Contents

11.1 Normal Pressure Hydrocephalus Syndrome Today 159
11.2 Diagnosing Normal Pressure Hydrocephalus. Guidelines and Potential Mistakes 161
11.3 The Ideal Valve for NPH Patients 162
11.4 Improvement After Shunting in NPH Patients.................... 163
11.5 Mortality and Complication Rates 164
11.6 Towards a Near-Zero Shunt Infection Rate 165
11.7 Avoiding Overdrainage in NPH Patients. Facts and Fiction 167
11.8 Problems Related to the Use of Gravitational Devices and Antisiphon Mechanisms 169
11.9 Overlooked Causes of Lack of Improvement After Shunting. The Problem of Intra-abdominal Pressure 171
11.10 Late Worsening in Shunted NPH Patients. Causes and Diagnoses 172
11.11 Keypoints 172
References 173

M.A. Poca, MD, PhD (✉) • J. Sahuquillo, MD, PhD
Department of Neurosurgery and Neurotraumatology Research Unit, Vall d'Hebron University Hospital and Vall d'Hebron Research Institute, Universitat Autònoma de Barcelona, Barcelona, Spain
e-mail: pocama@neurotrauma.net; sahuquillo@neurotrauma.net

11.1 Normal Pressure Hydrocephalus Syndrome Today

Normal pressure hydrocephalus (NPH) is a treatable cause of motor and cognitive impairment in the elderly and has become more frequently diagnosed in recent years. In its complete clinical form, the syndrome is characterized by gait disturbances, progressive cognitive dysfunction, and sphincter disturbances in association with enlarged ventricles [1, 21]. In some patients, however, clinical manifestations are atypical (Parkinsonian syndrome or psychiatric manifestations) or incomplete [23, 52, 59, 64]. The basic clinical evaluation of patients with NPH includes neurological examination, neuropsychological tests, and assessment of the patient's functional status to identify the degree of dependence for daily life activities.

Despite the possibility of using sophisticated diagnostic tests, clinical symptoms continue to be the cornerstone for neurologists and neurosurgeons in the clinical evaluation of suspected NPH. Gait disorder is an early and prominent symptom of NPH [46, 59]. Nevertheless, the

C. Di Rocco et al. (eds.), *Complications of CSF Shunting in Hydrocephalus: Prevention, Identification, and Management*, DOI 10.1007/978-3-319-09961-3_11,

pattern of gait abnormality has not been clearly characterized. The severity of gait disturbance ranges from simple instability to a complete lack of balance, resulting in confinement to bed, with or without spasticity and sensory loss [52, 59]. This wide range of symptoms could contribute to the high variability in improvement after shunting reported in the literature. Gait abnormalities, however, are not the only motor disturbance present in patients with NPH [5, 23, 25, 33]. Additional abnormalities include slowing of all motor activities, including difficulty in performing fine motor tasks with the fingers, tremor of the hands, and dysgraphia [20, 66]. These patients may also present postural disturbances [5, 6] and frequently show extrapyramidal signs [33].

Despite nearly five decades of investigation, the pathological cause of idiopathic NPH (iNPH) remains unclear. Most evidence suggests that ventricular dilation is caused by impaired CSF resorption at the arachnoid granulations or impaired CSF conductance through the subarachnoid space. However, alterations of the viscoelastic properties of the brain have also been postulated as the most important causes of iNPH, especially in what is known as the "low-pressure" hydrocephalus [47]. Another hypothesis, supported by the frequently observed association between iNPH and arterial hypertension, diabetes mellitus, hypercholesterolemia, and arteriosclerotic vasculopathy [24, 26], postulates that ventricular dilation may be unrelated to CSF malabsorption and is instead secondary to periventricular microvascular disease, resulting in encephalomalacia and dilation of the cerebral ventricles. Momjian et al. demonstrated that the distribution of white matter cerebral blood flow (CBF) is different in NPH patients when compared with normal controls, with a more pronounced CBF reduction adjacent to the lateral ventricles and a logarithmic normalization with distance from the ventricles [43]. In a SPECT study, we demonstrated that CBF improves in specific regions located in frontal and parietal areas after surgery in iNPH patients [38]. The hypothesis that iNPH might be secondary to vascular encephalopathy, however, is still unproved and not uniformly accepted. What is most likely is that a combination of several of the abovementioned factors contributes to the physiopathology of iNPH. NPH symptoms have been ascribed to ischemia, stretching of the periventricular white matter, increased transmantle pressure, and the reduction of the periventricular CBF, among others.

Two main obstacles remain in the management of patients with suspected iNPH: the difficulty of making a correct diagnosis and the selection of an appropriate shunt to permit maximal clinical improvement with a minimal rate of complications. In the last few decades, different tests and diagnostic tools that combine ICP monitoring and CSF dynamics with neuroimaging studies and CSF removal strategies have been used. However, a standard protocol for the evaluation of patients with suspected iNPH is lacking, even after the recent publication of guidelines for the management of iNPH patients [34, 44]. In some centers, the decision to treat patients may be based only on clinical and neuroimaging studies, while in others further studies such as CSF dynamic studies or continuous ICP monitoring are required. It is important to note, however, that the best results reported are those in which the diagnosis was based on continuous ICP monitoring [17, 54].

It is now clear that in some patients with NPH syndrome mean ICP is not always normal, even when these patients have no symptoms of intracranial hypertension but show the classical symptoms of NPH syndrome. In some of these patients, continuous ICP monitoring shows either isolated episodes of intracranial hypertension—usually during rapid eye movement (REM) sleep—or even continuously elevated mean ICP. Although the term "normal pressure hydrocephalus," as first described by Hakim, continues to be used, the alternative term "adult chronic hydrocephalus," which does not indicate any ICP value or pathophysiological theories, is being increasingly adopted and better defines this complex and frequent syndrome.

The treatment of NPH syndrome has remained relatively unchanged since the early 1970s. The implantation of a ventriculoperitoneal or a ventriculoatrial shunt with a differential-pressure valve to drain excess CSF from the cerebral ventricles is still the treatment of choice. The best clinical results have been achieved with the use of low-pressure opening valves. However, some strategies have been adopted to reduce the complications associated with these devices. At present, high rates of improvement associated with very low mortality and morbidity rates have been reported.

11.2 Diagnosing Normal Pressure Hydrocephalus. Guidelines and Potential Mistakes

Suspicion of NPH syndrome requires the presence of compatible clinical symptoms and an increased ventricular size. However, older patients with suspected idiopathic NPH can also present associated morbidities, such as small vessel white matter disease with its associated cognitive burden, Alzheimer disease, Parkinsonism, or other subclinical neuronal degenerative processes, and cervical spondylotic myelopathy, among others, which can hinder the diagnosis of the entity and the decision of whether or not to use shunt therapy [32]. Stimulated by a consensus workshop held in San Antonio in September 2000, Marmarou et al. published in 2005 the guidelines for the diagnosis and management of the iNPH patients with the aim of providing the best evidence to support current clinical practice [35]. These guidelines cover 4 major topics: the clinical diagnosis of iNPH, the value of supplementary diagnostic tests, surgical management, and outcome. In 2012, Mori et al., supported by the Japanese Society of NPH and by the Japan Neurosurgical Society, published the second edition of their guidelines for management of iNPH (the first edition was published in May 2004 by the Japanese Society of NPH Guidelines Committee) [44]. In both cases, iNPH is classified into three diagnostic levels: "probable," "possible," or "unlikely" in the Marmarou guideline and preoperatively "possible" or "probable" and postoperatively "definite" in the Japanese guidelines. These subclassifications cause confusion in the management of these patients. On the other hand, it is important to note that a limiting factor of both guidelines is that their recommendations are based only on class III evidence (retrospectively collected data), which is suitable for validating management options but not for establishing guidelines or standards of care.

In the Marmarou guidelines, several controversial points are found in the algorithm for predicting shunt response in iNPH that can in fact delay the treatment of patients who may improve after shunting. The first is the requirement of the complete clinical triad. Patients with only two of the three classical symptoms are classified as possible iNPH; the guidelines recommend follow-up without any supplementary diagnostic testing [34]. However, the presence of an incomplete clinical triad is frequently associated with a high rate of improvement after shunting (84 %) when the diagnosis of iNPH was confirmed by ICP findings [54]. In the same algorithm of the guidelines, patients with the complete triad are studied in an outpatient clinic to perform a CSF tap test of 40–50 mL. If the response is positive, the authors consider it highly predictive of a favorable shunt response (72–100 %) and recommend surgical treatment; however, if the response is negative, they recommend performing an infusion test to calculate the resistance to CSF absorption (R_{out}) based on the low sensitivity of the test (26–61 %). If R_{out} is abnormally increased, the guidelines recommend treating the patient, but if it is normal, surgical treatment is ruled out [34]. In a recent study (unpublished results), we determined the sensitivity, specificity, and predictive values of R_{out} in predicting clinical improvement after shunting in 136 patients with iNPH who were monitored with continuous ICP and CSF dynamics studies. In this study, improvement after shunting was considered the gold standard in the diagnosis of NPH. Our results show that the use of R_{out} values—calculated using the Katzman and Hussey infusion test—to select iNPH for shunting is associated with a substantial false-negative rate that increases when the cutoff value of R_{out} is raised from 10 mmHg/mL/min (16.6 %) to 18 mmHg/mL/min (63.3 %). The take-home message for the clinician is that when R_{out} is abnormal, patients should undergo

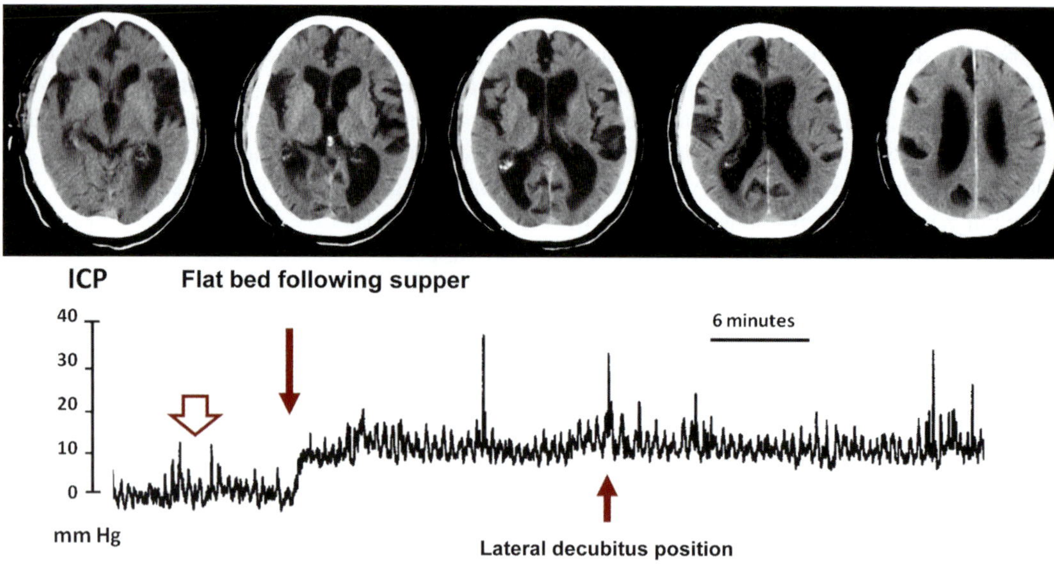

Fig. 11.1 Intracranial pressure (*ICP*) monitoring in a patient with idiopathic normal pressure hydrocephalus. Note that ICP values are negative when the bed is inclined 45° to allow the patient to eat (first part of the recording, *large arrow*). After returning the bed to a flat position, ICP values increased by a mean of 12 mmHg

shunting. However, if R_{out} is normal, additional tests should be performed before ruling out shunt therapy (unpublished study). In our experience, continuous ICP monitoring should be mandatory when the tap test is negative or R_{out} is within a normal range despite compatible clinical and radiological data. Several authors support the view that continuous ICP monitoring is the most useful diagnostic test in NPH [49, 58, 61].

11.3 The Ideal Valve for NPH Patients

The most important and neglected factor for optimizing outcome in patients with iNPH is valve selection. For many years, the selection of the most appropriate shunt for these patients has been controversial and continues to be an unresolved issue [4, 44]. The most appropriate shunt in these patients would be one that ensures the maximal clinical benefit with minimal shunt-related complications. The selection of the shunt hardware for implantation has traditionally been considered a secondary issue by most neurosurgeons. In the last decade, the appearance of a wide variety of different valves, shunt designs, and gravity-compensating devices in the neurosurgical market has made things far more complicated for the neurosurgeon, who now must choose among valves with different opening pressures, variable hydrodynamics, and adjustable valves with or without gravitational devices. Before this significant increase in shunt hardware, the most difficult decision for a neurosurgeon was whether a medium, high, or low opening pressure valve should be implanted. Bergsneider et al. [4] emphasized that there is insufficient evidence to recommend a specific pressure setting in valves for patients with iNPH. However, Boon et al. [7] and McQuarrie et al. [40, 41] reported more significant improvement rates when low-pressure valves rather than medium- or high-pressure valves were used in NPH patients. Moreover, Zemack and Romner [70] found that when adjustable valves (so-called "programmable" valves) with a medium opening pressure of 130 mm H_2O were used in iNPH patients, 53.6 % required a reduction in the opening pressure of the valve, with 46 % of patients improving after this modification [70].

In patients with secondary NPH syndrome, ICP is usually high, while in iNPH patients continuous ICP monitoring shows that mean ICP is frequently below 12 mmHg and in some patients may even be negative (Fig. 11.1). In these patients, medium- or high-pressure valves will function erratically. When the valve opening pressure is higher than the patient's mean ICP, the valve will open only during Valsalva maneuvers when the patient is upright (siphoning effect) and possibly during REM sleep and concomitant high-amplitude B-waves. We believe that low-pressure, low-resistance valves should always be implanted in these patients to avoid occult shunt underdrainage and the lack of improvement associated with medium- or high-pressure valves. Low-pressure valves, combined with a gravitational device, may permit a more homogeneous and physiological CSF drainage in these patients; this could explain the lower rate of subdural collections (hematomas and hygromas) found in our patients (<10 %) [50, 54, 64] in comparison with those of Boon et al. [7], who reported a rate of 71 %.

At present, the selection criteria used in our department to select a shunt in iNPH patients can be summarized as follows: (a) in low-risk patients (Evans Index <0.40 without anticoagulant therapy), a ventriculoperitoneal differential low-pressure, low-resistance valve associated with a gravitational device is used, and (b) in high-risk patients (Evans Index ≥0.40, severe cortical atrophy, or treatment with acenocoumarol or similar drugs), an adjustable valve, implanted together with an in-line gravity-compensating accessory, is the recommended system. In this latter group, we usually select an initial opening pressure of 100–110 mm H_2O. This opening pressure is progressively reduced over days or weeks, with a final opening pressure of between 30 and 50 mm H_2O, depending on preoperative ICP values and clinical changes. One of the main advantages of using adjustable valves in these patients is the possibility of temporarily increasing the opening pressure if the patient develops subdural effusions. In our opinion, the extra cost of this configuration compared with that of a simple differential-pressure valve with the same gravitational device is compensated by the possibility of manipulating the shunt without the need for further surgery. The pressure selected for the gravitational device may vary according to height and body mass index (BMI) [62]. Valves and gravitational devices should be of the ball-in-cone design, which have been shown to be much more reliable than silicon designs in laboratory studies [45]. We recommend the neurosurgeons develop a good understanding of the hydrodynamic characteristics of shunts that, ideally, have been tested in independent laboratories [12, 13].

11.4 Improvement After Shunting in NPH Patients

The clinical outcomes of treated NPH patients reported in the literature vary widely and depend on several factors: the type of patients treated (idiopathic versus secondary NPH and the degree of clinical deterioration before shunt placement), symptom duration, comorbidity, the tests used to establish the diagnosis of NPH (all of which are associated with a variable percentage of false negatives), and the type of hardware selected, among others. Significant improvement after shunting ranges from 29 to 96 % [22, 57, 69]. The largest percentages of improvement have usually been reported in small series of patients managed in single centers [50, 51, 57]. However, larger recent studies have consistently shown that a high percentage of patients improve after shunt placement [17, 39, 54] and that improvement persists several years after treatment [39, 56].

In several series of patients with iNPH, we showed that a high percentage of improvement and a low complications rate can be achieved by using a strict protocol for the study and treatment of these fragile patients [50, 54]. In the management protocol for iNPH, outcome was independently assessed by the neurosurgeon and an independent neuropsychologist using the NPH scale (Table 11.1) 6 months after shunting [64]. If discrepancies were found between the neurosurgeon and the neuropsychologist, the patient was reevaluated and the final score was assigned by consensus. Because a small change in the NPH scale score represents a substantial change in the patient's functional status, we defined moderate improvement as a one-point increase and marked improvement as an increase of at least two points.

In a series of 244 iNPH patients who were shunted, 1 patient died in the postoperative period from an acute respiratory infection and 3 patients

Table 11.1 Normal pressure hydrocephalus scale

	Score
I. Gait evaluation (GE)	
Patient is bedridden or unable to ambulate	1
Ambulation is possible with help	2
Independent walking is possible but unstable or the patient falls	3
Abnormal but stable gait	4
Normal gait	5
II. Cognitive functions (CF)	
Patient is in a vegetative or minimally conscious state	1
Severe dementia	2
Severe cognitive problems with behavior disturbances	3
Cognitive problems reported by the patient or family	4
Cognitive disturbances are only found by specific testing	5
III. Sphincter disturbances (SD)	
Urinary and fecal incontinence	1
Continuous urinary incontinence	2
Sporadic urinary incontinence	3
Urinary urgency	4
No objective or subjective sphincter dysfunction	5

Normal pressure hydrocephalus score = GE + CF + SD. Minimum possible score = 3 points. Maximum score = 15 points

died less than 6 months after surgery from causes unrelated to shunting (stroke, chronic respiratory disease, and myocardial infarction). Four patients (1.6 %) were lost to follow-up and therefore the final sample consisted of 236 patients. After shunting, an increase of 1 or more points in the total NPH scale score was found in 212 of the 236 evaluated patients (89.8 %), no improvement was found in 18 patients (7.6 %), while some worsening was observed in 6 patients (2.5 %). In the 212 patients who improved, improvement was moderate in 30 patients (an increase of 1 point in the NPH scale) and was marked in 182 (a median increase in the NPH scale of 4 points, min = 2, max = 11). In agreement with previous literature, greater improvement was observed in gait and sphincter control when compared to cognitive function [54]. Patients with the highest scores on the NPH scale (13 and 14) showed lower percentages of improvement than patients with scores of between 3 and 12 on the NPH scale. These lower percentages of improvement were probably due to the ceiling effect in the NPH scale: in patients with minor clinical symptoms and little functional deterioration, only small improvements are possible. In these patients the aim of surgery is not only to reverse the subtle symptoms they might present but, more importantly, to prevent further clinical and neuropsychological deterioration. Knowledge of these results is essential when discussing the expectations of surgery with patients and their caregivers.

11.5 Mortality and Complication Rates

Because of the potential morbidity associated with shunt implantation, many neurosurgeons have been reluctant to operate on iNPH patients. The complication rates reported in literature vary and are sometimes very high. A meta-analysis by Hebb and Cusimano [22] reported a mean complication rate of 38 % (range: 5–100 %), mostly shunt revisions (22 %; range: 0–47 %), and a 6 % mortality or permanent neurological deficit. The Dutch NPH study reported subdural effusions in 53 % of shunted patients, two-thirds of which spontaneously decreased or resolved [7]. In this series, two patients (0.8 %) died due to problems directly related to shunting (one in the early postoperative period and another at 6 months after surgery). This percentage is very low if we consider the age and the frequent comorbidity commonly found in iNPH patients. Rates of shunt revision of as high as 47 % have also been reported [27]. In Hebb and Cusimano's review, 22 % of patients required additional surgery [22]. The most frequent serious shunt-related complications are cerebral or subdural hematoma, shunt obstruction, and infection. Less serious adverse events include subdural hygromas that do not require evacuation, orthostatic headache, abdominal pain, and transitory hypoacousia or tinnitus, among others.

In our most recently published cohort of patients, mortality related to treatment was 0.4 % (1 of the 244 shunted patients died in the early

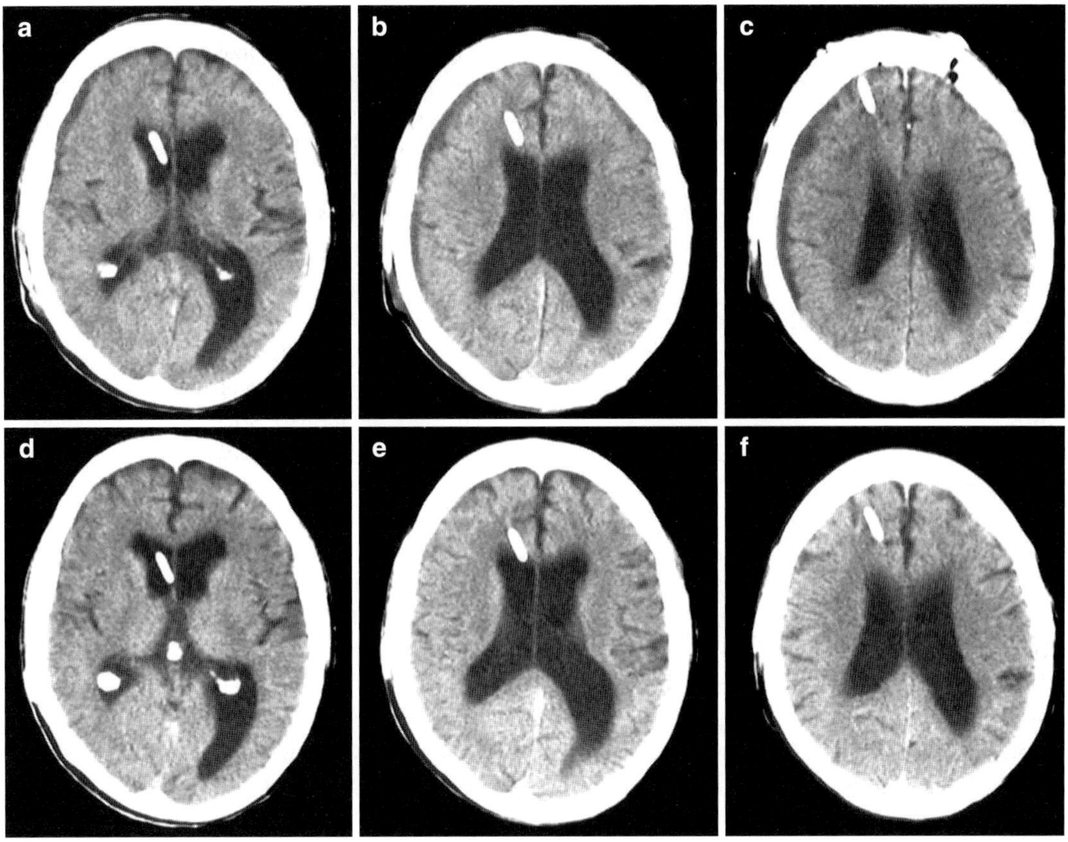

Fig. 11.2 CT scans from a patient with iNPH after shunting. The initial follow-up CT scan (1 week after surgery; *top images* **a–c**) showed a small hygroma that did not have a relevant mass effect through the hemisphere and did not require treatment. The hygroma completely resolved at 3.5 months after shunting (*bottom images* **d–f**)

postoperative period from an acute respiratory infection) [54]. Early (first month after shunting) or late (within 6 months of surgery) complications were found in less than 10 % of shunted iNPH patients. Only one patient had a shunt infection. Asymptomatic subdural collections found immediately after or at 6 months after surgery were not considered complications because they did not require treatment (Fig. 11.2). However, if we include these collections in the complication rate, the total percentage would increase to 13.8 % [54]; this is still a very low percentage when compared with outcomes reported in other series. This low percentage could be due not only to the use of shunts that include a gravitational device but also by our surgical management protocol, which combines several measures before, during, and after shunt placement [50, 51]. Table 11.2 outlines the complications in this cohort of 244 treated patients.

11.6 Towards a Near-Zero Shunt Infection Rate

CSF shunt infection remains 1 of the major causes of morbidity in the treatment of both pediatric and adult hydrocephalus and occurs in 3–15 % of patients [8, 9, 39]. Recently published studies of large series of patients, however, reported relatively low infection rates (1–6 %) [11, 17, 54]. The hardware used does not significantly modify the risk of infection [44], although several studies have demonstrated the modest efficacy of antibiotic-impregnated shunt systems

Table 11.2 Clinical improvement and complications in iNPH ($n = 236$)

	Patients	(%)
Clinical improvement		
Increase of 1 point in the total NPH scale *(moderated improvement)*	30	12.7
Increase of >1 point in the total NPH scale *(marked improvement)*	182	77.1
No improvement	18	7.6
Some worsening	6	2.5
Improvement in everyday activities scale ($n = 195$)	114	58.5
Reduction in the degree of disability assessed by the RDRS-2 ($n = 206$) From a median of 32 (IQR: 16.25, min: 19, max: 60) before surgery to a median of 26 (IQR: 12, min: 18, max: 54) after shunting ($W = -12701.0$, $p < 0.001$)		
Mortality and early and late complications		
Mortality	1	0.4
Early complications ($n = 244$)	13	5.3
Subdural hematoma	4	5.3
Shunt malfunction	2	0.8
Systemic complications	4	1.6
Postural hypoacousia	1	0.4
Parenchymal hematoma	1	0.4
Hemorrhagic complication when the burr hole was performed	1	0.4
Late complications ($n = 236$)	15	6.4
Asymptomatic hygromas	8	3.4
Subdural hematomas (3 acute and 3 chronic)	6	2.5
Distal catheter infection	1	0.4

iNPH idiopathic normal pressure hydrocephalus, *RDRS-2* rapid disability rating scale-2, *IQR* interquartile range

in reducing infections in both pediatric and adult patients [18, 19, 48, 60]. In fact, improvements in surgical technique and surgical experience may be the factors that contribute most to reducing the rate of infection and other shunt-related complications.

The low rates of infection and other complications reported in our series could be explained, in part, by the following surgical management protocol used in our department [50, 54].

- One dose of sulfamethoxazole (1,600 mg) and trimethoprim (320 mg) is used as antibiotic prophylaxis during anesthesia induction, followed by three additional doses every 12 h.
- The head, thorax, and abdomen are washed twice (once in the ward and again after anesthesia induction).
- The surgical field is painted with iodine solution and covered with iodine-soaked gauze strips for at least 3 min.
- The ventriculostomy is always made using a frontal approach with a curved incision centered on the burr hole (10.5 cm from the nasion and 2.5–3 cm from the midline).
- The dura mater is always opened by making a small 3- or 4-mm dural perforation after coagulating the dura with low-intensity monopolar coagulation and adhering it to the arachnoid by the same process. Whenever possible, the maximum diameter of the dural perforation is limited to the maximum diameter of the ventricular catheter.
- To clean the catheter lumen of brain debris and as an additional measure to prevent infection, an intraventricular bolus of vancomycin (20 mg) is administered in all patients.
- The distal catheter is always introduced in the peritoneal cavity by open dissection through a small laparotomy. A percutaneous trocar is never used.
- When the surgical procedure is finished, moderate abdominal compression is applied using a girdle. This abdominal compression is maintained during the day and is removed at night for 3–4 weeks.
- Ambulation is started on the third day after shunting.
- In patients with gravitational valves or devices, beds are inclined at 30–45° for the first postoperative week to reduce the flow though the shunt and avoid overdrainage. At hospital discharge, the patients are advised to maintain this bed position at home until the first follow-up visit, which is routinely performed 2–3 months after surgery.

Using this protocol, the infection rate in NPH-shunted patients is less than 1 % [50, 54]. This percentage does not justify the routine use of antibiotic-impregnated shunt systems.

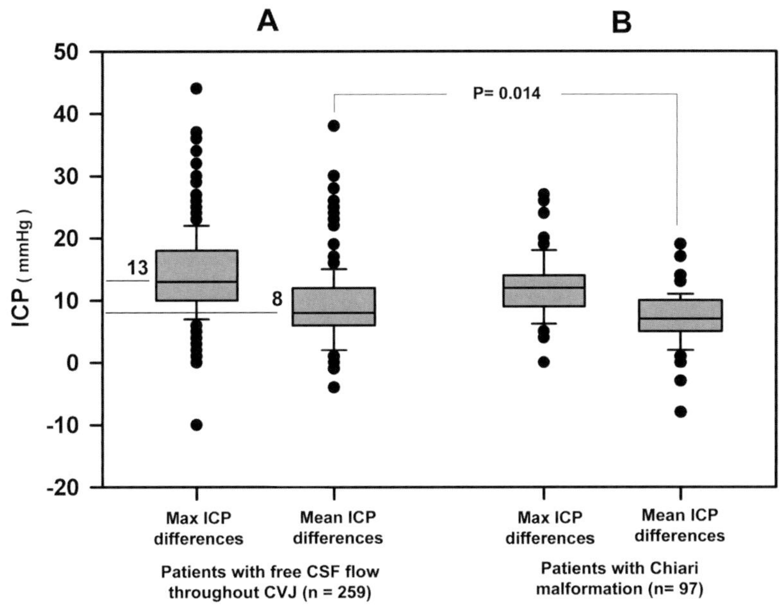

Fig. 11.3 Box-and-whisker plots showing the maximum and mean ICP differences obtained in (**a**) 259 patients with free CSF flow throughout the craniovertebral junction (*CVJ*) and (**b**) 97 patients with Chiari malformations. In all patients ICP was continuously monitored after changing body position (from supine to sitting position). In the first group, the median of the maximum (differences between mean ICP in the supine position and the lowest ICP values recorded after changing body position) and the mean ICP differences (differences between mean ICP in the supine position and mean ICP recorded while the patient remained in sitting position during 3 h) were 13 mmHg (interquartile range: 10–17) and 8 mmHg (interquartile range: 5–11), respectively. *Max* maximum

11.7 Avoiding Overdrainage in NPH Patients. Facts and Fiction

Complications due to shunt overdrainage still have an unreasonably high prevalence in high-risk patients such as those with iNPH. Overdrainage is directly related to the hydrodynamic profile of shunts and is caused by the negative hydrostatic pressure distal to the valve when the patient assumes the erect position. Orthostatic headache, diplopia, tinnitus, and chronic subdural effusions are the most frequent phenomena related to overdrainage in adults, while ventricular catheter block, slit ventricle syndrome, subdural hematoma, trapped fourth ventricle, and acquired Chiari I malformation have been frequently reported in children [36, 37]. Between 10 and 30 % of shunt revisions have been attributed to overdrainage in NPH patients.

Under normal circumstances, when a supine subject sits or stands up, ICP falls to subatmospheric values [29]. ICP reduction with even slightly negative values is a well-known physiological phenomenon demonstrated in humans in pivotal clinical studies [29–31]. Head elevation physiologically decreases ICP by displacing CSF into the spinal canal and by improving cerebral venous drainage thought the opening of alternative venous channels in the posterior circulation that remain closed when patients are recumbent [29, 31, 68]. In a large series of patients in whom ICP was monitored before shunting, we showed that ICP values are significantly reduced after changing from a supine to a sitting or upright position. However, this ICP reduction is significantly greater in patients with free CSF flow through the craniospinal junction when compared to those with Chiari malformations (Fig. 11.3).

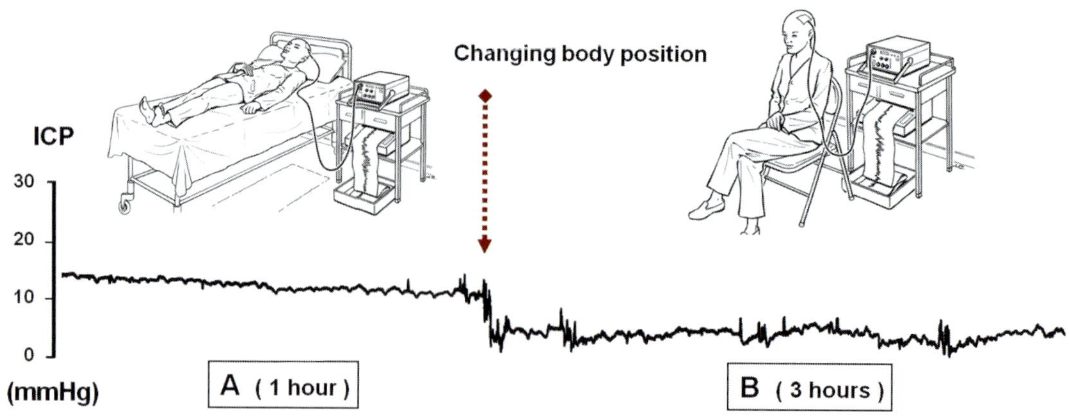

Fig. 11.4 Posture-related ICP changes. The ICP profile after postural changes was very similar in all the patients studied and showed a maximal decrease immediately after patients were seated, with a subsequent moderate recovery followed by stabilization

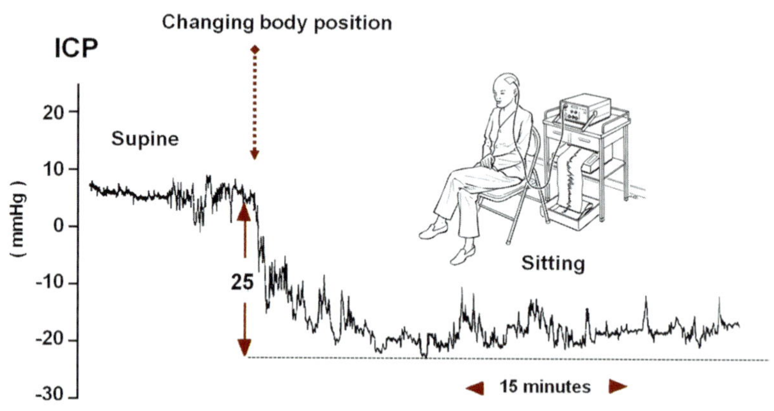

Fig. 11.5 ICP recording of a patient in whom a classical differential low-pressure valve was implanted. In this patient, ICP dropped suddenly by 25 mmHg when placed in sitting position. These values remained very low and the patient reported headaches

This finding reinforces the theory that CSF displacement into the spinal canal is hampered in this latter group of patients [53]. ICP profile after postural changes was very similar in all the patients, showing a maximal decrease immediately after patients assume the sitting position, with a subsequent moderate recovery followed by stabilization (Fig. 11.4). The median of the maximum ICP differences (differences between mean ICP in the supine position and the lowest ICP values recorded after changing body position) was 13 mmHg (interquartile range: 10–17 mmHg), and the median of the mean ICP differences (differences between mean ICP in the supine position and mean ICP recorded while the patient remained in sitting position during 3 h) was 8 mmHg (interquartile range: 5–11 mmHg) [53].

ICP reduction after changes in body position may also occur in patients with high ICP [16]. To prevent or help to improve intracranial hypertension, various degrees of head elevation have been used as a routine maneuver in the management of neurocritical patients. This physiological phenomenon is magnified, however, in patients in whom a classical differential pressure valve has been implanted. In these patients, ICP values of less than −20 mmHg may be observed when the patient changes to a vertical body position (Fig. 11.5), unless a mechanism to compensate or eliminate what has been called the "siphoning effect" is used [3, 10]. This nonphysiological gradient is a direct consequence of the gravitational changes induced by the hydrostatic fluid column between the tips of the ventricular and the distal catheters. In the supine position, the closing pressure of the valve is the main factor that controls flow in shunts. However, when the patient is upright, hydrostatic pressure in the distal catheter keeps the valve open continuously, even when intraventricular pressure becomes negative [63]. Under these circumstances, the hydrodynamics of the shunt (R_{shunt}) is the main factor controlling CSF flow until the valve is closed again. In the absence of gravitational devices, when the patient is in an upright position the flow can continue as long as the ventricles contain drainable CSF. A common—but mistaken—strategy to avoid problems related to overdrainage has been the use of medium- or high-pressure valves. However, as Aschoff has stated (personal communication), the problems of overdrainage are related to gravity and therefore have to be prevented by gravitational devices, not by upgrading the opening pressure of the valve. The belief that upgrading the opening pressure of a valve avoids overdrainage is not entirely correct because the opening pressure of a valve only controls flow when the patient is recumbent. There is strong evidence that the use of medium- or high-pressure valves does not exclude the possibility of subdural effusions (hygromas or hematomas). Boon et al. reported a 34 % incidence of subdural effusions in a group of patients with medium-pressure valves [7]. The use of adjustable valves can reduce, but not exclude, nonphysiological flow rates while the patient is upright and the possibility of complications related to hyperdrainage [2].

Since the introduction of the first antisiphon device by Portnoy et al. in 1973 [55], various devices have been developed to compensate for the gravitational effect of the negative hydrostatic pressure induced when the patient stands and control shunt overdrainage. Both antisiphon and gravitational devices reduce the rate of CSF drainage in differential pressure valves when the patient is sitting or standing. Antisiphon mechanisms are based on a subcutaneous membrane that responds to negative pressure inside the shunt while gravitational devices upgrade the opening pressure of the system to control the gravitational effect that an upright position causes. Both designs have been used as separate devices added in series to the distal catheter or they have been already incorporated into the valve. Both types of hardware significantly reduce the incidence of shunt overdrainage. In a recent multicenter randomized trial in patients with iNPH (SVASONA study), patients were treated with either a programmable gravitational valve (proGAV, Aesculap-Miethke, Potsdam, Germany) or a programmable non-gravitational valve (CMPV, Codman and Shurtleff, Johnson and Johnson, Raynham, Massachusetts, USA). In a 1-year follow-up, the authors showed that the use of a gravitational valve significantly reduced the incidence of overdrainage complications while maintaining the same treatment efficacy [28]. In that study, both valves were initially implanted with an opening pressure of 100 mm H_2O and adjusted 3 months after surgery to 70 mm H_2O [28]. However, caution should be taken when using gravitational devices with medium- or high-pressure valves because they may induce underdrainage.

11.8 Problems Related to the Use of Gravitational Devices and Antisiphon Mechanisms

The use of gravitational devices incorporated into the valve or added in series into the distal catheter produces a more physiological CSF drainage through the shunt, reducing overdrainage complications. However, the use of these devices requires knowledge of several aspects that can potentially reduce efficacy or even produce underdrainage. The association of an antisiphon or a gravity-compensating device in series with medium- or high-pressure shunts, which reduces CSF drainage when the patient is upright, may increase the possibility of underdrainage, especially if the patient is obese; in this group of patients, intra-abdominal pressure is usually above 0 mmHg [62]. There are other potential problems associated with the use of antisiphon and gravity-compensating devices. Malfunction

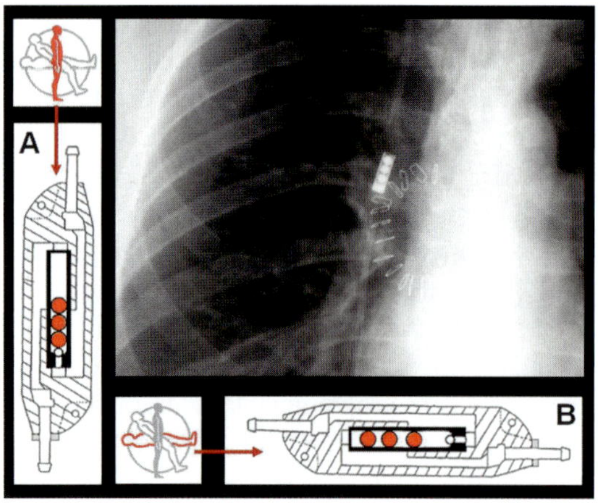

Fig. 11.6 Gravity-compensating accessory containing three stainless steel balls (medium pressure) in a ruby ball-in-cone mechanism. When the patient is upright, the opening pressure of the shunt system increases (**a**) due to the weight of the balls, and when the patient is in supine position, the pressure is theoretically equal to 0 mmHg because the balls fall away (**b**)

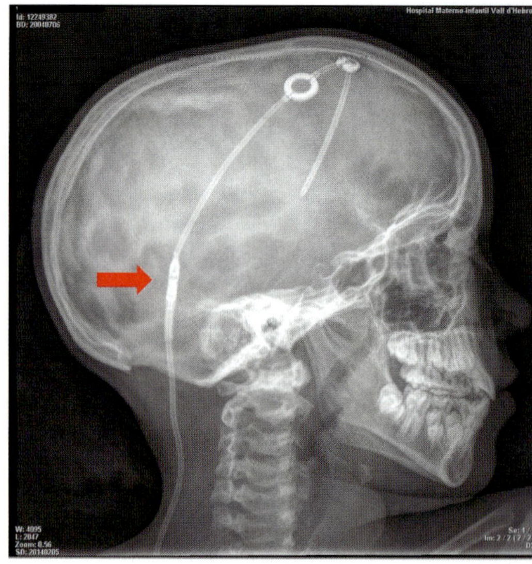

Fig. 11.7 Skull radiography showing a PaediGAV gravity-assisted valve (Aesculap AG, Potsdam, Germany) of 9/19 mm H_2O implanted in a pediatric patient with hydrocephalus. Observe the vertical orientation of the device (*red arrow*)

can also occur when gravitational devices become misaligned with the vertical position after implantation, while CSF drainage can be hampered when subcutaneous pressure increases over the membrane of an antisiphon device [2]. By design, gravitational devices are much more robust and reliable than antisiphon devices. In addition, antisiphon devices can induce ICP recording abnormalities when the patient is sitting or standing [63].

The basic mechanism used in antisiphon devices is increased resistance of the shunt (R_{shunt}). Gravitational devices upgrade the opening pressure of the valve through the movement of inbuilt metallic balls when the patient moves from the recumbent to the sitting or standing position (Fig. 11.6). Consequently, the correct function of any gravitational device depends on an adequate vertical implantation. Any degree of deviation from the vertical axis equal to or more than 45° may eliminate the effect of the device (Christoph Miethke, personal communication, 2004). Although retroauricular implantation of the gravitational valve is common, especially in pediatric patients (Fig. 11.7), correct vertical alignment should always be ensured because the movement of the head with relation to the body axis may compromise the functioning of the device. In adults for whom body growth is not a factor, we prefer to implant the gravitational devices based on ball technology in the thorax (Fig. 11.6) to avoid or minimize this problem.

Antisiphon mechanisms, based on a subcutaneous membrane, have been used as a separate device added to the distal catheter or, more frequently, incorporated into the valve. These devices may reduce overdrainage associated with postural changes. However, CSF drainage can be hampered when the subcutaneous pressure increases over the membrane [14]. When these devices are used, clinical deterioration after a transient improvement should serve as a warning to the clinician of the possibility of antisiphon malfunction. In general, caution should be exercised when antisiphon devices are used in patients with iNPH, even when this device is combined with a differential low-pressure valve. Progressive subcutaneous scarring over the membrane of the antisiphon may overpressurize the device and produce functional underdrainage of the shunt [15], which may cause B-waves or marked ICP irregularities in some patients when sitting or

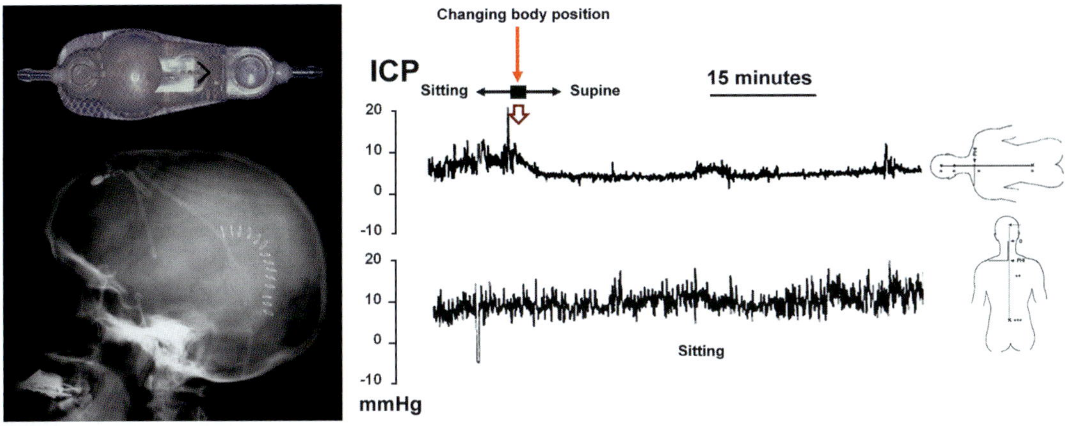

Fig. 11.8 (*Left*) Patient with an adult chronic hydrocephalus secondary to aqueductal stenosis shunted with a Delta valve (performance level 0.5). (*Right*) ICP was normal while the patient was supine (*upper chart*). Observe the immediate normalization of the ICP recording induced by the patient when changing from a sitting to a supine position (*arrows*). The ICP recording was clearly abnormal after the patient had returned to sitting position for 2 h, without significant changes in mean ICP (*bottom chart*) (Figure modified from Sahuquillo et al. [63])

standing (Fig. 11.8) [63]. This can induce occult shunt dysfunction with a subsequent lack of improvement or clinical worsening. We believe that in patients with iNPH, low-pressure valves associated with gravitational devices that are not sensitive to scarring or external pressures are superior to any antisiphon design.

11.9 Overlooked Causes of Lack of Improvement After Shunting. The Problem of Intra-abdominal Pressure

Classically, intra-abdominal pressure (IAP) has been considered to be of little importance due to the traditional idea that this value is close to zero. Nevertheless, in overweight patients (Fig. 11.9) and in pregnant women, IAP can be higher, interfering with correct shunt function. IAP is one of the four factors that determine perfusion pressure (PP) in a ventriculoperitoneal shunt. PP is expressed as the difference between inflow pressure (P1), calculated by adding ICP and the hydrostatic pressure (HP) values, and outflow pressure (P2), the sum of the closure pressure (CP) of the valve and IAP [PP=P1 – P2=(ICP+HP) – (CP+IAP)]. An elevated IAP may decrease the PP of the shunt and induce a significant flow reduction, preventing the shunt from opening when the PP is equal to or less than 0. Several case reports of shunt dysfunction with neurological worsening or even coma secondary to a significant increase in IAP have been reported [42, 62].

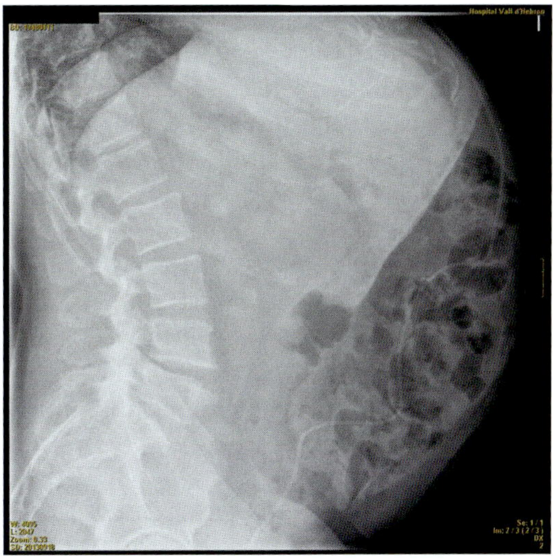

Fig. 11.9 Abdominal radiography of an obese patient who showed a shunt dysfunction due to high abdominal pressure. A Polaris adjustable valve with an opening pressure of 70 mm H_2O, combined with a gravity-compensating accessory, was initially used. The patient improved after the gravity-compensating accessory was removed

The classical idea that IAP is atmospheric (0 mmHg) or slightly subatmospheric (<0 mmHg) was first contradicted by Sugerman et al. in 1997 [67]. He determined the IAP in 84 morbidly obese patients and in 5 normal individuals and found that an increased sagittal abdominal diameter was associated with an increased IAP. These results were corroborated in a posterior study by Sanchez et al. in 2001 [65]. Those authors found that BMI was positively related to IAP measured using a transurethral bladder catheter (Foley), which showed that IAP reached pressures of higher than 8 mmHg in obese and morbidly obese patients [65]. In a study in which IAP was directly measured in the peritoneal cavity during shunt surgery in 60 patients with hydrocephalus of different etiologies, we demonstrated that BMI is a good estimator of IAP [62]. We also found a strong linear correlation between BMI and IAP. The mean IAP obtained in our study was 4 mmHg in obese patients, 3 mmHg in overweight patients, and 1 mmHg in patients with a normal BMI. Therefore, the assumption of an IAP of around 0 mmHg can only be considered in patients with a normal BMI who are recumbent. Due to the high prevalence of overweight and obesity in developed countries, neurosurgeons should take IAP into account when selecting the most adequate shunt to be implanted. This is especially important for patients with NPH syndrome in whom normal or even subatmospheric ICP can be found and in whom a significant increase in IAP increases the risk of underdrainage.

11.10 Late Worsening in Shunted NPH Patients. Causes and Diagnoses

McGirt et al. reviewed 10 years of clinical data in their center involving a diagnostic protocol with CSF pressure monitoring and controlled CSF drainage to recommend CSF shunting in the treatment of 132 patients with iNPH. Of the 99 patients who initially responded to CSF shunting, 9 patients (9 %) had late deterioration 10±6 months after their initial improvement, despite no evidence of shunt malfunction [39]. The long-term response rate was 75 % after a significant follow-up period (mean: 18 months) [39]. Incorrect valve selection or shunt malfunction should be suspected in patients with positive diagnostic criteria who failed to improve after surgery. Worsening after initial improvement may be due to added comorbidities, a shunt with insufficient CSF drainage, or shunt dysfunction, as well as significant weight gain and the possibility of occult shunt underdrainage due to high IAP. The assessment of shunt malfunction by manual exploration of the chamber valve, shunt radiographs, or radionuclide shunt studies may be misleading. In this clinical scenario, continuous ICP monitoring allows shunt function to be studied in vivo. This test may be especially important if ICP has also been monitored before shunting because mean ICP values and recording characteristics (amplitude, pathological ICP waves, ICP differences during postural changes, etc.) may be compared.

11.11 Keypoints

Several points, summarized below, may be considered in the diagnosis and treatment of iNPH patients to avoid false negatives in the diagnosis, reduce complications, and improve success rates after treatment.

1. Although the complete clinical triad is the most frequent form of presentation, the absence of the complete syndrome should not rule out NPH or the possibility of improvement after shunting. Parkinsonism, other motor symptoms and signs, and, in some patients, psychiatric symptoms may also be present.
2. Patients with iNPH may present a wide variability in the ventricular size and in the width of the cortical sulci and sylvian fissure size. Patients with obliterated cortical sulci show better cognitive and functional responses to shunting, supporting the positive predictive value of this radiological sign. However, patients with normal or enlarged cortical sulci, including that mimicking brain atrophy, may improve significantly after surgery. Consequently, cortical atrophy does not rule out a diagnosis of NPH or the possibility of improvement after shunting.

3. CSF withdrawal (tap test) and the calculation of the R_{out} are associated with a substantial rate of false negatives and therefore have a low predictive value. Consequently, when these tests are positive, patients should be shunted. However, when negative in patients with suspected NPH, additional tests should be used (lumbar CSF drainage for several days or continuous ICP monitoring) before excluding these patients from surgery.
4. The use of continuous ICP monitoring for diagnosis provides important information that can also be used later if patients do not improve after surgery or show late clinical deterioration: ICP recordings before and after shunting can be compared.
5. The use of differential low-pressure valves has been associated with greater rates of improvement after shunting in iNPH patients. The use of these valves is safe if caution is taken to protect the patient from overdrainage by implanting a gravitational device in the shunt system.
6. The use of adjustable valves in high-risk patients has several benefits: (a) the possibility of progressively reducing the opening valve pressure after surgery, (b) the possibility of transitory increase of the opening pressure in cases of subdural effusions, and (c) the possibility of late reduction of the opening pressure in cases of late worsening.
7. Infection and other complications can be drastically reduced by using a strict management protocol. Surgical technique and surgical experience are also important factors.
8. Today, high rates of improvement and low rates of complications are possible in patients with iNPH. This should encourage neurologists to refer these patients to neurosurgical departments, and neurosurgeons should not be reluctant to treat these frequent and fragile patients. Successful surgery significantly improves quality of life in these patients and at the same time reduces the burden on their family and caregivers.

Acknowledgments We gratefully acknowledge Sabrina Voss for editorial assistance as well as the nurses of the Neurosurgery Department, especially María Jesus Peñarrubia and Maria Asunción Muns, for their collaboration in the studies performed. The authors of this chapter have no conflicts of interest with regard to the manufacturers or distributors of the devices mentioned in the text.

References

1. Adams RD, Fisher CM, Hakim S et al (1965) Symptomatic occult hydrocephalus with "normal" cerebrospinal fluid pressure. A treatable syndrome. N Engl J Med 273:117–126
2. Aschoff A, Kremer P, Benesch C et al (1995) Overdrainage and shunt technology. A critical comparison of programmable, hydrostatic and variable-resistance valves and flow- reducing devices. Childs Nerv Syst 11:193–202
3. Barami K, Sood S, Ham SD et al (2000) Postural changes in intracranial pressure in chronically shunted patients. Pediatr Neurosurg 33:64–69
4. Bergsneider M, Black PM, Klinge P et al (2005) Surgical management of idiopathic normal-pressure hydrocephalus. Neurosurgery 57:S29–S39
5. Blomsterwall E, Bilting M, Stephensen H et al (1995) Gait abnormality is not the only motor disturbance in normal pressure hydrocephalus. Scand J Rehabil Med 27:205–209
6. Blomsterwall E, Svantesson U, Carlsson U et al (2000) Postural disturbance in patients with normal pressure hydrocephalus. Acta Neurol Scand 102:284–291
7. Boon AJ, Tans JT, Delwel EJ et al (1998) Dutch normal-pressure hydrocephalus study: randomized comparison of low- and medium-pressure shunts. J Neurosurg 88:490–495
8. Borgbjerg BM, Gjerris F, Albeck MJ et al (1995) Risk of infection after cerebrospinal fluid shunt: an analysis of 884 first-time shunts. Acta Neurochir (Wien) 136:1–7
9. Chapman PH, Borges LF (1985) Shunt infections: prevention and treatment. Clin Neurosurg 32:652–664
10. Cook SW, Bergsneider M (2002) Why valve opening pressure plays a relatively minor role in the postural ICP response to ventricular shunts in normal pressure hydrocephalus: modeling and implications. Acta Neurochir Suppl 81:15–17
11. Cordero TN, Roman Cutillas AM, Jorques Infante AM et al (2013) [Adult chronic idiopathic hydrocephalus-diagnosis, treatment and evolution. Prospective study]. Neurocirugia (Astur) 24:93–101
12. Czosnyka Z, Czosnyka M, Richards HK et al (2002) Laboratory testing of hydrocephalus shunts – conclusion of the U.K. Shunt evaluation programme. Acta Neurochir (Wien) 144:525–538
13. Czosnyka ZH, Czosnyka M, Pickard JD (2002) Shunt testing in-vivo: a method based on the data from the UK shunt evaluation laboratory. Acta Neurochir Suppl 81:27–30
14. da Silva MC, Drake JM (1990) Effect of subcutaneous implantation of anti-siphon devices on CSF shunt function. Pediatr Neurosurg 16:197–202

15. Drake JM, da Silva MC, Rutka JT (1993) Functional obstruction of an antisiphon device by raised tissue capsule pressure. Neurosurgery 32:137–139
16. Durward QJ, Amacher AL, Del Maestro RF et al (1983) Cerebral and cardiovascular responses to changes in head elevation in patients with intracranial hypertension. J Neurosurg 59:938–944
17. Eide PK, Sorteberg W (2010) Diagnostic intracranial pressure monitoring and surgical management in idiopathic normal pressure hydrocephalus: a 6-year review of 214 patients. Neurosurgery 66:80–91
18. Eymann R, Chehab S, Strowitzki M et al (2008) Clinical and economic consequences of antibiotic-impregnated cerebrospinal fluid shunt catheters. J Neurosurg Pediatr 1:444–450
19. Farber SH, Parker SL, Adogwa O et al (2011) Effect of antibiotic-impregnated shunts on infection rate in adult hydrocephalus: a single institution's experience. Neurosurgery 69:625–629
20. Fisher CM (1982) Hydrocephalus as a cause of disturbance of gait in the elderly. Neurology 32:1358–1363
21. Hakim S, Adams RD (1965) The special clinical problem of symptomatic hydrocephalus with normal cerebrospinal fluid pressure. Observations on cerebrospinal fluid hydrodynamics. J Neurol Sci 2: 307–327
22. Hebb AO, Cusimano MD (2001) Idiopathic normal pressure hydrocephalus: a systematic review of diagnosis and outcome. Neurosurgery 49:1166–1184
23. Ishii M, Kawamata T, Akiguchi I et al (2010) Parkinsonian symptomatology may correlate with CT findings before and after shunting in idiopathic normal pressure hydrocephalus. Parkinsons Dis. doi:10.4061/2010/201089
24. Koto A, Rosenberg G, Zingesser LH et al (1977) Syndrome of normal pressure hydrocephalus: possible relation to hypertensive and arteriosclerotic vasculopathy. J Neurol Neurosurg Psychiatry 40:73–79
25. Krauss JK, Regel JP, Droste DW et al (1997) Movement disorders in adult hydrocephalus. Mov Disord 12:53–60
26. Krauss JK, Regel JP, Vach W et al (1996) Vascular risk factors and arteriosclerotic disease in idiopathic normal-pressure hydrocephalus of the elderly. Stroke 27:24–29
27. Larsson A, Wikkelso C, Bilting M et al (1991) Clinical parameters in 74 consecutive patients shunt operated for normal pressure hydrocephalus. Acta Neurol Scand 84:475–482
28. Lemcke J, Meier U, Muller C et al (2013) Safety and efficacy of gravitational shunt valves in patients with idiopathic normal pressure hydrocephalus: a pragmatic, randomised, open label, multicentre trial (SVASONA). J Neurol Neurosurg Psychiatry 84:850–857
29. Loman J, Myerson A, Goldman D (1935) Effects of alterations in posture on the cerebrospinal fluid pressure. Arch Neurol Psychiat 33:1279–1295
30. Magnaes B (1976) Body position and cerebrospinal fluid pressure. Part 1: clinical studies on the effect of rapid postural changes. J Neurosurg 44:687–697
31. Magnaes B (1976) Body position and cerebrospinal fluid pressure. Part 2: Clinical studies on orthostatic pressure and the hydrostatic pressure indifferent point. J Neurosurg 44:698–705
32. Malm J, Graff-Radford NR, Ishikawa M et al (2013) Influence of comorbidities in idiopathic normal pressure hydrocephalus – research and clinical care. A report of the ISHCSF task force on comorbidities in INPH. Fluids Barriers CNS 10:22. doi:10.1186/2045-8118-10-22
33. Mandir AS, Hilfiker J, Thomas G et al (2007) Extrapyramidal signs in normal pressure hydrocephalus: an objective assessment. Cerebrospinal Fluid Res 4:7. doi:10.1186/1743-8454-4-7
34. Marmarou A, Bergsneider M, Klinge P et al (2005) The value of supplemental prognostic tests for the preoperative assessment of idiopathic normal-pressure hydrocephalus. Neurosurgery 57:S17–S28
35. Marmarou A, Bergsneider M, Relkin N et al (2005) Development of guidelines for idiopathic normal-pressure hydrocephalus: introduction. Neurosurgery 57:S1–S3
36. Martinez-Lage JF, Perez-Espejo MA, Almagro MJ et al (2005) Syndromes of overdrainage of ventricular shunting in childhood hydrocephalus. Neurocirugia (Astur) 16:124–133
37. Martinez-Lage JF, Ruiz-Espejo AM, Almagro MJ et al (2009) CSF overdrainage in shunted intracranial arachnoid cysts: a series and review. Childs Nerv Syst 25:1061–1069
38. Mataro M, Poca MA, Salgado-Pineda P et al (2003) Postsurgical cerebral perfusion changes in idiopathic normal pressure hydrocephalus: a statistical parametric mapping study of SPECT images. J Nucl Med 44:1884–1889
39. McGirt MJ, Woodworth G, Coon AL et al (2005) Diagnosis, treatment, and analysis of long-term outcomes in idiopathic normal-pressure hydrocephalus. Neurosurgery 57:699–705
40. McQuarrie IG, Saint-Louis L, Scherer PB (1984) Treatment of normal pressure hydrocephalus with low versus medium pressure cerebrospinal fluid shunts. Neurosurgery 15:484–488
41. McQuarrie IG, Scherer PB (1982) Treatment of adult-onset obstructive hydrocephalus with low- or medium- pressure CSF shunts. Neurology 32: 1057–1061
42. Mirzayan MJ, Koenig K, Bastuerk M et al (2006) Coma due to meteorism and increased intra-abdominal pressure subsequent to ventriculoperitoneal shunt dysfunction. Lancet 368:2032
43. Momjian S, Owler BK, Czosnyka Z et al (2004) Pattern of white matter regional cerebral blood flow and autoregulation in normal pressure hydrocephalus. Brain 127:965–972
44. Mori E, Ishikawa M, Kato T et al (2012) Guidelines for management of idiopathic normal pressure hydrocephalus: second edition. Neurol Med Chir (Tokyo) 52:775–809
45. Oikonomou J, Aschoff A, Hashemi B et al (1999) New valves: new dangers? 22 valves (38 probes) designed

in the 'nineties in ultralong-term tests (365 days)'. Eur J Pediatr Surg 9(Suppl 1):23–26
46. Ojemann RG, Fisher CM, Adams RD et al (1969) Further experience with the syndrome of "normal" pressure hydrocephalus. J Neurosurg 31:279–294
47. Pang DL, Altschuler E (1994) Low-pressure hydrocephalic state and viscoelastic alterations in the brain. Neurosurgery 35:643–655
48. Pattavilakom A, Xenos C, Bradfield O et al (2007) Reduction in shunt infection using antibiotic impregnated CSF shunt catheters: an Australian prospective study. J Clin Neurosci 14:526–531
49. Pickard JD, Teasdale G, Matheson M et al (1980) Intraventricular pressure waves. The best predictive test for shunting in normal pressure hydrocephalus. In: Shulman K, Marmarou A, Miller JD et al (eds) Intracranial pressure IV. Springer, Berlin, pp 498–500
50. Poca MA, Mataro M, Matarin M et al (2004) Is the placement of shunts in patients with idiopathic normal-pressure hydrocephalus worth the risk? Results of a study based on continuous monitoring of intracranial pressure. J Neurosurg 100:855–866
51. Poca MA, Mataro M, Matarin M et al (2005) Good outcome in patients with normal-pressure hydrocephalus and factors indicating poor prognosis. J Neurosurg 103:455–463
52. Poca MA, Sahuquillo J, Busto M et al (1996) Clinical management of patients with normal pressure hydrocephalus syndrome. Ann Psychiatry 6:273–292
53. Poca MA, Sahuquillo J, Topczewski T et al (2006) Posture-induced changes in intracranial pressure: a comparative study in patients with and without a cerebrospinal fluid block at the craniovertebral junction. Neurosurgery 58:899–906
54. Poca MA, Solana E, Martinez-Ricarte FR et al (2012) Idiopathic normal pressure hydrocephalus: results of a prospective cohort of 236 shunted patients. Acta Neurochir Suppl 114:247–253
55. Portnoy HD, Schulte RR, Fox JL et al (1973) Anti-siphon and reversible occlusion valves for shunting in hydrocephalus and preventing post-shunt subdural hematomas. J Neurosurg 38:729–738
56. Pujari S, Kharkar S, Metellus P et al (2008) Normal pressure hydrocephalus: long-term outcome after shunt surgery. J Neurol Neurosurg Psychiatry 79:1282–1286
57. Raftopoulos C, Massager N, Baleriaux D et al (1996) Prospective analysis by computed tomography and long-term outcome of 23 adult patients with chronic idiopathic hydrocephalus. Neurosurgery 38:51–59
58. Reilly P (2001) In normal pressure hydrocephalus, intracranial pressure monitoring is the only useful test. J Clin Neurosci 8:66–67
59. Relkin N, Marmarou A, Klinge P et al (2005) Diagnosing idiopathic normal-pressure hydrocephalus. Neurosurgery 57:S4–S16
60. Richards HK, Seeley HM, Pickard JD (2009) Efficacy of antibiotic-impregnated shunt catheters in reducing shunt infection: data from the United Kingdom Shunt Registry. J Neurosurg Pediatr 4:389–393
61. Rosenfeld JV, Siraruj S (2001) In normal pressure hydrocephalus, intracranial pressure monitoring is the only useful test. J Clin Neurosci 8:68–69
62. Sahuquillo J, Arikan F, Poca MA et al (2008) Intra-abdominal pressure: the neglected variable in selecting the ventriculoperitoneal shunt for treating hydrocephalus. Neurosurgery 62:143–149
63. Sahuquillo J, Poca MA, Martinez M et al (1994) Preventing shunt overdrainage in hydrocephalus: are anti-siphon devices really physiological? In: Nagai H, Kamiya K, Ishii S (eds) Intracranial pressure IX. Springer, Tokyo, pp 83–86
64. Sahuquillo J, Rubio E, Codina A et al (1991) Reappraisal of the intracranial pressure and cerebrospinal fluid dynamics in patients with the so-called "normal pressure hydrocephalus" syndrome. Acta Neurochir (Wien) 112:50–61
65. Sanchez NC, Tenofsky PL, Dort JM et al (2001) What is normal intra-abdominal pressure? Am Surg 67:243–248
66. Soelberg Sorensen P, Jansen EC, Gjerris F (1986) Motor disturbances in normal-pressure hydrocephalus. Special reference to stance and gait. Arch Neurol 43:34–38
67. Sugerman H, Windsor A, Bessos M et al (1997) Intra-abdominal pressure, sagittal abdominal diameter and obesity comorbidity. J Intern Med 241:71–79
68. Toole JF (1968) Effects of change of head, limb and body position on cephalic circulation. N Engl J Med 279:307–311
69. Vanneste J, Augustijn P, Dirven C et al (1992) Shunting normal-pressure hydrocephalus: do the benefits outweigh the risks? A multicenter study and literature review. Neurology 42:54–59
70. Zemack G, Romner B (2002) Adjustable valves in normal-pressure hydrocephalus: a retrospective study of 218 patients. Neurosurgery 51:1392–1400

Complications Specific to the Type of CSF Shunt: Atrial Shunt

12

Luca Massimi and Concezio Di Rocco

Contents

12.1 **Introduction** 177

12.2 **Complications Unique to Atrial Shunts** 178

12.2.1 Pulmonary Thromboembolism and Its Consequences 178

12.2.2 Thrombosis 180

12.2.3 Endocarditis 181

12.2.4 Cardiac Tamponade 181

12.2.5 Shunt Nephritis 182

12.3 **Complications Shared with VPS** 183

12.3.1 Septicemia 183

12.3.2 Misplacement/Migration of the Distal Catheter 183

References 184

L. Massimi, MD, PhD (✉)
Pediatric Neurosurgery,
A. Gemelli Hospital, Institute of Neurosurgery,
Catholic University Medical School,
Largo A. Gemelli, 8, 00168 Rome, Italy
e-mail: lmassimi@email.it

C. Di Rocco, MD
Pediatric Neurosurgery, Institute of Neurosurgery,
Catholic University Medical School,
Largo A. Gemelli, 8, 00168 Rome, Italy

Pediatric Neurosurgery,
International Neuroscience Institute,
Hannover, Germany
e-mail: cdirocco@rm.unicatt.it

12.1 Introduction

Thanks to the development of sophisticated and reliable ventriculoperitoneal shunts (VPS) and to the wide and still increasing diffusion of neuroendoscopy, the use of ventriculoatrial shunts (VAS) is currently limited to selected cases in many Centers, namely, those where the two previous treatments failed. VPS actually are burdened by a lower rate of severe complications and revisions [4], and they are more easy to be placed and revised so that they have replaced VAS as gold standard treatment for hydrocephalus starting from the 1970s [22, 24]. Moreover, VPS do not need to be periodically lengthened to follow the body growth, which is a significant advantage over VAS in children. Neuroendoscopy, on the other hand, offering the possibility to completely avoid shunting prostheses, is used whenever possible, sometimes after the removal of a previous VAS [40]. On these grounds, there are only few papers currently focusing on the complications of VAS, which generally report on isolated cases. Indeed, the clinical series consisting of patients with this type of CSF shunt are often little and/or dated, and most of the available data refers to papers written during the VAS era, that is, about four decades ago.

The complications of VAS can be divided into two groups: those proper of VAS, as cardiopulmonary complications and shunt nephritis, and those shared with VPS but with a peculiar course, such as catheter displacement and infections. In

C. Di Rocco et al. (eds.), *Complications of CSF Shunting in Hydrocephalus: Prevention, Identification, and Management*, DOI 10.1007/978-3-319-09961-3_12,

this chapter, both types of complications will be addressed.

12.2 Complications Unique to Atrial Shunts

12.2.1 Pulmonary Thromboembolism and Its Consequences

Thromboembolic complications of VAS may present as silent pulmonary embolization or as pulmonary vascular occlusive disease, pulmonary hypertension, or even right heart failure. Therefore, the exact incidence of these complications is hard to be established, mainly because of the undiagnosed cases or because of the difficulties in recognizing the clinical onset of the disease. However, a 0.4 % rate of clinically evident lung embolism and a 0.3 % rate of pulmonary hypertension are now universally accepted [18, 32, 40]. The autoptic investigations, instead, point out significantly higher figures, the frequency of pulmonary embolism ranging around 60 % while that of pulmonary hypertension around 6 % [13, 39].

Pulmonary embolization is caused by the detachment of emboli from a partial or complete thrombosis of the superior vena cava or right atrium. Such a thrombosis is thought to result from the presence of a foreign body (the shunting catheter) into these vascular cavities. However, the incidence of thromboembolism in patients with VAS is higher than in patients with other foreign bodies (e.g., cardiac pacemaker) [28]. Therefore, several hypotheses have been formulated to explain such a greater rate: (1) Concomitant presence of infection: The frequency of thromboembolism is increased in patients who experienced septicemia [31]. However, based on autoptic observations, some authors concluded that sepsis is not a necessary condition for embolization although the histological changes are more severe in cases of septic emboli (inflammatory process extended to the adventitia and the surrounding tissues) than in cases of bland emboli [14]. (2) Atrial ulceration due to a mechanical injury by the tip of the shunting catheter, leading to a chronic endocarditis followed by atrial thrombosis [30]. (3) Chemical injury by the CSF against the endothelium of the lung vessels, with subsequent thrombosis in situ and pulmonary hypertension [32]. (4) Thromboplastic-like activity by some CSF components [15, 35]. On the other hand, the age of the patient, the shunt material, and the location of the atrial catheter do not seem to influence the occurrence of thromboembolic complications [14, 17].

Pulmonary thromboembolism is generally an early complication (days or months after the shunt placement), thought it can also occur later on (even years after the shunt implantation) [18, 19, 28]. As mentioned before, it can remain asymptomatic in some patients, namely, those with microembolization where the small emboli are lysed before occluding pulmonary arteries or are not able to completely obstruct the arterial lumen [14]. In symptomatic cases, pulmonary embolism is complicated by respiratory symptoms and pulmonary hypertension (revealed by accentuation of the second heart sound and by the murmurs due to pulmonary or tricuspid valve insufficiency) leading, in turn, to cor pulmonale and, eventually, to irreversible right heart failure. On the other hand, chronic non-thromboembolic pulmonary hypertension is exceptional and it is induced by repeated infections [1]. Pulmonary hypertension accounts for almost all the deaths occurring after thromboembolic complications [11, 32, 34]. Sleigh death in asymptomatic cases or in patients with chronic thromboembolic pulmonary hypertension has been also reported [13, 30].

The diagnostic work-up includes: (1) arterial blood gas analysis, seeking for hypoxia; (2) chest X-rays, looking for cardiomegaly and dilatation of the proximal pulmonary arteries (Fig. 12.1) (a pulmonary angiogram can confirm the dilatation and/or obstruction of the pulmonary vessels); (3) ventilation-perfusion lung CT scan, to find the signs of embolization (multiple subsegmental perfusion defects); (4) electrocardiogram, usually showing right ventricle hypertrophy and right axis deviation (Fig. 12.2); (5) echocardiography, which can provide information on the dilatation of the right heart, the right ventricle hypertrophy, the estimated pulmonary artery pressure, the tricuspidal insufficiency, and the possible presence of atrial/vena cava thrombosis (Fig. 12.3); and (6) cardiac catheterization, to confirm and to establish the severity of the pulmonary hypertension.

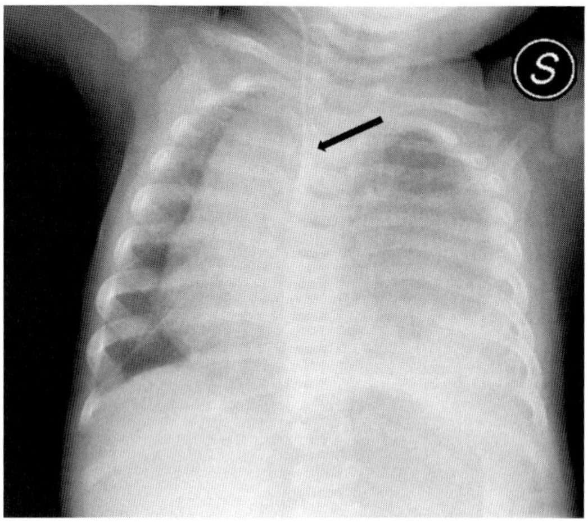

Fig. 12.1 Hypertrophy of the right cardiac cavities with right deviation of the heart in a child with a VAS positioned at T4 level (*arrow*) who developed pulmonary embolism and hypertension

The surgical management consists of the removal of the VAS, to be performed as early as possible and to be converted into VPS or other shunts (e.g., ventriculo-gallbladder or ventriculo-bladder shunt), or endoscopic treatment. The medical treatment is first based on pharmacological thrombolysis, then on diuretic and anticoagulant drugs. Medical therapies including vasodilators and prostacyclin analogues can be used in the attempt of reducing the pulmonary vascular resistance [3]. Unfortunately, the prognosis of pulmonary hypertension complicating VAS is often dismal, with a 50–100 % rate of mortality [28, 39]. Reduction of the risk of shunt colonization, elective revision of the shunt if a migration into the superior vena cava is detected, periodic checkup screening to exclude atrial thrombosis or initial signs of pulmonary hypertension (chest X-rays, electrocardiography, echocardiography), and, according to some authors [35], anti-aggregation drug prophylaxis, can be

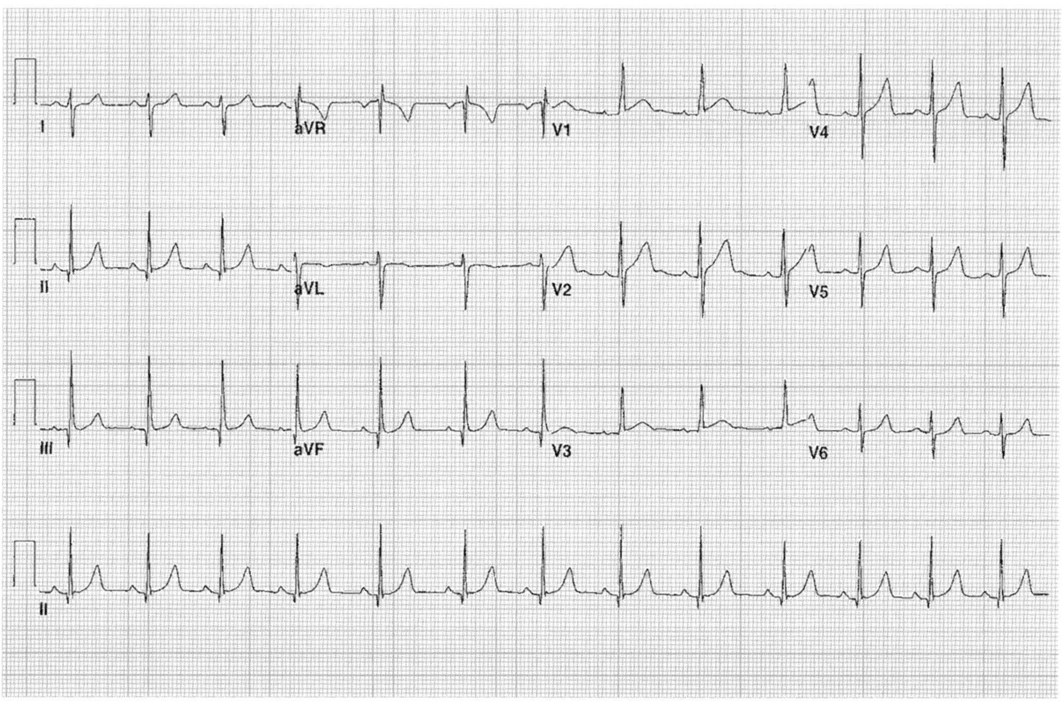

Fig. 12.2 Electrocardiogram showing the signs of right hypertrophy and right deviation of the cardiac axis in a patient with cor pulmonale

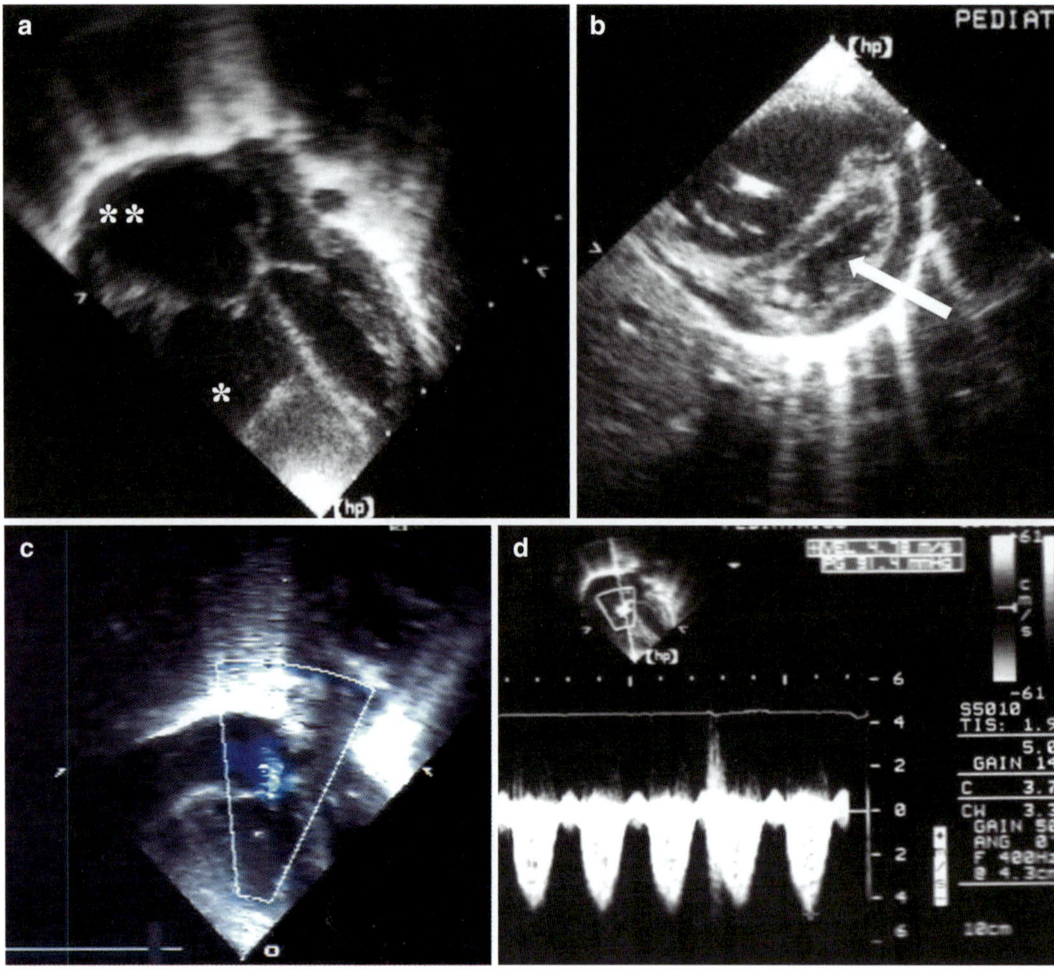

Fig. 12.3 Echocardiographic signs in a case of pulmonary hypertension: (**a**) severe enlargement of the right ventricle (*asterisk*) and atrium (*double asterisk*); (**b**) hypertrophy of the right ventricle with shift of the ventricular septum (*arrow*) toward the left ventricle; (**c**) blood regurgitation through the tricuspid valve; (**d**) pulmonary hypertension: the overall value is about 100 mmHg resulting from the gradient through the tricuspid valve (91.4 mmHg) plus the atrial pressure (10 mmHg)

attempted to reduce the risk of thromboembolic complications.

12.2.2 Thrombosis

The formation of clots inside the right atrium, possibly extending to the pulmonary artery and/or the superior vena cava/internal jugular vein, is a quite common complication of VAS. Actually, the frequency on autoptic series ranges around 60–100 % [9]. However, the clinical evidence is lower, ranging from 2 to 50 % [37]. The phenomenon is macroscopically described as fibrinous material with attached clots surrounding the tip of the atrial catheter [13]. The clot is usually attached to the atrial wall, with a portion floating free.

The pathogenesis and the consequences of atriovenous thrombosis are reported in the previous paragraph. In addition, the risk of enlargement of the thrombus up to the intracranial sinuses or the tricuspid valve has to be taken into account (Fig. 12.4). This phenomenon is also favored by remnants of the distal catheter left in place for a long time because they are undetected or hard to remove [7]. The diagnostic management consists of chest X-rays and echocardiography, completed

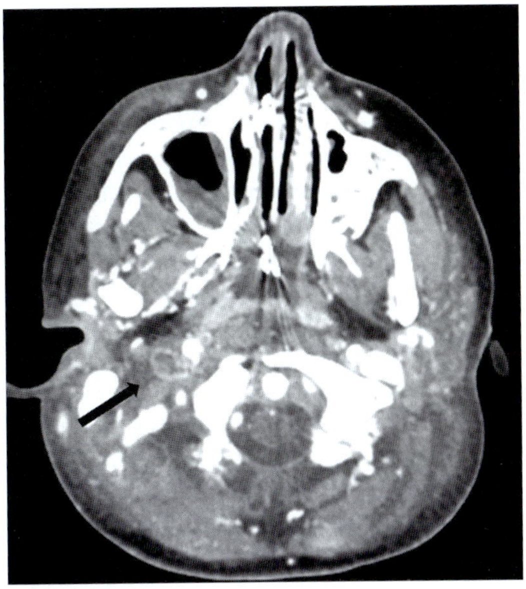

Fig. 12.4 Angio-CT scan of the brain showing a filling defect of the right jugular bulb (*arrow*) in a patient whose VAS was removed because of jugular/vena cava thrombosis

by transesophageal ultrasounds, D-dimer test, and high-resolution CT scan, to confirm the diagnosis and to exclude pulmonary embolization. Moreover, it is important to rule out factors inducing thrombophilia (e.g., homozygous factor V Leiden mutation or intake of oral contraceptives). The treatment includes anticoagulation therapy, antibiotic prophylaxis (to prevent endocarditis), and removal of the shunt. A thoracocentesis may be required to confirm the diagnosis or in the case of abundant pleural transudate [37].

12.2.3 Endocarditis

Endocarditis in VAS occurs as a result of the combination of atrial thrombus and bacteremia [43]. Indeed, the clinical history usually discloses previous, recurrent infections (e.g., urinary tract or bronchial tubes). Fever, asthenia, skin purpuric rash, and presence of cardiac murmur are the main clinical signs/symptoms. It is worth noting that the cardiac murmur can be poorly appreciated or even absent in the early phases of infective endocarditis [6]. The diagnostic work-up includes transthoracic and/or transesophageal ultrasounds, which show the typical atrial floating vegetation, and blood examinations and cultures, which demonstrate the signs of bacteremia or sepsis. The cultures from all the possible sites of contamination have to be obtained to identify the primary site of infection.

The management of VAS-related endocarditis is based on: (1) prompt antibiotic therapy administration, to hinder the infection; (2) anticoagulant treatment, to prevent pulmonary embolization; (3) removal of the shunt, to eliminate the source of the thrombosis and/or the infection; and, if needed, (4) removal of the atrial clot by cardiac surgery, to prevent tricuspid obstruction and/or pulmonary embolization (especially if the atrial clot is detached after the neurosurgical removal of the VAS) [6].

12.2.4 Cardiac Tamponade

This is a rare, late complication of VAS resulting from the progressive erosion of the myocardium leading to atrial perforation and pericardial effusion. In the series of 455 patients with VAS reported by Forrest and Cooper, cardiac tamponade occurred in three cases (0.6 %) [16]. The authors noticed that, in two out those three patients, the atrial erosion was probably due to an undesirable position of the tip of the atrial catheter, which was entangled in the pectinate muscles of the right atrium. Actually, the perforation of the myocardium is thought to result from an increased stiffness of the tip of the atrial catheter, due to its abnormal position or to a clot filling and stiffening it [9]. Exceptionally, the myocardial damage can be provoked intraoperatively by the forceful introduction of the atrial catheter with a stylet into a thrombotic jugular vein [36]. In all these instances, the cardiac tamponade is related to the blood pericardial effusion due to the bleeding from the perforation site. However, some unusual cases of tamponade due to the CSF accumulating into the pericardium and coming from a migrated atrial catheter perforating the cardiac walls have been described [12, 23]. Mastroianni et al. even reported on a 48-year-old woman whose pericardial tamponade resulted from a disconnected remnant of VAS perforating the right

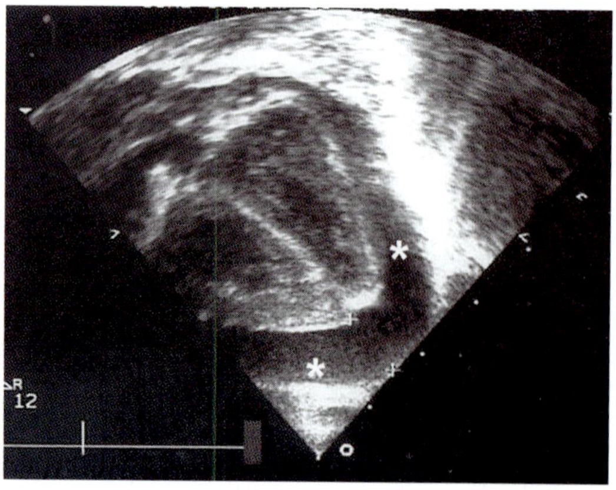

Fig. 12.5 Cardiac tamponade in a young child because of severe circumferential pericardial effusion (*asterisks*)

ventricle and draining CSF, thanks to a fibrin sheath still connecting it with the proximal part of the shunt [27].

Cardiac tamponade is a life-threatening condition that requires an emergency management to prevent low cardiac output and cardiac arrest. Dyspnea, respiratory distress, tachycardia, swelling of the jugular veins, softened hear sounds, and, finally, signs of shock are the most common clinical signs. Chest X-rays show an enlarged pericardial shadow and clear lung fields, while chest CT scan can also demonstrate a pericardial and pleural effusion other than the position of the shunting catheter. Echocardiography points out the circumferential pericardial effusion with a compression of the right heart cavities during the diastole (Fig. 12.5). Laboratory signs of multiorgan failure can be appreciated in the late phases. The patients are monitored and stabilized in an intensive care unit; then, a pericardiocentesis or, if this is unfeasible or ineffective, an open cardiosurgical (sternotomy) evacuation of the pericardial effusion with surgical repair of the atrial or ventricular perforation and extraction/replacement of the shunt are performed.

12.2.5 Shunt Nephritis

This complication is a result of the colonization of the VAS by a low-virulence microorganism. The chronic infection is usually sustained by *Staphylococcus epidermidis* or, less frequently, by *Staphylococcus aureus*, *Propionibacterium acnes*, *Listeria monocytogenes*, and *Pseudomonas aeruginosa* [9]. Such a persistent infection induces an immune-complex disease through a chronic hyperantigenemia and hyperglobulinemia with deposition of complements, immunoglobulins, and immune complexes on the glomerular basement membranes [39]. In more detail, the persistent antigenemia due to the long-lasting immunization of the host against the low-virulence bacterium (the bacterium proliferates by adhering to the shunt and continuously releases its antigens) leads to the continuous formation of antigen-antibody complexes in antibody excess, with secondary activation of the complement system and deposits in the glomerular capillary wall, cytokine release, and subsequent membranoproliferative or focal proliferative glomerulonephritis. The histologic analysis of autoptic kidney specimens actually points out mesangial cell proliferation with widening of the mesangial matrix, granular deposits, and thickening of the glomerular basement membrane [26]. The immunofluorescence observation of the deposits reveals the presence of bacterial antigen, complements, IgM, IgG, and fibrinogen [44].

Shunt nephritis is a rare, usually late complication, occurring several months/years after the VAS placement [38]. Infants and children are more prone to develop it than adolescents and adults because of the higher risk of shunt infection by coagulase-negative staphylococci. The early clinical picture is characterized by fever, anemia, hepatosplenomegaly, and signs of septicemia (including positive blood cultures). Afterward, a nephritic syndrome (arterial hypertension, proteinuria, azotemia) or, less commonly, a nephrotic syndrome appears (severe proteinuria, hypoproteinemia, body edema). The diagnosis is obtained by demonstrating the renal impairment, with a glomerular filtration rate decreased up to 20–45 ml/min, associated with hypocomplementemia and high serum levels of cryoglobulins and bacterial antibodies. Shunt removal and the antibiotic therapy are generally able to stop the nephritis and to restore a normal renal function in most cases; otherwise, immunosuppressive drugs can be added in the severe or refractory forms. It has been sporadically observed that the complement activation is not interrupted by the shunt removal and replacement, thus suggesting the persistence of the antigen somewhere (e.g., inside the ventricles) as activating factor [41]. Shunt nephritis can be prevented by periodic blood examinations aiming at monitoring the renal function and, in suspected cases, the C3 and C4 levels. The prevention of this complication is mandatory because, though rarely, fatal cases have been reported [44].

12.3 Complications Shared with VPS

12.3.1 Septicemia

Septicemia is the most common complication of VAS, its frequency ranging from 10 to 15 % of cases [5]. According to the review by Luthardt on 1540 published cases during the VAS era, its incidence was actually 13.5 % [25]. Septicemia also accounts for the highest rate of mortality among VAS complications, especially in infants and/or immunodepressed patients [10]. Indeed, sepsis in VAS is complicated, other than by the multiorgan failure due to the action of the microorganism, also by the possible occurrence of shunt malfunction and thrombosis around the cardiac catheter followed by the aforementioned cardiopulmonary complications. Once again, coagulase-negative staphylococci are the most frequently involved in the infectious process [2]. *Staphylococcus aureus* is usually associated with a highly virulent and widely diffused infection so that the clinical course may be acute or fulminating. Differently, *Staphylococcus epidermidis*, which is also the most frequently involved bacterium, shows a more indolent and chronic course. The clinical picture is characterized by fever, signs and symptoms of progressive anemia, lethargy, splenomegaly, and, later on, petechiae, hemorrhages, and multiorgan failure. Laboratory investigations point out leukocytosis and positive blood cultures. Bacteremia in infected VAS is more frequently detected than in colonized VPS [33].

The management consists of adequate support and monitoring of the patient (who is referred to the intensive care unit, if necessary), immediate removal of the shunt replaced by an external ventricular drainage, and appropriate antibiotic drug administration.

12.3.2 Misplacement/Migration of the Distal Catheter

The misplacement of VAS is a result of an incorrect placement of the shunt or the consequence of its migration because of the patient's growth or because of a mechanical complication (rupture or disconnection of the atrial catheter). The wrong placement of the distal catheter is defined by the position of its tip above the T4 level or into the subclavian vein or too deeply inside the atrium or even in the right ventricle. This complication can exceptionally follow an involuntary displacement of the catheter by a central venous catheter introduced through the basilic vein [8]. In the first instance (tip in the vena cava or in the subclavian vein), the misplacement is followed by a thrombosis within the catheter with subsequent shunt malfunction [9]. In the second one (too long distal catheter), the thrombosis involves the atrium with subsequent risk of pulmonary embolization, tricuspid valve obstruction, endocarditis, and infections. Infection and dysfunction of the pulmonary valve have been described as specific consequences of this complication [20]. Furthermore, persistent extrasystoles leading to permanent cardiac arrhythmia have been reported in some cases [21]. The misplacement of the distal catheter can be avoided by using an intraoperative fluoroscopic control during the shunt progression into the atrium coupled with electrocardiogram feedback for extrasystoles. Should the postoperative X-ray control show an incorrect position, the VAS has to be quickly replaced.

Migration of the catheter into the vena cava/jugular vein/subclavian vein following the patient's growth is encountered in children or still growing adolescents, where it represents also the most common cause of VAS malfunction (Fig. 12.6). To avoid this complication, an elective lengthening of

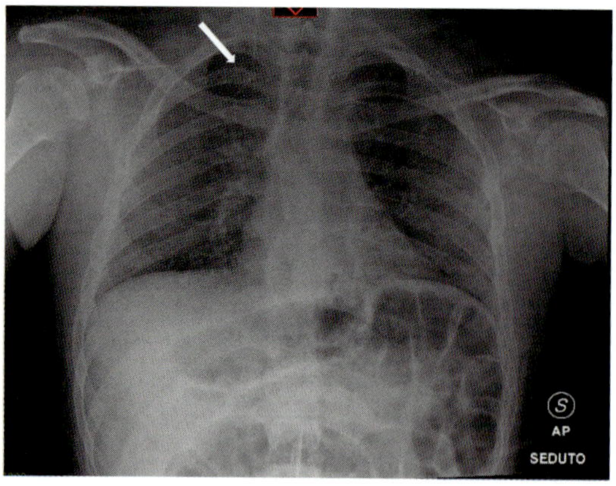

Fig. 12.6 Distal catheter shortening (because of the patient's growth) and migration into the right subclavian vein (*arrow*) in an adolescent

the shunt each 12–18 months, according to the patient's age, was propounded [16].

Although currently uncommon, thanks to the improvement in the shunt design and in the surgical technique, the migration can also originate from the detachment of the distal catheter. The disconnected catheter usually migrates into the right heart cavities, favored by the venous flow and the negative intrathoracic pressure, causing thromboembolic complications or heart perforation (with cardiac tamponade) [27] other than shunt malfunction. More rarely, the migration site is represented by the pulmonary artery [29]. In all these instances, the migrated catheter has to be removed soon by endovascular retrieval [42] or, if unfeasible, by thoracotomic surgery.

References

1. Amelot A, Bouazza S, George B, Bresson D (2014) Causative role of infection in chronic non-thromboembolic pulmonary hypertension following ventriculo-atrial shunt. Br J Neurosurg 28: 559–561
2. Bayston R, Rodgers J (1994) Role of serological tests in the diagnosis of immune complex disease in infection of ventriculoatrial shunts for hydrocephalus. Eur J Clin Microbiol Infect Dis 13:417–420
3. Benedict N, Seybert A, Mathier MA (2007) Evidence-based pharmacologic management of pulmonary arterial hypertension. Clin Ther 29:2134–2153
4. Borgbjerg BM, Gjerris F, Albeck MJ, Hauerberg J, Børgesen SV (1998) A comparison between ventriculo-peritoneal and ventriculo-atrial cerebrospinal fluid shunts in relation to rate of revision and durability. Acta Neurochir (Wien) 140:459–465
5. Buchard KW, Monir LB, Slotman GJ, Gann DS (1984) Staphylococcus epidermidis sepsis in surgical patients. Arch Surg 119:96–100
6. Chaw HY, Buxton N, Wong PS (2004) Staphylococcal endocarditis with a ventriculo-atrial shunt. J R Soc Med 97:182–183
7. Chiu GA, Nisar K, Shetty S, Baldwin AJ (2010) Remnants of a 35-year-old ventriculo-atrial shunt presenting as orofacial pain. Ann R Coll Surg Engl 92:W15–W17
8. Dean DF (1980) Knotted ventriculoatrial catheter. J Neurosurg 52:407–409
9. Di Rocco C, Iannelli A (1987) Complications of CSF shunting. In: Di Rocco C (ed) The treatment of infantile hydrocephalus, vol 2. CRC, Boca Raton, pp 79–153
10. Di Rocco C, Massimi L, Tamburrini G (2006) Shunt versus endoscopic third ventriculostomy in infants: are there different types and/or rates of complications? Childs Nerv Syst 22:1573–1589
11. Drucker MH, Vanek VW, Franco AA, Hanson M, Woods L (1984) Thromboembolic complications of ventriculoatrial shunts. Surg Neurol 22:444–448
12. El-Eshmawi A, Onakpoya U, Khadragui I (2009) Cardiac tamponade as a sequela to ventriculoatrial shunting for congenital hydrocephalus. Tex Heart Inst J 36:58–60
13. Emery JL, Hilton HB (1961) Lung and heart complications of the treatment of hydrocephalus by ventriculoauriculostomy. Surgery 59:309–314
14. Erdohazi M, Eckstein HB, Crome L (1966) Pulmonary embolization as a complication of ventriculo-atrial shunts inserted for hydrocephalus. Dev Med Child Neurol 11:36–44
15. Farvea BE, Paul RN (1967) Thromboembolism and cor pulmonale complicating ventriculovenous shunt. JAMA 199:668–671
16. Forrest DM, Cooper DGW (1968) Complications of ventriculo-atrial shunts: a review of 455 cases. J Neurosurg 29:506–512
17. Friedman S, Zita-Gozum G, Chatten J (1964) Pulmonary vascular changes complicating ventriculo-vascular shunting for hydrocephalus. J Pediatr 64: 305–314
18. Grover SK, Puri R, Wong TLD, Dundon BK, Tayeb H, Steele PM (2010) Ventriculo-atrial shunt induced severe pulmonary arterial hypertension: a time for routine screening? Intern Med J 40:386–391
19. Haasnoot K, van Vught AJ (1992) Pulmonary hypertension complicating a ventriculo-atrial shunt. Eur J Pediatr 151:748–750
20. Hougen TJ, Emmanoulides GC, Moss AJ (1975) Pulmonary valvular dysfunction in children with ventriculovenous shunts for hydrocephalus: a previously unreported correlation. Pediatrics 55:836–841

21. Huber ZA (1981) Complications of shunt operations performed in 206 children because of communicating hydrocephalus. Zentralbl Neurochir 42:165–168
22. Keucher TR, Mealey J (1979) Long-term results after ventriculoatrial and ventriculoperitoneal shunting for infantile hydrocephalus. J Neurosurg 50:179–186
23. Jorro Barón F, Casanovas A, Guaita E, Bolasell C, Rombolá V, Debaisi G (2012) Cardiac tamponade as a complication of ventriculo atrial shunt. Arch Argent Pediatr 110:e1–3 (Article in Spanish)
24. Little JR, Rhoton AL, Mellinger JF (1972) Comparison of ventriculoperitoneal and ventriculoatrial shunts for hydrocephalus in children. Mayo Clin Proc 47: 396–401
25. Luthardt T (1970) Bacterial infections in ventriculo-atrial shunt systems. Dev Med Child Neurol 12: 110–113
26. Marini G, Gabriele PW, Tanghetti B, Castellani A, Olivetti G, Zunin E (1977) Membrano-proliferative glomerulonephritis associated with infected ventriculo-atrial shunt. Mod Probl Paediatr 18:207–210
27. Mastroianni C, Chauvet D, Ressencourt O, Kirsch M (2013) Late ventriculo-atrial shunt migration leading to pericardial cerebrospinal fluid effusion and cardiac tamponade. Interact Cardiovasc Thorac Surg 16:391–393
28. Milton CA, Sanders P, Steele PM (2001) Late cardiopulmonary complication of ventriculo-atrial shunt. Lancet 358:1608
29. Nguyen HS, Turner M, Butty SD, Cohen-Gadol AA (2010) Migration of a distal shunt catheter into the heart and pulmonary artery: report of a case and review of the literature. Childs Nerv Syst 26:1113–1116
30. Normand J, Guillot B, Tabib A, Loire R, Joffre B, Lapras C (1981) Coeur pulmonaire chronique post-embolique de l'enfant après mise en place d'une derivation ventriculo-atriale pour hydrocéphalie-aspects anatomique. Pediatrie 36:283–289 (Article in French)
31. Nugent GR, Lucas R, Judy M, Bloor BM, Warden H (1966) Thrombo-embolic complications of ventriculo-atrial shunts. J Neurosurg 24:34–42
32. Pascual JMS, Prakash UBS (1993) Development of pulmonary hypertension after placement of a ventriculoatrial shunt. Mayo Clin Proc 68:1177–1182
33. Schoenbaum SC, Gardner P, Shillito J (1975) Infections of cerebrospinal fluid shunts: epidemiology, clinical manifestations and therapy. J Infect Dis 131:543–552
34. Sleigh G, Dawson A, Penny WJ (1993) Cor pulmonale as a complication of ventriculo-atrial shunts reviewed. Dev Med Child Neurol 35:74–78
35. Stuart M, Stockman J, Murphy S, Schut L, Ames M, Urmson J, Oski F (1972) Shortened platelet lifespan in patients with hydrocephalus and ventriculojugular shunts: results of preliminary attempts at correction. J Pediatr 80:21–25
36. Tsingoglou S, Eckstein HB (1971) Pericardial tamponade by Holter ventriculo-atrial shunts. J Neurosurg 35:695–699
37. Tonn P, Gilsbach JM, Kreitschmann-Andermahr I, Franke A, Blindt R (2005) A rare but life-threatening complication of ventriculo-atrial shunt. Acta Neurochir (Wien) 147:1303–1304
38. Vella J, Carmody M, Campbell E, Browne O, Doyle G, Donohoe J (1995) Glomerulonephritis after ventriculo-atrial shunt. QJM 88:911–918
39. Vernet O, Rilliet B (2001) Late complications of ventriculoatrial or ventriculoperitoneal shunts. Lancet 358:1569–1570
40. Wu XJ, Luo C, Liu Z, Hu GH, Chen JX, Lu YC (2011) Complications following ventriculo-peritoneal and subsequent ventriculo-atrial shunting resolved by third ventriculostomy. Br J Neurosurg 25:300–302
41. Wyatt RJ, Walsh JW, Holland NH (1981) Shunt nephritis. J Neurosurg 55:99–107
42. Xu B, Chotai S, Yang K, Feng W, Zhang G, Li M, Qi S (2012) Endovascular intervention for repositioning the distal catheter of ventriculo-atrial shunt. Neurointervention 7:109–112
43. Yavuzgil O, Ozerkan F, Erturk U, Islekel S, Atay U, Buket S (1999) A rare cause of right atrial mass: thrombus formation and infection complicating a ventriculoatrial shunt for hydrocephalus. Surg Neurol 52:54–55
44. Zamora I, Lurbe A, Alvarez-Garijo A, Mendizabal S, Simon J (1984) Shunt nephritis: a report on five children. Childs Brain 11:183–187

Complications of Peritoneal Shunts

13

José Hinojosa

Contents

13.1 **Introduction** 187

13.2 **Epidemiology** 188

13.3 **Physiopathology of Nonfunctional Abdominal Complications of Shunt Catheters** 188

13.4 **Sterile Ascites** 189

13.5 **Pseudocyst** 190

13.6 **Anal Extrusion. Bowel Perforation** 193

13.7 **Bladder Perforation** 194

13.8 **Other Infrequent Complications** 195
13.8.1 Migration 195
13.8.2 Intestinal Volvulus 196
13.8.3 Abdominal Wall Perforation 196
13.8.4 Abdominal Metastasis 197

13.9 **Options for Catheter Placement After Peritoneal Dysfunction** 197

References 200

J. Hinojosa, MD
Pediatric Neurosurgical Unit,
Hospital Universitario 12 de Octubre,
Madrid 28041, Spain
e-mail: jose.hinojosa@salud.madrid.org

13.1 Introduction

Diversion of CSF fluid for the treatment of hydrocephalus constitutes a standard technique in neurosurgery, and it is one of the most frequent procedures performed in a neurosurgical unit [9, 10, 21, 22, 29, 32, 65]. The peritoneal cavity is the most common site for cerebrospinal fluid (CSF) absorption. It was first used by Ferguson in 1898, through a lumboperitoneal shunt system, and later popularized by authors like Nulsen and Spitz (1952), Holter or Pudenz (1956) [18, 65]. In spite of the spread of endoscopic third ventriculostomies for the treatment of obstructive hydrocephalus, ventriculoperitoneal shunting remains the elective technique for most of the cases of communicating hydrocephalus, which nowadays still stand as the first cause of hydrocephalus for the vast majority of patients. Ventriculoperitoneal shunting usually provide immediate relief of intracranial hypertension, and it is simple to be performed [47]. Unfortunately, the complication rate is relatively high, mostly related to infection and mechanical failure (obstruction, fracture of the distal catheter, or pseudocysts) [4, 9, 10, 21, 45, 66, 69].

Abdominal complications are relatively frequent after VP and lumboperitoneal CSF shunting and account for up to 25 % of noninfectious complications [1, 4, 9, 18, 21, 22, 26, 39, 43, 50]. They can present with a variety of signs and symptoms. Complications of the procedure include ascites, shunt infection, metastases of

C. Di Rocco et al. (eds.), *Complications of CSF Shunting in Hydrocephalus: Prevention, Identification, and Management*, DOI 10.1007/978-3-319-09961-3_13,

brain tumors, pleural effusion, pneumothorax, intestinal obstruction, perforation of a hollow viscus (such as the bladder and bowel), volvulus, and migration of the distal catheter [2, 4, 10, 12, 13, 15, 18, 24, 27, 39, 45, 59, 66, 70, 77]. Although some of these complications are merely mechanical (disconnection, fracture, migration), many others include an inflammatory and/or infectious etiology, and are potentially hazardous if left undiagnosed [10, 12, 72, 80]. All of them have been related as "nonfunctional abdominal complications of the distal catheter" [47], due to the fact that they share a common pathophysiological origin in the presence of a functioning shunt.

Due to the high variety of possibilities that may complicate an abdominal shunt, awareness about the different pathological entities and prompt recognition will render best results in their treatment and prognosis.

13.2 Epidemiology

In a review of the literature performed by de Aquino et al., they found abdominal complications to be a common problem after ventriculoperitoneal shunting [18]. Prevalence is as high as 47 % (more frequent in males than in females). It may happen at any age, but seems to be more frequent in younger children than in eldest or adults, who are affected only in 10 % of all the cases. The age of the first VP shunt on each patient varied from a few days to 58 years but in 66.7 % of the patients, they were less than 1 year old (usually between the first and tenth month of life).

The lapse of time between the first VP shunt and its complication occurred in the 1st year after VP shunt implantation in 57.5 % of the patients, and only 20 % beyond the 3rd year after shunting [18, 22].

Grosfeld et al. reported an intra-abdominal complication rate of 24 % in a series of 185 children treated by VP shunting procedures [32].

Intra-abdominal fluid collections are also relatively uncommon complications of CSF peritoneal shunts. Abdominal pseudocysts are more frequent among them, and in a study by Salomao et al. 18 cases of abdominal pseudocysts were reported [71]. In their series with positive CSF cultures they found a 44.4 % rate of shunt components infection and positive cultures of the peritoneal end of the catheter in 61 %.

13.3 Physiopathology of Nonfunctional Abdominal Complications of Shunt Catheters

Complication rate after peritoneal shunting is high, mostly related to infection (at CNS, peritoneum, or shunt components) [10, 18, 22, 66], or due to obstruction (of the proximal catheter by choroids plexus, ventricular wall, cerebral parenchyma, blood, and other debris) [2, 9, 11, 34, 52, 83].

Although the silicon elastomer is considered an inert material and designed to remain in the body for very long periods, the fact is that catheters may fracture in its long trajectory at the subcutaneous tissue by mechanical trauma, by a biodegradation process [10, 18, 20, 31], or by the formation of a bacterial biofilm on the catheter surface [26]. Many abnormalities found on this surface can be responsible for bacterial adhesion. There is also evidence that CSF proteins are absorbed at the catheters and act as another responsible factor for biodegradation and bacterial adhesion [18].

Pathophysiology of peritoneal fibrosis has been studied in animal models and humans undergoing continuous abdominal peritoneal dialysis [40]. Ultrafiltration of CSF at the peritoneum follows an osmotic pressure gradient facilitated by hydrostatic pressure mechanisms. Higher pressure of CSF at peritoneum helps the passage of fluid through micropores at the membrane. Molecular studies in chronic peritoneal dialysis models confirm the presence of small pores, which are responsible for the flow of low molecular weight substances such as urea, creatinine, glucose, as well as the presence of large pores, which are responsible for the flow of high molecular weight substances. Larger pores, called "aquapores," would facilitate the passage of substances with higher molecular weight.

Success of the ultrafiltrating process (and thus of the CSF resorption in the abdominal cavity) depends on the functional integrity of the peritoneal membrane and of the vascular mesothelium. Absorption rate of the peritoneal fluid through the lymphatics ranges from 0.5 to 1.5 ml/min, with the peak absorption occurring through diaphragmatic lymphatics, especially at the subdiaphragmatic region, where there are open intracellular channels "stomata." These are conducted to the mediastinal lymphatic and localized before the right lymphatic duct, so it can then reach the right internal jugular and subclavian veins (see the reference paper by de Aquino et al.) [18] Continuous exposure of the peritoneal membrane to the CSF fluid can result in significant changes on its morphology and ultrastructure with a potential risk of peritoneal fibrosis.

Abnormalities in the morphology and ultrastructure of the peritoneal membrane occur especially at the peritoneal mesothelium, with an increased development of the wrinkled endoplasmic reticulum and a decrease in membrane microvilli (responsible for the increase in its surface area), micro-pinocytic vesicles, and changes on the submesothelial layer, leading to a sclerosis effect on the connective tissue (see Krediet and de Aquino et al.) [18, 40]. Glucose present in the CSF fluid could be potentially toxic to the mesothelial cells and be responsible for vascular changes in the peritoneal membrane.

On the other hand, and acting as a summatory mechanism, the presence of foreign bodies inside the peritoneal cavity activates macrophages and monocytes, which stimulate mesothelial cells to produce immunomediators (interleukins or IL) [18]. These initial IL, such as IL-β1, TNF-α, PGE-2, and prostacyclin 2 (PGI-2), activate IL-6 and IL-8, which attract neutrophils to the inflammatory site. It is postulated that IL-β1 yielded by monocytes and macrophages may have an important role in physiopathology of peritoneal fibrosis and can increase collagen synthesis to an elevated level of procollagen in fibroblasts [18]. Peritoneal fibroblasts would respond to inflammatory stimuli by increasing the extracellular matrix compounds, potentially contributing to the development of peritoneal fibrosis. Fibrosis reaction around the distal catheters and structures together with bowel peristaltic movements and increased intra-abdominal pressure would act as a constant source of mechanical pressure that would lead to necrosis and ultimate serosal perforation of viscus at the site of the anchoring [12, 19, 27, 58, 73]. As it will be explained later, the weakness of certain peritoneal areas and the umbilical end of the vitellointestinal duct or the patent processus vaginalis into the scrotum could act as a facilitating mechanism for perforation [6, 49, 58, 81].

13.4 Sterile Ascites

Sterile ascites is a complication rarely reported [2, 9, 16, 17, 32, 43, 75, 83]. In the majority of cases, the pathological collection of CSF in the peritoneum occurs within a pseudocyst, due to infection from a shunt and posterior peritonitis that causes the pathological accumulation of abdominal CSF [9, 26, 83]. In sterile ascites, on the other hand, CSF is not loculated but accumulated in the peritoneal cavity. It is defined by negative Gram stains from the ascitic fluid as well as negative viral and bacterial cultures [16, 75].

Ascites usually results from a concurrent illness such as cirrhosis, congestive heart failure, nephrosis, or disseminated carcinomatosis. To explain the development of sterile ascites after abdominal shunting, different pathological pathways have been recalled.

1. Immune responses from a shunt material breakdown causing inflammatory reaction could lead to fibrosis of the peritoneal layer and abnormal resorption at the serosa level [10, 18, 31].
2. Prior abdominal surgeries or multiple shunt revisions may cause adhesions or preclude resorption due to a malabsorptive peritoneum [9, 32].
3. Elevated CSF protein levels from CNS pathology, such as infection or neoplastic processes, which could increase oncotic forces within the peritoneum [2, 75, 83].
4. CSF overproduction from diffuse villous hyperplasia or papilloma of the choroid plexus [11].

Patients with ascites usually have delayed symptoms of underdrainage on presentation [21, 32].

Physical examination may show abdominal distension and tenderness, usually with little signs of defense. Findings include altered abdominal contour, fluid wave, or dullness to percussion. Abdominal perimeter is high and dilated abdominal wall veins may be seen as a sign of ascites.

Diagnostic imaging consists of abdominal ultrasound, which shows diffuse collection, without loculation or septae and excludes signs of thrombosis in the hepatic vessels. Abdominal CT scans show single, usually large, nonloculated peritoneal fluid collection surrounding the catheter but usually no thickened omentum or peritoneum or other signs of inflammation.

Peritoneal centesis is the diagnostic modality of choice and can provide information regarding the source of the ascites.

In the absence of these potential causative issues, the shunt should be externalized to confirm that the ascites is a result of excessive CSF accumulation. So far, CSF cultures remain the most reliable method to rule out infection [57, 71]. However, growths of microorganisms in the shunt components in the absence of positive cultures in CSF are often attributed to contamination. Extending cultures longer for up to 14 days is recommended to effectively exclude most organisms including slow growing anaerobes such as *Propionibacterium acnes*, before infection is definitively ruled out.

Treatment After diagnosis, the peritoneal catheter is externalized and the patient remains under antibiotics (e.g., vancomycin and ceftazidime) until CSF cultures are proven negative and infection is ruled out. Antibiotics are kept for 24 h after definitive insertion in a new cavity [83]. Due to the high protein accumulation and CSF formation in some pathological entities, atrium is usually the selected one, and ventriculoatrial shunting commonly resolves the problem [2, 11, 51, 78].

Summary Sterile ascites should always be a diagnosis of exclusion. Standard workup must include analysis of the ascitic fluid including cellularity, protein levels, glucose, and cultures as well as cytology to exclude malignancy. Imaging consists of abdominal CT and cranial MRI to rule out associated pathologies. Once malignancy and infection have been ruled out and abdominal pathology resolved, the shunt can be safely converted to a VA shunt.

13.5 Pseudocyst

Pseudocysts are loculated intra-abdominal fluid collections developing around the distal end of the peritoneal catheter [52, 60]. The occurrence of a pseudocyst after peritoneal CSF diversion was first described by Harsh [33]. Since then, a frequency of around 0.7–10 % has been reported in the literature. Pseudocyst can occur any time between several weeks and several years after the initial shunting procedure [21, 22].

The exact cause of cerebrospinal fluid abdominal pseudocysts is not completely understood, but risk factors seem to be related to inflammatory processes. Several predisposing factors have been described: acute shunt infection, a past history of cerebrospinal fluid infection, multiple shunt revisions, previous abdominal surgery, and central nervous system tumors [9, 10, 21, 26, 29, 34, 39, 69]. It is agreed that an inflammatory process, either infectious or sterile, is a frequent predisposing factor. Bacterial infection of the shunt system preceded the pseudocyst formation in as much as 73 % of the reported cases [71], but the incidence of infection could be higher if cultures of CSF were maintained over 14 days or processed for anaerobic germs. The inflammatory process has an important role in pseudocyst formation: inflamed intestinal serosal surfaces, fibrous tissue without epithelial lining, fibrous tissue with acute inflammation, and granulomatous tissue with fibroblasts, collagen bundles, and scattered inflammatory cells have been found in the histological examination [18, 29, 34, 39, 52]. All these figures turn the wall of the pseudocyst into an inflammatory surface that is unable to absorb cerebrospinal fluid.

The time from a shunting procedure to the development of abdominal cerebrospinal fluid pseudocyst ranges from few days to several years.

In a paper from Santos de Oliveira et al., this period extended from 10 days to 15 years [57]. Often, abdominal pseudocysts tend to occur within 6 months of the last intra-abdominal surgical intervention. It has been suggested that smaller pseudocysts tend to be infected, and larger pseudocysts tend to be sterile [61, 71]. However, this could not be proven and one study from Roitberg et al. found no statistically significant link between infection and pseudocyst size [69]. Infection rates varied between 17 and 80 % (average of 42 %) in 128 reviewed cases [52]. *Staphylococcus epidermidis* is the most frequent responsible organism, but other coagulase negative staphylococci may be found such as *S. capitis* or *S. hominis*, as well as Gram negatives like *Propionibacterium acnes* [52, 61, 69].

Symptoms related to the occurrence of an abdominal cyst include vomiting, distension, abdominal pain, fever, and/or abdominal mass. It is often accompanied by signs and symptoms of shunt dysfunction due to the nonreabsorption of CSF loculated inside the cyst such as fontanel bulging, somnolence, headaches, vomiting, or seizures.

Allergic reactions are another potential cause of the sterile inflammation leading to pseudocyst formation [18, 34]. In cases of repetitive pseudocysts in a patient in whom shunt infection has been reasonably ruled out, the possibility of allergic reaction against any of the components of the catheter must be borne in mind. Increase in peripheral eosinophils and serum IgE levels, as well as an eosinophilic infiltrate of the pseudocyst walls may alert about this possibility [18, 39].

There is an open debate about which of the components of the shunt would be responsible for the immunological reaction. Silicone elastomers and gels have been extensively studied due to the widespread use of breast implants. Three different and independent investigation groups have concluded that there is no convincing evidence to support or lend biologic plausibility to an association of silicone breast implants with immune-related human health conditions. They further indicate that there is insufficient or flawed evidence that silicones can elicit an immunotoxic response, trigger a specific immune reaction, or amplify an autoimmune-like disease [39]. Previous reports of specific antisilicone antibodies could have been misdiagnosed due to a different level of circulating albumin and a nonspecific adsorption of the IgG fraction [31].

Other sources of antigenic stimulation have been considered. The ethylene oxide (ETO), a gas used to sterilize medical devices, including VP shunts, is a highly reactive alkylating agent that can react with endogenous proteins to create a neo-antigen. IgE antibodies specifically directed toward ETO protein conjugates, and the presence of an ETO metabolite (ethylene chlorohydrin) in the CSF have been found for as long as 4 months after the last shunt revision in patients with elevated eosinophil counts, who underwent multiple shunt revisions without evidence of an infection.

Another possible antigen source is barium sulfate, the radiopaque agent included in the manufacture of VP shunts to allow for visualization of the shunt by x-rays, latex the material used in the fabrics of surgical gloves, or antibiotics such as vancomycin or gentamycin, frequently used by some surgeons to impregnate catheters during surgery for VP shunting [31].

"Silicone" allergy has been treated with corticosteroids, but reactions recurred upon removal of the medication. Changing the shunt system made of the usual silicone elastomer to one made of polyurethane or made of 'extracted silicone' elastomer usually solves the problem. "Extracted silicone" elastomers are manufactured through an industrial process that retrieves the small percentage of unbounded silicone oil from the catheters leaving only pure solid silicone elastomer, thus making immune reaction less likely to reappear (Medtronic Neurosurgery).

Diagnosis Any patient that carries a VP shunt and complains of abdominal pain or distension is potentially a candidate to suffer a pseudocyst. Diagnostic tools include CSF sampling from the shunt reservoir and aspirate from the cyst to be sent to the laboratory. CSF is evaluated for signs of infection.

Laboratory tests should include Gram stain, culture, glucose, protein, and cell counts.

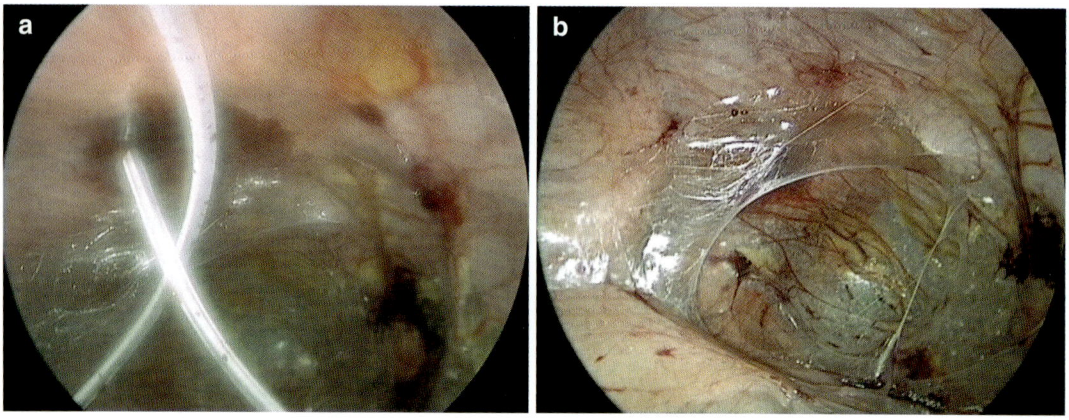

Fig. 13.1 Pseudocyst. Peritoneal catheter is withdrawn from the pseudocyst (**a**) and repositioned in functional peritoneum under laparoscopic assistance (**b**)

Shunt infection is defined after a positive culture of either cerebrospinal fluid or abdominal fluid.

Plain radiographs may show the shunt tube coiled in a soft tissue mass displacing adjacent bowel loops. Abdominal ultrasound or CT

Treatment Several techniques have been used, usually with good results. Pseudocysts have been treated traditionally with surgical shunt externalization, antibiotics for presumed or documented infection, and a second surgical procedure for shunt reinsertion.

The presence or absence of infection must be established before definitive treatment can be carried out. Usually, it is assumed that there is concurrent infection that requires shunt externalization or external ventricular drain. Identification of cerebrospinal fluid infection precludes prompt reinsertion into the peritoneum.

Pseudocysts have traditionally been treated with surgical shunt externalization, connecting the distal catheter to a collecting sterile bag, antibiotics for presumed or documented shunt infection [71], and a second surgical procedure for shunt reinsertion either in the peritoneal cavity or in a new location such as pleura or cardiac atrium through a jugular vein [51]. In the past, ultrasound guided paracentesis followed by radical excision of the cyst walls through exploratory laparotomy and insertion of the distal catheter in a new location inside the peritoneal cavity was the choice elected. Recently, laparoscopic management of the pseudocyst, which involves excision of a portion of the cyst and repositioning the catheter within the peritoneal cavity, is preferred (Fig. 13.1). For some authors repositioning of the peritoneal catheter in the abdomen could lead to the recurrence of abdominal pseudocyst. However, shunt replacement back into the abdomen has been feasible in most cases and in the majority of the patients, contralateral peritoneal cavity is a reliable option. Peritoneal cavity can be used for shunting once the cyst had reabsorbed [1, 9, 29, 37, 41, 42, 44, 71]. To minimize the effects of peritoneal adhesions, the peritoneal catheter may be placed in a retrohepatic subdiaphragmatic position [41, 67, 71]. CSF diversion to ventriculo-omental bursa or lesser sac may be considered as another acceptable alternative technique to CSF shunting when the anterior peritoneum loses or decreases its CSF absorption capacity [23, 50] (see later). Only exceptionally, and after failure of the previous techniques, it is a necessary conversion to an atrial shunt [47, 77].

When there is a chance for it, endoscopic third ventriculostomy (ETV) is an excellent approach for selected cases of noncommunicating hydrocephalus. As it has been shown, for those patients that remain shunt dependent or ETV has failed, ventriculoperitoneal shunt can be safely reinserted in the majority of the cases.

13.6 Anal Extrusion. Bowel Perforation

Bowel perforation and anal extrusion of the distal portion of a VP shunt (AEVPS) is a rare mechanic complication of VP shunts. Wilson et al. described the first case reported in 1966 [81]. Since then, more than 100 cases of bowel perforation have been reported and the incidence of this complication is thought to be around 0,1–1 % [15, 19, 27, 49, 58, 63, 72, 81, 82]. In a retrospective review of their series in 2006, Vinchon and colleagues found 19 cases of bowel perforation due to VP shunt: only three of them developed anal extrusion of the catheter.

Pathophysiology and risk factors Pathogenesis and predisposing factors are not completely well understood. By definition, AEVPS involves a bowel perforation that has been produced through different mechanisms. Di Rocco suggested that bowel erosion results from inflammation caused by a preexisting shunt infection [21]. Interaction between mechanic trauma and inflammation following infection can lead to the bowel perforation [18, 19, 27, 43]. In the majority of the reported cases pathogenic agents suggest a peritoneal focus (e.g., *Escherichia coli*), but it is not uncommon to find organisms that are typically related with a perioperative contamination (*S. aureus* or *S. epidermidis*). Different authors suggest that some cases of bowel perforation can be linked to mechanisms of inflammation and rejection of an infected foreign body [18, 19, 34]. Intestinal developmental alterations can be a predisposing factor too: in a paper from Matsuoka et al. bowel perforation was related to a duplication of ileum terminalis that resulted in continuous irritation of a fixed point on the bowel's surface and finally perforation of the sigmoid colon [49]. Encasing fibrosis around the tube has been reported; this fibrosis may have an anchoring effect on the catheter, resulting in pressure and decubitus ulceration, which can lead to a perforation [6, 49]. It has been also reported that the weakness of certain peritoneal areas and the umbilical end of the vitellointestinal duct and the processus vaginalis into the scrotum might

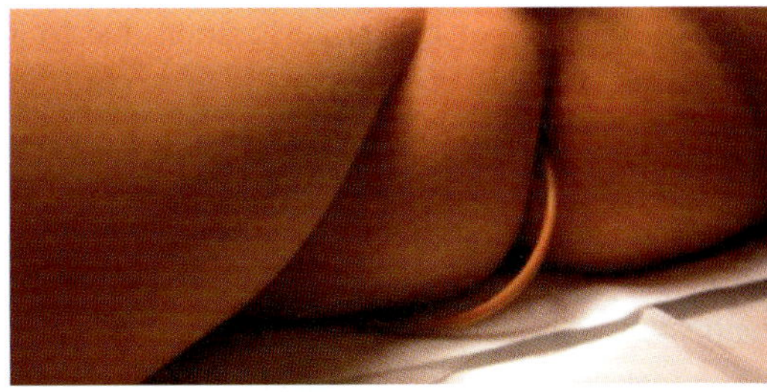

Fig. 13.2 Anal extrusion of peritoneal catheter

remain patent and act as a facilitating mechanism for perforation [59, 81]. Formerly it was believed that spring-coiled catheters were more prone to produce visceral perforations, as this kind of catheter had been implicated in more than the 50 % of the cases, and in cases of gastric and peroral migrations. However, many reports have shown that softer and more flexible silicon catheters can also produce bowel and other viscus perforation [21, 27, 63, 72].

No evidence has been found that the peritoneal opening technique (laparotomy versus trochar) when the shunt is positioned could be a risk factor for bowel perforation. Some authors consider that laparotomy is a safer technique; on the other hand, many papers find that trochar technique is at least as safe as laparotomy and it is not a risk factor for bowel perforation [78]. Perforations due to the trochar are described, but usually they are an operative, acute complication, not related to a chronic inflammatory process. Serious vascular damage has been reported during trochar insertion: for this reason, we favor mini-open laparotomy in opposition to trochar-guided insertion.

Other potential risk factors for bowel perforation could be suspected silicone allergy or weakness in the bowel wall resulting from deficient innervation like in children with myelomeningocele or congenital hydrocephalus [4, 12, 34]. It is not clear whether the length of the peritoneal catheter has any implication in hollow viscus perforations.

Diagnosis AEVPS is a pathognomonic sign of bowel perforation (Fig. 13.2), but it is infrequent (15.7 %). The absence of peritoneal signs is common in cases of bowel perforation due to a VP shunt. Clinical peritonitis is observed in 15–25 % of the cases. As much as 48 % of the cases can develop meningitis and/or ventriculitis. Abdominal radiology can be used when the diagnosis is not obvious. Abdominal CT scan with contrast and ultrasonography may show local inflammation signs and a thickened abdominal wall, but this exploration may result negative. In some cases with a high index of suspicion, it is possible to perform a shuntogram, which consists in the instillation of a contrast medium into the lower portion of the shunt, to demonstrate bowel perforation. Colonoscopy could be used to identify the point of the perforation [27, 49]. Cranial CT scan or MRI must complete the follow-up diagnostic studies. CSF sampling must be obtained from the shunt reservoir, from the tip of the catheter exposed or after externalization of the peritoneal end.

Treatment Bowel perforation has to be managed as a surgical emergency. If the patient does not show any symptom apart from the AEVPS, a conservative management is possible. The shunt can be cut in the abdominal surface, externalizing the proximal end and eliminating the distal end by a trans-anal traction. If the patient presents with clinical (peritoneal and/or meningeal) symptoms, imaging studies are needed to assess the presence of active hydrocephalus and localize the site of the bowel perforation. In this case, laparotomy or laparoscopy should be done in order to repair the intestinal perforation and retire the peritoneal end of the shunt [49, 82]. External ventricular drainage and antibiotic therapy is started until proven that CSF is not contaminated or, in case of CSF infection, that the infection has been defeated. After two or three consecutive negative CSF cultures, it is possible to replace the entire shunt system. Usually, new shunting to the peritoneum is an option, but atrial or pleural diversion is preferred when peritoneal positioning of the catheter is not feasible (e.g., big laparotomy, adhesions, or recurrent perforation).

Prognosis AEVPS is a rare but potentially severe complication of VP shunts. Children with no symptoms of perforation or meningitis show a better evolution. If intestinal perforation leads to a chemical or infectious peritonitis, or the patient suffers meningitis or ventriculitis after Gram-negative infection, then prognosis is bad. The highest mortality rates are shown in patients with abdominal complications [82].

13.7 Bladder Perforation

Bladder perforation by a peritoneal catheter is another rare complication of VPS [6, 15, 35, 53, 63]. This complication was first reported by Grosfeld in two patients, aged 3 months and 1 year, in 1974 [32]. Catheter removal, bladder repair, supra-pubic cystostomy, and antibiotic therapy resulted in recovery in each case. Around ten cases involving normal (nonaugmented) urinary bladder have been reported [6, 15, 35]. It has been also reported more commonly after abdominal repair of urinary bladder, during augmentative procedures for neurogenic bladder [53]. The location of the bladder, which lies in the extraperitoneal compartment, makes it a highly unlikely site of peritoneal catheter perforation, as the catheter must pass through the peritoneum into the extraperitoneal space and subsequently penetrate the bladder.

The mechanisms by which peritoneal catheters perforate hollow organs are not fully understood. An initial local inflammatory reaction around the tip of the catheter initiates its anchoring to the serosa of the hollow viscus [6, 19]. Calcifications occur at the distal tube in barium-impregnated catheters as sign of the fragmentation of the silicon polymers facilitating inflammation and anchoring [10]. Increase intra-abdominal pressure, peristaltic movements of the bowels, and CSF pulsation originates local pressure leading to necrosis and ultimate bladder perforation [6, 19, 63]. After entry into the urethra, final extrusion happens.

Shunt factors, which have been related to perforation, are sharp abdominal tip, long abdominal end of catheter, stiff consistency, barium coating of the catheter, or allergies to the shunt components (like silicon allergy). Initially, a higher tendency of perforation with spring-coiled catheters was reported. However, perforation may occur with any type of catheter.

Perforation of the bladder during trochar insertion or abdominal surgery can be prevented by draining the bladder before surgery. It is our policy to drain the bladder with a Foley catheter at the beginning of every surgery. If the patient is expected to have a long postoperative period (e.g., severe trauma or spinal cord tumor), Foley catheter is left in place. On the other hand, if shunting is a scheduled surgery, Foley is retired immediately after the procedure.

It has been reported that silicone rubber has a slight tendency to stick when it is in a dry state [35]. In distal independent catheters, the system may be flushed with saline. In unishunt systems, at least all components must be moisturized with saline and/or gentamycin dilution.

On examination, patients can be afebrile without neurological deficits or meningeal signs. Abdomen signs may be absent and peritoneal catheter can be seen coming out of the urethra with drops of CSF from the distal end. This can be explained because of a sealing effect of peritoneum around the catheter. If urine enters peritoneal cavity, patients may present with fever, abdominal pain, distension, and erythema of the abdominal wall between the umbilicus and the pubis. Diagnostic imaging must include again abdominal ultrasound and CT scanning.

Treatment In case that a bladder perforation occurs, it must be treated as an emergency. The shunt can be cut proximally and pulled out through the urethra. If no irritative signs are present or abdominal imaging excludes intraperitoneal complication (such as pneumoperitoneum or urinoma) a Foley catheter is placed and one may allow the bladder to heal on its own. However, at the lesser symptom of peritoneal defense, bladder can be approached extraperitoneally, repaired, and cystostomy or transient Foley catheter performed. In both cases, shunt is externalized proximally or external ventricular drainage left in place until CSF cultures are negative or peritoneum is ready to receive again the shunt in the opposite side.

Following a similar pathological pattern, perforation of the scrotum, umbilicus, and vagina has been also reported.

13.8 Other Infrequent Complications

Other rare complications of VP shunt surgery include migration, intestinal volvulus, abdominal wall perforation, or VPS-related abdominal metastases originating from brain tumors. Acute cholecystitis after subphrenic suprahepatic abscess among other bizarre complications is reported occasionally in literature.

13.8.1 Migration

Migration of the distal endings of the shunt components has been reported at different levels [24, 30, 44, 45, 59, 73]. In some cases, the weakness of the wall at anatomical preexisting foramina or their failure to fuse permits the occurrence of this unusual complication. Factors related to the migrations are anchoring of shunt tube to a calcified point, abdominal wall contractions, increased intra-abdominal pressure, flexo-extension movements of head and neck, and also the retained memory of shunt tube [3, 4, 6, 19, 34, 45, 59, 63].

Martin et al. reported migration of the intra-abdominal catheter through the right vertebrocostal trigone (foramen of Bochdalek) into the right hemithorax. This resulted in hydrothorax that resolved after revision of the distal end of the shunt [45]. Symptomatic pleural effusion after VP shunt has been reported, even in the absence of intrathoracic migration [3]. In some cases, this has been caused after hypochondrial compression through diaphragm due to formation of a pseudocyst after placing the shunt catheter in the suprahepatic subphrenic space [30].

Not uncommon, mostly in premature and newborns, is to find the distal end of peritoneal catheter migrating to the scrotal sac. Communication between testicular albuginea and peritoneal cavity together with decubitus and elevated pressure that CSF exerts on the tubular pass, may lead to hydrocele, and entry of the tube in the scrotum.

Upward migration of distal catheter has been also reported to the breast [73], intrathoracic to the pleura [3], intracardiac [70], or even to the pulmonary artery. Thoracic trauma during placement of a shunt or direct trauma to vessels in the neck are mechanisms related to these complications [30, 46]. Migration of the distal catheter in the heart is a very rare complication of VP shunt that may be lethal, possibly causing pulmonary emboli, arrhythmia, sepsis, or cardiac insufficiency [70]. In all cases reported in literature, the catheter passed through a cervical vein into the jugular vein and ultimately into the heart. Erosion of the vein at the supraclavicular fossa related to a kinking in the catheter may be an alternative mechanism. For some authors, its frequency would be greater in children because of the thinner subcutaneous tissues in the neck. However, it has been hypothesized that it should be less likely in children below the age of 6 years for whom the tunneling devices are typically larger than subcutaneous veins of the neck.

To avoid this complication, tunneling the shunt too medial and too deep in the neck must be avoided. A vein perforated by the shunt passer may be difficult to detect intraoperatively unless profuse venous bleeding is found during subcutaneous tunneling [46].

Diagnosis is easy on simple XRs but CT scanning is advisable to delineate the course of the catheter within the thoracic cavity and heart. Echocardiography may help to discard cardiac perforation, thrombus, or valvular lesions.

Removal of the migrated shunt into the vascular/cardiac flow can be performed: percutaneously under fluoroscopic guidance, by interventional radiology, and in the most complex cases, through open thoracotomy. In those cases where the catheter is completely detached inside the heart or the pulmonary artery, percutaneous transvenous retrieval with a variety of loop snare devices, can be used, and open thoracotomy reserved for the cases of failure of interventional radiology. In these cases, a new VP shunt is indicated.

When the catheter remains connected to the extrathoracic part and the entire distal catheter is in the venous circulation it can be withdrawn percutaneously under fluoroscopic guidance. Care must be taken to ensure that there is no erosion of the heart walls or entanglement with the valves. If echocardiogram or enhanced CT scan shows no injuries to cardiac valves, some authors believe that there is no increased risk of endocarditis in the eventuality of shunt infection [70].

13.8.2 Intestinal Volvulus

Knotting of the distal catheter around the bowel and/or volvulus around the tube is a rare complication that is reported from time to time. Abdominal pain, distension, tenderness and defense, tympanic percussion, and intestinal silence are signs to bear in mind. XRs and ultrasound will make proper diagnosis straight.

Treatment consists of exploratory laparotomy, usually under laparoscopic technique, but sometimes, the entanglement of the tube and the suffering of the intestine may be so severe as to make an open laparotomy necessary. Then, the shunt is externalized and connected to sterile bag until new diversion procedure is needed.

Volvulus is a serious condition that necessitates confirmation of the integrity of the bowel and peritoneum before a new VP shunt is inserted. Otherwise, alternatives to diversion are pleural space, right cardiac atrium, or suprahepatic infradiaphragmatic recess.

13.8.3 Abdominal Wall Perforation

As we have seen, tip of distal catheter may induce a chronic inflammation and localized pressure that will finally result in erosion [4]. The end of the tube together with the continuous effect of the CSF pulsations penetrates the wall and perforates it.

Patients with myelomeningocele are more susceptible to perforation due to a weak musculature and local infective adhesion [4]. Fibrosis around the peritoneal catheter is a risk factor of visceral wall perforation [18]. In premature patients or low-weight newborns, abscess and perforation through umbilicus is another reported complication.

Treatment Infection of the shunt components must be suspected after any perforation of a hollow viscus or abdominal walls. After proper cultures from CSF or purulent discharges are taken, broad-spectrum antibiotherapy is started; this must include typically gram-positives as well as gram-negative germs, which are not unusual in abdominal pathology related to shunting.

In case that peritonitis or peritoneal abscess is not suspected, distal catheter can be safely removed without laparotomy. The shunt must be removed by cutting the distal tube at the abdominal wall, externalizing the proximal edge and pulling the distal edge from the abdominal wall, without pulling the distal tip proximally, thus preventing the spread of the infection to the externalization site. Management includes shunt removal, external CSF drainage, and assessment for CSF infection followed by a new shunt device within the peritoneum.

13.8.4 Abdominal Metastasis

Extraneural metastases of primary brain tumors are rare and may occur through blood or lymphatic vessels [7, 13]. Spread through VPS can be facilitated by the direct connection established between cerebral ventricles and abdominal. It is also extremely rare, and less than 100 cases have been reported so far in literature [13, 64, 68].

The most frequent histological entities spreading through tube shunting are germinomas and endodermal sinus tumors in older patients (10–18 years of age), while medulloblastomas and astrocytomas are particularly common in the group of younger patients (below the age of 10). There is an overall male prevalence (1.9–1) a feature more pronounced in the older age group [68]. Mean interval between shunt operation and diagnosis of metastases is around one and a half year, but it may extend between 2 months and as late as 5 years after the first procedure. Occasionally, metastases have been diagnosed at autopsy [73].

Ultrasound or CT imaging of the abdomen might be considered as part of the routine follow-up in children with VPS who are being treated from brain tumors.

There are marked differences in prognosis with age and sex, in favor of older children and boys. But main prognostic factor affecting survival is histology of the tumor [7, 68, 74]. Not surprisingly, patients with germinomas and abdominal metastasis after shunting show better prognosis than those with a diagnosis of endodermal sinus tumor or glioblastoma.

Peritoneal metastases appear to respond well to systemic chemotherapy and/or radiation, but they must be considered a severe complication that may affect outcome.

13.9 Options for Catheter Placement After Peritoneal Dysfunction

After multiple distal failures, the peritoneal cavity is often deemed unsuitable for cerebrospinal fluid (CSF) diversion. Probably more than 30 % of patients with VP shunts will experience abdominal complications [1, 9, 18, 22]. Different places have been described when peritoneum is considered inadequate or impaired for CSF diversion, including right atrium of the heart, pleural space, or gall bladder among others. However, because of the benefits of VP over VA shunting (mostly a lower rate of severe complications) [25, 51, 78], many authors defend that every effort should be made to preserve the peritoneum as the place for the definitive distal catheter [1, 23, 37, 41, 62]. Potential complications of ventriculoatrial shunt malfunction are thromboemboli and infection, both life threatening [51, 78]. Thromboembolism occurs in 0.3 % of patients and is nearly always fatal [51]. Shunt nephropathy is also a potential risk long time recognized and reported in the past. The treatment of occluded or sluggish catheters is often anticoagulation that exposes the patient to severe bleeding risks, and revision of these catheters, when needed, is related to more complex procedures that include manipulation of central veins. Revision rates due to catheter outgrowth have been reported to be as high as 66 % [78].

For all these reasons, every effort must be made to find a functional peritoneum after previous shunt failures due either to infection or distal occlusion. Laparoscopy has been used as in the management of VP shunt complications since the 1970s, providing excellent visualization of the abdomen through a minimally invasive approach [1, 37, 41, 42]. Surgeon can examine the abdomen for adhesions, cysts, loculations, and laparoscopy can be used to clear distal obstructions, excise CSF pseudocysts, or successfully reposition the distal catheter in patients with previous multiple shunt revisions or distorted abdominal anatomy. Laparoscopy is an excellent tool in locating suitable peritoneal pockets of the peritoneum where the distal catheter can be successfully replaced [1, 41, 42]. Open laparotomy remains an alternative for abdominal exploration, in more complex cases where laparoscopy is not indicated or easy to perform due to multiple loculations or dense adhesions [50, 62].

An alternative approach to minimize the effects of peritoneal adhesions is the employment of "reserve pouches" inside the peritoneal cavity [9, 23, 50, 57, 62]. Typically, retrohepatic subdiaphragmatic recess has been successfully used after "lost peritoneum" [57]. Several reports emphasize the advantages: it is away from previous adhesions, which usually affect the anterior peritoneum; and it is the place where the absorption rate of the peritoneal fluid through the lymphatics is higher, due to concentration of lymphatic ducts, and the presence of intracellular channels ("stomata") at the diaphragmatic peritoneum. Rengachary described a transthoracic transdiaphragmatic VP shunt for patients with difficult access to the peritoneal cavity due to diffuse anterior peritoneal adhesion. In this approach, the catheter is inserted directly into the suprahepatic subdiaphragmatic space through the thoracic cavity [67].

Matushita et al. have regained an interesting alternative technique to keep the peritoneal cavity as the main receptacle of CSF absorption [50]. They proposed to insert the distal catheter in the omental bursa (the lesser peritoneal sac), through the foramen of Winslow, jointly with a pediatric surgeon. They denominated this technique of as ventriculo-omental bursa (VOB) shunting. Follow up of three of their patients for over 1 year showed no recurrence of the peritoneal malabsorption. Omental bursa and retroperitoneal space had been used in the past as a receptacle for CSF since 1956, by authors like Picasa [62], Dodge [23], or Kubo [41] (see the beautiful review by Matushita et al.).

The omental bursa, also termed lesser sac, constitutes an extension of the anterior peritoneal space located behind the caudate lobule of the liver and covered by the stomach. It communicates with the anterior peritoneal space, the greater sac, or peritoneal cavity, through a constriction between the liver and duodenum named the epiploic foramen or foramen of Winslow. In its vertical extension, the omental bursa may reach the left iliac fossa and become very compliant in acceptance of fluid absorption, particularly in children. In adults, owing to the adhesions between the layers of the gastrocolic omentum, the vertical extent of the omental bursa is usually more limited [50].

Ventriculopleural diversion is an option that has been popularized in the last years when the VP shunt is not feasible [47]. However, it must be emphasized that pleural absorption may not be effective in children younger than 5 years of age [57]. The coexistence of pulmonary disease may contraindicate this surgery due to the risk of respiratory insufficiency in case of large pleural effusion. Martinez-Lage et al. suggested that the new technology valves may overcome complications related to pleural effusions or hydrothorax after ventriculopleural shunting [47].

For some authors the gallbladder provides also an alternate reservoir for CSF diversion. In 1959, Smith described the gallbladder as a shunt site [76], and since then, it has been used as a "last resource" option after failures of other cavities. The gallbladder is a sterile receptacle, a non-essential organ, reabsorbs water and electrolytes, and the pressure inside the bladder allows for maintenance of intracranial pressure. Bile is believed to provide lytic action, preventing fibrous adhesions and may have the added effect of neutralizing the excess of proteins in CSF [56]. In our personal series, three cases shunted into the gall bladder reached adulthood without any further complication after several failures of shunting procedures to the peritoneum. In two cases, shunt was inserted through an open

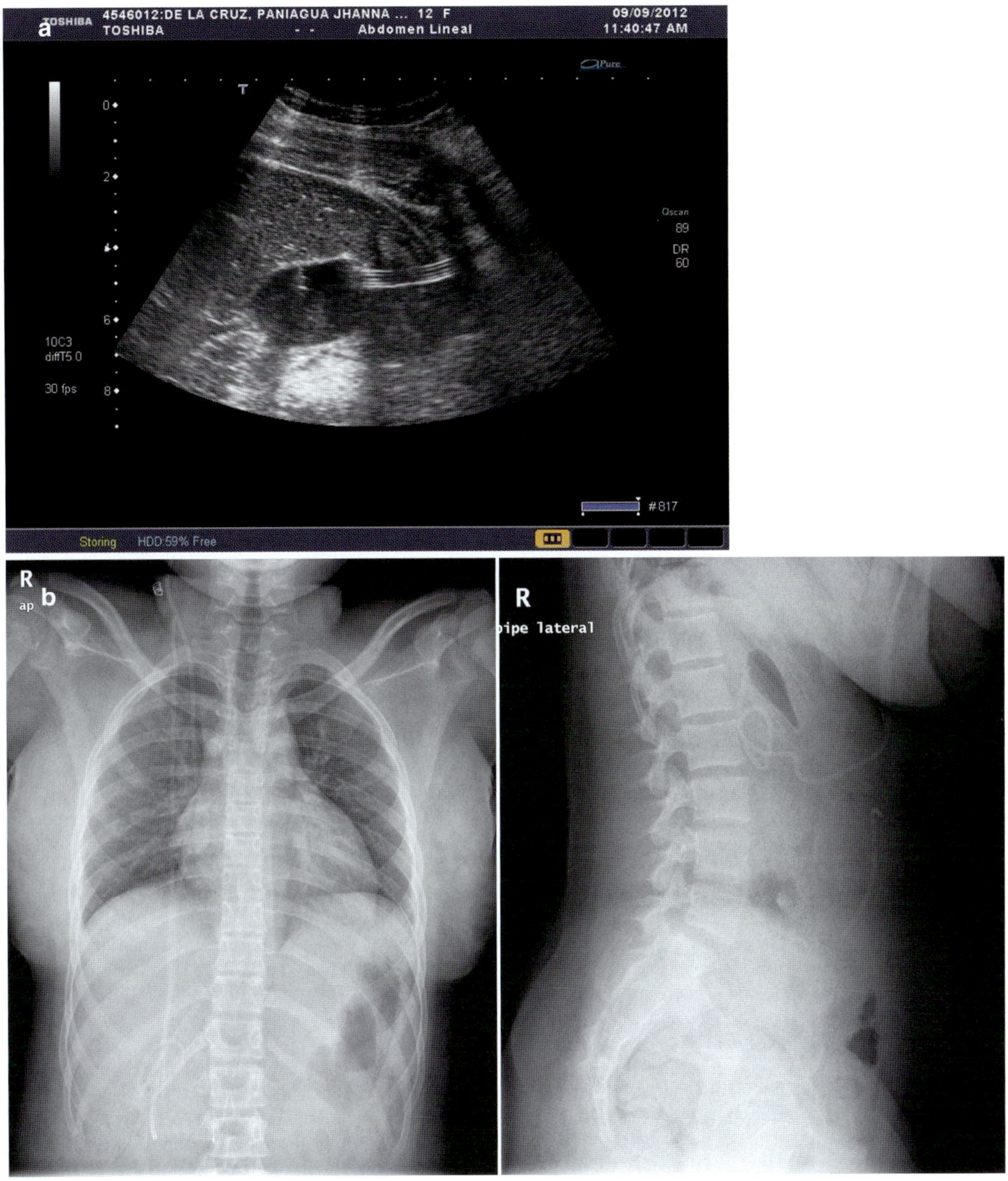

Fig. 13.3 VP shunt, with CSF derived to gall bladder. (**a**) Ultrasound shot showing distal catheter inside the gall bladder. (**b**) XR shows abandoned peritoneal catheter and distal catheter inside the gall bladder

laparotomy (Fig. 13.3), while in the last patient, laparoscopy was sufficient for insertion of the catheter inside the gallbladder and a purse-string suture to secure it to the wall.

Ventriculo-gallbladder shunt is an attractive alternative to peritoneal shunting [36, 48, 55, 75] in children with high protein levels in CSF, like in hydrocephalus secondary to tumors, where the lytic action of bile can potentially break down the high level of proteins present in the CSF [56]. Biliary sphincter tone and relatively high gallbladder pressures (10–20 cm H_2O) would function against the siphon phenomenon, preventing slit ventricle. But this may be also a point for shunt dysfunction [55, 79]. There have been cases reported for mortality and morbidity associated with meningitis and ventriculitis due to reflux of the bile into the CSF [5, 8]. Olavarria, Tomita et al., remember that the distal slit valve for the gallbladder should be avoided as it may be kinked and opened by the gallbladder contraction [56]. Finally, it must be remembered that, though bile is usually sterile in children, infection rates may be as high as 30 % or higher in adults [48].

References

1. Acharya R, Ramachandran CS, Singh S (2001) Laparoscopic management of abdominal complications in ventriculoperitoneal shunt surgery. J Laparoendosc Adv Surg Tech A 11(3):167–170
2. Adegbite AB, Khan M (1982) Role of protein content in CSF ascites following ventriculoperitoneal shunting. Case report. J Neurosurg 57(3):423–425
3. Adeolu AA, Komolafe EO, Abiodun AA, Adetiloye VA (2006) Symptomatic pleural effusion without intrathoracic migration of ventriculoperitoneal shunt catheter. Childs Nerv Syst 22:186–188
4. Aras M, Altaş M, Serarslan Y, Akçora B, Yılmaz A (2013) Protrusion of a peritoneal catheter via abdominal wall and operated myelomeningocele area: a rare complication of ventriculoperitoneal shunt. Childs Nerv Syst 29:1199–1202
5. Barami K, Sood S, Ham S, Canady A (1998) Chemical meningitis from bile reflux in a lumbar-gallbladder shunt. Pediatr Neurosurg 29:328–330
6. Barker GM, Läckgren G, Stenberg A, Arnell K (2006) Distal shunt obstruction in children with myelomeningocele after bladder perforation. J Urol 176:1726–1728
7. Berger MS, Baumeister B, Geyer JR, Milstein J, Kanev PM, LeRoux PD (1991) The risks of metastases from shunting in children with primary central nervous system tumors. J Neurosurg 74:872–877
8. Bernstein RA, Hsueh W (1985) Ventriculocholecystic shunt: a mortality report. Surg Neurol 23:31–37
9. Bhasin RR, Chen MK, Pincus DW (2007) Salvaging the "lost peritoneum" after ventriculoatrial shunt failures. Childs Nerv Syst 23:483–486
10. Boch AL, Hermelin E, Sainte-Rose C, Sgouros S (1998) Mechanical dysfunction of ventriculoperitoneal shunts caused by calcification of the silicone rubber catheter. J Neurosurg 88:975–982
11. Britz GW, Kim DK, Loeser JD (1996) Hydrocephalus secondary to diffuse villous hyperplasia of the choroid plexus. Case report and review of the literature. J Neurosurg 85(4):689–691
12. Brownlee JD, Brodkey JS, Schaefer IK (1998) Colonic perforation by ventriculoperitoneal shunt tubing: a case of suspected silicone allergy. Surg Neurol 49:21–24
13. Campbell AN, Chan HSL, Becker LE, Daneman A, Park TS, Hoffman HJ (1984) Extracranial metastases in childhood primary intracranial tumors. A report of 21 cases and review of the literature. Cancer 53: 974–981
14. Casey KF, Vries JK (1989) Cerebral fluid overproduction in the absence of tumor or villous hypertrophy of the choroid plexus. Childs Nerv Syst 5(5):332–334
15. Chen TH, Lin MS, Kung WM, Hung KS, Chiang YH, Chen CH (2011) Combined ventriculoperitoneal shunt blockage, viscus perforation with migration into urethra, presenting with repeated UTI. Ann R Coll Surg Engl 93:151–153
16. Chidambaram B, Balasubramaniam V (2000) CSF ascites: a rare complication of ventriculoperitoneal shunt surgery. Neurol India 48(4):378–380
17. Dean D, Keller I (1972) Cerebrospinal fluid ascites: a complication of ventriculoperitoneal shunt. J Neurol Neurosurg Psychiatry 35:474–476
18. de Aquino HB, Carelli EF, Borges Neto AG, Pereira CU et al (2006) Nonfunctional abdominal complications of the distal catheter on the treatment of hydrocephalus: an inflammatory hypothesis? Experience with six cases. Childs Nerv Syst 22:1225–1230
19. De Jong L, Van Der Aa F, De Ridder D, Van Calenbergh F (2011) Extrusion of a ventriculoperitoneal shunt catheter through an appendicovesicostomy. Br J Neurosurg 25:115–116
20. DiLuna ML, Johnson ML, Bi WL, Chiang VL, Duncan CC (2006) Sterile ascites from a ventriculoperitoneal shunt: a case report and review of the literature. Childs Nerv Syst 22:1187–1193
21. Di Rocco C (1987) Complications unique to peritoneal shunts. In: The treatment of infantile hydrocephalus, vol 2. CRC Press, Boca Raton, pp 129–139
22. Di Rocco C, Marchese E, Velardi F (1994) A survey of the first complication of newly implanted CSF devices for the treatment of nontumoral hydrocephalus. Childs Nerv Syst 10:321–327
23. Dodge HW, Remine WH, Leaens MD (1957) The treatment of hydrocephalus by spinal subarachnoid-omental bursa shunt. Minn Med 40:227–230
24. Dominguez CJ, Tyagi A, Hall G, Timothy J, Chumas PD (2000) Subgaleal coiling of the proximal and distal components of a ventriculo-peritoneal shunt. An unusual complication and proposed mechanism. Childs Nerv Syst 16:493–495
25. Eichler I (1986) Complications following implantation of ventriculo–atrial and ventriculoperitoneal shunts. Zentralbl Neurochir 47(2):161–166
26. Ersahin Y, Mutluer S, Tekeli G (1996) Abdominal cerebrospinal fluid pseudocysts. Childs Nerv Syst 12:755–758
27. Ferreira PR, Bizzi JJ, Amantea SL (2005) Protrusion of ventriculoperitoneal shunt catheter through the anal orifice. A rare abdominal complication. J Pediatr Surg 40:1509–1510
28. Gattuso P, Carson HJ, Attal H, Castelli MJ (1995) Peritoneal implantation of meningeal melanosis via ventriculoperitoneal shunt: a case report and review of the literature. Diagn Cytopathol 13:257–259

29. Gaskill SJ, Marlin AE (1989) Pseudocysts of the abdomen associated with ventriculoperitoneal shunts: a report of twelve cases and a review of the literature. Pediatr Neurosci 15:23–27
30. Gaudio R, De Tommasi A, Occhiogrosso M, Vailati G (1988) Respiratory distress caused by migration of ventriculoperitoneal shunt catheter into the chest cavity: report of a case and review of the literature. Neurosurgery 23:768–769
31. Goldblum RM, Pyron D, Shenoy M (1998) Modulation of IgG binding to silicone by human serum albumin. FASEB J 12(Part II):5967
32. Grosfeld JL, Cooney DR, Smith J, Campbell RL (1974) Intra- abdominal complications following ventriculoperitoneal shunt procedures. Pediatrics 54:791–796
33. Harsh GR III (1954) Peritoneal shunt for hydrocephalus: utilizing the fimbria of the fallopian tube for entrance to the peritoneal cavity. J Neurosurg 11:284–294
34. Hashimoto M, Yokota A, Urasaki E, Tsujigami S, Shimono M (2004) A case of abdominal CSF pseudocyst associated with silicone allergy. Childs Nerv Syst 20:761–764
35. Kataria R, Sinha VD, Chopra S, Gupta A, Vyas N (2013) Urinary bladder perforation, intra-corporeal knotting, and per-urethral extrusion of ventriculoperitoneal shunt in a single patient: case report and review of literature. Childs Nerv Syst 29:693–697
36. Ketoff J, Klein R, Maukkassa K (1997) Ventricular cholecystic shunts in children. J Pediatr Surg 32: 181–183
37. Khosrovi H, Kaufman HH, Hrabovsky E, Bloomfield SM, Prabhu V, el-Kadi HA (1998) Laparoscopic-assisted distal ventriculoperitoneal shunt placement. Surg Neurol 49(2):127–134 (discussion 134–125)
38. Kimura N, Namiki T, Wada T, Sasano N (1984) Peritoneal implantation of endodermal sinus tumor of the pineal region via a ventriculo-peritoneal shunt. Cytodiagnosis with immunocytochemical demonstration of alpha-fetoprotein. Acta Cytol 28:143–147
39. Klykken PC (2005) Abdominal CSF pseudocyst. Childs Nerv Syst 21:1018–1019
40. Krediet RT (1999) The peritoneal membrane in chronic peritoneal dialysis. Kidney Int 55:341–356
41. Kubo S, Ueno M, Takimoto H, Karasawa J, Kato A, Yoshimine T (2003) Endoscopically aided retroperitoneal placement of a lumboperitoneal shunt. Technical note. J Neurosurg 98:430–433
42. Kurschel S, Eder HG, Schleef J (2005) CSF shunts in children: endoscopically-assisted placement of the distal catheter. Childs Nerv Syst 21(1):52–55
43. Longstreth GF, Buckwalter NR (2001) Sterile cerebrospinal fluid ascites and chronic peritonitis. N Engl J Med 345(4):297–298
44. Lourie H, Bajwa S (1985) Transdiaphragmatic migration of a ventriculo-peritoneal catheter. Neurosurgery 17:324–326
45. Martin LM, Donaldson-Hugh ME, Cameron MM (1997) Cerebrospinal fluid hydrothorax caused by transdiaphragmatic migration of a ventriculoperitoneal catheter through the foramen of Bochdalek. Childs Nerv Syst 13:282–284
46. Martinez-Lage JF, Poza M, Izura V (1993) Retrograde migration of the abdominal catheter as a complication of ventriculoperitoneal shunts: the fish hook sign. Childs Nerv Syst 9:425–427
47. Martinez-Lage JF, Torres J, Campillo H, Sanchez-del-Rincon I, Bueno F, Zambudio G, Poza M (2000) Ventriculopleural shunting with new technology valves. Childs Nerv Syst 16:867–871
48. Martínez-Lage JF, Girón O, López A, Martínez-Lage L, Roqués JL, Almagro MJ (2008) Acute cholecystitis complicating ventriculo-peritoneal shunting: report of a case and review of the literature. Childs Nerv Syst 24:777–779
49. Matsuoka H, Takegami T, Maruyama D, Hamasaki T, Kakita K, Mineura K (2008) Transanal prolapse of a ventriculoperitoneal shunt catheter. Neurol Med Chir (Tokyo) 48:526–528
50. Matushita H, Cardeal D, Campos Pinto F, Pereira Plese JP, Santos de Miranda J (2008) The ventriculoomental bursa shunt. Childs Nerv Syst 24:949–953
51. Milton C, Sanders P, Steele P (2001) Late cardiopulmonary complication of ventriculo–atrial shunt. Lancet 358:1608
52. Mobley LW III, Doran SE, Hellbusch LC (2005) Abdominal pseudocyst: predisposing factors and treatment algorithm. Pediatr Neurosurg 41:77–83
53. Murthy KVR, Reddy SJ, Prasad DV (2009) Perforation of the distal end of the ventriculoperitoneal shunt into the bladder with calculus formation. Pediatr Neurosurg 45:53–55
54. Newton HB, Rosenblum MK, Walker RW (1992) Extraneural metastases of infratentorial glioblastoma multiforme to the peritoneal cavity. Cancer 69:2149–2153
55. Novelli PM, Reigel DH (1997) A closer look at the ventriculo-gallbladder shunt for the treatment of hydrocephalus. Pediatr Neurosurg 26:197–199
56. Olavarria G, Reitman AJ, Goldman S, Tomita T (2005) Post-shunt ascites in infants with optic chiasmal hypothalamic astrocytoma: role of ventricular gallbladder shunt. Childs Nerv Syst 21:382–384
57. Oliveira RS, Barbosa A, Moraes Villela YA, Machado HR (2007) An alternative approach for management of abdominal cerebrospinal fluid pseudocysts in children. Childs Nerv Syst 23:85–90
58. Oshio T, Matsumura C, Kirino A (1991) Recurrent perforations of viscus due to ventriculoperitoneal shunt in a hydrocephalic child. J Pediatr Surg 26: 1404–1405
59. Park CK, Wang KC, Seo JK, Cho BK (2000) Transoral protrusion of a peritoneal catheter: a case report and literature review. Childs Nerv Syst 16:184–189
60. Parry SW, Schuhmacher JF, Llewellyn RC (1975) Abdominal pseudocysts and ascites formation after ventriculoperitoneal shunt procedures. Report of four cases. J Neurosurg 43(4):476–480
61. Pathi R, Sage M, Slavotinek J, Hanieh A (2004) Abdominal cerebrospinal fluid pseudocyst. Australas Radiol 48:61–63
62. Picasa JA (1956) The posterior-peritoneal shunt technique for the treatment of internal hydrocephalus in infants. J Neurosurg 13:289–293

63. Pohlman GD, Wilcox DT, Hankinson TC (2011) Erosive bladder perforation as a complication of ventriculoperitoneal shunt with extrusion from the urethral meatus: case report and literature review. Pediatr Neurosurg 47:223–226
64. Pollack IF, Hurtt M, Pang D, Albright AL (1994) Dissemination of low-grade intracranial astrocytomas in children. Cancer 73:2869–2878
65. Pudenz RH (1980) The surgical treatment of hydrocephalus—an historical review. Surg Neurol 15:15–26
66. Rainov N, Schobess A, Heidecke V, Burkert W (1994) Abdominal CSF pseudocysts in patients with ventriculo–peritoneal shunts. Report of fourteen cases and review of the literature. Acta Neurochir 127:73–78
67. Rengachary SS (1997) Transdiaphragmatic ventriculoperitoneal shunting: technical case report. Neurosurgery 41:695–697
68. Rickert CR (1998) Abdominal metastases of pediatric brain tumors via ventriculo-peritoneal shunts. Childs Nerv Syst 14:10–14
69. Roitberg BZ, Tomita T, McLone DG (1998) Abdominal cerebrospinal fluid pseudocyst: a complication of ventriculoperitoneal shunt in children. Pediatr Neurosurg 29:267–273
70. Ruggiero C, Spennato P, De Paulis D, Aliberti F, Cinalli G (2010) Intracardiac migration of the distal catheter of ventriculoperitoneal shunt: a case report. Childs Nerv Syst 26:957–962
71. Salomao JF, Leibinger RD (1999) Abdominal pseudocysts complicating CSF shunting in infants and children. Report of 18 cases. Pediatr Neurosurg 31: 274–278
72. Sathyanarayana S, Wylen EL, Baskaya MK et al (2000) Spontaneous bowel perforation after ventriculoperitoneal shunt surgery: case report and a review of 45 cases. Surg Neurol 54:388–396
73. Shafiee S, Nejat F, Raouf SM, Mehdizadeh M, El Khashab M (2011) Coiling and migration of peritoneal catheter into the breast: a very rare complication of ventriculoperitoneal shunt. Childs Nerv Syst 27: 1499–1501
74. Shibasaki T, Takeda F, Kawafuchi J, Suzuki Y, Yanagisawa S (1977) Extra- neural metastases of malignant brain tumors through ventriculo-peritoneal shunt. Report of two autopsy cases and review of the literature. Neurosurgery (Tokyo) 5:71–79
75. Shuper A, Horev G, Michovitz S, Korenreich L, Zaizov R, Cohen IJ (1997) Optic chiasm glioma, electrolyte abnormalities, nonobstructive hydrocephalus and ascites. Med Pediatr Oncol 29(1):33–35
76. Smith GW, Moretz WH, Pritchard WL (1958) Ventriculo-biliary shunt, a new treatment for hydrocephalus. Surg Forum 9:701–705
77. Taub E, Lavyne MH (1994) Thoracic complications of ventriculoperitoneal shunts: case report and review of the literature. Neurosurgery 34:181–183
78. Vernet O, Campiche R, de Tribolet N (1993) Long-term results after ventriculoatrial shunting in children. Childs Nerv Syst 9(5):253–255
79. Wang GM, Fu SL, Ge PF, Fan WH, Li GM, Meng FK, Luo YN (2011) Use of a new type of trocar for the surgical treatment of hydrocephalus: a simple and effective technique. J Int Med Res 39(3):766–771
80. West K, Turner MK, Vane DW, Boaz J, Kalsbeck J, Grosfeld JL (1987) Ventricular gallbladder shunts: an alternative procedure in hydrocephalus. J Pediatr Surg 22:609–612
81. Wilson CB, Bertan V (1966) Perforation of the bowel complicating peritoneal shunt for hydrocephalus. Report of two cases. Am Surg 32:601–603
82. Yousfi MM, Jackson NS, Abbas M et al (2003) Bowel perforation complicating ventriculoperitoneal shunt: case report and review. Gastrointest Endosc 58: 144–148
83. Yukinaka M, Nomura M, Mitani T, Kondo Y, Tabata T, Nakaya Y et al (1998) Cerebrospinal ascites developed 3 years after ventriculoperitoneal shunting in a hydrocephalic patient. Intern Med 37(7):638–641

Complications Specific to Lumboperitoneal Shunt

14

Ignacio Jusué-Torres, Jamie B. Hoffberger, and Daniele Rigamonti

Contents

14.1 **Mechanical Failure (40 %)** 205
14.2 **Overdrainage (20 %)** 206
14.3 **Spinal Deformities (16 %)** 207
14.4 **Infection (9 %)** 207
14.5 **Mechanical-Induced Pain (8 %)** 207
14.6 **CSF Leakage (3 %)**.................. 207
14.7 **Others** 207
14.8 **Special Situation: Pregnancy**.......... 207
Conclusions................................ 208
References................................. 208

I. Jusué-Torres, MD • J.B. Hoffberger, MD
D. Rigamonti, MD (✉)
Department of Neurosurgery,
The Johns Hopkins University School of Medicine,
Baltimore, MD, USA
e-mail: ijusuet1@jhmi.edu; hydrocephalus@jhmi.edu; dr@jhmi.edu

For the past half-century, the lumboperitoneal shunt (LP shunt) has been the leading surgical treatment for idiopathic intracranial hypertension (IIH) [1, 2]. More recently in Japan, this procedure has been offered in the management of Normal Pressure Hydrocephalus (NPH) [3]. In some institutions, the LP shunt comprises up to 40 % of all cerebrospinal fluid (CSF) shunting [4]. One of the reasons that LP shunt is used when treating patients with IIH is because it is difficult to place a ventricular catheter in ventricles that are usually small, in this condition [5]. Furthermore, the avoidance of an intracranial procedure with LP shunt spares the small risk of intracranial hemorrhage while passing a catheter through the brain parenchyma. It is to be remembered, however, that given the pathogenetic mechanism of IIH, LP shunt and optic nerve fenestration (ONF) are symptomatic treatment while reducing patients weight (diet, bariatric surgery, etc.) and/or dural sinus stenting intervene on the cause itself of IIH and therefore should be offered first.

The LP shunt has been associated with higher failure rates compared to ventriculoperitoneal shunts [6–13]. There are many possible causes for postoperative LP shunt complications and consequently surgical revision. These include obstruction, overdrainage, mechanical failure, catheter migration, catheter fracture, abdominal complications, lumbo-spinal complications, infections, and other less common complications (see Fig. 14.1). Understanding the different

C. Di Rocco et al. (eds.), *Complications of CSF Shunting in Hydrocephalus: Prevention, Identification, and Management*, DOI 10.1007/978-3-319-09961-3_14,

Fig. 14.1 Indication for shunt revision in adults older than 17 years old (Adapted from data from Youman's book [14, 15])

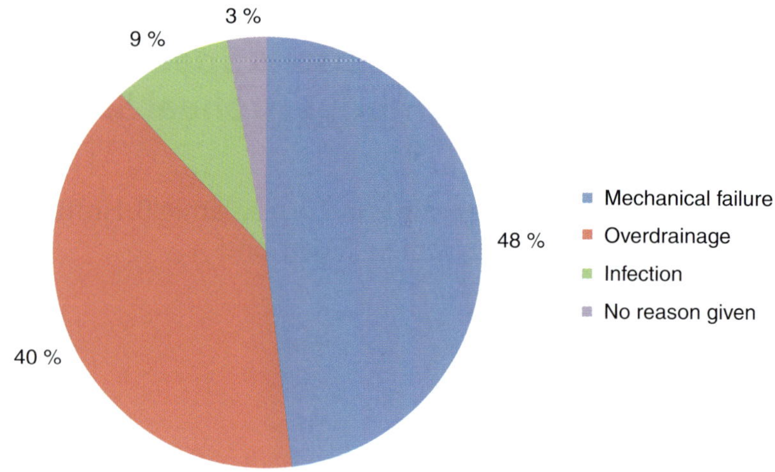

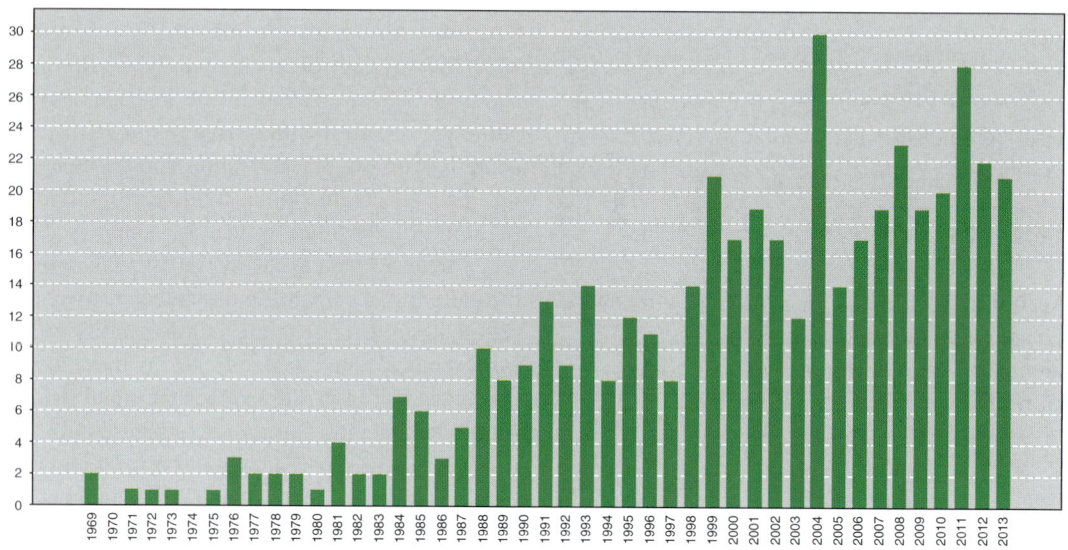

Fig. 14.2 Number of papers referenced by year of publication in Web of Knowledge containing the words "lumboperitoneal shunt" in title or abstract

causes of postoperative LP shunt complications is a crucial step in improving health care for our patients. The purpose of this chapter is to describe the complications derived from the LP shunt insertion.

During the first decade of the twentieth century, the initial attempts of LP shunt showed a very high perioperative mortality rate [1, 16]. Finally, in 1949, a successful LP shunt procedure was reported by Cone et al. [17]. Later the substitution of polyethylene catheters by silastic catheters in 1967 was associated with a dramatic decline in obstruction and shunt fracture rate [8, 18].

The literature confirms that complication and surgical revision rates after CSF shunting with the LP shunt vary considerably among different studies [1, 7, 12, 19–35]. Possible explanations for this discrepancy include different cohort sizes of the studies as well as the propensity to underreport poor outcomes.

For this reason, we conducted a comprehensive review of the literature with the intention to establish overall reported complications rates derived from the LP shunt. From 1971 through 2013, we identified 602 published papers that reported the use of the LP shunt to treat CSF disorders (see Fig. 14.2). Out of those, 72 manuscripts reported on complications related to the LP shunt [1, 4, 7, 12, 16, 18–29, 31–79]. These 72 studies reviewed a total of 2,871 patients who were treated with an LP shunt. A total of 853 patients (30 %) developed at least one complication. Forty-eight percent (n=402) of the patients who had a complication underwent surgical revision.

Out of the 30% of patients who developed a complication, 40 % had mechanical failure; 20 % had overdrainage derived complications including acquired tonsillar herniation or subdural collections; 16 % had spinal deformities; 9 % had infection which includes meningitis, discitis, and peritonitis; 8 % had mechanical-induced pain including radiculopathy or back pain; and 3 % had CSF leakage (see Table 14.1 and Fig. 14.3). These complications represent 94 % of all reported complicated LP shunt surgeries.

Table 14.1 Complications postlumboperitoneal shunt reported in the literature (n and %) with percentage of complications in relationship to the total reported

Lumboperitoneal shunt reported (n=2,871)	n	(%)	n=853 (%)
Obstruction	206	(7.18)	24.15
Spinal deformities	130	(4.53)	15.24
Shunt migration	111	(3.87)	13.01
Overdrainage	84	(2.93)	9.85
Infection	72	(2.51)	8.44
Tonsillar herniation	47	(1.64)	5.51
Radiculopathy	43	(1.50)	5.04
Subdural collection	34	(1.18)	3.99
CSF leakage	22	(0.77)	2.58
Back pain	20	(0.70)	2.34
Disconnection or fracture	14	(0.49)	1.64
Abdominal pain	7	(0.24)	0.82
Pneumoencephalus	5	(0.17)	0.59
Pseudomeningocele	5	(0.17)	0.59
Syringomyelia	5	(0.17)	0.59
Spontaneous abortion	5	(0.17)	0.59
Hydrocele	5	(0.17)	0.59
Wound dehiscence	4	(0.14)	0.47
Intraparenchymal hematoma	3	(0.10)	0.35
Seizure	3	(0.10)	0.35
Preterm delivery	2	(0.07)	0.23
Subarachnoidal hemorrhage	1	(0.03)	0.12
Venous sinus thrombosis	1	(0.03)	0.12
Abdominal hemorrhage	1	(0.03)	0.12
Myelopathy	1	(0.03)	0.12
Gastrointestinal perforation	1	(0.03)	0.12
Catheter malposition	1	(0.03)	0.12
Pulmonar embolus	1	(0.03)	0.12
Ileus	1	(0.03)	0.12
Total of complications reported	**853**	**(29.71)**	**100**

14.1 Mechanical Failure (40 %)

According to the data derived from the studies that reported complications in the use of the LP shunt, 40 % of all complications reported are due to mechanical failure of the shunt [1, 7, 12, 14, 15, 19, 24, 26, 29, 32–35, 37, 40, 53, 54, 56, 62, 65, 73, 78, 80]. This complication typically presents with recurrence of preoperative clinical symptoms. It can be due to *shunting obstruction* (either along catheters or inside the valve), *catheter migration, catheter disconnection or catheter fracture* and *catheter malposition*. LP shunt obstruction is an insufficient CSF flow diversion inadequate to compensate the intracranial hypertension. Unfortunately, *shunt obstruction*, although suspected, is usually confirmed only after surgical revision. Obstruction can occur in any location of the shunt system, including the lumbar catheter, the valve, or the distal catheter. Surgical management is required and during the procedure each element of the shunt system should be individually tested for malfunction.

Disconnection or catheter fracture often has a subtle clinical presentation [1, 12, 32, 56, 81]. Many disconnections or fractures are found incidentally during follow-up routine visits or during radiological studies required for other purposes. However, catheter disconnection typically occurs shortly after surgical shunt placement. The most useful and sensitive imaging studies to demonstrate disconnection of catheter fracture are the shunt series. This complication requires surgical management, either urgent or elective depending on the clinical status of the patient. Both disconnection and shunt fracture are progressively decreasing its rates as the catheter materials improve with time. Similarly, *catheter migration* happens when an appropriately placed catheter

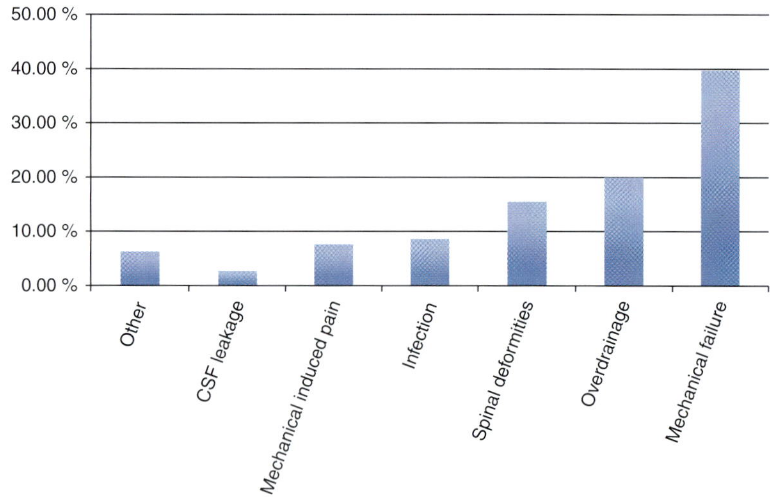

Fig. 14.3 Bar plot of the most reported LP shunt complications represented by their percentage from the total of reported complications

moves from its intraperitoneal location to an extraperitoneal position where CSF no longer drains or the drainage is severely compromised. This complication is managed by repositioning the migrated catheter. Anticipation of possible problems from tethering should be addressed at the time of the initial shunt placement [1, 7, 12, 18, 19, 21, 23, 24, 26, 32, 33, 35, 49, 50, 53, 60, 65, 78, 80, 82–86]. Unfortunately, the avoidable surgical catheter malposition happens and when this occurs management is identical to catheter migration cases [38].

14.2 Overdrainage (20 %)

CSF overdrainage causes intracranial hypotension. It usually presents with intense headache which typically resolves when patients switch from vertical to horizontal position. Secondary intracranial hypotension has been reported as the number one complication in some studies [15]. The apparent decline in those rates when looking into the literature review may be due to a better prevention and avoidance by a more appropriate valve system selection [7, 18, 19, 21, 23, 25, 27, 29, 32, 33, 35, 37, 38, 40, 49, 69, 73, 78, 87]. Treatment of overdrainage requires surgical valve replacement with a valve with more resistance or adding an antisiphon device to the shunting system.

Chronic overdrainage may lead to a secondary *tonsillar herniation or acquired Chiari Malformation type I*, and sometimes even requiring decompressive posterior fossa craniectomy [7, 22, 24, 26–28, 47, 54, 60, 73, 88–90]. A vigilant postoperative follow-up policy may reduce the rate of post-LP shunt tonsilar herniation by increasing the rates of LP shunt revision in patients with symptoms of overdrainage post-LP shunt sparing decompressive posterior fossa craniectomies.

Significant CSF overdrainage may result in the formation of *subdural collections* due to the collapse of the brain and accumulation of fluid or blood around the brain [19, 21–23, 26, 29, 30, 32, 41, 53, 76, 91, 92]. Most commonly, benign cerebrospinal fluid collections are observed, however, subdural hematomas are possible. This complication has been reported mainly associated to NPH. It is exceptional in IIH [40, 76]. Three approaches could be proposed for extra-axial fluid collections. First, it may be possible to manage these collections conservatively if they are small and do not cause brain compression or herniation. A second option is to treat the overdrainage by replacing the valve with one with more resistance or inserting an antisiphon device. The third option is to drain the extra-axial fluid collection either alone or in combination with changing the valve. Drainage may be accomplished by a burr hole and a temporary drain or via a subdural catheter that is spliced into the existing shunt system below the valve. This complication is best prevented by avoidance of overdrainage.

14.3 Spinal Deformities (16 %)

This spinal group of complications includes spinal scoliosis, lumbar lordosis, or the combination of both of them. We believe that spinal deformity complications may be overrepresented in comparing it to the rest of LP shunt complications. During our review we found a lack of uniformity reporting spinal deformity complications. In some of the manuscripts reviewed, all of the spinal deformity complications were reported as a group, while others reported each spinal deformity complication independently [20, 24]. This complication is intrinsically related to patients in their infancy through adolescence, when many developmental changes occur in a small amount of time, and it is highly associated with patients that already have syringomyelia. Syringomyelia may be responsible for the spinal deformity and spasticity of the posterior spinal muscles may be a cause of hyperlordosis.

14.4 Infection (9 %)

Infection rates reported include meningitis, discitis, and peritonitis [1, 7, 19, 21–27, 29, 32, 33, 35–40, 49, 56, 60, 73, 78]. It is surprising that the sum of these three complications is much lower than similarly reported in other type of shunting systems. The difference in infection rates between different shunting systems is not well known and difficult to assess.

14.5 Mechanical-Induced Pain (8 %)

Post-LP shunt back pain and radiculopathy have been underestimated and underreported [1, 7, 19, 21, 22, 24–26, 38, 41, 49, 69]. Radiculopathy leads to significant patient limitation in quality of life and work performance. This is due to direct spinal root irritation by the lumbar catheter. The treatment for this complication is surgical revision with repositioning of the lumbar catheter.

14.6 CSF Leakage (3 %)

CSF leak is one of the most feared complications due to the fact that once CSF leak develops it is difficult to fix [1, 23, 25–27, 56, 65, 71, 87, 93]. When CSF leak happens, it is advisable to completely remove the shunting system, possibly insert an external CSF drainage at a different location and wait until the patient has healed before further surgical treatment. The presence of infection will delay the insertion of a new system usually until after the completion of an appropriate course of antibiotic treatment and until confirmation of CSF sterility a few days after antibiotic discontinuation. Sometimes the CSF leakage persists and direct repair of the durotomy becomes necessary.

14.7 Others

Each of the following complications represents less than 1 % and together total 6 % of all complications reported in the literature. They are pneumocephalus [22, 23, 38, 94], seizure [29, 95], subarachnoid hemorrhage [96], venous sinus thrombosis [96], pseudomeningocele [33, 35, 44, 97], wound dehiscence [1, 23, 26, 29], syringomyelia [28, 98], myelopathy [22], hydrocele [1, 99], abdominal pain [23, 25, 49, 73], abdominal hemorrhage [100], and gastrointestinal perforation [36].

14.8 Special Situation: Pregnancy

Clinical management of women in their reproductive age should take into consideration possible pregnancies. When women with IIH become pregnant they present a special challenge [101]. Their symptomatology might deteriorate and if they do not have a shunt they may need to undergo surgery for an LP shunt during pregnancy putting them at risk of preterm delivery and spontaneous abortion [102]. If they have a shunt already, special spinal anesthetic management might become necessary during delivery.

Conclusions

The LP shunt is prone to different types of complications, as outlined earlier, but remains a valuable tool in the management of CSF diseases. Insertion of LP shunt is recommended in patients with IIH who are failing medical and ophthalmological treatment. LP shunts use is limited for NPH. However in Japan there has been an increased use for this purpose. The high rate of postoperative complications as well as the frequent need for multiple shunt revisions has plagued the procedure for many years. Progress in preventing short- and long-term shunt complications requiring surgical revision has been slow to occur over the last several decades.

References

1. Eisenberg HM, Davidson RI, Shillito JJ (1971) Lumboperitoneal shunts: review of 34 cases. J Neurosurg 35(4):427–431
2. Pudenz RH (1981) The surgical treatment of hydrocephalus—an historical review. Surg Neurol 15(1): 15–26
3. Mori E, Ishikawa M, Kato T et al (2012) Guidelines for management of idiopathic normal pressure hydrocephalus: second edition. Neurol Med Chir (Tokyo) 52(11):775–809
4. Yamashiro S, Hitoshi Y, Yoshida A, Kuratsu J (2012) Historical considerations of the predominance of lumboperitoneal shunt for treatment of adult communicating hydrocephalus in Kumamoto, Japan. Clin Neurol Neurosurg 114(7):1115–1116
5. Gallia GL, Rigamonti D, Williams MA (2006) The diagnosis and treatment of idiopathic normal pressure hydrocephalus. Nat Clin Pract Neurol 2(7): 375–381
6. Choux M, Genitori L, Lang D, Lena G (1992) Shunt implantation: reducing the incidence of shunt infection. J Neurosurg 77(6):875–880
7. McGirt MJ, Woodworth G, Thomas G, Miller N, Williams M, Rigamonti D (2004) Cerebrospinal fluid shunt placement for pseudotumor cerebri-associated intractable headache: predictors of treatment response and an analysis of long-term outcomes. J Neurosurg 101(4):627–632
8. Kestle J, Drake J, Milner R et al (2000) Long-term follow-up data from the Shunt Design Trial. Pediatr Neurosurg 33(5):230–236
9. Browd SR, Ragel BT, Gottfried ON, Kestle JRW (2006) Failure of cerebrospinal fluid shunts: part I: obstruction and mechanical failure. Pediatr Neurol 34(2):83–92
10. Browd SR, Gottfried ON, Ragel BT, Kestle JRW (2006) Failure of cerebrospinal fluid shunts: part II: overdrainage, loculation, and abdominal complications. Pediatr Neurol 34(3):171–176
11. Stein SC, Guo W (2008) Have we made progress in preventing shunt failure? A critical analysis. J Neurosurg Pediatr 1(1):40–47
12. Sinclair AJ, Kuruvath S, Sen D, Nightingale PG, Burdon MA, Flint G (2011) Is cerebrospinal fluid shunting in idiopathic intracranial hypertension worthwhile? A 10-year review. Cephalalgia 31(16): 1627–1633
13. Toma AK, Papadopoulos MC, Stapleton S, Kitchen ND, Watkins LD (2013) Systematic review of the outcome of shunt surgery in idiopathic normal-pressure hydrocephalus. Acta Neurochir 155(10):1977–1980
14. O'Kane MC, Richards H, Winfield P, Pickard JD (1997) The United Kingdom Shunt Registry. Eur J Pediatr Surg 7(Suppl 1):56
15. Keong NC, Czosnyka M, Czosnyka Z, Pickard JD (2011) Clinical evaluation of adult hydrocephalus. In: Youmans neurological surgery, vol 1, 6th edn. Elsevier Saunders, Philadelphia
16. Vander Ark GD, Kempe LG, Smith DR (1971) Pseudotumor cerebri treated with Lumbar-peritoneal shunt. JAMA 217(13):1832–1834
17. Jackson IJ (1951) A review of the surgical treatment of internal hydrocephalus. J Pediatr 38(2):251–258
18. Spetzler RF, Wilson CB, Grollmus JM (1975) Percutaneous lumboperitoneal shunt. Technical note. J Neurosurg 43(6):770–773
19. Selman WR, Spetzler RF, Wilson CB, Grollmus JW (1980) Percutaneous lumboperitoneal shunt: review of 130 cases. Neurosurgery 6(3):255–257
20. McIvor J, Krajbich JI, Hoffman H (1988) Orthopaedic complications of lumboperitoneal shunts. J Pediatr Orthop 8(6):687–689
21. Philippon J, Duplessis E, Dorwling-Carter D, Horn YE, Cornu P (1989) Lumboperitoneal shunt and normal pressure hydrocephalus in elderly subjects. Rev Neurol 145(11):776–780
22. Aoki N (1990) Lumboperitoneal shunt: clinical applications, complications, and comparison with ventriculoperitoneal shunt. Neurosurgery 26(6):998–1003; discussion 1003–1004
23. Brunon J, Motuo-Fotso MJ, Duthel R, Huppert J (1991) Treatment of chronic hydrocephalus in adults by lumboperitoneal shunt. Results and indications apropos of 82 cases. Neurochirurgie 37(3):173–178
24. Chumas PD, Kulkarni AV, Drake JM, Hoffman HJ, Humphreys RP, Rutka JT (1993) Lumboperitoneal

shunting: a retrospective study in the pediatric population. Neurosurgery 32(3):376–383; discussion 383
25. Rosenberg ML, Corbett JJ, Smith C et al (1993) Cerebrospinal fluid diversion procedures in pseudotumor cerebri. Neurology 43(6):1071–1072
26. Duthel R, Nuti C, Motuo-Fotso MJ, Beauchesne P, Brunon J (1996) Complications of lumboperitoneal shunts. A retrospective study of a series of 195 patients (214 procedures). Neurochirurgie 42(2):83–89
27. Burgett RA, Purvin VA, Kawasaki A (1997) Lumboperitoneal shunting for pseudotumor cerebri. Neurology 49(3):734–739
28. Johnston I, Jacobson E, Besser M (1998) The acquired Chiari malformation and syringomyelia following spinal CSF drainage: a study of incidence and management. Acta Neurochir 140(5):417–427; discussion 427–418
29. Chang CC, Kuwana N, Ito S (1999) Management of patients with normal-pressure hydrocephalus by using lumboperitoneal shunt system with the Codman Hakim programmable valve. Neurosurg Focus 7(4):e8
30. Kamiryo T, Hamada J-i, Fuwa I, Ushio Y (2003) Acute subdural hematoma after lumboperitoneal shunt placement in patients with normal pressure hydrocephalus. Neurol Med Chir (Tokyo) 43(4):197–200
31. Yadav YR, Pande S, Raina VK, Singh M (2004) Lumboperitoneal shunts: review of 409 cases. Neurol India 52(2):188–190
32. Wang VY, Barbaro NM, Lawton MT et al (2007) Complications of lumboperitoneal shunts. Neurosurgery 60(6):1045–1048; discussion 1049
33. Barcia-Marino C, Gonzalez-Bonet LG, Salvador-Gozalbo L, Goig-Revert F, Rodriguez-Mena R (2009) Lumboperitoneal shunt in an outpatient setting for the treatment of chronic hydrocephalus in adults. A study and follow-up of 30 cases. Rev Neurol 49(6):300–306
34. Jia L, Zhao Z-x, You C et al (2011) Minimally-invasive treatment of communicating hydrocephalus using a percutaneous lumboperitoneal shunt. J Zhejiang Univ Sci B 12(4):293–297
35. Bloch O, McDermott MW (2012) Lumboperitoneal shunts for the treatment of normal pressure hydrocephalus. J Clin Neurosci 19(8):1107–1111
36. Brook I, Johnson N, Overturf GD, Wilkins J (1977) Mixed bacterial meningitis: a complication of ventriculo-and lumboperitoneal shunts: report of two cases. J Neurosurg 47(6):961–964
37. Johnston I, Paterson A, Besser M (1981) The treatment of benign intracranial hypertension: a review of 134 cases. Surg Neurol 16(3):218–224
38. Bret P, Hor F, Huppert J, Lapras C, Fischer G (1985) Treatment of cerebrospinal fluid rhinorrhea by percutaneous lumboperitoneal shunting: review of 15 cases. Neurosurgery 16(1):44–47
39. Huppert J, Bret P, Lapras C, Fischer G (1987) Lumboperitoneal shunt in persistent or recurrent fistulae of the base of skull. Apropos of 20 cases. Neurochirurgie 33(3):220–223
40. Johnston I, Besser M, Morgan MK (1988) Cerebrospinal fluid diversion in the treatment of benign intracranial hypertension. J Neurosurg 69(2): 195–202
41. Aoki N (1989) Lumboperitoneal shunt for the treatment of postoperative persistent collection of subcutaneous cerebrospinal fluid (pseudomeningocele). Acta Neurochir 98:32–34
42. Park TS, Cail WS, Broaddus WC, Walker MG (1989) Lumboperitoneal shunt combined with myelotomy for treatment of syringohydromyelia. J Neurosurg 70(5):721–727
43. Lundar T, Nornes H (1990) Pseudotumour cerebri-neurosurgical considerations. Acta Neurochir Suppl 51:366–368
44. Dhiravibulya K, Ouvrier R, Johnston I, Procopis P, Antony J (1991) Benign intracranial hypertension in childhood: a review of 23 patients. J Paediatr Child Health 27(5):304–307
45. Angiari P, Corradini L, Corsi M, Merli GA (1992) Pseudotumor cerebri. Lumboperitoneal shunt in long lasting cases. J Neurosurg Sci 36(3):145–149
46. Chen IH, Huang CI, Liu HC, Chen KK (1994) Effectiveness of shunting in patients with normal pressure hydrocephalus predicted by temporary, controlled-resistance, continuous lumbar drainage: a pilot study. J Neurol Neurosurg Psychiatry 57(11): 1430–1432
47. Payner TD, Prenger E, Berger TS, Crone KR (1994) Acquired Chiari malformations: incidence, diagnosis, and management. Neurosurgery 34(3):429–434; discussion 434
48. Sgouros S, Malluci C, Walsh AR, Hockley AD (1995) Long-term complications of hydrocephalus. Pediatr Neurosurg 23(3):127–132
49. Eggenberger ER, Miller NR, Vitale S (1996) Lumboperitoneal shunt for the treatment of pseudotumor cerebri. Neurology 46(6):1524–1530
50. Aoki N, Oikawa A, Sakai T (1997) Isolated ophthalmological manifestations due to malfunction of a lumboperitoneal shunt: shortening of the spinal catheter in three pediatric patients. Childs Nerv Syst 13(5):264–267
51. Cinciripini GS, Donahue S, Borchert MS (1999) Idiopathic intracranial hypertension in prepubertal pediatric patients: characteristics, treatment, and outcome. Am J Ophthalmol 127(2):178–182
52. García-Uria J, Ley L, Parajón A, Bravo G (1999) Spontaneous cerebrospinal fluid fistulae associated with empty sellae: surgical treatment and long-term results. Neurosurgery 45(4):766–773; discussion 773–764
53. Kang S (1999) Efficacy of lumbo-peritoneal versus ventriculo-peritoneal shunting for management of chronic hydrocephalus following aneurysmal subarachnoid haemorrhage. Acta Neurochir 142(1): 45–49
54. Levy EI, Scarrow AM, Firlik AD et al (1999) Development of obstructive hydrocephalus with lumboperitoneal shunting following subarachnoid hemorrhage. Clin Neurol Neurosurg 101(2):79–85
55. Hebb AO, Cusimano MD (2001) Idiopathic normal pressure hydrocephalus: a systematic review of

diagnosis and outcome. Neurosurgery 49(5):1166–1184; discussion 1184–1166
56. Salman MS, Kirkham FJ, MacGregor DL (2001) Idiopathic "benign" intracranial hypertension: case series and review. J Child Neurol 16(7):465–470
57. Lesniak MS, Clatterbuck RE, Rigamonti D, Williams MA (2002) Low pressure hydrocephalus and ventriculomegaly: hysteresis, non-linear dynamics, and the benefits of CSF diversion. Br J Neurosurg 16(6): 555–561
58. Lueck C, McIlwaine G (2002) Interventions for idiopathic intracranial hypertension. Cochrane Database Syst Rev (3):CD003434
59. Rekate HL, Wallace D (2003) Lumboperitoneal shunts in children. Pediatr Neurosurg 38(1):41–46
60. Karabatsou K, Quigley G, Buxton N, Foy P, Mallucci C (2004) Lumboperitoneal shunts: are the complications acceptable? Acta Neurochir 146(11):1193–1197
61. McGirt MJ, Woodworth G, Thomas G, Miller N, Williams M, Rigamonti D (2004) Frameless stereotactic ventriculoperitoneal shunting for pseudotumor cerebri: an outcomes comparison versus lumboperitoneal shunting. Neurosurgery 55(2):458
62. Torbey MT, Geocadin RG, Razumovsky AY, Rigamonti D, Williams MA (2004) Utility of CSF pressure monitoring to identify idiopathic intracranial hypertension without papilledema in patients with chronic daily headache. Cephalalgia 24(6):495–502
63. Woodworth GF, McGirt MJ, Elfert P, Sciubba DM, Rigamonti D (2005) Frameless stereotactic ventricular shunt placement for idiopathic intracranial hypertension. Stereotact Funct Neurosurg 83(1):12–16
64. Ferguson SD, Michael N, Frim DM (2007) Observations regarding failure of cerebrospinal fluid shunts early after implantation. Neurosurg Focus 22(4):1–5
65. Kavic SM, Segan RD, Taylor MD, Roth JS (2007) Laparoscopic management of ventriculoperitoneal and lumboperitoneal shunt complications. JSLS 11(1):14–19
66. Lehman RM (2008) Complications of lumboperitoneal shunts. Neurosurgery 63(2):E376
67. Ulivieri S, Oliveri G, Georgantzinou M et al (2009) Long-term effectiveness of lumboperitoneal flow-regulated shunt system for idiopathic intracranial hypertension. J Neurosurg Sci 53(3):107–111
68. Oluigbo CO, Thacker K, Flint G (2010) The role of lumboperitoneal shunts in the treatment of syringomyelia. J Neurosurg Spine 13(1):133–138
69. Toma AK, Dherijha M, Kitchen ND, Watkins LD (2010) Use of lumboperitoneal shunts with the Strata NSC valve: a single-center experience. J Neurosurg 113(6):1304–1308
70. Udayakumaran S, Roth J, Kesler A, Constantini S (2010) Miethke DualSwitch Valve in lumboperitoneal shunts. Acta Neurochir 152(10):1793–1800
71. Yadav YR, Parihar V, Agarwal M, Bhatele PR, Saxena N (2012) Lumbar peritoneal shunt in idiopathic intra cranial hypertension. Turk Neurosurg 22(1):21–26
72. Yadav YR, Parihar V, Sinha M (2010) Lumbar peritoneal shunt. Neurol India 58(2):179–184
73. Abubaker K, Ali Z, Raza K, Bolger C, Rawluk D, O'Brien D (2011) Idiopathic intracranial hypertension: lumboperitoneal shunts versus ventriculoperitoneal shunts – case series and literature review. Br J Neurosurg 25(1):94–99
74. Kanazawa R, Ishihara S, Sato S, Teramoto A, Kuniyoshi N (2011) Familiarization with lumboperitoneal shunt using some technical resources. World Neurosurg 76(3–4):347–351
75. Stranjalis G, Kalamatianos T, Koutsarnakis C, Loufardaki M, Stavrinou L, Sakas DE (2012) Twelve-year hospital outcomes in patients with idiopathic hydrocephalus. (null). Acta Neurochir Suppl 113:115–117, Springer, Vienna
76. Tarnaris A, Toma AK, Watkins LD, Kitchen ND (2011) Is there a difference in outcomes of patients with idiopathic intracranial hypertension with the choice of cerebrospinal fluid diversion site: a single centre experience. Clin Neurol Neurosurg 113(6):477–479
77. Chern JJ, Tubbs RS, Gordon AS, Donnithorne KJ, Oakes WJ (2012) Management of pediatric patients with pseudotumor cerebri. Childs Nerv Syst 28(4): 575–578
78. El-Saadany WF, Farhoud A, Zidan I (2012) Lumboperitoneal shunt for idiopathic intracranial hypertension: patients' selection and outcome. Neurosurg Rev 35(2):239–244
79. Niotakis G, Grigoratos D, Chandler C, Morrison D, Lim M (2013) CSF diversion in refractory idiopathic intracranial hypertension: single-centre experience and review of efficacy. Childs Nerv Syst 29(2): 263–267
80. Yoshida S, Masunaga S, Hayase M, Oda Y (2000) Migration of the shunt tube after lumboperitoneal shunt–two case reports. Neurol Med Chir (Tokyo) 40(11):594–596
81. Anthogalidis EI, Sure U, Hellwig D, Bertalanffy H (1999) Intracranial dislocation of a lumbo-peritoneal shunt-catheter: case report and review of the literature. Clin Neurol Neurosurg 101(3):203–206
82. Alleyne CH Jr, Shutter LA, Colohan AR (1996) Cranial migration of a lumboperitoneal shunt catheter. South Med J 89(6):634–636
83. Satow T, Motoyama Y, Yamazoe N, Isaka F, Higuchi K, Nabeshima S (2001) Migration of a lumboperitoneal shunt catheter into the spinal canal–case report. Neurol Med Chir (Tokyo) 41(2):97–99
84. Rodrigues D, Nannapaneni R, Behari S et al (2005) Proximal migration of a lumboperitoneal unishunt system. J Clin Neurosci 12(7):838–841
85. Solaroglu I, Okutan O, Beskonakli E (2005) Foraminal migration of a lumboperitoneal shunt catheter tip. J Clin Neurosci 12(8):956–958
86. Kimura T, Tsutsumi K, Morita A (2011) Scrotal migration of lumboperitoneal shunt catheter in an adult–case report. Neurol Med Chir (Tokyo) 51(12): 861–862
87. Liao YJ, Dillon WP, Chin CT, McDermott MW, Horton JC (2007) Intracranial hypotension caused by leakage of cerebrospinal fluid from the thecal sac after lumboperitoneal shunt placement. J Neurosurg 107(1):173–177
88. Sullivan LP, Stears JC, Ringel SP (1988) Resolution of syringomyelia and Chiari I malformation by

ventriculoatrial shunting in a patient with pseudotumor cerebri and a lumboperitoneal shunt. Neurosurgery 22(4):744–747
89. Huang WY, Chi CS, Shian WJ, Mak SC, Wong TT (1995) Lumboperitoneal shunt complicated with chronic tonsillar herniation: a case report. Zhonghua Yi Xue Za Zhi (Taipei) 55(5):417–419
90. Deginal A, Manoj TK, Parthiban J, Vinodan K, Rao ANS (1998) Radiculopathy – a complication in lumbo-peritoneal shunt. Neurol India 46(1):78–79
91. Aoki N, Mizutani H (1988) Acute subdural hematoma due to minor head trauma in patients with a lumboperitoneal shunt. Surg Neurol 29(1):22–26
92. Barash IA, Medak AJ (2013) Bilateral subdural hematomas after lumboperitoneal shunt placement. J Emerg Med 45(2):178–181
93. Sood S, Gilmer-Hill H, Ham SD (2008) Management of lumbar shunt site swelling in children. J Neurosurg Pediatr 1(5):357–360
94. Muthukumar N, Palaniappan P, Gajendran R (1996) Tension pneumocephalus complicating lumboperitoneal shunt. J Indian Med Assoc 94(12):457, 459
95. Garcia ME, Morales IG, Fernandez JM, Giraldez BG, Sacoto DD, Bengoechea PB (2013) Episodes of loss of consciousness in a patient with a background of cerebral venous thrombosis. Epileptic Disord 15(2): 175–180
96. Castillo L, Bermejo PE, Zabala JA (2008) Unusual complications of the lumboperitoneal shunt as treatment of benign intracranial hypertension. Neurologia (Barcelona, Spain) 23(3):192–196
97. Ohba S, Kinoshita Y, Tsutsui M et al (2012) Formation of abdominal cerebrospinal fluid pseudocyst. Neurol Med Chir (Tokyo) 52(11):838–842
98. Fischer EG, Welch K, Shillito J Jr (1977) Syringomyelia following lumboureteral shunting for communicating hydrocephalus. Report of three cases. J Neurosurg 47(1):96–100
99. Pollak TA, Marcus HJ, James G, Dorward N, Thorne L (2011) Adult hydrocoele complicating a lumboperitoneal shunt. Br J Neurosurg 25(5):647–648
100. Samandouras G, Wadley J, Afshar F (2002) Life-threatening intra-abdominal haemorrhage following insertion of a lumboperitoneal shunt. Br J Neurosurg 16(2):192–193
101. Tang RA, Dorotheo EU, Schiffman JS, Bahrani HM (2004) Medical and surgical management of idiopathic intracranial hypertension in pregnancy. Curr Neurol Neurosci Rep 4(5):398–409
102. Landwehr JB Jr, Isada NB, Pryde PG, Johnson MP, Evans MI, Canady AI (1994) Maternal neurosurgical shunts and pregnancy outcome. Obstet Gynecol 83(1):134–137

15 Complications Specific to Pleural Type of CSF Shunt

Marcelo Galarza and Patricia Martínez

Contents

15.1	**Introduction**	213
15.2	**Pneumothorax and Subcutaneous Emphysema**	216
15.2.1	Prevention	216
15.2.2	Identification	216
15.2.3	Management	217
15.3	**Pleural Effusions, Empyema, and Fibrothorax**	217
15.3.1	Prevention	218
15.3.2	Identification and Specific Management	218
15.4	**Overdrainage**	222
15.5	**Migration**	222
15.6	**Proximal and Distal Obstructions**	223
15.7	**Disconnection and Coiling**	223
15.8	**Cerebrospinal Fluid Galactorrhea**	224
15.9	**Tumor Spread Through the Shunt Tubing**	224
15.10	**Cardiac Tamponade**	224
	References	225

M. Galarza, MD, MSc (✉)
Regional Department of Neurosurgery, "Virgen de la Arrixaca" University Hospital, Murcia, Spain

Regional Service of Neurosurgery, Hospital Universitario Virgen de la Arrixaca, E-30120, El Palmar, Murcia, Spain
e-mail: marcelo.galarza@carm.es, galarza.marcelo@gmail.com

P. Martínez, MD
Department of Thoracic surgery, "Virgen de la Arrixaca" University Hospital, Murcia, Spain
e-mail: patr2238@separ.es

Abbreviations

CSF	Cerebrospinal fluid
VPS	Ventriculoperitoneal shunt
VAS	Ventriculoatrial shunt
VPL	Ventriculopleural shunt

15.1 Introduction

When ventriculoperitoneal shunt (VPS) or ventriculoatrial shunt (VAS) is no longer suitable or is not an initial valid alternative for cerebrospinal fluid (CSF) diversion, VPL is usually the next option to consider. VPL drainage is seldom considered as an alternative route for CSF drainage owing to the feared complications of pleural effusion [2, 6, 7]. However, some series document the feasibility and safety of VPL and subdural-pleural shunting [1, 16, 21, 34, 39, 40, 45]. A few authors have even used VPL shunting as the first option for treating hydrocephalus [39]. The most frequent complication of pleural shunts is symptomatic tension hydrothorax causing respiratory distress [1, 2, 6, 43]. Some reports argue that pleural effusion is an age-related event [46]; accordingly the use of VPL shunting has been discouraged especially

C. Di Rocco et al. (eds.), *Complications of CSF Shunting in Hydrocephalus: Prevention, Identification, and Management*, DOI 10.1007/978-3-319-09961-3_15,

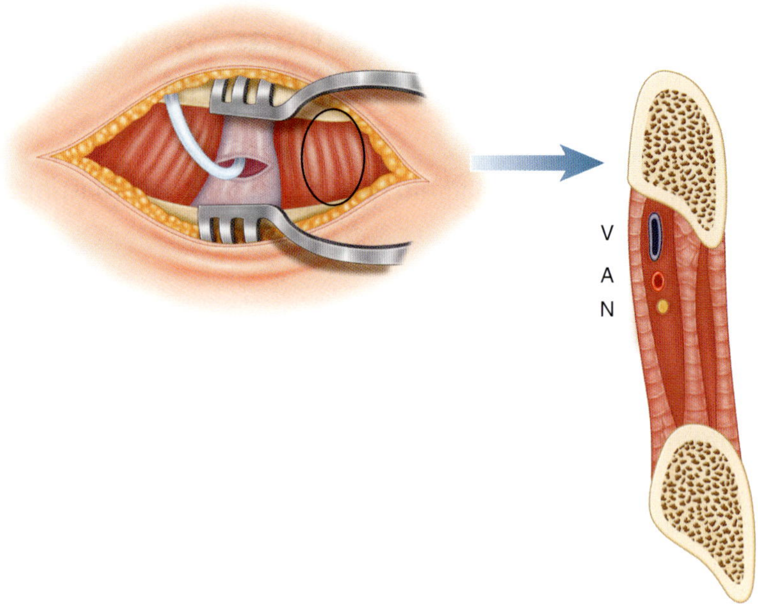

Fig. 15.1 Drawing showing the pleural step of a VPL shunt technique. A small transverse skin incision is made in the third to the fifth anterior intercostal space, and the distal catheter of the shunt is passed to the thoracic incision through the subcutaneous tissue. The pectoralis major and the intercostal muscles are split to expose the pleura. Care is taken to avoid the costal nerve, according to the rib anatomy (*n* nerve, *a* artery, *v* vein)

in children [33]. In contrast, other authors have demonstrated that the diversion of CSF to the pleural cavity constitutes a valid alternative in children as young as 3 years old [21, 34].

Insertion technique of VPL is essential to avoid initial complications and to prevent near future malfunctions. Our technique is not different to what is previously reported [31]. All children are operated on under general anesthesia and with orotracheal intubation. The cranial part of the surgical procedure did not differ from the techniques commonly used for peritoneal shunting. The ventricular catheter is introduced posterior parietal-occipital, inferior and posterior to the parietal boss, and well away from the sensorimotor cortex, with the tip being directed toward the frontal horn. After shaving, the patient is placed with the neck extended and the head turned away from the side to be shunted. Shunts are usually placed on the right side to avoid the dominant hemisphere areas. The scalp incision is made through the skin and galea, and a C-shaped flap is centered on the chosen burr hole site. The scalp is held open by a self-retaining retractor. A tunneling device is used to create a subcutaneous tunnel between the cranial and the thoracic incisions. The chosen shunt is passed into the subcutaneous tunnel, and the tunneler is removed. A small transverse skin incision is made in the third to the fifth anterior intercostal space. The distal catheter of the valve is passed down from the cranial to the thoracic incision through the subcutaneous tissue. Care is taken to avoid the costal nerve, according to the rib anatomy (Fig. 15.1). The costal nerve, if injured, can later develop chronic neuritis. The pectoralis major and the intercostal muscles are split to expose the pleura. The anesthetist deflates the lungs, and the parietal pleura is incised for a length of approximately 3 mm. At this point, the ventricular catheter is inserted, and a good flow of CSF confirms appropriate placement. The CSF pressure is checked by a manometer connected to the ventricular catheter if necessary. The CSF is collected for cell count, Gram's stain, protein, and glucose. The ventricular catheter is cut to an appropriate length and connected to the distal valve and tubing. The CSF flow is checked at the distal end. The catheter is then finally introduced into the pleural cavity. The lungs are inflated, the muscles approximated, and the skin closed. A chest radiograph was taken at the end of the operation. The patient is observed in the pediatric intensive care unit for 6 h and then returned to the neurosurgical ward. Children are discharged home on the fifth to seventh day. A repeat chest radiograph and a computerized tomography scan are performed before discharge.

Alternatively, the transdiaphragmatic route was reported by Rengachary in [42], as a substitute path to the peritoneum through the pleural cavity. We do not have experience with this route.

From a historical perspective, the VPL was initially described by Heile in [15]. An initial attempt to drain CSF into the thoracic duct and pleural cavity was reported by Ingraham and Sears [18]. Later, a series of VPL by Ransohoff in 1954 [40] and 1963 [41], Fein and Rovit [8], Venes (1979) [45] and Hoffmann (1983) [19] gave support to this option. Nonetheless, some reports on complications of VPL shunting have obscured the benefits of its use in daily clinical practice.

Although reported early, the first up to standard series of VPL shunting in the management of hydrocephalus was reported by Ransohoff in 1954. He pointed out that the procedure was relatively simple and that the pleural surfaces tended to absorb CSF well. Pleural effusions were not a significant problem in the initial six patients that he reported.

Nixon in 1962 [37] indicated that many surgeons had encountered problems, particularly pleural effusions, with VPL shunts and recommended the use of valves to avoid that complication, with good results in three patients.

The series of Jones et al. included, from 1969 to 1979, an initial series of 29 children, and later, from 1979 to 1982, a further series of 52 other patients received VPL shunts.

In 1979, Venes and Shaw described their technique for insertion of a pleural shunt, using a trocar to pass the tube to the pleural cavity. They mentioned a 10–20 % risk of a pneumothorax following VPL shunt insertion.

Further serial cases were reported by Hoffman et al. [16], giving support to this option, although not exempted from complications.

Megison and Benzel [33] have carried out a retrospective study of 88 pleural shunting procedures. There was a 7 % complication rate related to the use of the pleural space as the shunt finishing point. Complications at the pleural end included shunt obstruction, either functional or structural; pleural effusion; pneumothorax; and other technical problems. There were no deaths associated with shunt dysfunction or other complications. VPL shunting for hydrocephalus, when used with appropriate precautions and with careful patient selection, is a viable alternative for the treatment of adult hydrocephalus. Although the complications that are unique to this procedure are pneumothorax and pleural effusion, they were encountered infrequently in this series. The authors concluded that VPL shunting may be indicated when other routes are not available.

Piatt [39] reported that the survival of simple ventriculopleural shunts in his series was not significantly different from that of simple ventriculoperitoneal shunts in patients of comparable age with a comparable recent shunt revision history.

Table 15.1 shows the listed cases of reported complications in the literature, including cases from our personal series.

From here, we will discuss the possible complications that we may find with this technique.

Table 15.1

Associated complications in the pleura related to hydrocephalus and to pleural shunts	Reference
Tension pneumothorax	[16]
Tension hydrothorax	[2]
Tension hydrothorax related to subdural-pleural shunt	[6]
Recurrent pleural effusion	[33]
Empyema	[19]
Disconnection	[39]
Migration	[20]
Dislodged/coiling	[34]
Pleural adhesions	[45]
Peritoneal effusion	[47]
Costal neuritis	Personal series
Cerebrospinal fluid galactorrhea	[35]
Hydrothorax related to ventriculoperitoneal shunt	[13]
Pleurisy with clear liquid due to ventriculoatrial shunt	[10]
Infarction pneumonia due to ventriculoatrial shunt	[44]
Cardiac tamponade and heart failure	[50]
Fibrothorax child	[49]
Glial tumor metastases	[46]
Fibrothorax adult	[22]

15.2 Pneumothorax and Subcutaneous Emphysema

A pneumothorax (pl. pneumothoraces) is an abnormal collection of air or gas in the pleural space that separates the lung from the chest wall and which may interfere with normal breathing. Pneumothorax is also defined as the presence of any air inside the chest, and it can be made during the procedure of inserting the catheter through the thorax wall to the pleural cavity (Fig. 15.2). Subcutaneous emphysema develops when the air migrates into the subcutaneous space. It may also be found in the physical examination of patients with serious pulmonary disease.

Usually the surgical technique employs either a thoracoscopic approach [26] or, usually, an intercostal incision to introduce the catheter inside the thorax. This latter technique may predispose for the development of a pneumothorax.

15.2.1 Prevention

Prevention is related to anesthesia events. Continuous feedback within the surgical and anesthetist team is essential. General anesthesia with orotracheal intubation, with no attempts to spontaneous breathing in order to avoid cough, avoiding nitrous oxide and providing hand ventilation to deflate the lung when the surgeon enters the parietal pleura are anesthetic management details for preventing complications such as pneumothorax and subcutaneous emphysema [14].

A positive pressure sustained ventilation administered by the anesthesiologist is used during approximation of the previously spread muscles with a single absorbable stitch. This minimizes the retention of air in the pleural space [33].

In general, no purse-string suture is needed at the pleural entry site [31, 38].

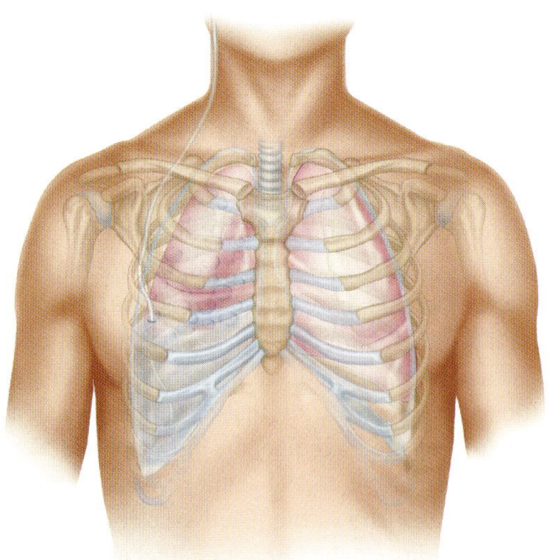

Fig. 15.2 Schematic drawing showing a pneumothorax or presence of any air inside the chest

15.2.2 Identification

Physical exploration reveals crepitus at palpation, if there is associated subcutaneous emphysema, and thoracic auscultation shows decreased breath sounds. Chest radiograph is the standard procedure for the diagnosis of pneumothorax. It should be upright and preferably in the posteroanterior projection. If the patient cannot be upright, a lateral decubitus view with the suspect side positioned up may be helpful. Radiographs obtained in exhalation may accentuate the pneumothorax, but most of the thoracic surgeons have not found this technique useful enough in most clinical situations to warrant the double radiographic exposure. In general, the percentage of collapse is underestimated with the X-ray chest. It is feasible to find air in the subcutaneous space at X-ray when subcutaneous emphysema appears.

Computed tomography of the lungs gives an excellent evaluation of pneumothorax, but the cost-effectiveness of such a procedure must be questioned [28].

The physiologic consequences of a pneumothorax range from little, such as 10 % of collapse in a young person, to life-threatening, such as tension pneumothorax in an older patient with an already compromised cardiopulmonary function aggravated by mediastinal shift and compression of the contralateral lung [9].

15.2.3 Management

A small pneumothorax in a healthy patient can be observed and followed until its reabsorption. Supplying extra oxygen to such patients theoretically hastens the resolution of the pneumothorax, but the true cost-effectiveness of such treatment can be questioned. Kircher and Swartzel [23] estimated that 1.5 % of the air is reabsorbed over each 24-h period.

Simple aspiration is particularly useful in a smaller pneumothorax with a delayed diagnosis, when the passage of time suggests that the process will be self-limited.

Thoracocentesis is indicated when a wait and see conduct is not an option. A tube thoracostomy should be carried out for pneumothoraces over 30 % to hasten recovery or in cases of lesser degrees of lung collapse for those patients with symptoms of associated disorders, such as heart or chronic pulmonary disease. We prefer to insert tube thoracostomy of 24–28-F catheter directed toward the apex. Rarely, this iatrogenic pneumothorax requires a more aggressive surgical option, like videothoracoscopic approach or even thoracotomy. The complications of thoracocentesis include aggravation of pneumothorax, which may be seen in 3–20 % of patients, hemothorax, pulmonary edema, intrapulmonary hemorrhage, and hemoptysis. Other rare events are vagal inhibition, air embolism, subcutaneous emphysema, bronchopleural fistula, empyema, seeding of a needle tract with malignant cells, and puncture of the liver or spleen.

Subcutaneous emphysema is directly related to the pneumothorax and usually resolves itself when pneumothorax is resolved [9]. There is no need for a specific approach.

15.3 Pleural Effusions, Empyema, and Fibrothorax

The presence of a pleural collection of fluid observed on chest radiographs of patients with VPL shunting (Fig. 15.3a) should be of no concern in the absence of respiratory symptoms [21]. In our opinion [31], the finding of small hydrothoraces in otherwise asymptomatic patients indicates that the shunt is functioning. However, we consider that patients with VPL shunts must be regularly followed up in view of the reports on

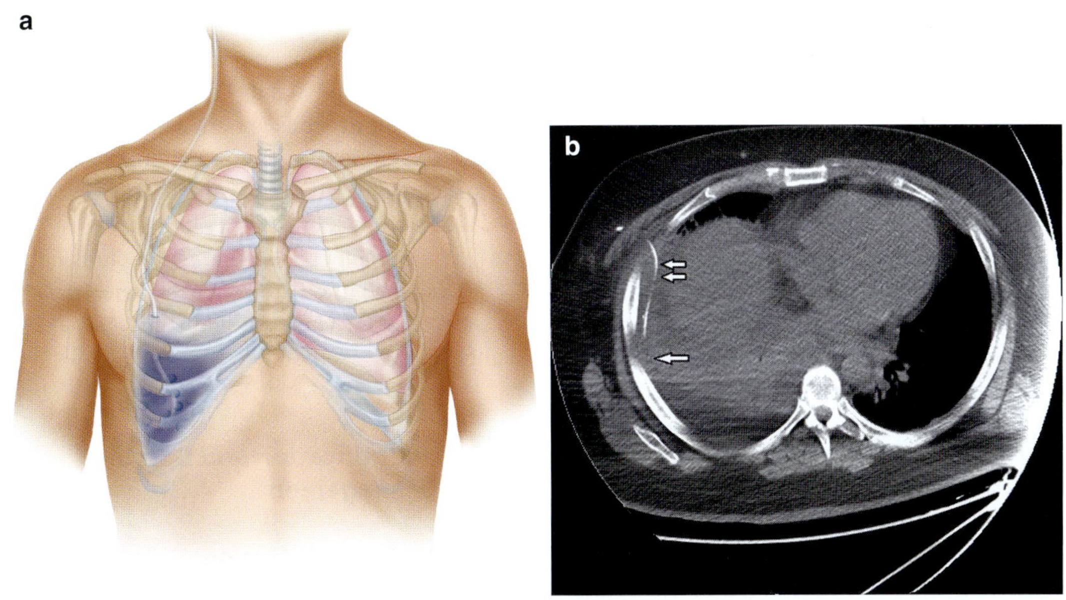

Fig. 15.3 (**a**, **b**) Pleural collection of fluid observed on the chest radiographs of patients with VPL shunting is shown in this schematic drawing. Fluid collection (*single arrow*) secondary to CSF drainage of a VPL shunt in the pleural space depicted in this thorax computed tomography. The distal catheter is in close relationship (*double arrow*)

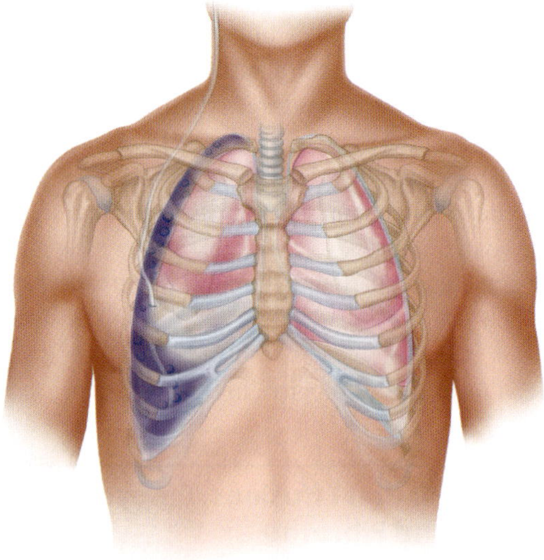

Fig. 15.4 Schematic drawing showing a symptomatic tension hydrothorax causing respiratory distress

tension pleural effusions that can appear at any time, as a result of changes in the valve pressure or in the absorption capability of the pleural cavity [21, 25]. Still, the most frequent blunt complication of pleural shunts is symptomatic tension hydrothorax causing respiratory distress [2] (Fig. 15.4).

When pleural effusions are not resolved, fibrotic changes may develop. However, severe fibrotic change in the pleural cavity is an unusual complication of ventriculopleural shunts, and only two cases of a fibrothorax have been described [22, 49]. Although these cases do not warrant abandonment of the pleura as a potential site for CSF drainage, they raise awareness about this complication.

The development of fibrotic changes in the pleura is believed to be related to the chemical composition of CSF, an immune-related mechanism, or on the other hand, related to a low-grade infection. The length of time required to produce these severe changes appears to be quite variable. It is not clear whether the antisiphon devices will be able to prevent this complication, and a long-term follow-up of patients with these devices may help detect the development of fibrosis.

15.3.1 Prevention

Megison and Benzel [33] warned about the use of VPL shunting in adults with pulmonary disease. The ventilator reserve must be considered with particular care especially in meningomyelocele patients with kyphoscoliosis and in cases of Chiari malformation. In all these cases the burden of a pleural fluid effusion in an already-restricted ventilatory capacity might precipitate a frank respiratory failure [39].

Jones et al. [21] have achieved the use of an antisiphon device connected with the valve, with the aim of preventing the formation of clinically significant CSF pleural effusions. The authors reported that only 1 of 52 children developed a symptomatic hydrothorax that required conversion to a ventriculoperitoneal shunt

Nevertheless, the use of antisiphon devices in children frequently induces symptoms of underdrainage, owing to the narrow margins that these devices achieve for effectively controlling raised intracranial pressure [31].

Ventriculopleural shunts can be associated with debilitating scenarios, and caution should be exerted in their use in debilitated or immunocompromised patients, to avoid the occurrence of severe fibrotic changes in the pleural cavity with lung entrapment [22].

The general management consists of evaluation of pleural fluid and its drainage, supplemental oxygen, intravenous volume replacement, and the consideration of empiric antibiotics to cover coexistent infections. A comprehensive shunt evaluation with careful observation or revision of the ventriculopleural shunt is recommended. Removing the intrapleural shunt catheter must be considered, only if an infection has been demonstrated.

15.3.2 Identification and Specific Management

15.3.2.1 Pleural Effusion

Fluid collection in the pleural space decreases lung volume, increases intrathoracic pressure, and leads to irritation and chest pain (Fig. 15.3b). On

Table 15.2 Mechanisms of pleural effusions

Mechanisms of pleural effusions
Increased systemic hydrostatic pressure
Decreased oncotic pressure in the microcirculation
Increased pleural microcirculation permeability
Increased pulmonary interstitial fluid
Obstruction of lymphatic drainage
Flow of liquid from walls or other sources: peritoneum, retroperitoneum, cerebrospinal space, external catheters
Reduction of the negative pressure in the pleural space
Thoracic vascular rupture
Rupture of the thoracic duct

examination, patients may demonstrate tachypnea, hypoxia, hypotension, dullness to percussion of the involved hemithorax, decreased chest wall expansion, and jugular venous distention.

Pleural fluid accumulates relatively slowly, allowing for the body to compensate with alterations in intravascular volume and reflex tachycardia [25].

Once a critical volume and pressure has been reached within the hemithorax, decreased venous return and hypotension ensues [48].

Pleural effusions develop due to the alterations in dynamics of net pleural fluid production and absorption. There are many possible mechanisms involved (Table 15.2). The mechanisms for accumulation of pleural effusions with ventriculopleural shunts remain speculative. The presence of a shunt catheter in the pleural space may produce local irritant effects, inducing a chronic subclinical inflammatory response, as supported by the predominant lymphocytosis in the pleural fluid. Inflammation leads to increased pleural fluid production and impaired lymphatic flow, causing pleural fluid accumulation and lung collapse. This further reduces the pleural surface area, resulting in a decrease in the net absorption of the pleural fluid. Continuous addition of cerebrospinal fluid compounds the problem, leading to rapid accumulation of large pleural effusions [2].

Beta-2-transferrin level has been used as a novel diagnostic strategy. A sample of fluid, drained via tube thoracostomy, was sent for beta-2-transferrin level. This desialated isoform of transferrin is almost exclusively found in the CSF with only minimal amounts present in cochlear perilymph and in the aqueous and vitreous humor of the eye. Multiple studies have validated the use of beta-2-transferrin as a specific marker for CSF leakage with sensitivity and specificity approaching 100 and 95 %, respectively. Furthermore, Huggins and Sahn [17] report the use of beta-2-transferrin to identify the presence of a CSF pleural effusion in an elderly patient with a duropleural fistula. According to the authors, beta-2- transferrin has never been previously utilized to identity CSF hydrothorax in children with VP shunts.

Increased densities on chest radiography are frequently attributed to parenchymal infiltrates when they actually represent pleural fluid. Free pleural fluid is best demonstrated with lateral decubitus chest radiography, ultrasonography, or computed tomographic scans. The presence of loculated pleural fluid is best demonstrated with ultrasonography [9].

Thoracocentesis with a needle aspiration of the pleural fluid under local anesthesia may be indicated. If the fluid appears benign, is not loculated, and can be removed totally or nearly so, thoracocentesis may be all that is necessary to control the disease process. Leukocyte count, Gram stain, cultures, cytological studies, and glucose and LDH levels of the fluid should be carried out. If negative, resolution usually occurs. If the fluid is positive by biochemical evaluation, staining, or culture, pleural effusion has turned to an empyema, and close chest tube drainage is required [30].

Biochemical and microbiological analyses of pleural fluid can demonstrate that there is an intrapleural complication such as empyema. The appearance of pleural fluid and the levels of glucose, LDH, pH, and proteins (see Light's criteria [29]) with white blood cell count and the presence of microorganisms in the pleural fluid (Gram's stain) or in specific growth culture could indicate a complicated exudative pleural effusion that requires to be drained with a tube of thoracostomy.

An uncomplicated effusion is nonpurulent, has a negative Gram's stain result for bacteria, has negative results by culture, and is generally free flowing. Using biochemical parameters, Light and associates noted a pH greater than 7.30, a normal glucose level, and an LDH concentration less than 1,000 IU/L.

In case of loculated pleural effusion, the administration of intrapleural fibrinolytic agents such as urokinase may be required. Although chest tube drainage combined with enzymatic debridement is effective, some authors [24, 27, 29] have reported better results with the videothoracoscopic approach, reporting a higher success rate, shorter hospital stay, and less overall economic costs.

In our experience, a video-assisted thoracoscopy procedure for treating pleural effusion related with VPL shunts is rarely needed.

Rarely, VP shunts may develop pleural effusions. The tip of a VP shunt may be located intraabdominally, usually in the suprahepatic area or the pelvis. One case has been reported of a suprahepatic shunt perforating the diaphragm with a CSF collection in the pleural cavity. Still, according to some authors, VPL shunts are rarely used because of frequent pleural effusions, which may cause a decrease in the effectiveness of CSF shunts and respiratory compromise [12].

Third ventriculostomy was used as an alternative of cerebrospinal diversion in a case of hydrothorax due to ventriculopleural shunting in a child with spina bifida on chronic dialysis [11].

Acetazolamide was used to decrease cerebrospinal fluid production in chronically ventilated patients with ventriculopleural shunts [4].

Tonn et al. [44] reported a rare but life-threatening complication of ventriculoatrial shunt as infarction pneumonia and pleural effusion. They presented the case of a female patient with ventriculoatrial shunt insertion as long-term treatment for aqueductal stenosis who presented with recurrent episodes of dyspnea, chest pain, and unilateral pleural effusion. Diagnostic evaluation revealed a positive D-dimer test, bilateral basal infiltrates, and pleural effusion. Transesophageal echocardiography established the diagnosis of a thrombus in the right atrium. Laboratory testing for thrombophilia revealed a homozygous factor V Leiden mutation. A shunt revision was performed and resolved the malfunction.

A similar case was reported by Gerbeaux et al. in 1977 [10].

Specific management of pleural effusion that consists of a needle thoracocentesis is needed when a clinical infection is suspected, or it could be performed only if the pleural effusion measures more than 10 mm on lateral decubitus chest radiography [32].

15.3.2.2 Tension Hydrothorax

Tension hydrothorax is an emergency condition that requires prompt recognition and treatment to maximize chances for survival. The presentation of a hydrothorax is often subacute due to the slow accumulation of fluid in the hemithorax (Fig. 15.4). Hypotension, hypoxia, and tachycardia are signs of clinical decompensation and indicate that the collection of fluid in the pleural space has impaired cardiopulmonary function.

Davidson and Zito [6] reported also an acute tension hydrothorax in a patient with subdural-pleural shunting. He reported a 3-year-old child with a bilateral chronic subdural hematoma treated successfully with a subdural-pleural shunt. Two months later, the patient returned with severe respiratory embarrassment due to cerebrospinal fluid hydrothorax. By removing the shunt the hydrothorax was resolved.

Hadzikaric et al. [13] reported a case of cerebrospinal fluid tension hydrothorax as a rare complication of ventriculoperitoneal shunt. The case was a 16-month-old boy known to have congenital hydrocephalus and a Dandy-Walker cyst who presented with serious respiratory distress. Examination revealed right pleural effusion and congested throat. Thoracocentesis with drainage of the pleural cavity for 10 days failed to free the patient from pleural effusion. Following an intraperitoneal injection of Omnipaque, a chest X-ray was done, and samples of pleural fluid taken before and after the injection were compared on X-ray, revealing the presence of contrast in the postinjection pleural effusion. Changing the VP shunt for a ventriculoatrial shunt resulted in immediate complete disappearance of the pleural effusion and of the patient's chest symptoms. This was a rare occurrence.

Specific management consists when a tension hydrothorax must be treated immediately with a tube thoracostomy when clinical decompensation is noted. Emergency physicians should be aware of this potential complication and consider it in their differential diagnosis for cardiopulmonary distress in patients with a ventriculopleural shunt [48].

15.3.2.3 Thoracic Empyema and Fibrothorax

A thoracic empyema occurs when bacteria invade the normally sterile pleural space. The process was described by Andrews in 1962 (cited by Light [29]) as a continuum of three stages. Stage 1 is characterized by the presence of an exudative effusion from increased permeability of the inflamed and swollen pleural surfaces. This stage corresponds to the uncomplicated effusion and is initially sterile.

With bacterial invasion, the process blends into fibrinopurulent stage 2, true empyema or Light's (Light 1980 [30]) complicated pleural effusion; it is composed of white blood cells greater than 500 cells per μL, protein level greater than 2.5 g/dL, pH less than 7.2, and LDH levels greater than 1,000 IU/L. Heavy fibrin deposition takes places on both pleural surfaces, particularly the parietal pleura. The effusion becomes purulent, with a white blood cell count above 15,000 cells per μL. Biochemically, the pH decreases to levels below 7.0, the glucose decreases to less than 50 mg/dL, and the LDH increases to greater than 1,000 IU/L.

Stage 3 begins as early as 1 week after infection with collagen organization and deposition on both pleural surfaces and entrapment of the underlying lung. This process is mature in 3–4 weeks, and the organized collagen on the pleural surface is termed a peel [32].

Usually, thoracic empyema is a cause of a generalized and systemic infection (Fig. 15.5). It could aggravate the patient clinical situation and later can develop a sepsis with lethal consequences, if it is not promptly and correctly treated.

As shunt infection is a known complication of ventriculopleural shunting, a high index of suspicion must be maintained for infection in both the CSF and any associated pleural effusion when these patients present with fevers without another obvious source. Early sampling of the CSF and pleural fluid will direct prompt institution of antimicrobial therapy and shunt exteriorization, which may prevent the development of frank empyema [19].

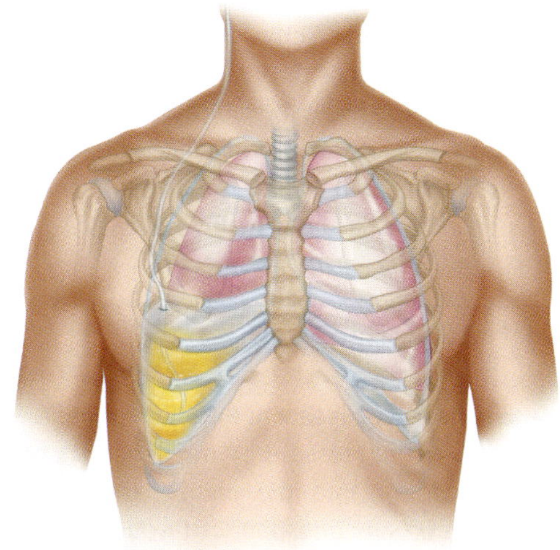

Fig. 15.5 Schematic design of a case of thoracic empyema secondary to VPL shunt. Usually it is a cause of a generalized and systemic infection

For the development of fibrothorax, chronic condition is essential and is characterized by dense fibrosis, contraction and trapping of the lung, atelectasis, and reduction of the size of the hemithorax. Fibrothorax with invasion of the chest wall and narrowing of the intercostal spaces may be thought of as the end stage of this process [32, 49].

The specific management of empyema and fibrothorax consists basically of two techniques. Video-assisted thoracoscopy (VATS) allows adhesiolysis and debridement of pleural cavity. Nowadays, it is considered to be the primary modality for treating complicated empyema after initial therapy, with or without chest tube drainage, in many institutions.

Although VATS has the advantages of better exposure and patient tolerance, open thoracostomy with debridement is an effective approach to treat empyema and fibrothorax. Empyemectomy is rarely performed. Extrapleural dissection of the parietal surface and the sac from the lung, just as in decortication of a chronically collapsed and trapped lung, requires undesirable and unnecessary lung resection very often [32].

As this complication is rarely seen, only two cases were reported. Yellin et al. in 1992 [49] reported open thoracostomy and decortication. In this case, the shunt had to be removed, and decortication had to be performed to alleviate severe respiratory symptoms in the child. Another similar case was reported by Khan and Kahlil in 2008 [22].

15.4 Overdrainage

An interesting issue is that of the changes induced in the intracranial pressure by the dynamics of a valve that drains into the pleura. Intrapleural pressures are subatmospheric throughout the respiratory cycle, which probably induces a continuous sucking effect of the CSF that could decrease the intracranial pressure. At least theoretically, VPL shunting should produce symptoms and signs of CSF overdrainage in all patients treated by this technique. In 1998, Munshi recorded the intraventricular pressures with a telemetric sensor in patients with VPL shunts. Four patients with ventriculopleural shunts were monitored telemetrically while supine and at increments of head elevation to 90°. Their findings indicated that the negative intrapleural pressures generated during the respiratory cycle tend to generate intraventricular pressures that are consistently lower than those observed with peritoneal shunting. This observation suggests that VPL shunts may be appropriate for patients requiring very low intraventricular pressures in order to resolve their hydrocephalic symptoms [36]. This event was partially reflected by a similar case reported by Chiang et al. [5].

Using an antisiphon device attached to the valve probably prevents this untoward effect. In fact, several authors have stressed the importance of placing such a device in cases with CSF drainage into the pleural cavity [21, 36].

Antisiphon devices are believed to prevent this complication by preventing overdrainage. Short-term follow-up of patients with VPL shunts for as long as 2.5 years has shown good results from these devices in preventing the occurrence of pleural effusions [31].

The use of antisiphon devices in children frequently induces symptoms of underdrainage

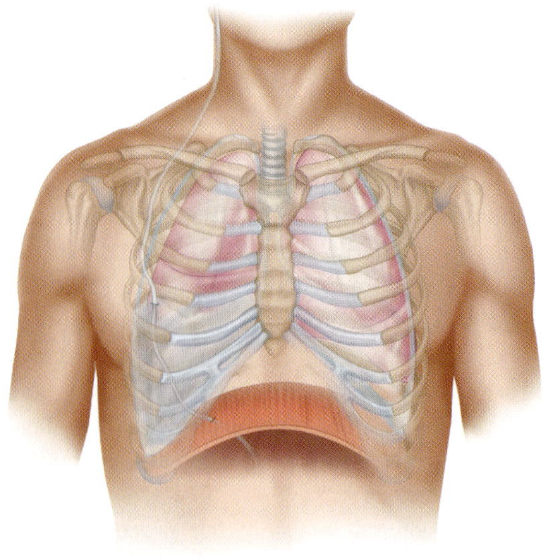

Fig. 15.6 Schematic design of a case of a transdiaphragmatic migration of a VPL shunt

[21], owing to the narrow margins that these devices achieve for effectively controlling raised intracranial pressure. The good results obtained in the cases reported by Martínez-Lage et al. [31] could well be attributed to the fact that their valves were not of the standard differential-pressure type.

It would be reasonable to expect that the use of an externally adjustable shunt, by regulating the pressure settings of the valve to the patient's needs, will be capable of avoiding both the siphoning effects on the ventricles and the formation of significant collections of CSF within the pleura [31].

15.5 Migration

Migration of ventriculoperitoneal shunts into the pleural cavity has also been noted in association with the growth of the patient, with resultant pleural effusion. Johnson and Maxwell [20] reported a delayed case, while Pearson et al. [38] reported a migration of the distal catheter between the ribs and pleura with subsequent dysfunction.

We have seen a case of a transdiaphragmatic migration of a VPL shunt (Fig. 15.6) as well as a rare migration of the distal catheter from the pleural space to the cardiac atrium through the pulmonary vein (Fig. 15.7). Another migration reported is from the pleural space to the mediastinum with ensuing pericardiac effusion. These two later cases are extremely rare occurrences.

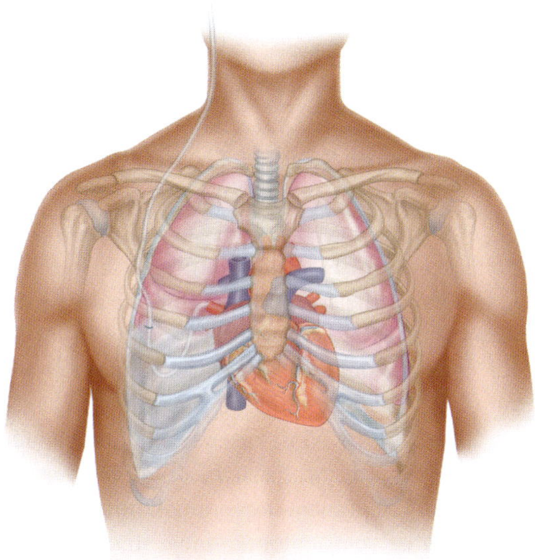

Fig. 15.7 Schematic drawing showing a rare migration of the distal catheter from the pleural space to the cardiac atrium through the pulmonary vein

15.6 Proximal and Distal Obstructions

Pleural inflammatory process associated to pleural effusion and fibrin deposits over the pleural surfaces can produce distal catheter obstruction. This complication is associated with a catheter malfunctioning and pleural effusion, with or without an infection.

Management consists of removing the catheter inside the pleura and replacing it if necessary.

15.7 Disconnection and Coiling

Disconnection is a fairly common complication, directly related to the surgical technique. Their management consists in reconnecting both ends surgically.

We have seen two cases of coiling of the distal catheter in the pleural space. An excessive length of the distal catheter may have contributed to this complication (Fig. 15.8a, b).

a

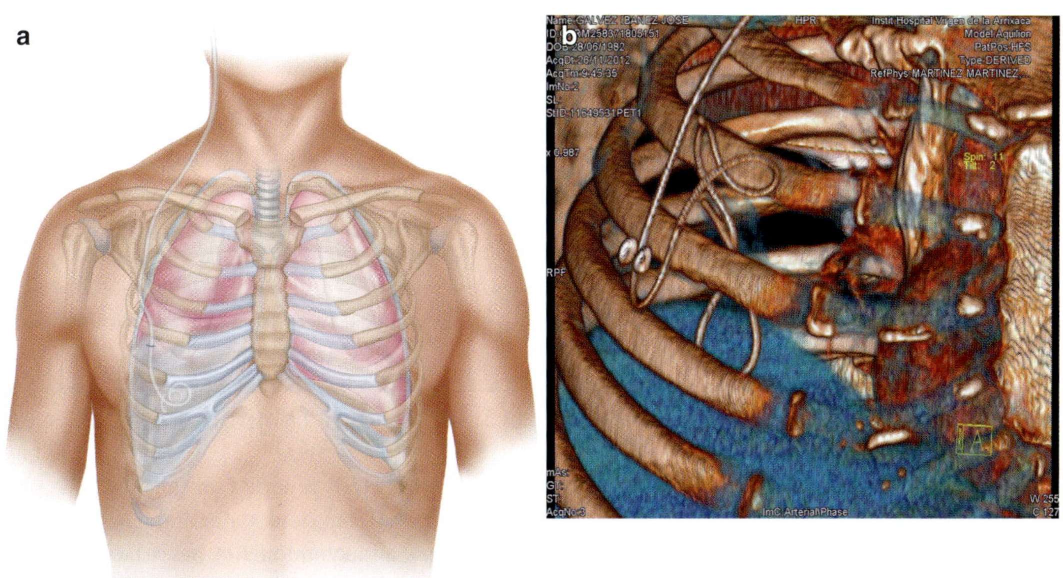

Fig. 15.8 (**a**, **b**) Schematic design showing coiling of the distal catheter in the pleural space. An excessive length of the distal catheter may have contributed to this complication as we have seen in this 3-D thorax computed tomography

15.8 Cerebrospinal Fluid Galactorrhea

When a migration of catheter takes place or even in association with pleural effusion, the cerebrospinal fluid could spread around nearer tissues such as the breast. Continued drainage of the cerebrospinal fluid into the subcutaneous and breast tissue led to the development of breast enlargement and drainage via the nipple. Also, it is collected inside until drained spontaneously through the nipple or is surgically drained. This extremely rare complication is related to the pleural end of the catheter retracted out of the pleural cavity [35].

Regarding our experience, we have recently treated a case that simulated abscess mastitis in a young male treated with ventriculopleural shunt due to a ventriculoperitoneal shunt failure. He presented an asymptomatic loculated pleural effusion with initial fibrotic changes that stopped the normal CSF reabsorption, so the CSF continued flowing to the issues around (adipose tissue of the breast) simulating an abscess mastitis (Fig. 15.9).

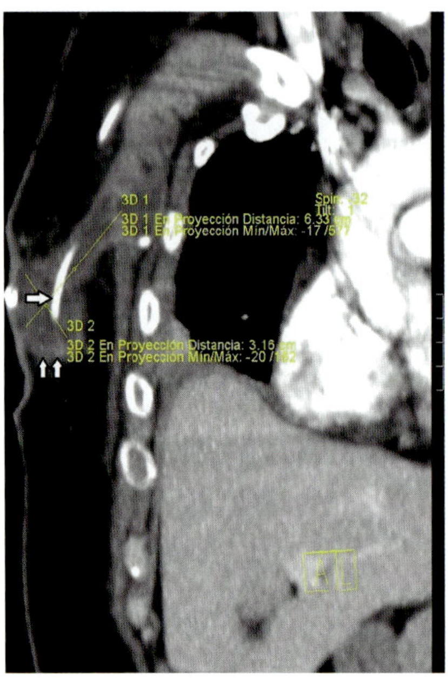

Fig. 15.9 Thorax computed tomography showing an abscess mastitis (*double arrow*) flowing to the adipose tissue of the breast from the distal catheter of a VPL shunt (*single arrow*)

It was surgically drained, microbiological cultures were taken, and the shunt catheter was externalized.

Management included CSF microbiological cultures, systemics antibiotics, and removing the shunt catheter with surgical drainage of the damaged area. A third ventriculostomy was performed to alleviate his hydrocephalic symptoms.

15.9 Tumor Spread Through the Shunt Tubing

Shunts as an artificial anastomosis can provide the means for the spreading of tumor cells by the cerebrospinal fluid. The first spreading of tumor cells via a shunt was reported in 1954 by Ransohoff, and interestingly, it was a ventriculopleural shunt [40]. Most cases from there include seeding of posterior fossa medulloblastoma or other highly malignant intracranial tumor spreading through a ventriculoperitoneal shunt. Further nearly 100 cases of the world literature with shunt-associated metastasizing of brain tumors were reported. The extraneural spreading of tumor cells through shunt tubes must be considered as a possible complication of the shunting procedure.

Other authors have described the spreading of tumor cells from ventricles to the pleural space [46].

Brust et al. [3] reported a case of glial tumor metastases through a ventriculopleural shunt resulting in massive pleural effusion.

Specific management consists of chemotherapy and/or radiotherapy, if they are indicated.

If a tension hydrothorax occurs, thoracocentesis or even chest tube drainage is recommended.

15.10 Cardiac Tamponade

Zaman et al. [50] reported an unusual case of a patient with a ventriculopleural shunt presenting with signs and symptoms of heart failure due to massive pericardial effusion. Imaging revealed the distal shunt catheter end within the middle mediastinum to have migrated from the pleural space. The patient underwent a shunt revision procedure resulting in complete resolution of the presenting pathology. This complication is extremely rare, and we have only seen a similar case once.

In sum, VPL is an accepted shunt technique in neurosurgical scenarios. Although technically feasible and relatively simple, it is not exempted from specific complications. It can be used when the peritoneum is not feasible. The avoidance of complications is directly related to the shunting insertion technique, including anesthesiologist facts and proper selection of the patient. Prevention of malfunction is also related to the abovementioned factors and to intrinsic factors of the shunt components. Nonetheless, as in any shunt procedure, there is still too much to gain knowledge of.

References

1. Arsalo A, Louhimo I, Santavuori P, Valtonew S (1977) Subdural effusion: results after treatment with subdural pleural shunts. Childs Brain 3:79–86
2. Beach C, Manthey DE (1998) Tension hydrothorax due to ventriculopleural shunting. J Emerg Med 16:33–36
3. Brust JC, Moiel RH, Rosenberg RN (1968) Glial tumor metastases through a ventriculo-pleural shunt. Resultant massive pleural effusion. Arch Neurol 18(6):649–653
4. Carrion E, Hertzog JH, Medlock MD, Hauser GJ, Dalton HJ (2001) Use of acetazolamide to decrease cerebrospinal fluid production in chronically ventilated patients with ventriculopleural shunts. Arch Dis Child 84(1):68–71
5. Chiang VL, Torbey M, Rigamonti D, Williams MA (2001) Ventriculopleural shunt obstruction and positive-pressure ventilation. Case report. J Neurosurg 95(1):116–118
6. Davidson RI, Zito J (1982) Acute cerebrospinal fluid hydrothorax: a delayed complication of subdural-pleural shunting. Neurosurgery 10:503–505
7. Detwiler PN, Porter RW, Rekate HL (1999) Hydrocephalus – clinical features and management. In: Choux M, Di Rocco C, Hockley A, Walker M (eds) Pediatric neurosurgery. Churchill- Livingstone, London, pp 253–274
8. Fein JM, Rovit RL (1973) The ventriculo-pleural fenestration shunt. Surg Neurol 1(4):205–208
9. Fry WA, Paape K (2000) Pneumothorax. In: Shields TW (ed) General thoracic surgery, vol 1. Lippincott Williams & Wilkins, Philadelphia, pp 675–679
10. Gerbeaux J, Baculard A, Laugier J, Combe P, Grimfeld A, Van Effenterre R (1977) Pleurisy with clear liquid. Rare complication of ventriculo-cardiac shunt: Pudenz valve [Article in French]. Ann Med Interne (Paris) 128(3):289–294
11. Grunberg J, Rébori A, Verocay MC, Ramela V, Alberti R, Cordoba A (2005) Hydrothorax due to ventriculopleural shunting in a child with spina bifida on chronic dialysis: third ventriculostomy as an alternative of cerebrospinal diversion. Int Urol Nephrol 37(3):571–574
12. Gupta AK, Berry M (1994) Ventriculo-peritoneal shunt presenting with recurrent pleural effusion: report of a new complication. Pediatr Radiol 24:147
13. Hadzikaric N, Nasser M, Mashani A, Ammar A (2002) CSF hydrothorax–VP shunt complication without displacement of a peritoneal catheter. Childs Nerv Syst 18(3–4):179–182, 2001
14. Haret DM, Onisei AM, Martin TW (2009) Acute-recurrent subcutaneous emphysema after ventriculopleural shunt placement. J Clin Anesth 13:352–354
15. Heile B (1914) Sur chirurgischen Behandlung des Hydrocephalus internus durch Ableitung der Cerebrospinalflüssigkeit nach der Bauchhöhle und nach der Pleurakuppe. Arch Klin Chir 105:501–516
16. Hoffman HJ, Hendrick EB, Humphreys RP (1983) Experience with ventriculopleural shunts. Childs Brain 10:404–413
17. Huggins JT, Sahn SA (2003) Duro-pleural fistula diagnosed by beta-2- transferrin. Respiration 70: 423–425
18. Ingraham FD, Sears RA (1949) Further studies on the treatment of experimental hydrocephalus; attempts to drain the cerebrospinal fluid into the pleural cavity and the thoracic duct. J Neurosurg 6(3):207–215
19. Iosif G, Fleischman J, Chitkara R (1991) Empyema due to ventriculopleural shunt. Chest 99:1538–1539
20. Johnson MC, Maxwell MS (1995) Delayed intrapleural migration of a ventriculoperitoneal shunt. Childs Nerv Syst 11:348–350
21. Jones RF, Currie BG, Kwok BC (1988) Ventriculopleural shunts for hydrocephalus: a useful alternative. Neurosurgery 23:753–755
22. Khan TA, Khalil-Marzouk JF (2008) Fibrothorax in adulthood caused by a cerebrospinal fluid shunt in the treatment of hydrocephalus. J Neurosurg 109:478–479
23. Kircher LT Jr, Swartzel RL (1954) Spontaneous pneumothorax and its treatment. J Am Med Assoc 155(1):24–29
24. Krasna MJ (1996) Introduction to thoracoscopic surgery: indications, basic techniques, and instrumentation. Semin Laparosc Surg 3(4):201–210
25. Küpeli E, Yilmaz C, Akçay S (2010) Pleural effusion following ventriculopleural shunt: case reports and review of the literature. Ann Thorac Med 5(3): 166–170
26. Kurschel S, Eder HG, Schleef J (2003) Ventriculopleural shunt: thoracoscopic placement of the distal catheter. Surg Endosc 17:1850
27. Landreneau RJ, Keenan RJ, Hazelrigg SR, Mack MJ, Naunheim KS (1996) Thoracoscopy for empyema and hemothorax. Chest 109(1):18–24

28. Lesur O, Delorme N, Fromaget JM, Bernadac P, Polu JM (1990) Computed tomography in the etiologic assessment of idiopathic spontaneous pneumothorax. Chest 98(2):341–347
29. Light RW (2000) Physiology of pleural fluid production and benign pleural effusion. In: Shields TW (ed) General thoracic surgery, vol 1. Lippincott Williams & Wilkins, Philadelphia, pp 687–693
30. Light RW, Girard WM, Jenkinson SG, George RB (1980) Parapneumonic effusions. Am J Med 69(4): 507–512
31. Martínez-Lage JF, Torres J, Campillo H, Sanchez-del-Rincón I, Bueno F, Zambudio G, Poza M (2000) Ventriculopleural shunting with new technology valves. Childs Nerv Syst 16:867–871
32. McLaughlin JS, Krasna MJ (2000) Parapneumonic empyema. In: Shields TW (ed) General thoracic surgery, vol 1. Lippincott Williams & Wilkins, Philadelphia, pp 703–708
33. Megison DP, Benzel EC (1988) Ventriculo- pleural shunting for adult hydrocephalus. Br J Neurosurg 2: 503–505
34. Milhorat TH (1972) Hydrocephalus and the cerebrospinal fluid. Williams & Wilkins, Baltimore, pp 208–210
35. Moron MA, Barrow DL (1994) Cerebrospinal fluid galactorrhea after ventriculo- pleural shunting: case report. Surg Neurol 42:227–230
36. Munshi I, Lathrop D, Madsen JR, Frim DM (1998) Intraventricular pressure dynamics in patients with ventriculopleural shunts: a telemetric study. Pediatr Neurosurg 28:67–69
37. Nixon HH (1962) Ventriculoperitoneal drainage with a valve. Dev Med Child Neurol 4:301–302
38. Pearson B, Bui CJ, Tubbs RS, Wellons JC III (2007) An unusual complication of a ventriculopleural shunt. J Neurosurg 106(5 suppl):410
39. Piatt JH Jr (1994) How effective are ventriculopleural shunts? Pediatr Neurosurg 21:66–70
40. Ransohoff J (1954) Ventriculopleural anastomosis in treatment of midline obstructional masses. J Neurosurg 11:295–301
41. Ransohoff J, Marini G, Shulman K (1963) The ventriculo-pleural shunt. Minerva Neurochir 12: 68–70, Italian
42. Rengachary SS (1997) Transdiaphragmatic ventriculoperitoneal shunting: technical case report. Neurosurgery 41(3):695–697; discussion 697–8
43. Sanders DY, Summers R, Derouen L (1997) Symptomatic pleural collection of cerebrospinal fluid caused by a ventriculoperitoneal shunt. South Med J 90:831–832
44. Tonn P, Gilsbach JM, Kreitschmann-Andermahr I, Franke A, Blindt R (2005) A rare but life-threatening complication of ventriculo-atrial shunt. Acta Neurochir (Wien) 147(12):1303–1304
45. Venes JL, Shaw RK (1979) Ventriculopleural shunting in the management of hydrocephalus. Childs Brain 5:45–50
46. Wakamatsu T, Matsuo K, Kawano S, Teramoto S, Matsumara H (1971) Glioblastoma with extracranial metastasis through ventriculopleural shunt: case report. J Neurosurg 34:697–701
47. Willison CD, Kopitnik TA, Gustafson R, Kaufman HH (1992) Ventriculoperitoneal shunting used as a temporary diversion. Acta Neurochir (Wien) 115:62–68
48. Wu TS, Kuroda R (2011) Tension hydrothorax in a pediatric patient with a ventriculopleural shunt. J Emerg Med 40(6):637–639
49. Yellin A, Findler G, Barzilay Z, Simansky DA, Lieberman Y (1992) Fibrothorax associated with a ventriculopleural shunt in a hydrocephalic child. J Pediatr Surg 27:1525–1526
50. Zaman M, Akram H, Haliasos N, Bavetta S (2011) Cardiac tamponade and heart failure secondary to ventriculo-pleural shunt malfunction: a rare presentation. BMJ Case Rep pii: bcr1220092548. doi:10.1136/bcr.12.2009.2548

Complications Specific to Rare Type Procedures of CSF Shunting

16

Bernard Trench Lyngdoh

Contents

16.1 **Introduction** ... 227
16.2 **Ventriculocholecysto Shunt** ... 228
16.3 **Ventriculosubgaleal Shunt** ... 228
16.4 **Ventriculosinus Shunts** ... 229
16.5 **Ventriculoureteral Shunt** ... 230
References ... 231

B.T. Lyngdoh, MD
Department of Neurosurgery, Woodland Hospital, Shillong, Meghalaya, India
e-mail: bernitl@yahoo.com

16.1 Introduction

Hydrocephalic patients can exhibit varied medical problems, from the neonates that are underweight with acute meningitis/ventriculitis or intraventricular hemorrhage to the chronic infections such as tuberculosis that can occur in any age group, rendering some of them difficult to manage by the ventriculoperitoneal (VP) shunt, ventriculoatrial (VA) shunt, and endoscopic third ventriculostomy (ETV) procedures.

The regular procedures may be contraindicated when required parameters for their use are lacking, such as CSF characteristics, poor absorptive surface of the peritoneum secondary to associated infection or repeated abdominal surgeries (Fig. 16.1), local or systemic infections, and general condition. Much of these are encountered in the pediatric population.

Tubercular meningitis (TBM) is a major concern in developing nations. It is gradually becoming a global problem with rising immunocompromised status.

In such situations, temporary diversions are required to tide over the situation. Procedures such as ventricular taps, repeated lumbar punctures, or the exteriorized ventricular or lumbar drains are more risky and labored with inadequate CSF diversion or ventricular decompression.

Here we discuss a few procedures performed when the distal receptor site becomes unavailable. They provide a continuous temporary diversion while the receptor site heals. Many have reported

C. Di Rocco et al. (eds.), *Complications of CSF Shunting in Hydrocephalus: Prevention, Identification, and Management*, DOI 10.1007/978-3-319-09961-3_16,

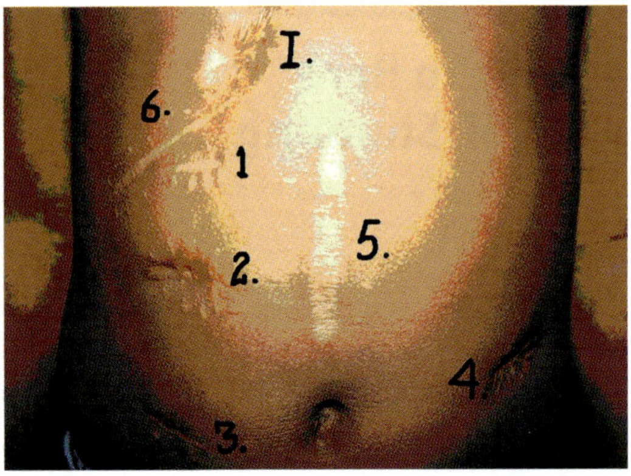

Fig. 16.1 Multiple abdominal scars indicate the prolonged morbidity. Scars *1–5* are the revisions due to blocked lower end secondary to pseudocyst formation. Scar "*I*" indicates scar formation due to retrograde CSF filling of the shunt track and erosion with infection. Scar *6* is the standard right subcostal incision used for the ventriculocholecysto shunt

the usefulness of these procedures in an otherwise recalcitrant situation. Some patients with these procedures are still in follow-up and do not require a conversion procedure [14, 22, 25].

These procedures include ventriculocholecysto (VC) shunt, ventriculosubgaleal (VSG) shunt, ventriculosinus shunt, and ventriculoureteral shunt.

These procedures are performed mainly when the routine procedures fail, making them temporary. They are technically more demanding, and with failure or complications, their revisions may be difficult or even impossible. Here we discuss their merits and complications and how they could be managed.

16.2 Ventriculocholecysto Shunt

It is the diversion of CSF from the ventricles to the gallbladder. It was introduced by Yarzagaray in 1958 [29] and recently modified by Lyngdoh [22].

The gallbladder is the preferred distal site as it is a sterile environment; its major activity is to remove water and electrolytes. The water flux rate is about 25 ml/h, with 90 % of water being removed in this process [29]. The CSF absorption is more physiological. The valves of gallbladder prevent reflux and maintain a constant pressure for CSF drainage.

The fundus of the gallbladder is exposed via standard right subcostal incision and two purse string sutures applied around the proposed site of the puncture, an inner one around the proposed opening and the other surrounding the inner purse string. The distal end of the shunt catheter with its slit valve is cut 7 cm from the distal tip and then reconnected over a connector, this being secured by silk sutures to prevent dislodgement. A stab puncture is made on the proposed site of the fundus, just enough to pass the catheter; bile sample for checking pressure and for culture may be taken with a needle prior to this [29]. The catheter is introduced to the level of the connector. The inner purse string is tightened snugly around the connector and to the serosa of the gallbladder within the outer purse string suture. This prevents dislodgement of the lower end. Finally, the outer purse string is tied to invert the whole complex [25]. A 20 cm length of catheter tubing is left within the peritoneum for the child's growth.

Using this shunt, CSF diversion was achieved for a 6-year follow-up [29, 31], while others, still on follow-up, have a functioning shunt [22]. Those that did require revision at a later time were diverted to the peritoneum, which had healed and regained its absorptive power [29].

Blockage due to high resistance to outflow from the cystic duct has caused failure within a few weeks in cases and with revision, infection developed. Revision to the gallbladder was thought to be impractical [25]. Retrograde flow of bile causing ventriculitis has been reported and could be fatal, some reversible with ventricular lavage. Cholangitis, infections of the biliary pathways, and cholelithiasis are not seen [29]. MR cholangiogram, at follow-up, does confirm that there is a small "hydrops" of the gallbladder (Fig. 16.2) [25, 29].

16.3 Ventriculosubgaleal Shunt

There is renewed interest in the diversion of CSF from the ventricular system to a pouch created in the subgaleal space, termed ventriculosubgaleal (VSG) shunt.

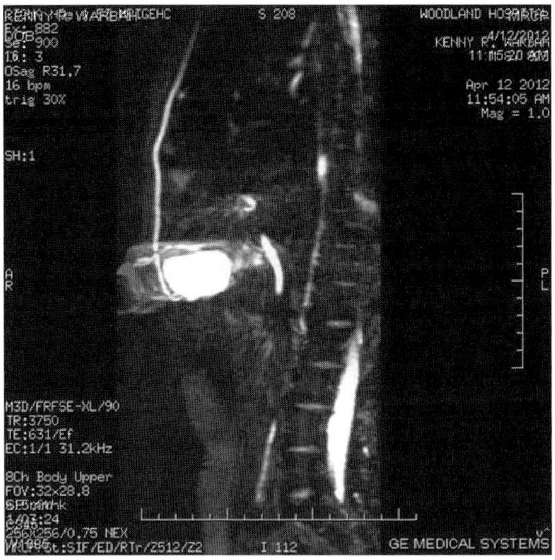

Fig. 16.2 Follow-up MR cholangiogram after 3.4 years showing the distal shunt tube in the gall bladder. There is a small "hydrops" of the gall bladder (Lyngdoh and Islam [22])

Von Mikulicz was probably the first to use this technique in 1893 [6]. The technique was improved and used since its initial description by many [5, 7, 8, 15, 16, 21, 26, 27].

It has been most beneficial for premature infants and neonates suffering intraventricular hemorrhage (IVH), meningitis with or without ventriculitis, and multiple congenital anomalies, for example, meningomyelocele with a colostomy for imperforate anus. There is a poor absorption from the peritoneum of the premature child.

Temporary diversion of CSF via a VSG shunt provides regular decompression of the ventricle system. It is a more attractive option than the other forms of temporary diversions in premature infants with hydrocephalus [18]. Other methods of temporary diversions can create more complications. The child suffers "puncture porencephaly" with repeated ventricular taps [17]. Repeated lumbar punctures are time-consuming and do not drain sufficiently; spinal osteomyelitis have been reported [3]. An external ventricular drain cannot be kept for a prolonged period of time. All these procedures have the risk of introducing infection.

The lateral ventricle is cannulated with a ventricular catheter via the standard coronal site and connected with a right-angled connector to 3 cm of shunt tubing with distal slit valves. The valves ensure unidirectional flow of fluid and debris. The connector is fixed to the dura. A subgaleal pocket is created with blunt dissection in the anterolateral and posterolateral directions from the coronal site. The catheter is then placed in the created pouch [17]. The space may get filled; this can then be tapped at intervals of a few days.

Conversion to a ventriculoperitoneal shunt could be done at 9.2 weeks; some did not require it [28]. It is the treatment of choice for neonatal hydrocephalus not suitable for a VP shunt at some centers [17].

Complications like wound leakage require the removal of the shunt. Other complications are similar to placement of a ventricular catheter such as acute hemorrhage following sudden decompression of the ventricles. This can be fatal. Dislodgement and intraventricular migration of the ventricular catheter. Many have reported no VSG shunt infection [17, 26, 27, 28]. Sklar, in 1992, reported a 10 % infection rate [30].

16.4 Ventriculosinus Shunts

In the past 35 years, several reports have described the superior sagittal sinus as a physiological and easily accessible site for distal catheter placement [1, 4, 19, 33].

More recently, El-Shafei demonstrated the success of the shunts into the sinus [7]. This evolved from his theoretical conclusion [9–13] that "CSF shunts should deliver the drained excess CSF from the ventricles into the upper end of the internal jugular vein (IJV) or into a dural sinus against the direction of blood flow such as a retrograde Ventriculo jugular shunt (RVJ) and retrograde Ventriculo sinus shunt (RVS). The dynamics of flow in theses shunts depend entirely on its being a watertight connection that allows no leakage of CSF"[10].

Here we shall describe the RVS shunt.

RVS shunt can be placed in any age group, a simpler and shorter procedure, minimally invasive [12, 13]. It can be used in the treatment of hydrocephalus regardless of the cause, type, degree, or duration, provided that diversion is indicated and with great success. Cerebral mantle of less than 1.0 cm in infants suffering advance-communicating hydrocephalus is a strict contraindication [14].

Valveless ventricular catheters were used, either through an anterior (anterior to the coronal suture) or a posterior parietal approach, the latter being preferred [14]. The ventricular end was introduced into the anterior horn of the lateral ventricle such that no CSF leaks from around the catheter at the dural hole and the catheter's venous end into the superior sagittal sinus, for a suitable distance, against the direction of blood flow [14].

With experience, this has proved to be a successful procedure as follow-up of up to 15 years and 4 months (mean 6 years 3 months) were recorded. 95.78 % patients benefited from this shunt [14].

Failures and complications that occurred with this procedure were due to:

CSF leakage because of dural injury and improper sealing of the dural hole around the catheter. Distal catheter impaction in a narrow superior sagittal sinus of an infant, superior sagittal sinus occlusion secondary to faulty ligature application (iatrogenic). Receding of the intrasinus catheter. Receding of the intraventricular catheter into the brain parenchyma following regression of ventriculomegaly. A 5 % infection rate. CSF leak is prevented by ensuring that the dural opening is circular and smaller than the ventricular catheter diameter. Making it fit snugly. Not to use a needle to search the superior sagittal sinus in infants. Introduced a longer catheter segment (5 cm) into the sinus of infants to prevent receding during head growth.

16.5 Ventriculoureteral Shunt

First reports of using the ureter for CSF diversion were by Matson [24] in 1951. Then, operations involved nephrectomies to achieve viable anastomosis between the shunt tubing and the urinary system. With the evolution of ventriculoperitoneal and ventriculoatrial shunts, urinary tract as a site for distal catheter placement was not favored.

There are, however, case reports of the urinary tract being used [2, 20, 25, 32].

Repeated revision of the distal sites, the peritoneum in particular, renders these sites nonabsorptive due to adhesions. Distal sites less frequently used are generally more challenging to access and more likely to be associated with complications, which can be serious [25]. Revision is difficult with such site being impossible to reuse.

There are three reported techniques for a ventriculoureteral (VU) shunt.

Smith's [32] technique is more favored. After ruling out urinary tract infection, the right ureter is transected 10 cm from the bladder and the distal end of the shunt tubing is connected to the distal ureteral stump via a connector. The distal end of the shunt tubing is then anchored to the psoas muscle without any constricting suture on the ureter. The proximal end of the ureter is reimplanted into the bladder medial to the original stump through a submucosal tunnel. The psoas hitch is applied to prevent tension on the shortened ureter.

Behrendt and Nau [2] describe a method where the shunt tubing is inserted into the renal pelvis, securing it with a purse string suture. Irby [20] describes a method where the shunt tubing was connected into the left ureter and then a uretero-ureterostomy was done.

Smith's technique has the advantage in that only one ureter is manipulated [20] and the shunt tubing is kept out of the urinary stream, which may decrease the likelihood of encrustation and infection [25]. Absence of vesicoureteral reflux or obstruction and the presence of a normal bladder is a prerequisite to this procedure. The procedure is contraindicated in cases of neurogenic bladder [32].

Complications such as dislodgement of the shunt tubing has been reported; protrusion of the shunt tubing from the urethral meatus has been reported too [23]. Revision is clearly a very difficult task due to severe scarring and distortion of anatomy. This may lead to further complications if revision is attempted.

References

1. Becker DP, Jane JA, Nulsen FE (1965) Investigation of sagittal sinus for venous shunt in hydrocephalus. Surg Forum 16:440–442
2. Behrendt H, Nau HE (1987) Ventriculo-renal shunt in the therapy of hydrocephalus (in German). Urologe A 26:331–333
3. Bergman I, Wald E, Meyer J, Painter M (1983) Epidural abscess and vertebral osteomyelitis following serial lumber punctures. Pediatrics 72:476–480
4. Borgesen SE, Gjerris F, Agerlin N (2002) Shunting to the sagittal sinus. Acta Neurochir Suppl (Wien) 81: 11–14
5. Dardenne G (1964) Le traitement par le drainage ventriculaire sous-cutane des fistules de liquid cephalorachidienpostoperatoiresrebelles. Acta neurol Psychiatr belg 64:1202–1211
6. Davidoff L (1929) Treatment of hydrocephalus. Arch Surg 18:1737–1762
7. Dereynaeker A (1948) De l'utilite du drainage ventriculairepreoperatoiredans les tumeurs de la fosse posterieure chez l'enfant. Acta Neurol Psychiatr Belg 48:68–78
8. Dogliotti A (1938) Sempliceprocedimento per la derivazionesottocutanea del liquor ventriculare. Arch Ital Chir 51:749–752
9. El-Shafei IL (1985) Ventriculo-jugular shunt against the direction of blood flow: a new approach for shunting the cerebrospinal fluid to the venous circulation. Childs Nerv Syst 1:200–207
10. El-Shafei IL (1987) Ventriculo-jugular shunt against the direction of blood flow II. Theoretical and experimental basis for shunting the cerebrospinal fluid against the direction of blood flow. Child Nerv Syst 3:285–291
11. El-Shafei IL, El-Rifaii MA (1987) Ventriculo-jugular shunt against the direction of blood flow. I. role of the internal jugular vein as an antisiphonage device. Childs Nerv Syst 3:282–284
12. El-Shafei IL, El-Shafe HI (2001) The retrograde ventriculo-sinus shunt: concept and technique for treating hydrocephalus by shunting the cerebrospinal fluid to the superior sagittal sinus against the direction of blood flow. Preliminary report. Childs Nerv Syst 17:457–465
13. El-Shafei IL, El-Shafe HI (2005) The retrograde ventriculo-sinus shunt (El-Shafei RVS shunt): rationale, evolution, surgical technique and long term results. Pediatr Neurosurg 41:305–317
14. El-Shafei IL, El-Shafe HI (2010) The retrograde ventriculovenous shunts: the El-Shafei retrograde ventriculojugular and ventriculosinus shunts. Pediatr Neurosurg 46:160–171
15. FerreiraN,CorreaJ(1972)Derivacaoliquoricaventriculosubcutaneanaterapeuticacirurgica das fistulas liquoricaspos-operatoriasrebeldes. Neurobiologica 35: 97–104
16. Fischer R (1967) Surgery of the congenital anomalies. In: Walker A (ed) A history of neurological surgery. Hafner Publishing, New york, pp 339–341
17. Fulmer BB, Grabb PA, Oakes W, Jerry W (2000) Neonatal ventriculosubgaleal shunts. J Neurosurg 47(1):80–84
18. Gurtner P, Bass T, Gudeman S, Gudeman S, Penix J, Philput C, Schinco F (1992) Surgical management of post hemorrhagic hydrocephalus in 22 low birth weight infants. Childs nerv Syst 8:198–202
19. Hash CJ, Shenkin HA, Crowder LE (1979) Ventricle to sagittal sinus shunt for hydrocephalus. Neurosurgery 4:394–400
20. Irby PB III, Wolf JS Jr, Schaeffer CS, Stoller ML (1993) Long term follow up of ventriculoureteral shunts for treatment of hydrocephalus. Urology 42:193–197
21. Koljubakin S (1924) Die operative therapie der hirnwassersucht. Arch Klin Chir Berl 128:151–161
22. Lyngdoh BT, Islam MS (2012) Ventriculocholecysto shunt: a solution to recurrent shunt complications in comorbid post-tubercular hydrocephalus with tubercular adhesive peritonitis. Acta Neurochir 154(12):2267–2270
23. Mador DR, Marshall FC (1981) Ventriculoureteral shunts for hydrocephalus without nephrectomy. J Urol 126:418
24. Matson DD (1951) Ventriculo-ureterostomy. J Neurosurg 8:398–404
25. Ohaegbulam C, Peters C, Goumnerova L (2004) Multiple successful revisions of a ventriculoureteral shunt without nephrectomy for the treatment of hydrocephalus: case report. Neurosurgery 55:E1027–E1031
26. Perret G, Graf C (1977) Subgaleal shunt for temporary ventricle decompression and subdural drainage. J Neurosurg 47:590–595
27. Perret G, Graf C (1978) Subgaleal shunt for ventricular and subdural drainage. J Neurosurg 49:474–475 (letter)
28. Rahman S, Teo C, Morris W, Lao D, Boop FA (1995) Ventriculosubgaleal shunt: a treatment option for progressive post hemorrhagic hydrocephalus. Childs Nerv Syst 11:650–654
29. Raimondi AJ (1998) Hydrocephalus. In: Raimondi AJ (ed) Theoretical principles-art of surgical techniques. (Pediatric neurosurgery). Springer, Berlin/Heidelberg/New York, pp 549–619
30. Sklar F, Adegbite A, Shapiro K, Miller K (1992) Ventriculosubgaleal shunts: management of posthemorrhagic hydrocephalus in premature infants. Pediatr Neurosurg 18:263–265
31. Smith GW, Moretz WH, Pritchard WL (1958) Ventriculo-biliary shunt. A new treatment of hydrocephalus. Surg Forum 9:701–705
32. Smith JA Jr, Lee RE, Middleton RG (1980) Ventriculoureteral shunt for hydrocephalus without nephrectomy. J Urol 123:224–226
33. Wen HL (1982) Ventriculo-superior sagittal sinus shunt for hydrocephalus. Surg Neurol 17:432–434

17 Cranio-cerebral Disproportion as a Late Complication

Concezio Di Rocco and Paolo Frassanito

Contents

17.1 **Introduction** 233

17.2 **Pathogenesis of ACCD: A Three Actors Drama** 234

17.2.1 The Shunt 235

17.2.2 The Brain 236

17.2.3 The Skull 237

17.3 **Diagnosis** 238

17.4 **Prevention** 240

17.5 **Treatment** 241

Conclusions 245

References 245

C. Di Rocco, MD (✉)
Pediatric Neurosurgery,
International Neuroscience Institute,
Hannover, Germany

Pediatric Neurosurgery, Institute of Neurosurgery,
Catholic University Medical School,
Largo A. Gemelli 8, 00168 Rome, Italy
e-mail: profconceziodirocco@gmail.com

P. Frassanito, MD
Pediatric Neurosurgery, Institute of Neurosurgery,
Catholic University Medical School,
Largo A. Gemelli 8, 00168 Rome, Italy
e-mail: paolo.frassanito@gmail.com

17.1 Introduction

As a broad definition cranio-cerebral disproportion (CCD) identifies all types of mismatch between the volume of the skull and its contents. These mismatches commonly occur in pathological conditions characterized by an excessive volume of the cerebrospinal fluid (CSF) (e.g., hydrocephalus) or, considerably more rarely, of the brain (e.g., macrocephaly, hemimegalencephaly). They also may take place in case of an excessively small skull unable to accommodate the growing brain (e.g., some forms of craniosynostosis). However, as a complication of extra-thecal CSF shunts, CCD refers to an acquired condition where the chronic CSF subtraction from the cranio-spinal theca exerted by the shunt results in a diminished force for the calvarial growth. The phenomenon finally leads to an abnormally small skull insufficient to guarantee the normal growth of the brain in infancy or, in subsequent ages, the compensation for the transitory volumetric increase of the intracranial content which occurs in specific physiological conditions. In this chapter, the definition ACCD (acquired cranio-cerebral disproportion) will be utilized to refer to this particular type of acquired mismatch which is occurring nearly always in subjects who had undergone the placement of an extra-thecal CSF shunting apparatus in infancy or early childhood [1]. Due to the nearly constant evidence of slit-like lateral cerebral ventricles in patients with ACCD, the misleading term of slit ventricle syndrome (SVS) has been

C. Di Rocco et al. (eds.), *Complications of CSF Shunting in Hydrocephalus: Prevention, Identification, and Management*, DOI 10.1007/978-3-319-09961-3_17,

frequently used in an interchangeable fashion with secondary ACCD in the literature. SVS consists of a clinical symptomatology of headache, vomiting, and impaired consciousness mimicking a malfunctioning CSF shunt. It was described by Becker and Nulsen in the early 1960s [2] as due to an inadequate drainage of CSF secondary to excessively small lateral cerebral ventricles in shunted hydrocephalic subjects. Unfortunately, SVS remains a poorly understood clinical entity, as this definition might apply to various pathological states and because small-sized ventricles are quite common in hydrocephalic children harboring CSF shunt drainage systems [3]. As most of these children do not exhibit any clinical manifestations, some authors advised to abandon this confusing term [4], while others proposed the definition of noncompliant ventricle syndrome [5] which obviously refers to those conditions in which a malfunctioning CSF shunt is not associated to dilation of the lateral cerebral ventricles because of an acquired abnormal rigidity of their walls. A restricted use of this definition has been advocated with the aim of excluding those conditions that could be explained on the base of an intermittent CSF shunt malfunctioning due to an overdraining or partially obstructed CSF shunt device and those pathological conditions still characterized by small-sized lateral cerebral ventricles which occur in unshunted subjects (e.g., pseudotumor cerebri) [6]. Consequently, SVS would strictly define the association of symptoms of raised intracranial pressure in patients with the radiological evidence of a working shunt. This condition may be isolated or associated to ACCD that may be eventually considered a subgroup of SVS.

17.2 Pathogenesis of ACCD: A Three Actors Drama

A shunt that works "too well" may end up with complications secondary to chronic drainage of the CSF [7]. This group of complications includes subdural hygromas, postshunting craniosynostosis, SVS, and ACCD, which probably share common pathogenetic mechanisms, though still not completely understood [8].

SVS became the subject of great interest in the 1980s when the wide availability of neuroimaging investigations led to recognize that a large percentage of operated hydrocephalic patients presented very small slit-like ventricles. Signs and symptoms of raised intracranial pressure such as headache, vomiting, and drowsiness finally progress to coma and eventually death in case of the classical CSF shunt obstruction. On the contrary, if these signs and symptoms appear to fade away spontaneously or following the medical treatment, the etiology was hypothesized to depend on an intermittent CSF shunt dysfunction. The typical course of the complication would have been characterized firstly by the ventricular walls of the slit-like ventricles abutting on the tip of the endoventricular catheter and causing its transient obstruction. Secondly, the immediately following ventricular dilation, due to the temporary blockage of the shunt, would have allowed, according to the proposed pathogenetic mechanism, the shunt to work again so compensating for the increased intracranial pressure and explaining the intermittent clinical manifestations [9]. The hypothesis was challenged since the beginning, as the propounded condition would end up in the definitive obstruction of the shunt and its overt shunt malfunction more likely than resulting in a prolonged intermittent clinical symptomatology. Furthermore, in the clinical practice, all possible states of patency of the shunt had been found besides ventricular catheters partially obstructed by ependymal or gliotic debris in patients undergoing CSF shunt revision, most of them having been found to harbor still unobstructed devices. However, the most compelling evidence against the theory is that up to 60–70 % of children with shunted hydrocephalus present slit-like ventricles at the CT scan control, that is an anatomical situation apt to favor the "intermittent" obstruction of the endoventricular catheter, but only a minority of them, less than 1 % of the cases, actually presents clinical manifestations of a malfunctioning CSF shunt [6].

Data about ACCD available in the literature are poor since a significant proportion of the affected patients were actually included in the misleading category of SVS. The prevalence of

Table 17.1 Synopsis of the main features differentiating symptomatic CSF overdrainage from SVS and ACCD

Features		CSF overdrainage	SVS	ACCD
Clinical features	Age at shunt placement	Not related	<3 years	<3 years
	Shunt valve pressure	Usually low	Not related	Not related
	Delay to clinical onset (from shunt placement)	Short	Medium–long	Long
	Symptoms related to posture	Yes	No	No
	Course of symptoms	Continuous	Intermittent	Intermittent
Radiological features	Slit-like ventricles	Yes	Yes	Yes
	Other signs of acute overdrainage (e.g., subdural hygroma/hematoma)	Yes	No	No
	Subarachnoid spaces	Well represented	Represented	Effaced
	Crowded posterior cranial fossa	No	No	Yes (+/– Chiari)
	Bone modifications	No	No	Yes

SVS widely ranges from 1 %, that is found in papers including only symptomatic SVS [6], to 37 %, that is found in case of exclusively radiological definition of SVS [10]. For the same reason, that is the missed identification of ACCD from the cases of symptomatic SVS, the specific characteristics and the specific pathogenetic mechanisms of the condition have been the subject only of a few studies. Probably, SVS and ACCD may be considered a continuum of the same condition sharing a common pathogenesis. The events dynamically leading to this intriguing complications of shunted hydrocephalic subjects may be represented like a drama played by three actors, namely, the shunt, the brain, and the skull.

17.2.1 The Shunt

The extra-thecal CSF shunt device is undoubtedly the actor in the leading role of the drama. Its presence and its action are necessary for the development of the ACCD. Thus, it is easy to understand why the CSF shunt devices received so much interest by the researchers.

The insertion of a CSF draining system induces an intracranial hypotension due to the rapid subtraction of CSF from the ventricular system. This intracranial hypotension, which occurs immediately after the operation, generally fades away after some days or weeks due to natural adaptation of the organism to the new "physiological" equilibrium between CSF fluid production and its artificially enhanced reabsorption. However, the secondary intracranial hypotension determined by the shunt may fail to be compensated without clinical disturbances in case of excessive CSF drainage especially when the apparently adequate draining action of the shunt device is exacerbated by the "suction" effect added by the upright position of the infant. The strict temporal relation between the appearance of clinical signs and symptoms of an excessively low intracranial pressure and the insertion of shunt usually leads to the prompt recognition of the overdrainage and to its immediate correction.

More difficult can be the recognition of CSF overdrainage when its clinical manifestations occur late, that is months or years after the CSF shunt placement. The clinical features of these complications differ from those revealing a CSF overdrainage in the early postoperative period not only for the longer temporal interval but also for the frequently absent relation with the posture and for its common intermittent nature (Table 17.1). Accurate neurological evaluation and repeated neuroimaging studies may be then necessary to recognize the etiology of the symptoms and for the differential diagnosis from other conditions, also presenting with headache, vomiting, and eventually some degree of consciousness impairment, namely migraine. The presence of slit-like ventricles may contribute to the diagnosis with, however, the already mentioned limit of the large proportion of shunted hydrocephalic children with small-sized ventricle and no clinical disturbances.

Even more difficult to recognize early is the subtle "overdrainage" that takes places for years without any clinical complaint. Although not yet sufficiently investigated it is quite likely that in several shunted patients the chronic depletion of CSF from the intra-thecal space exerted by the CSF draining device may result not only in a lower intracranial pressure but also in a diminished intracranial CSF volume, a phenomenon of which slit lateral cerebral ventricles are the most typical heralds at the neuroimaging controls. Indeed, while CT or MR investigations easily detect the volumetric reduction of the lateral cerebral ventricles, in the clinical practice less attention is usually paid to the concomitant reduction in size of the cerebral cisterns and of the subarachnoid spaces of the cerebral convexities. This type of phenomenon is so common that a progressive reduction in size of the cerebral lateral ventricle volume, which is not accompanied by an increase of the volume of the peripheral subarachnoid spaces, rather by its reduction, is accepted as a "normal" effect of the CSF shunt and the evidence of a satisfactorily working extra-thecal CSF draining apparatus. To understand the impact of this type of event in the genesis of an ACCD it is necessary to call into the play the remaining two actors of the drama.

17.2.2 The Brain

The brain is the supporting actor of the drama, accounting for the occurrence of the clinical manifestations in symptomatic cases. Actually, when this actor is not able to perform, namely, in case of atrophy, ACCD is an exceptional event. The intrinsic role of the brain in the genesis of the complication here considered is further demonstrated by the rare occurrence of ACCD in patients shunted in adult age, although in such patients the gradient of the hydrostatic pressure, that is the main factor favoring overdrainage, is higher than in children. In other terms, a necessary factor for the establishment of an ACCD is a brain able to expand in order to compensate for an abnormal volumetric reduction of the ventricles, cisternal, and peripheral subarachnoid spaces. Such an expansion can be a real cerebral growth, as it occurs in the first years of life. More commonly, in subsequent ages, the main cause for the brain to occupy the space, made available by the reduced volume of the ventricles and subarachnoid spaces, is the turgor of the brain determined by the dilation of the cerebral veins associated to the chronically low intracranial pressure related to the continuous depletion of CSF by the extra-thecal CSF shunt device. In the long run, the phenomenon will progressively account for further volumetric reduction of the CSF space that is the disappearance of the peripheral subarachnoid spaces and slit-like ventricles, easily detected on the neuroimaging studies. The increased elastance of the brain, the dilation of the cerebral venous structures, and the volumetric reduction of the CSF space will then account for the reduced ability of the patients to compensate for transient increases in intracranial pressure and for the reduced possibility of the ventricular system to enlarge. Actually, the attention of scientists has been longtime focused on the last aspect, that is on the excessively small ventricular cavities apparently unable to enlarge even when the clinical manifestations of the patients seemed to indicate a CSF shunt malfunctioning. The most shared interpretation was that the chronic drainage of CSF would have led to rigid ventricular walls, thereby preventing the ventricles to dampen any increase in intraventricular volume. Based upon animal studies, it was also suggested that the long-standing presence of a ventricular catheter could have promoted subependymal gliosis, which also contributed to the rigidity of the ventricular walls [11]. However, ex vivo studies have documented that the degree of subependymal gliosis is no different in subjects with dilated or nondilated ventricles at shunt malfunction [12].

Thus, the noncompliant ventricles should be considered the effect of the dynamic unbalance created by the long-standing action of the shunt device rather than the cause of the clinical manifestations presumed to depend on an intermittent and transitory malfunctioning of the CSF shunt apparatus.

The role of a possibly impaired venous outflow in ACCD is still matter of discussion. Albeit in some cases overt stenosis of the main venous sinuses may be identified [13], a venous outflow impairment has been hypothesized and recently attributed to a condition defined as "capillary absorption laziness" [14]. At the moment, however, it is not possible to draw any definitive conclusion on the subject, as a venous outflow impairment in ACCD could be either the cause or the effect of the increased cerebral pressure, resulting in both cases in a modification of the viscoelastic properties of the brain and in its subsequent decreased ability to compensate for increases in intracranial volume [15].

Finally, it is interesting to note how the size of the ventricles has received so much attention, while so scant attention has been paid to the volume of the subarachnoid spaces. Although in SVS there is dissociation between the low intraventricular pressure and the high subarachnoid pressure, the volume of the subarachnoid spaces still allows some degree of brain compliance. On the other side, in case of ACCD the nearly complete obliteration of the cisternal and peripheral CSF space would prevent any physical possibility for the brain to increase its volume so resulting in a more severe pathological condition.

17.2.3 The Skull

The third actor involved in the drama is the skull. As Hoffman observed in 1976, the placement of the CSF shunt may dramatically decrease the pressure exerted by the growing brain, thus arresting the growth of the skull. As a consequence, "when brain volume has increased to occupy the space provided by diminished ventricular size, the neurocranium must enlarge, but this may not readily occur after a period of arrested growth. The result is a state of cephalocranial disproportion as brain volume exceeds the available [intracranial] space" [16]. The phenomenon described by the author is what actually leads to a secondary "craniosynostosis." It occurs mainly in infants and in the first months after the placement of a CSF shunting device. A more subtle "overdrainage" which persists for years and even the mere presence of the shunt also diminishes the pressure forces of the intracranial content which act on the calvarium and assure the physiological equilibrium between bone absorption and formation. Dampened CSF pulses and chronically low mean intracranial pressure result in excessive deposition of lamellar bone at the inner surface of the calvarium. The phenomenon represents a reactive change of the skull aimed at compensating the reduced volume of the intracranial content. In some patients, however, it results in the excessive reduction of the volume of the subarachnoid spaces which in normal condition assure to the brain the possibility to expand or, more in general, to accommodate the physiological volumetric changes related to the cerebrovascular dynamics. Thickened skull vault, prematurely fused cranial sutures, hyperpneumatosis of the air sinus cavities, and impacted posterior fossa constitute the radiological evidences of the effect of the long-standing intracranial fluid subtraction determined by the extra-thecal CSF shunt device.

This bone "compensation" phase can last several years without clinical symptoms. However, the brain compliance and the possibility of the cerebral ventricle to enlarge diminish progressively during such a phase until the reduced cranial volume and the concomitant changes in cerebrovascular compliance result in a symptomatic ACCD.

In conclusion, the interaction of three actors is essential for the drama to take place. However, the role of a single actor may be prevalent in a given subject so reminding what can happen when a single actor plays alone that is the skull in cases of osteopetrosis or craniosynostosis, the brain in case of pseudotumor cerebri, and the shunt in case of CSF overdrainage. All these conditions are characterized by CCD, the etiology of which is, however, easy to be recognized. Only the ACCD is multifactorial and difficult to be diagnosed in its early stages, as it requires years to fully establish.

When the role of one actor is prevalent different complications may occur before or during the establishment of a condition of CCD. For example, the mismatch between the volume of

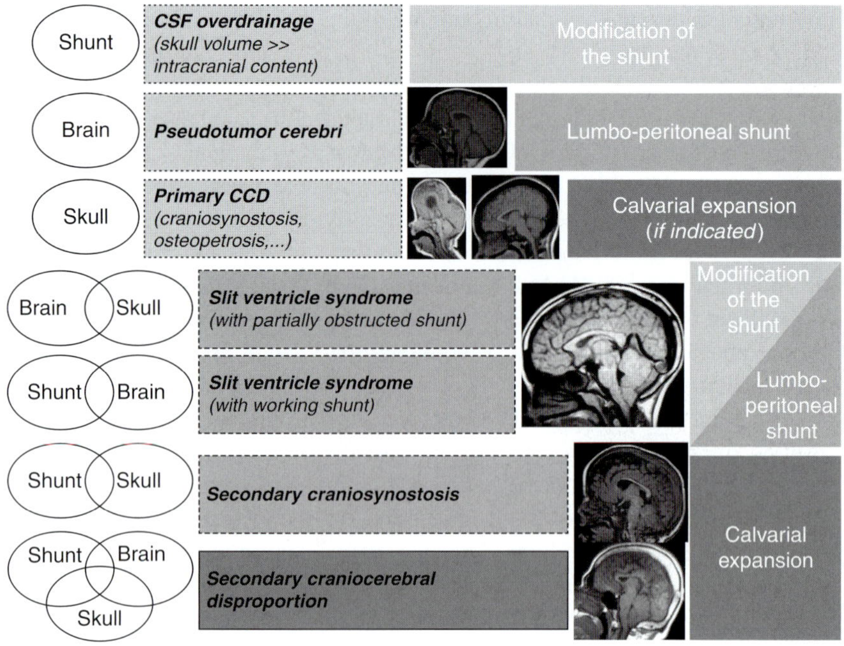

Fig. 17.1 Synopsis of the pathogenesis of ACCD and possibly related syndromes, according to the prevailing action of the shunt, the brain, and the skull *(see the text for further details)*

the brain and that of skull caused by an overdraining CSF shunt may be complicated by the occurrence of subdural hematomas. Two actors playing together may result in brain turgor and SVS (with working shunt) without any role of the skull, while the last actor may be particularly involved when an atrophic brain is not able to expand sufficiently. In the last occurrence, the action of the extra-thecal CSF shunt may induce over-riding and premature fusion of the cranial sutures with the development of microcrania, as described by Faulhauer and Schmitz [17]. Finally, the partial failure of the first actor, that is the CSF shunt device, while the two remaining actors still play, is clinically translated by the intermittent clinical manifestations of a partially obstructed ventricular catheter, the surgical revision of which usually results only in a relief of the symptoms (Fig. 17.1).

17.3 Diagnosis

The clinical history is usually that of a subject with a hydrocephalus shunted before the age of 2–3 years, albeit anecdotal cases of ACCD following shunting of an endocranial arachnoid cyst have been described [18–20].

As headache is often the first complaint, the diagnostic algorithms aim at differentiating between headache independent from the shunt from headache due to shunt malfunction, SVS with working shunt, and ACCD [5]. In case of migraine, an appropriate medical treatment often solves the diagnostic dilemma. Similarly, headache disappears after CSF shunt surgical revision in case of shunt malfunction. This result is persistent in time, at least until the next shunt malfunctioning, so confirming the direct relation between the headache and the shunt failure. On the other hand, the differential diagnosis between SVS and ACCD requires the integration of clinical and instrumental data because of the characteristic intermittence of the symptoms and the frequent illusory improvement which follows the revision of the shunt. Even the analysis of the clinical manifestations may be difficult as patients complain of chronic, debilitating headaches that in some cases are prevalent in the nuchal region, so heralding the possible descent of the cerebellar tonsils into the upper cervical canal (Fig. 17.2). In general, the clinical manifestations are progressively worsening and may impact considerably on the social life and on the well-being of the patient. In some cases the diagnosis is unnecessarily delayed by the hypothesis of

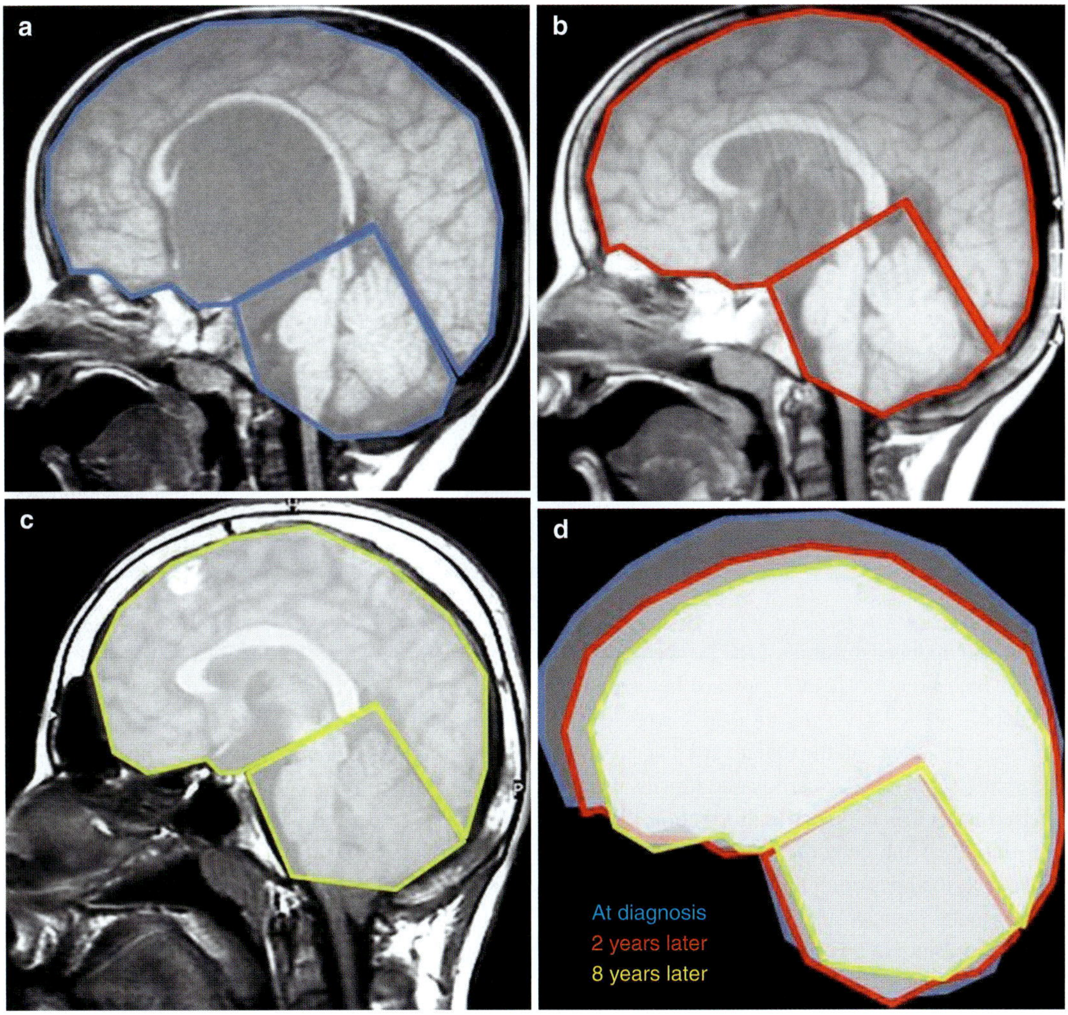

Fig. 17.2 MRI examinations of a 5-month-old boy affected by a large suprasellar arachnoid cyst, in particular at diagnosis (**a**), 2 and 8 years after placement of a cysto-ventriculo-peritoneal shunt (**b**, **c**, respectively). Rendering of the progressive restriction of the supratentorial and infratentorial compartment volumes (**d**)

psychological or merely "functional" disturbances. The clinical picture may be further complicated by additional signs and symptoms of intermittent abnormal elevations in ICP, such as diplopia, ataxia, dizziness, and lethargy. It is worth to note in order to emphasize the need of a prompt diagnosis that acute neurologic deterioration secondary to ACCD evolving rapidly to sudden death has also been described [1].

Collapsed ventricles and absent or small volume subarachnoid spaces, together with a thickened vault of the skull are the usual neuroimaging findings of ACCD (Fig. 17.3). In particular, skull X-ray films or bone window images on the CT scan may document the progressive thickening of the cranial vault, due to the deposition of laminated bone at the inner surface of the skull, the typical appearance of the "copper beaten skull," the presence of "thumbprintings," and hyperpneumatosis of the air sinus cavities. Parenchymal window images on the CT scan or MRI studies show slit-like ventricles, lack of CSF signal over the convexities following the obliteration of the cortical subarachnoid spaces, effacement of the cisterns, and, often, a crowded posterior fossa (with or without cerebellar tonsillar herniation) [1]. Cranial volumetric studies may confirm the global reduction in size of the inner cranial volume in a high percentage of the patients and, in several cases,

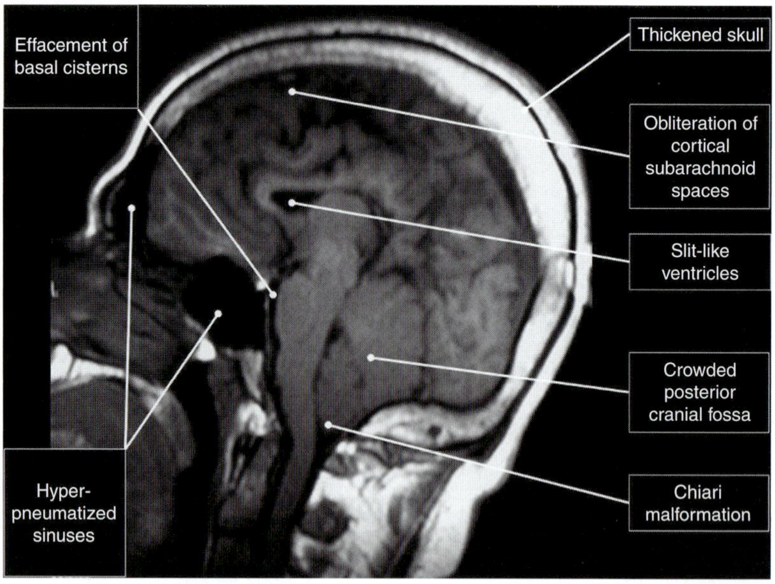

Fig. 17.3 Main radiological findings of ACCD

a markedly reduced volume of the posterior cranial fossa which accounts for the upward herniation of the upper cerebellar vermis into the cistern of the great vein of Galen and the downward displacement of the inferior cerebellar vermis and tonsils, usually referred to as Chiari type I malformation [20, 21]. The impact of the cerebrovascular structures contained in a small posterior cranial fossa may be exacerbated in the younger subjects by the robust growth of the cerebellum in postnatal life [22].

To summarize, the peculiar modifications of the calvarium, together with the evidence of effaced subarachnoid spaces are essential to differentiate ACCD from SVS.

Although the association of the clinical manifestations mimicking those of a malfunctioning CSF shunt and the just mentioned radiological findings usually drives the correct diagnosis, the use of ICP monitoring has been advocated by some authors. This examination may rule out an increased intracranial pressure while documenting the presence of plateau waves, thereby confirming the reduced compliance of the brain [1].

17.4 Prevention

As ACCD is the inherent complication of a working extra-thecal CSF shunt, the only reliable prevention would be avoiding the placement of such a type of device. Indeed, it is what is happening in several cases of hydrocephalus nowadays managed endoscopically. When endoscopic third ventriculostomy is not possible, prevention of ACCD is mainly based on the choice of a CSF apparatus apt to reduce the risk of overdrainage. Unfortunately, in spite of the many currently available devices, the overall clinical experience indicates that the "perfect" draining system does not exist yet. However, some manufacturing companies claim a better function of their own products as the result of a specific attention paid to avoid an excessive drainage. The common target of these CSF shunt devices is avoiding or at least limiting the effect of the hydrostatic pressure associated to the standing position of the patients. The research has been mainly addressed at controlling the flow of the CSF through the valve of the shunting apparatus in order to maintain it as constant as possible independently from the position of the patient and the value of the intracranial CSF pressure or at providing a valve which restricts the passage of CSF when the subject is standing so preventing the siphoning effect. The currently available types of apparatus are considerably more effective than the previous antisiphon devices, which could be added to the extra-thecal CSF draining system and depended on the direct effect of the atmosphere pressure. Actually, the function of these devices, which were placed along the course of the distal catheter of the shunt system, could be impaired by local structural changes of the overlying skin during the course of time.

17.5 Treatment

The treatment of an established ACCD is not easy, thus further stressing the need to prevent it.

The difficulties in differentiating the condition from other types of inadequate CSF drainage in operated hydrocephalic subjects coupled with the still incompletely understood pathogenetic mechanisms justify the numerous and different approaches that have been adopted in facing this complication.

Some approaches are utilized simply to impede further progression of the cerebro-cranial disproportion and aim at re-establishing a normal ventricular volume while limiting the presumed overdrainage of the valve apparatus. Upgrading of the pressure opening value of the CSF shunt apparatus [2] or adding to the *in situ* CSF shunt system an antisiphon device [23, 24] are the most common examples of such a policy, the results of which remain nevertheless controversial [25, 26]. A more physiological approach is represented by the attempts to correct the condition and its progression by performing an endoscopic third ventriculostomy and removing the existing CSF extra-thecal shunting device. However, the small size of the lateral and third cerebral ventricles and the noncompliant brain limit such an option to a few selected cases [27]. A more complex physiopathogenetic interpretation accounts for other surgical approaches which hypothesize different levels of pressure within the ventricles (low pressure) and the subarachnoid spaces (high pressure) and aim at removing fluid from the peripheral spaces. In the clinical practice, the most utilized surgical maneuver based on such a theory is the placement of a lumbo-peritoneal CSF shunt, in nearly all the cases leaving the ventriculo-peritoneal shunt in site. Those surgeons who favor such a type of treatment emphasize the good success of lumbo-peritoneal CSF shunt in cases of SVS or pseudotumor cerebri and the clinical and functional similarities that these conditions share with ACCD, namely, the young age, the inadequate CSF drainage, and the turgor of the brain with its diminished compliance [4, 28, 29]. However, the long-term efficacy of lumbo-peritoneal shunting has been questioned [1]. Main concern is that the chronic drainage of the subarachnoid spaces would eventually cause a worsening of the ACCD and favor the caudal descent of the cerebellar tonsils into the upper cervical canal, a feared complication of lumbo-peritoneal CSF shunting.

Also the attempts to treat ACCD with the procedures utilized to treat SVS were not successful. In 1974 Epstein introduced the subtemporal craniectomy with the aim of favoring ventricular expansion so allowing the intraventricular catheter of the CSF shunt system still to work also in cases of brain transitory swelling [30]. Unfortunately, this procedure has unreliable outcomes in the clinical practice, as the impact of the atmospheric pressure is increased by the partial removal of cranial vault, so actually favoring overdrainage and finally eliminating the ventricular dilation which can occur immediately after the operation. A modified technique including opening of the dura and arachnoid layer has been recently proposed, resulting in the dilation of slit-like ventricles after surgery but burdened by the same risk, that is the exposition to the atmospheric pressure accounting for the failures which ensue the utilization of the Epstein's procedure [31].

A further option to control the clinical manifestations of ACCD and avoid its further progression is a procedure which we utilized in a few patients with success. This procedure consists of diverting a proportion of the CSF drained by the extra-thecal CSF draining system into the cervical subarachnoid space by means of a catheter connected to the distal catheter of the shunting device with a Y connector and reaching the spinal subarachnoid space. The rationale is to not deplete the intrathecal CSF volume while leaving the existing device to compensate for the abnormally elevated mean and pulse pressure. Indeed, the role of excessively large CSF pulsations as those which likely occur in the presence of a poorly compliant brain and a skull, the volume of which is reduced for the secondary inner hyperostosis, is probably insufficiently considered at the light of experimental studies unequivocally demonstrating their role in inducing a ventricular dilation [32].

A second type of approach to treat ACCD does not take into account the harbored CSF shunt device but the secondary "hypoplastic" skull. The surgical technique utilized for expanding the cranial vault and, consequently, the intracranial volume vary in the different neurosurgical centers. All these techniques, however, are favored by the improvement in manipulating the cranial bone determined by the recent progresses in the treatment of craniosynostosis [33] (Fig. 17.4). The anterior frontal bone displacement that is the creation of a free bone flap which is replaced in a more advanced position has the advantage of correcting also the cosmetic defect that in some subjects is produced by the secondary retrusion and modified angulation of the frontal bone on the skull base. The bilateral outward expansion of the parietal bone, with a greenstick fracture at their base or, in some cases, with the aid of bone distractors is also effective though less rewarding cosmetically [34, 35]. Finally, the posterior expansion of the occipital region and the enlargement of the posterior cranial fossa are preferred in cases where these sectors of the skull are particularly thickened so to reduce the intracranial volume significantly. It is in such occurrence that ACCD determinates the caudal descent of the cerebellar tonsils and the upward displacement of the superior cerebellar vermis to occupy the prevermian cistern and the cistern of the great vein of Galen. The secondary impact of the cerebral, cerebellar, and vascular structures within the reduced occipital and posterior cranial fossa is resolved by the posterior displacement of the occipital bone and suboccipital squama which can be obtained by in groove movement of these bones or by means of springs or distractors. In case where the cranial vault is extensively thickened the desired increase in intracranial volume may be obtained by simply drilling the inner surface and the diploe of the pathologically modified bone which then can be replaced in its previous position (Fig. 17.5).

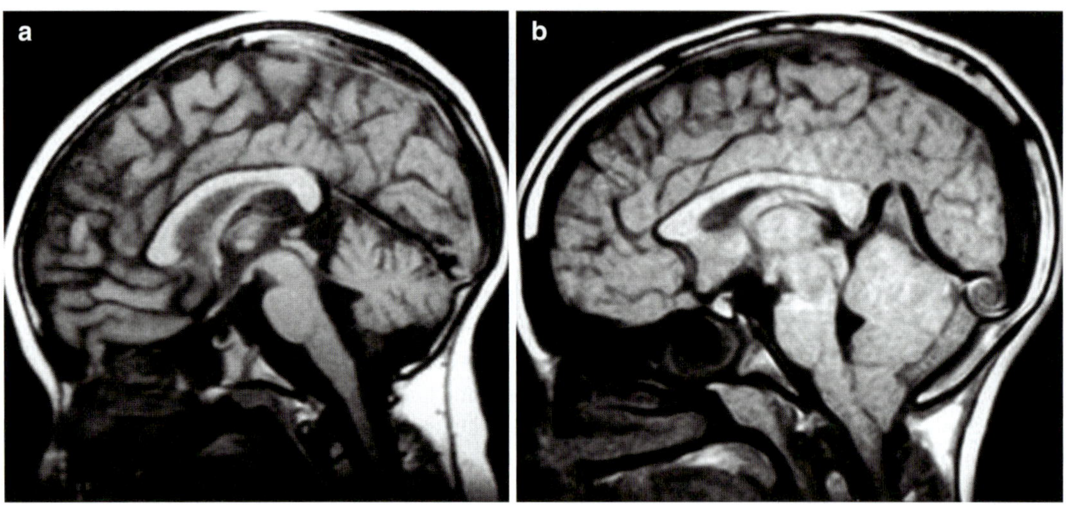

Fig. 17.4 Evolution toward ACCD in the follow-up MRI examinations of a patient shunted in the first year of life for congenital hydrocephalus, in particular 1 year (**a**), 4 years (**b**), 7 years after shunting (**c**). Biparietal expansion was performed to treat ACCD (**d**). Intraoperative picture and CT scan 3D reconstruction showing the bone flaps kept in the expanded position by means of two autologous bone grafts (respectively **e** and **f**, *arrows*). MRI confirming the results of the calvarial expansion, in particular the reduction in the caudal dislocation of the cerebellar tonsils (**g**)

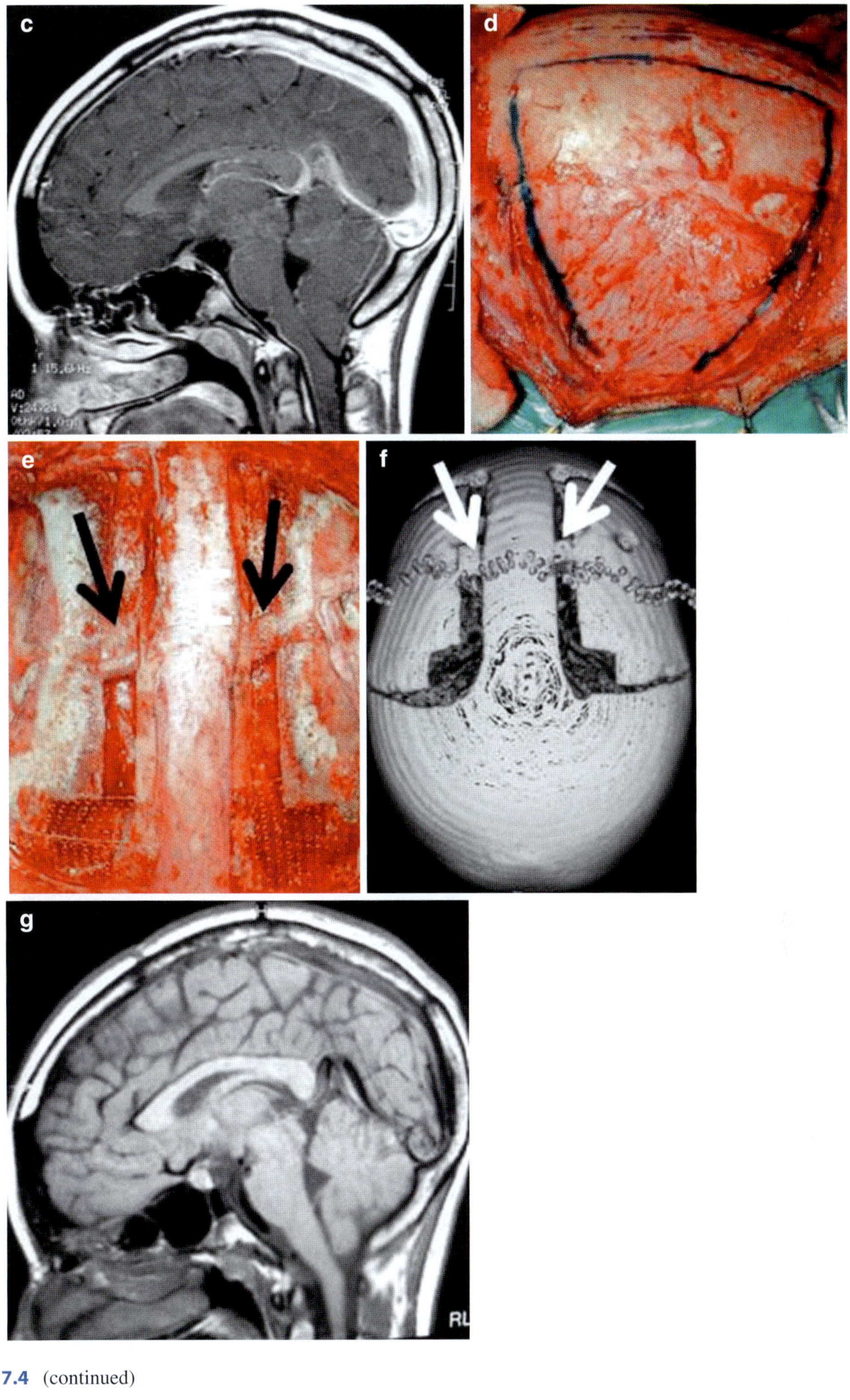

Fig. 17.4 (continued)

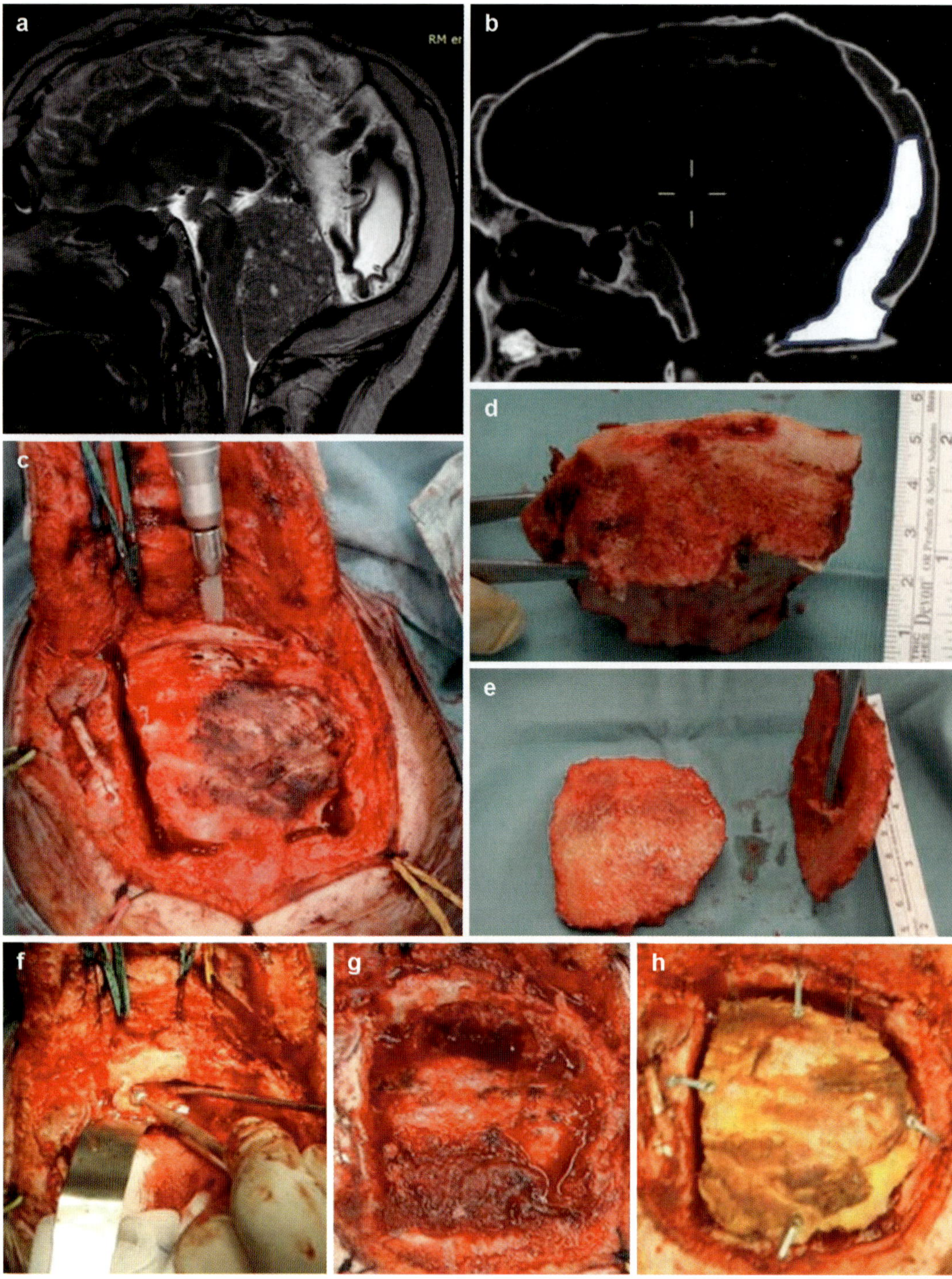

Fig. 17.5 18-year-old boy shunted in the first year of life, who underwent calvarial expansion 10 years later to treat ACCD. Seven years after cranial expansion he started to complain of debilitating nuchal headache. Sagittal MRI showing prevailing posterior cranial fossa ACCD (**a**). Sagittal CT scan showing the augmentation of intracranial space *(white area)*, after occipital calvarial expansion (**b**). The main steps of the surgical procedure: craniotomy performed with the aid of the oscillating saw (**c**), due to the hyperostosis of the calvarial bone (**d**), splitting of the bone flap (**e**), internal decompression of the suboccipital bone and the foramen magnum by means of high speed drill and bone rongeurs (**f**, **g**), and fixation of the outer layer of the bone flap (**h**)

Conclusions

ACCD is a late complication of the management of hydrocephalus based on the placement on an extra-thecal CSF shunt device. The genesis is multifactorial with the contribution of the chronic action of the shunt and the secondarily induced changes in brain compliance and intracranial volume. In the first phases of its development, ACCD should be considered an expected outcome of a functioning shunt which, however, successively becomes a clinical complication when the reduced volume of the cerebral ventricles, peripheral CSF spaces, and skull interferes with the normal CSF dynamics and exposes the subject to intermittent pathological increases in intracranial pressure. Avoiding the placement of an extra-thecal CSF shunt device whenever possible remains the best prevention. When this is not possible, the appropriate choice of the CSF shunt device might contribute at reducing the risk of its occurrence. Once established, ACCD may be controlled by modifying the functional characteristics of the harbored CSF device, by using a different CSF shunt system, or creating a new way for the CSF drainage. However, in most cases the enlargement on the intracranial volume with technical procedures similar to those commonly adopted in the management of craniosynostosis appears as the most effective and reliable therapeutic maneuver.

References

1. Sandler AL, Goodrich JT, Daniels LB 3rd, Biswas A, Abbott R (2013) Craniocerebral disproportion: a topical review and proposal toward a new definition, diagnosis, and treatment protocol. Childs Nerv Syst 29(11):1997–2010
2. Becker DP, Nulsen FE (1968) Control of hydrocephalus by valve-regulated venous shunt: avoidance of complications in prolonged shunt maintenance. J Neurosurg 28(3):215–226
3. Rekate HL (1993) Classification of slit-ventricle syndromes using intracranial pressure monitoring. Pediatr Neurosurg 19(1):15–20
4. Sood S, Barrett RJ, Powell T, Ham SD (2005) The role of lumbar shunts in the management of slit ventricles: does the slit-ventricle syndrome exist? J Neurosurg 103(2 Suppl):119–123
5. Olson S (2004) The problematic slit ventricle syndrome. A review of the literature and proposed algorithm for treatment. Pediatr Neurosurg 40(6):264–269
6. Di Rocco C (1994) Is the slit ventricle syndrome always a slit ventricle syndrome? Childs Nerv Syst 10(1):49–58
7. Walker ML, Fried A, Petronio J (1993) Diagnosis and treatment of the slit ventricle syndrome. Neurosurg Clin N Am 4(4):707–714
8. Cheok S, Chen J, Lazareff J (2014) The truth and coherence behind the concept of overdrainage of cerebrospinal fluid in hydrocephalic patients. Childs Nerv Syst 30(4):599–606
9. Epstein F, Lapras C, Wisoff JH (1988) 'Slit-ventricle syndrome': etiology and treatment. Pediatr Neurosci 14(1):5–10
10. Serlo W, Heikkinen E, Saukkonen AL, von Wendt L (1985) Classification and management of the slit ventricle syndrome. Childs Nerv Syst 1(4):194–199
11. Oi S, Matsumoto S (1986) Morphological findings of postshunt slit-ventricle in experimental canine hydrocephalus. Aspects of causative factors of isolated ventricles and slit-ventricle syndrome. Childs Nerv Syst 2(4):179–184
12. Del Bigio MR (2002) Neuropathological findings in a child with slit ventricle syndrome. Pediatr Neurosurg 37(3):148–151
13. Bateman GA (2013) Hypertensive slit ventricle syndrome: pseudotumor cerebri with a malfunctioning shunt? J Neurosurg 119(6):1503–1510
14. Jang M, Yoon SH (2013) Hypothesis for intracranial hypertension in slit ventricle syndrome: new concept of capillary absorption laziness in the hydrocephalic patients with long-term shunts. Med Hypotheses 81(2):199–201
15. Pang D, Altschuler E (1994) Low-pressure hydrocephalic state and viscoelastic alterations in the brain. Neurosurgery 35(4):643–655; discussion 55–6
16. Hoffman HJ, Tucker WS (1976) Cephalocranial disproportion. A complication of the treatment of hydrocephalus in children. Childs Brain 2(3):167–176
17. Faulhauer K, Schmitz P (1978) Overdrainage phenomena in shunt treated hydrocephalus. Acta Neurochir (Wien) 45(1–2):89–101
18. Lazareff JA, Kelly J, Saito M (1998) Herniation of cerebellar tonsils following supratentorial shunt placement. Childs Nerv Syst 14(8):394–397
19. Di Rocco C, Tamburrini G (2003) Shunt dependency in shunted arachnoid cyst: a reason to avoid shunting. Pediatr Neurosurg 38(3):164
20. Di Rocco C, Velardi F (2003) Acquired Chiari type I malformation managed by supratentorial cranial enlargement. Childs Nerv Syst 19(12):800–807
21. Osuagwu FC, Lazareff JA, Rahman S, Bash S (2006) Chiari I anatomy after ventriculoperitoneal shunting: posterior fossa volumetric evaluation with MRI. Childs Nerv Syst 22(11):1451–1456
22. Knickmeyer RC, Gouttard S, Kang C, Evans D, Wilber K, Smith JK et al (2008) A structural MRI study of human brain development from birth to 2 years. J Neurosci 28(47):12176–12182

23. Portnoy HD, Schulte RR, Fox JL, Croissant PD, Tripp L (1973) Anti-siphon and reversible occlusion valves for shunting in hydrocephalus and preventing post-shunt subdural hematomas. J Neurosurg 38(6):729–738
24. Gruber RW, Roehrig B (2010) Prevention of ventricular catheter obstruction and slit ventricle syndrome by the prophylactic use of the Integra antisiphon device in shunt therapy for pediatric hypertensive hydrocephalus: a 25-year follow-up study. J Neurosurg Pediatr 5(1):4–16
25. Drake LA, Shear NH, Arlette JP, Cloutier R, Danby FW, Elewski BE et al (1997) Oral terbinafine in the treatment of toenail onychomycosis: North American multicenter trial. J Am Acad Dermatol 37(5 Pt 1): 740–745
26. Major O, Fedorcsak I, Sipos L, Hantos P, Konya E, Dobronyi I et al (1994) Slit-ventricle syndrome in shunt operated children. Acta Neurochir (Wien) 127(1–2): 69–72
27. Baskin JJ, Manwaring KH, Rekate HL (1998) Ventricular shunt removal: the ultimate treatment of the slit ventricle syndrome. J Neurosurg 88(3): 478–484
28. Pudenz RH, Foltz EL (1991) Hydrocephalus: overdrainage by ventricular shunts. A review and recommendations. Surg Neurol 35(3):200–212
29. Le H, Yamini B, Frim DM (2002) Lumboperitoneal shunting as a treatment for slit ventricle syndrome. Pediatr Neurosurg 36(4):178–182
30. Epstein FJ, Fleischer AS, Hochwald GM, Ransohoff J (1974) Subtemporal craniectomy for recurrent shunt obstruction secondary to small ventricles. J Neurosurg 41(1):29–31
31. Roth J, Biyani N, Udayakumaran S, Xiao X, Friedman O, Beni-Adani L et al (2011) Modified bilateral subtemporal decompression for resistant slit ventricle syndrome. Childs Nerv Syst 27(1):101–110
32. Di Rocco C, Pettorossi VE, Caldarelli M, Mancinelli R, Velardi F (1978) Communicating hydrocephalus induced by mechanically increased amplitude of the intraventricular cerebrospinal fluid pressure: experimental studies. Exp Neurol 59(1):40–52
33. Weinzweig J, Bartlett SP, Chen JC, Losee J, Sutton L, Duhaime AC et al (2008) Cranial vault expansion in the management of postshunt craniosynostosis and slit ventricle syndrome. Plast Reconstr Surg 122(4): 1171–1180
34. Martinez-Lage JF, Ruiz-Espejo Vilar A, Perez-Espejo MA, Almagro MJ, Ros de San Pedro J, Felipe Murcia M (2006) Shunt-related craniocerebral disproportion: treatment with cranial vault expanding procedures. Neurosurg Rev 29(3):229–235
35. Sandler AL, Daniels LB 3rd, Staffenberg DA, Kolatch E, Goodrich JT, Abbott R (2013) Successful treatment of post-shunt craniocerebral disproportion by coupling gradual external cranial vault distraction with continuous intracranial pressure monitoring. J Neurosurg Pediatr 11(6):653–657

Epilepsy as a Late Complication 18

Mehmet Turgut and Ahmet Tuncay Turgut

Contents

18.1 **Introduction** 247

18.2 **Incidence of Epilepsy in Patients with Hydrocephalus** 248

18.3 **Influence of Etiology of Hydrocephalus Upon Epilepsy** 249

18.4 **Influence of Intracranial Shunting Procedure Upon Development of Epilepsy in Hydrocephalic Patients** 250

18.5 **Causative Factors for Epilepsy in Patients Who Underwent Shunting Procedure for Hydrocephalus** 251

18.5.1 Sex and Age of Patient at Time of Shunt Surgery 251

18.5.2 Number of Shunt Revisions 252

18.5.3 Shunt Location and Shunt Systems Used 252

18.5.4 Shunt Malfunction 252

18.5.5 Shunt Infection 253

18.5.6 Slit Ventricle Syndrome 253

18.5.7 Cortical Malformation 253

18.5.8 Intracranial Hemorrhage 253

18.5.9 Hyponatremia Due to Abdominal Pseudocyst 254

18.5.10 Episodes of Raised Intracranial Pressure 554

18.5.11 Intracranial Hypotension Related with Body Posture 554

18.6 **Time of Occurrence of Epileptic Seizure After Shunting Procedure** 254

18.7 **EEG Changes in Hydrocephalic Patients with/Without Shunting** 254

18.7.1 EEG Findings in Hydrocephalus 254

18.7.2 Focal EEG Changes in Hydrocephalic Patients with Shunting 255

18.8 **Relationship Between Mental or Physical Disability and Occurrence of Seizures in Shunted Hydrocephalus** 256

18.9 **Postoperative Hydrocephalus After Hemispherectomy in Patients with Epilepsy** 256

18.10 **Outcome of Hydrocephalic Patients with Epilepsy** 257

18.11 **Future Treatment Options** 257

Conclusion 257

References 258

M. Turgut, MD, PhD
Department of Neurosurgery, Adnan Menderes University School of Medicine, Aydın, Turkey
e-mail: drmturgut@yahoo.com

A.T. Turgut, MD (✉)
Department of Radiology, Ankara Training and Research Hospital, Ankara TR-06590, Turkey
e-mail: ahmettuncayturgut@yahoo.com

18.1 Introduction

Hydrocephalus has an incidence ratio of 1–3 cases/1,000 children in the population [20, 27], while epilepsy has an incidence ratio of 4–9 cases/1,000 children in the population [27]. Nowadays, surgery is the treatment of choice for congenital or acquired hydrocephalus and

C. Di Rocco et al. (eds.), *Complications of CSF Shunting in Hydrocephalus: Prevention, Identification, and Management*, DOI 10.1007/978-3-319-09961-3_18,

occurrence of epilepsy after shunting procedures is a well-known problem, but our knowledge concerning its mechanism is very limited [11, 16, 20, 22, 23, 27, 34, 36, 38, 42, 43, 47].

In the present chapter, we will review the relationship between hydrocephalus and epilepsy as a complication of shunt placement in detail to provide a useful information for the families of the patients, as well as neurosurgeons and neurologists, about the outcome of postoperative hydrocephalic patients.

18.2 Incidence of Epilepsy in Patients with Hydrocephalus

It is now widely accepted that epilepsy is frequently seen in children with hydrocephalus, although its mechanism is not clear [3]. In the current literature, there are conflicting reports as to the prevalence of epilepsy in hydrocephalus, ranging from 9 to 65 % [11, 16, 20, 22, 23, 27, 34, 36, 38, 42, 43, 47].

Based on results of a retrospective analysis of a total of 200 children with hydrocephalus, Hosking [22] reported that seizures developed in 30 % of the cases during a follow-up period of 5-year. Afterwards, Blaauw [4] published a retrospective review of 323 hydrocephalic children and he found that epileptic seizures were developed in 34 % of the patients with hydrocephalus caused by various etiologies including hemorrhage and infections. Also, Leggate et al. [30] found that seizures developed in 16 % of 56 hydrocephalic patients. In similar, Saukkonen and von Wendt [42] also reported that epileptic seizures developed in 80 of 168 patients (48 %) during the follow-up period of about 9 years. In 1992, an incidence of epileptic seizures as 49 % of the patients was reported in a series of 68 patients with congenital hydrocephalus [36]. In a retrospective review of 464 patients with hydrocephalus, Piatt and Carlson [38] reported that 12 % of patients had epilepsy at the time of diagnosis of hydrocephalus (Fig. 18.1).

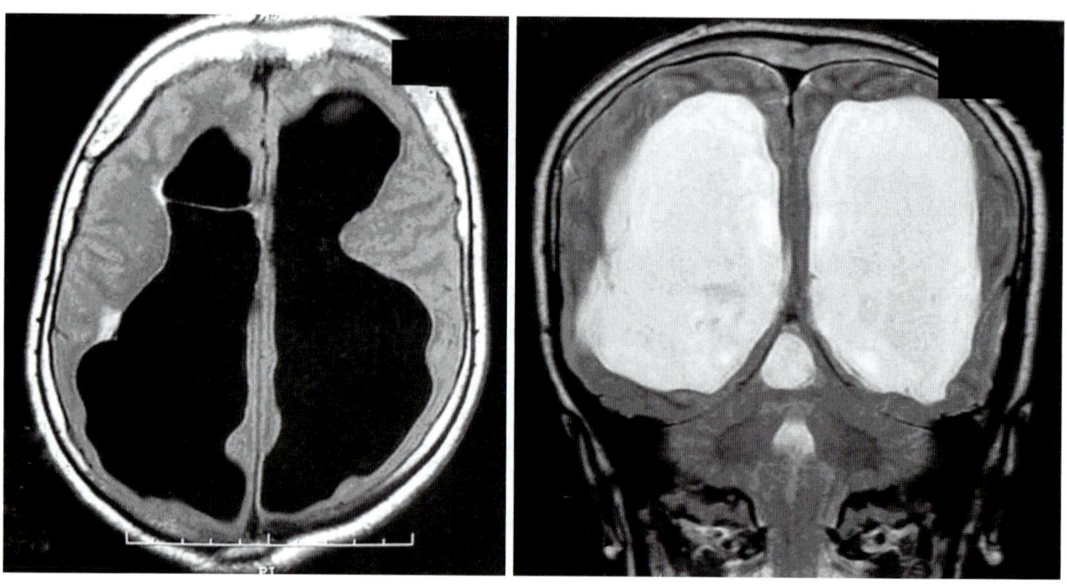

Fig. 18.1 MR scans of a 28-year-old woman with a history of learning difficulties at childhood and recent episodic diffuse headache that had lasted for almost 3 months as well as additional generalized seizure 1 month prior to admission revealed a chronic (no active) hydrocephalus. The patient was treated conservatively by antiepileptic drug (valproate) without any ventriculoperitoneal shunt insertion and had a good outcome during 15 months follow-up (Courtesy of Ali Akhaddar MD, Rabat, Morocco)

18.3 Influence of Etiology of Hydrocephalus Upon Epilepsy

In the current literature, there is general agreement that the etiology of hydrocephalus may play a critical role in the development of epilepsy, albeit the results are conflicting [4, 22, 24, 36, 38]. Piatt and Carlson [38] suggested that the cause of the hydrocephalus was correlated with the risk of development of epilepsy. Etiological categories of hydrocephalus are summarized as follows: hemorrhage, infection, intracranial tumor, myelomeningocele, other congenital malformations such as aqueduct stenosis, arachnoidal cyst, Dandy–Walker malformation, and idiopathic [20] (Fig. 18.2).

The highest incidence of epilepsy was found in cases who had posthemorrhagic and postinfectious hydrocephalus, etiologies known to be associated with complex brain pathology and low functional status. In 1974, Hosking [22] reported that hydrocephalus was developed secondary to either neonatal intracranial hemorrhage or meningitis. Afterwards, Blaauw [4] found that seizures associated with hydrocephalus were more frequent in the patients with shunt infections.

Notably, hydrocephalus associated with various congenital anomalies including myelomeningocele or arachnoidal cysts carried a far higher incidence of epilepsy [28]. In 1978, Lorber et al. [34] reported that 49 % of the hydrocephalic patients associated with a morphological lesion of the central nervous system (CNS) had epilepsy and they suggested that epileptic seizures were frequently seen in patients with physical or mental disabilities. Then, Noetzel and Blake [36] found that, in a long-term follow-up on 68 hydrocephalic patients, mental retardation and malformations of the CNS correlated with seizure occurrence. Also, Keene and Ventureyra [27] reported that the risk of seizures in hydrocephalic children associated with motor or intellectual impairment was increased due to underlying brain abnormalities.

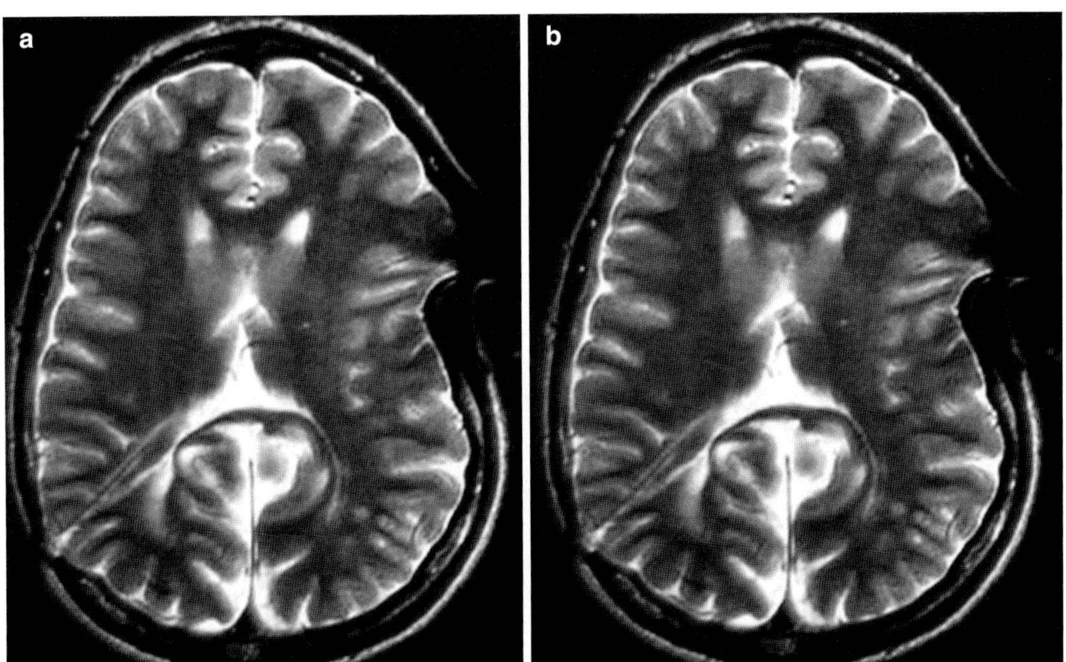

Fig. 18.2 (**a**, **b**) MR scans of a 19-year-old young lady with bilateral shunts and partial agenesis of corpus callosum with recent memory changes, decreased school performance, and automatisms. EEG identified temporal lobe epilepsy (Courtesy of Jogi V. Pattisapu, MD, Orlando, FL)

In a series of ten hydrocephalic children with tuberous sclerosis and intraventricular subependymal giant cell astrocytomas, Di Rocco et al. [14] reported that seven patients underwent direct surgical excision of the lesion, but the remaining three patients underwent a ventriculoperitoneal (VP) shunting and then removal of the intraventricular tumor. In addition, Di Rocco et al. [14] found that the surgical tumor removal was followed by a significant improvement in the epilepsy and they concluded that the surgical removal of the intraventricular tumors is the most appropriate treatment in patients with tuberous sclerosis and associated hydrocephalus.

Interestingly, as a cause of neonatal epilepsy with hydrocephalus, β-mannosidosis, which results from a deficiency of β-mannosidase, is an extremely rare disorder in humans [6]. Broomfield et al. [6] suggested that it should be considered in the differential diagnosis of neonatal seizures and subsequent hydrocephalus during follow-up, whereas others reported that there was no association between occurrence of epileptic seizures and the underlying etiology of the hydrocephalus [12, 27, 42]. In these patients, clinical findings such as altered skull morphology and intractable seizures develop in the neonatal period.

18.4 Influence of Intracranial Shunting Procedure Upon Development of Epilepsy in Hydrocephalic Patients

In neurosurgery, various shunting techniques known as ventriculo-atrial (VA) and VP are the standard treatment for hydrocephalus in both children and adults. Some authors reported that patients undergoing shunt surgery are at high risk of developing epilepsy as a surgical complication, but relation of the hydrocephalus and the shunting operation with the development of epilepsy is still controversial [28, 33, 40].

Today, it is accepted that there is an increased incidence of epilepsy risk after placement of the ventricular catheter, ranging from 5 to 58 % [5, 10, 12, 23, 24, 27, 28, 43]. To date, many authors reported large clinical series of seizure disorder following intracranial shunt insertion for hydrocephalus. In 1986, Stellman et al. [43] studied a total of 202 shunted hydrocephalic children, congenital or acquired origin, and they found an incidence of seizure disorder as 39 %. Of the 207 shunted hydrocephalic patients reported by Dan and Wade [12], 9.4 % had epilepsy. Besides, Johnson et al. [24] found that 38 % of the 817 children with shunted hydrocephalus had epilepsy. In a review of 182 patients, Klepper et al. [28] reported that shunt-related epilepsy was developed in 12 % patients. In a retrospective review of 197 patients with shunted hydrocephalus, Keene and Ventureyra [27] found that 17 % of hydrocephalic patients developed seizures.

Several authors investigated the role of shunting procedure upon the development of epilepsy in hydrocephalic patients. In a review of 92 patients with hydrocephalus, Ines and Markand [23] found that the incidence of epilepsy was high in the shunted group (65 % in the shunted group, while 18 % in the nonshunted group). Retrospectively, Venes and Deuser [47] found that 24 patients of 93 patients with hydrocephalus had epileptic seizures before the shunting procedure, but epilepsy developed following the procedure in only 5 patients. Afterwards, in a study of 168 shunt-treated hydrocephalic children, Saukkonen et al. [42] found that 48 % of the patients had epileptic seizures: 22 % of patients had epilepsy prior to the shunting procedure, and 26 % had epilepsy following the shunting procedure. Moreover, Klepper et al. [28] found that 37 (20 %) of the 182 patients developed epilepsy, 15 patients (8 %) before shunt insertion, and 22 patients (12 %) after intracranial shunting.

From an etiologic point of view, some authors investigated the effect of hydrocephalus upon the development of epilepsy in shunt-treated patients. In a retrospective study of 315 shunted hydrocephalic children, Lorber et al. [34] found that only 4 hydrocephalic patients with congenital etiology had seizures before the shunt placement, while seizures were related to the shunt device in 15 patients. Then, Klepper et al. [28] reported that epilepsy developed in 37 (20 %) of 182 patients with shunt insertion for hydrocephalus due to various etiologies including posthemorrhagic (5 %), postinfectious

(4 %), myelomeningocele (2 %), and aqueduct stenosis (0 %). In a retrospective study of 802 children with hydrocephalus, Bourgeois et al. [5] reported that 32 % of the patients had epileptic seizure, possibly owing to such episodes of raised ICP or the presence of a shunt device as an epileptogenic focus. Further, Kao et al. [26] found that postmeningitis hydrocephalic patients showed the highest incidence of epilepsy as 40 %, possibly due to its high shunt revision rate.

In clinical practice, the findings confirming the effect of shunting in development of epilepsy are: (a) the development of epilepsy following surgery; (b) focal discharges at the site of the shunt in electroencephalography (EEG); and (c) the existence of contralateral seizures [10, 23, 42, 47]. Besides, Ines and Markand [23] reported that all of the shunted patients who had epilepsy developed them after the shunting procedure and left-sided focal epilepsy was the most frequent focal motor seizures in the patients with shunt placement on the right side [23]. Based on their observation upon seizures involving the body side contralateral to the shunt placement, Copeland et al. [10] noted that development of seizures was possibly due to the surgical shunting procedure.

18.5 Causative Factors for Epilepsy in Patients Who Underwent Shunting Procedure for Hydrocephalus

Especially in shunted hydrocephalic children, it is commonly recognized that epileptic seizures occur as a result of shunting procedures, surgical complications due to these procedures, or the hydrocephalus itself. In this section, we will focus on increased risk of epilepsy following placement of shunt device, possibly related with the sex of patients and the age of patient at time of shunt placement, number of shunt revision procedures, shunt location (frontal, parietal) and shunt systems used, shunt malfunction, shunt infection, slit ventricle syndrome (SLVS), cortical malformation, intracranial hemorrhage, hyponatremia due to abdominal pseudocyst, episodes of raised intracranial pressure (ICP), and intracranial hypotension related with body posture in detail (Table 18.1).

Table 18.1 Causative factors for epilepsy in shunted hydrocephalic patients

Cause of epilepsy
Gender and age of patient
Number of shunt revision
Shunt location and shunt systems used
Shunt malfunction
Shunt infection
Slit ventricle syndrome
Cortical malformation
Intracranial malformation
Hyponatremia due to abdominal pseudocyst
Episodes of raised intracranial pressure
Intracranial hypotension related with body posture

18.5.1 Sex and Age of Patient at Time of Shunt Surgery

Studies suggested that there was no link between gender of the patients and occurrence of epilepsy in hydrocephalic patients [28]. On the other hand, there is now compelling evidence that age of the patient at the time of shunting procedure may be an important factor. It has been shown that children younger than 2 years of age have a high risk of epilepsy in contrast to older ones, possibly due to an increased risk of shunt malfunction [40]. As expected, early shunting as a well-known determinant of risk in cases with shunt obstruction was associated with a higher risk for epilepsy [10, 28, 40]. Accordingly, Dan and Wade [12] also found that postshunt seizures developed in 9 % of 207 patients with ventricular shunts, ranging from 15 % in infants to 7 % in patients over 50 years of age. Based on the results of their retrospective series, Noetzel and Blake [36] noted that risk factors for development of epileptic seizure in patients with shunted hydrocephalus included age at time of shunting. However, there was no correlation between the occurrence of epileptic seizures and the age of the patient at the time of initial shunt procedure [27, 38].

18.5.2 Number of Shunt Revisions

In a previous study, it has been reported that epilepsy developed in 24 % patients with shunt revision, in contrast to 6 % patients without shunt revision [12]. According to the results of a retrospective study, Noetzel and Blake [36] noted that risk factors for development of epilepsy in patients with shunted hydrocephalus included the total number of shunt revisions. Then, Johnson et al. [24] reported that a shunt revision was done in 3 % of admissions to the emergency unit of the hospital for epilepsy, and 1 % of shunt revisions was complicated with epilepsy.

In the existence of multiple shunt revisions, epilepsy is more common owing to traumatic injury to the brain tissue during the intracranial shunting for hydrocephalus [4, 10, 12, 22, 23, 24, 34, 36, 38, 40, 42, 43, 47]. Importantly, Heinsbergen et al. [20] found that patients with more than two shunt revisions have a high incidence of epileptic seizure. Especially in patients with postmeningitis hydrocephalus, higher shunt revision rates were reported compared with those due to other etiological types of hydrocephalus [26].

Nevertheless, others suggested that there was no correlation between risk of development of epileptic seizures and the number of shunt revisions [27, 28, 38, 42]. In a review of 168 shunt-treated children for hydrocephalus, Saukkonen et al. [42] found that there was no correlation between epileptic seizure and number of shunt revisions. They agree that multiple shunt revisions had no influence on the incidence of epilepsy and thus the total number of shunt revisions did not differ between the epileptic and nonepileptic groups [27, 28, 38, 42].

18.5.3 Shunt Location and Shunt Systems Used

Numerous studies have underlined that anatomic location of shunt insertion is important for the development of epilepsy [10, 12, 22, 23, 34, 36, 38, 40, 42, 43, 47]. In 1986, Dan and Wade [12] reported that 6 % of 168 cases who had shunt

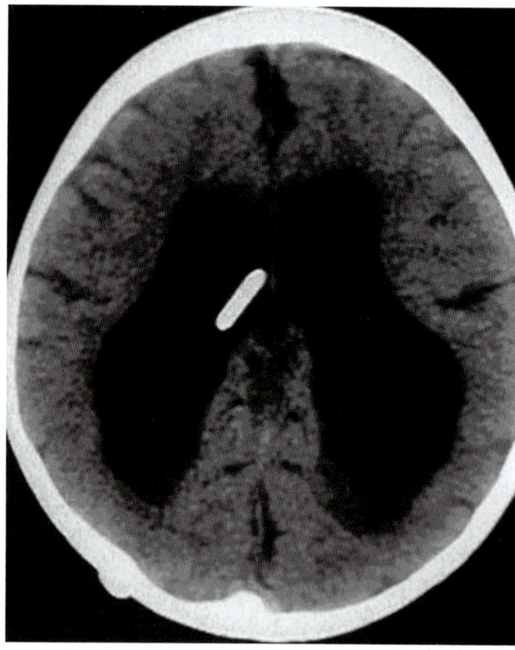

Fig. 18.3 CT scan of a 4-year-old girl with acute symptoms of headaches and generalized seizure presenting with enlarged ventricles due to shunt malfunction. The last surgical procedure was the original shunt insertion which was performed 3 years earlier (Courtesy of Jogi V. Pattisapu, MD, Orlando, FL)

placement in the parietal region had epilepsy, in contrast to 55 % of 11 patients who had undergone shunting procedure in the frontal region. Nevertheless, others found that the location of the burr hole for the shunt insertion and shunt device, frontal and parietal areas, did not correlate with the occurrence of focal or generalized seizures [24, 27, 43, 47].

Further studies investigating the role of the shunt systems as a foreign body upon development of epilepsy revealed that there is no difference between the epileptic and nonepileptic groups [28, 40].

18.5.4 Shunt Malfunction

It is logical to suggest that shunt malfunction may be related with epileptic seizure (Fig. 18.3). In a review of 200 hydrocephalic children, 10 patients had a seizure due to a blocked shunt device [22]. Faillace and Canady [18] retrospectively reviewed

15 patients with hydrocephalus who had an epileptic seizure at the time of shunt malfunction and they found that there had been no history of epilepsy in 8 patients. They suggest that as a rule, shunt malfunction should be considered, if a new or recurrent epileptic seizure develops after shunt insertion for hydrocephalus [18].

On the other hand, epilepsy was not generally associated with shunt malfunction in some series [4, 19, 27, 34, 36, 38, 42, 43]. Thus, they concluded that the existence of epileptic seizure alone was not a reliable indicator of a shunt malfunction [19].

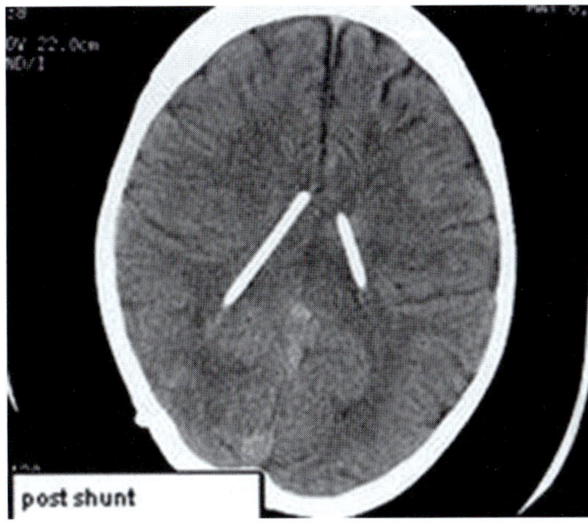

Fig. 18.4 CT scan of a 32-month-old boy with rapid ventricular decompression and absence-type seizures 5 weeks after shunt revision revealed collapsed ventricles (Courtesy of Jogi V. Pattisapu, MD, Orlando, FL)

18.5.5 Shunt Infection

Numerous retrospective studies reported that the risk of development of epileptic seizures was significantly increased in cases with shunt and/or cerebrospinal fluid (CSF) infection [10, 22, 24, 36, 37, 40, 43, 45]. In a review of 168 shunt-treated hydrocephalic children, however, Saukkonen et al. [42] found that there was no link between epileptic seizure and existence of shunt infection. Likewise, Piatt and Carlson [38] reported that there was no correlation between risk of development of epileptic seizures and a history of shunt infection. No matter in what way, shunt infection should be considered as a general rule, if an epileptic seizure develops after shunt insertion for hydrocephalus.

18.5.6 Slit Ventricle Syndrome

Typically, SLVS, which is characterized by very small ("slit-like") ventricles in computed tomography (CT) or magnetic response imaging (MRI), occurs as a result of collapse of the ventricles due to overdrainage of the CSF in minority of patients after shunt placement or revision (Fig. 18.4). As a cause of epilepsy after shunting, it was observed in only three of 182 patients with hydrocephalus, corresponding with the 0.9–3.3 % incidence in the current literature [41, 42]. After shunting procedure, epilepsy developed in 44 % of patients in the SLVS group, in contrast to 6 % of those in the non-SLVS group [41]. Out of 141 hydrocephalic patients treated with shunting, epilepsy developed in 31 those with SLVS, but 7 those with normal or dilated ventricles during the follow-up period [42]. More importantly, the same authors found that epilepsy decreased in patients with the SLVS after treatment [41]. Thus, one may suggest that serial EEG evaluation is useful in the follow-up of the patients after shunting.

18.5.7 Cortical Malformation

According to the results of their retrospective series, Noetzel and Blake [36] noted that risk factors for development of epileptic seizure in patients with shunted hydrocephalus included the existence of neuroradiological findings of cortical malformation. Nowadays, it is generally known that histopathological etiology of epilepsy such as cortical dysplasia, hemimegalencephaly, and Rasmussen encephalitis is the most important determinant for development of hydrocephalus [37].

18.5.8 Intracranial Hemorrhage

Epileptic seizure is believed to be a common presenting symptom in neonates, children, and adults with intracranial hemorrhage. Talwar et al. [45] noted that 3 patients out of 81 children had epileptic seizures possibly due to intracranial hemorrhage during the VP shunt revision surgery as a surgical complication. Likewise, Johnson et al. [24] also pointed out that epilepsy was more frequent in patients with acute intracranial bleeding.

18.5.9 Hyponatremia Due to Abdominal Pseudocyst

Interestingly, Buyukyavuz et al. [7] firstly reported a case of hyponatremic seizure caused by intra-abdominal pseudocyst formation as a complication of the VP shunt. As far as we know, there is no documented case of this condition in the current literature to date.

18.5.10 Episodes of Raised Intracranial Pressure

Interestingly, in a retrospective study of 802 children with hydrocephalus, Bourgeois et al. [5] reported that 32 % of the children had epileptic seizure, possibly owing to such episodes of raised ICP or the presence of a shunt device as an epileptogenic focus.

18.5.11 Intracranial Hypotension Related with Body Posture

Interestingly, Agrawal and Durity [1] described a child with a VP shunting who presented with epileptic seizures related with posture of the child, possibly due to intracranial hypotension.

18.6 Time of Occurrence of Epileptic Seizure After Shunting Procedure

In 1981, Copeland et al. [10] reported that 58 % of the cases developed epilepsy following the shunt placement within the first month. In similar, Dan and Wade [12] found a higher incidence of epileptic seizure in patients with multiple ventricular catheter revisions with a decreasing risk of seizures from 5 % in the post-shunt 1st year to 1 % after the 3rd year of shunting. Johnson et al. [24] found that 22 % of the 817 children with shunted hydrocephalus had first epileptic attack following the initial shunt placement, whereas 38 % of all patients had at least one epileptic seizure.

Based on their long-term follow-up retrospective study, Saukkonen et al. [42] reported that 14 % of the patients had seizures following the insertion of the shunt within the first 6 months; 25 % of the patients developed epilepsy within the 1st year, 40 % of the patients had epileptic seizure within 2 years, and the remaining 61 % of the patients developed epilepsy following shunting within 2–15 years. Afterwards, in a retrospective review of 464 patients with hydrocephalus, Piatt and Carlson [38] reported that 12 % of patients developed epileptic seizures at the time of diagnosis of hydrocephalus and the risk of epilepsy was 2 % following the shunt placement for each year and 33 % of the patients by 10 years following the shunt surgery.

18.7 EEG Changes in Hydrocephalic Patients with/Without Shunting

18.7.1 EEG Findings in Hydrocephalus

To date, many authors have reported a significantly higher rate of EEG abnormalities, such as generalized slow-wave activity, unilateral or focal attenuation, and focal spike waves and/or sharp waves, in patients with hydrocephalus and seizures, in contrast to hydrocephalic patients without development of epilepsy [10, 12, 23, 36, 41, 42, 44, 45, 47] Also, Carballo et al. [8] reported a series of 9 cases with hydrocephalus and continuous spikes and waves during slow sleep (CSWS), related with epilepsy.

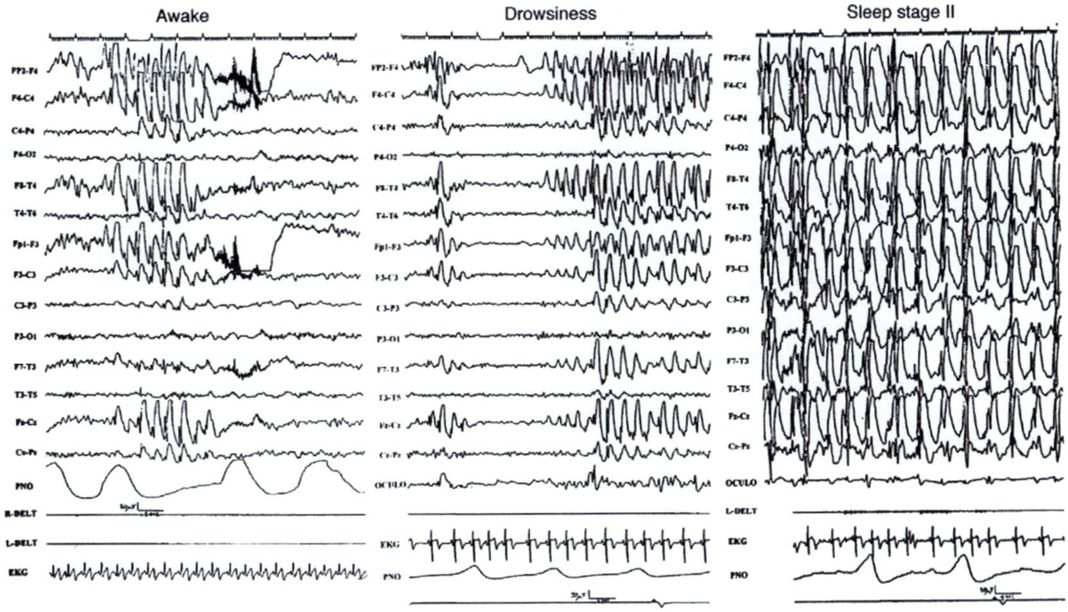

Fig. 18.5 EEG of a children with shunted hydrocephalus showing focal abnormalities (*left*), secondary bilateral synchrony (*centre*), continuous spikes and waves during sleep (*right*) (Reproduced with permission from Veggiotti et al. [46])

18.7.2 Focal EEG Changes in Hydrocephalic Patients with Shunting

So far, various focal epileptiform abnormalities have been described in children with cerebral ventricular shunting. Al-Sulaiman and Ismail [2] investigated the EEG abnormalities in 68 cases with hydrocephalus and they found focal or generalized findings in the shunted group including slow waves in 26 cases, epileptiform activity in 26, hypsarrhythmia in 4, and amplitude abnormalities in 2, giving a total ratio of abnormality above 90 %.

Besides, Veggiotti et al. [46] reported that focal EEG abnormalities were ipsilateral to the location of the shunt device in 95 % of children (Fig. 18.5). In general, it has been accepted that traumatic injury to the brain during the shunt procedure and the existence of an intracranial foreign material will result in focal epilepsy in contralateral side and EEG changes ipsilateral to the localization of the shunt [10, 12, 22, 23, 33, 34, 36, 38, 42, 43, 46, 47]. Ines and Markand [23] found that there was a high incidence of focal EEG abnormalities in the shunted hydrocephalic patients, about 50 % of the nonshunted hydrocephalic patients and almost all of the shunted hydrocephalic group, suggesting that the shunt as a kind of foreign body may be responsible for these findings. Likewise, Liguori et al. [33] evaluated the EEG findings in 40 patients with shunted hydrocephalus and epileptic seizures and they found that the frequencies of both specific and nonspecific EEG findings are higher on the shunted hemisphere (19 patients) compared to the unshunted side (8 patients), suggesting the presence of the intraventricular shunt catheter as a cause of the EEG focus.

Moreover, Saukkonen et al. [41] suggested that a kind of shunt malfunction should be suspected in patients with hydrocephalus, if any abnormal focal EEG finding develops after shunting procedure. Recently, Posar and Parmeggiani [39] described a case of an early-onset hydrocephalus causing partial epilepsy with a particular EEG finding, known as CSWS, possibly due to involvement of frontal, parietal, and occipital lobes.

In a series of 113 children with shunting, Saukkonen et al. [41] investigated the relationship between epilepsy and the EEG changes in the SLVS following shunting. The same authors found a generalized spike and sharp wave activity (SWA) in 81 % of 63 patients in the SLVS group, but in 54 % of patients of non-SLVS group following shunting procedure [41]. Importantly, the EEG findings disappeared in patients with the SLVS following treatment [41].

Nevertheless, current data is conflicting with regard to the effects of the intraventricular shunt catheter as a cause of the EEG focus. From a total of 168 shunted hydrocephalic patients, generalized SWA in EEG before shunting procedure was seen in 45 % of the patients, whereas partial epilepsy following shunting procedure was seen in 9 % of the patients [42]. Then, Veggiotti et al. [46] reported focal EEG abnormalities which were ipsilateral to the site of shunt in 95 % of children, confirming its possible role in the epilepsy. In contrast, however, Saukkonen et al. [42] reported that epileptic seizure had no correlation with the side of the shunt or with the side of the epileptic activity in the EEG.

Accordingly, Saukkonen et al. [41] reported that focal EEG changes are frequently seen within the first year of life in hydrocephalic children and a slow-wave focus may arise in an enlargement of the third ventricle or of the posterior fossa, not related with the direct effect of an intraventricular shunt catheter. Likewise, Klepper et al. [28] found that there were focal EEG abnormalities related to the anatomical location of the shunt in 14 of 16 (88 %) patients, while contralateral focal seizures and focal EEG abnormalities on the same side to the shunt device were present in only three patients (2 %). Based on their findings, Klepper et al. [28] suggested a minor effect of the surgical procedure for decision concerning epilepsy related with shunting in the presence of the following three criteria: (a) development of epilepsy in the postoperative period; (b) focal seizures contralateral to the site of shunt placement; and (c) presence of EEG changes which are ipsilateral to the site of the shunt device. In conclusion, they speculated that the epilepsy was determined by the cause of hydrocephalus rather than by the shunting procedure, an overestimated complication of intracranial shunting [28].

18.8 Relationship Between Mental or Physical Disability and Occurrence of Seizures in Shunted Hydrocephalus

Some authors pointed out various risk factors, including mental or physical disability, for development of epileptic seizure in patients with shunted hydrocephalus [29, 36, 40]. Stellman et al. [43] found that epileptic seizures frequently developed owing to various shunt-related problems in children with mental or physical disability. Later, Keene and Ventureyra [27] observed that epilepsy developed in patients with hydrocephalus associated with motor and/or cognitive disability, suggesting the importance of encephalopathy as an etiological factor instead of hydrocephalus.

18.9 Postoperative Hydrocephalus After Hemispherectomy in Patients with Epilepsy

From a surgical point of view, there are various hemispherectomy procedures – anatomical, functional, and modified – and the modified approach has some advantages in pediatric patients with hemispheric cortical dysplasia with small and/or malformed ventricles [9, 25]. In a series of 9 children with hemimegalencephaly who underwent surgical procedure for intractable epilepsy, Di Rocco et al. [15] reported a dramatic improvement in the seizures following hemispherectomy in all children. Afterwards, Di Rocco et al. [13] reported that there were a total of 5 children with a secondary hydrocephalus in a series of 15 children operated with hemimegalencephaly.

Unfortunately, a high incidence of hydrocephalus following various cerebral hemispherectomy procedures in pediatric patients with intractable seizures is a well-known entity [9, 25, 31, 32]. Phung et al. [37] suggested several mechanisms leading to some changes in CSF bulk flow for development of hydrocephalus following various hemispherectomy procedures. In a retrospective review of their findings, Di Rocco et al. [13] found that the age factor appeared to play a critical role in the development of postoperative hydrocephalus, as all of five children with the complication were less than 9 months of age at the time of the hemispherectomy. In a recent review of the findings from a total of 736 patients who underwent hemispherectomy procedure, Lew et al. [32] reported that the hydrocephalus was seen as an early or late surgical complication in patients, ranging from the early postoperative period to 8.5 years following surgical procedure. More recently, the same authors reported that the use of Avitene caused a higher incidence of hydrocephalus following the surgery in cases with modified hemispherotomy, a safe surgical technique, in patients with epilepsy (56 % vs 18 %) [31].

18.10 Outcome of Hydrocephalic Patients with Epilepsy

As a general rule, the etiology of hydrocephalus is the decisive factor in determining the outcome in hydrocephalic patients with epilepsy. So far, numerous studies have been done upon the result of shunted hydrocephalic patients with epilepsy [20, 21, 26]. Based on the findings from their hydrocephalic patients treated with shunting, Saukkonen et al. [42] reported that epilepsy developed in all of the patients without any prophylactic antiepileptic treatment, whereas 68 % of those with prophylactic treatment remained free of seizures.

Afterwards, Heinsbergen et al. [20] found that hydrocephalic children, owing to various congenital malformation including spina bifida had better prognosis, in contrast to other ones. On the other hand, the outcome of the patients with hydrocephalus is poor in the presence of the following risk factors: (a) peri- and postnatal hemorrhage; (b) delay in drain insertion more than 1 month; (c) children less than 2 years old; and (d) concomitant pathology such as Dandy–Walker malformation, aqueduct stenosis, myelomeningocele, and arachnoid cyst ([35, 40], Heinsbergen et al. [20]).

Indeed, Bourgeois et al. [5] suggested that the presence of epilepsy itself is an important predictor of poor outcome in children who were operated using a kind of shunt device. As given above, it may be a sign of shunt malfunction in cases with hydrocephalus. Regarding the role of surgery and antiepileptic drugs, Faillace and Canady [18] observed that seizure activity stopped in patients after revision procedure for shunt malfunction and medical treatment.

18.11 Future Treatment Options

Even today, it is unfortunate to note that antiepileptic medical treatment is ineffective in most of the cases with postshunt epilepsy [40]. Furthermore, the shunting procedure to control hydrocephalus may cause a complication with high incidence [11, 17]. On the other hand, the choice of the surgical technique to prevent various shunt complications is still a subject of debate, although there is a general agreement on the effectiveness of the surgery in controlling the seizure disorder in hydrocephalic patients. As a result of understanding of the pathophysiology of hydrocephalus, it has been suggested that development of more physiological new surgical techniques such as endoscopic third ventriculostomy procedure in neurosurgical practice may be useful in the prevention of this problem in the future [17, 40]. Our management strategies based on case reports or case series are very limited to date. Therefore, it is suggested that a prospective study is needed to identify the factors predisposing to epileptic seizures in hydrocephalic patients undergoing shunt surgery and to improve the life quality of the patients [5]. As a consequence, we strongly believe that the relationship between the shunting procedure for hydrocephalus and the epilepsy may be disclosed with improved studies using animal models in future.

Conclusion

The topic of epilepsy in patients with hydrocephalus is very important because the incidence of epilepsy in children with shunting is reported to be high, up to 50 % of patients. In addition to the etiology of the hydrocephalus, shunt dysfunction or various shunt complications may cause epileptic seizures in patients with hydrocephalus. It is our opinion that appropriate knowledge of the mechanisms responsible for the development of epilepsy in shunted hydrocephalus together with forthcoming improvements in the management of hydrocephalus will doubtless contribute to decrease these complications in future. It is now evident that every neurosurgeon should know the problem of epilepsy in hydrocephalic patients because of high incidence of seizures in shunted patients.

References

1. Agrawal D, Durity F (2006) Seizure as a manifestation of intracranial hypotension in a shunted patient. Pediatr Neurosurg 42:165–167
2. Al-Sulaiman AA, Ismail HM (1998) Pattern of electroencephalographic abnormalities in children with hydrocephalus: a study of 68 patients. Childs Nerv Syst 14:124–126
3. Battaglia D, Pasca MG, Cesarini L, Tartaglione T, Acquafondata C, Randò T, Veredice C, Ricci D, Guzzetta F (2005) Epilepsy in shunted posthemorrhagic infantile hydrocephalus owing to pre- or perinatal intra- or periventricular hemorrhage. J Child Neurol 20:219–225
4. Blaauw G (1978) Hydrocephalus and epilepsy. Z Kinderchir 25:341–345
5. Bourgeois M, Sainte-Rose C, Cinalli G, Maixner W, Malucci C, Zerah M, Pierre-Kahn A, Renier D, Hoppe-Hirsch E, Aicardi J (1999) Epilepsy in children with shunted hydrocephalus. J Neurosurg 90: 274–281
6. Broomfield A, Gunny R, Ali I, Vellodi A, Prabhakar P (2013) A clinically severe variant of β-mannosidosis, presenting with neonatal onset epilepsy with subsequent evolution of hydrocephalus. JIMD Rep 11: 93–97
7. Buyukyavuz BI, Duman L, Karaaslan T, Turedi A (2012) Hyponatremic seizure due to huge abdominal cerebrospinal fluid pseudocsyt in a child with ventriculoperitoneal shunt: a case report. Turk Neurosurg 22:656–658
8. Caraballo RH, Bongiorni L, Cersósimo R, Semprino M, Espeche A, Fejerman N (2008) Epileptic encephalopathy with continuous spikes and waves during sleep in children with shunted hydrocephalus: a study of nine cases. Epilepsia 49:1520–1527
9. Cook SW, Nguyen ST, Hu B, Yudovin S, Shields WD, Vinters HV, Van de Wiele BM, Harrison RE, Mathern GW (2004) Cerebral hemispherectomy in pediatric patients with epilepsy: comparison of three techniques by pathological substrate in 115 patients. J Neurosurg 100(2 Suppl Pediatrics):125–141
10. Copeland GP, Foy PM, Shaw MDM (1982) The incidence of epilepsy after ventricular shunting operations. Surg Neurol 17:279–281
11. Corber J, Sillanpaa M, Greenwood N (1978) Convulsions in children with hydrocephalus. Z Kinderchir 25:346–351
12. Dan N, Wade M (1986) The incidence of epilepsy after ventricular shunting procedures. J Neurosurg 65: 19–21
13. Di Rocco C, Iannelli A (2000) Hemimegalencephaly and intractable epilepsy: complications of hemispherectomy and their correlations with the surgical technique. A report on 15 cases. Pediatr Neurosurg 33:198–207
14. Di Rocco C, Iannelli A, Marchese E (1995) On the treatment of subependymal giant cell astrocytomas and associated hydrocephalus in tuberous sclerosis. Pediatr Neurosurg 23:115–121
15. Di Rocco C, Iannelli A, Marchese E, Vigevano F, Rossi GF (1994) Surgical treatment of epileptogenic hemimegalencephaly (in Italian). Minerva Pediatr 46: 231–237
16. Dinopoulos A (2010) Hydrocephalus and epilepsy. In: Mallucci C, Sgouros S (eds) Cerebrospinal fluid disorders. Taylor & Francis, New York/London, pp 528–531
17. Drake JM, Kestle JR, Tuli S (2000) CSF shunts 50 years on past, present and future. Childs Nerv Syst 16: 800–804
18. Faillace W, Canady A (1990) Cerebrospinal fluid shunt malfunction signalled by new or recurrent seizures. Childs Nerv Syst 6:37–40
19. Hack C, Ennile B, Donat J, Kosnik E (1990) Seizures in relation to shunt dysfunction in children with meningomyelocele. J Pediatr 116:57–60
20. Heinsbergen I, Rotteveel J, Roeleveld N, Grotenhuis A (2002) Outcome in shunted hydrocephalic children. Eur J Paediatr Neurol 6:99–107
21. Hirsh JF (1994) Consensus statement. Long-term outcome in hydrocephalus. Childs Nerv Syst 10:64–69
22. Hosking G (1974) Hits in hydrocephalic children. Arch Dis Child 49:633–635
23. Ines D, Markand O (1977) Epileptic seizures and abnormal electroencephalographic findings in hydrocephalus and their relation to shunting procedure. Electroencephalogr Clin Neurophysiol 42:761–768
24. Johnson D, Conry J, O'Donnell R (1996) Epileptic seizures as a sign of cerebrospinal fluid shunt malfunction. Pediatr Neurosurg 24:223–228
25. Jonas R, Nguyen S, Hu B, Asarnow RF, LoPresti C, Curtiss S, de Bode S, Yudovin S, Shields WD, Vinters HV, Mathern GW (2004) Cerebral hemispherectomy: hospital course, seizure, developmental, language, and motor outcomes. Neurology 62:1712–1721
26. Kao CL, Yang TF, Wong TT, Cheng LY, Huang SY, Chen HS, Kao CL, Chan RC (2001) The outcome of shunted hydrocephalic children. Zhonghua Yi Xue Za Zhi (Taipei) 64:47–53

27. Keene DL, Ventureyra EC (1999) Hydrocephalus and epileptic seizures. Childs Nerv Syst 15:158–162
28. Klepper J, Büsse M, Strassburg HM, Sörensen N (1998) Epilepsy in shunt-treated hydrocephalus. Dev Med Child Neurol 40:731–736
29. Kulkarni AV, Donnelly R, Shams I (2011) Comparison of hydrocephalus outcome questionnaire scores to neuropsychological test performance. J Neurosurg Pediatr 8:396–401
30. Leggate J, Baxter P, Minnes R, Steers AJW (1988) Epilepsy following ventricular shunt placement. J Neurosurg 68:318–319
31. Lew SM, Koop JI, Mueller WM, Matthews AE, Mallonee JC (2014) Fifty consecutive hemispherectomies: outcomes, evolution of technique, complications, and lessons learned. Neurosurgery 74:182–195
32. Lew SM, Matthews AE, Hartman AL, Haranhalli N, Post Hemispherectomy Hydrocephalus Workgroup (2013) Posthemispherectomy hydrocephalus: results of a comprehensive, multiinstitutional review. Epilepsia 54:383–389
33. Liguori G, Abate M, Buono S, Pittore L (1986) EEG findings in shunted hydrocephalic patients with epileptic seizures. Ital J Neurol Sci 7:243–247
34. Lorber J, Sillanpää M, Greenwood N (1978) Convulsions in children with hydrocephalus. Z Kinderchir 25:346–351
35. Mori K, Shimada J, Kurisaka M, Sato K, Watanabe K (1995) Classification of hydrocephalus and outcome and treatment. Brain Dev 17:338–348
36. Noetzel MJ, Blake JN (1992) Seizures in children with congenital hydrocephalus. Neurology 42: 1277–1281
37. Phung J, Krogstad P, Mathern GW (2013) Etiology associated with developing posthemispherectomy hydrocephalus after resection-disconnection procedures. J Neurosurg Pediatr 12:469–475
38. Piatt J, Carlson C (1996) Hydrocephalus and epilepsy: an actuarial analysis. Neurosurgery 39:722–728
39. Posar A, Parmeggiani A (2013) Neuropsychological impairment in early-onset hydrocephalus and epilepsy with continuous spike-waves during slow-wave sleep: a case report and literature review. J Pediatr Neurosci 8:141–145
40. Sato O, Yamguchi T, Kittaka M, Toyama H (2001) Hydrocephalus and epilepsy. Childs Nerv Syst 17:76–86
41. Saukkonen AL, Serlo W, von Wendt L (1988) Electroencephalographic findings and epilepsy in the slit ventricle syndrome of shunt-treated hydrocephalic children. Childs Nerv Syst 4:344–347
42. Saukkonen AL, Serlo W, von Wendt L (1990) Epilepsy in hydrocephalic children. Acta Paediatr Scand 79:212–218
43. Stellman GR, Bannister CM, Hillier V (1986) The incidence of seizure disorder in children with acquired and congenital hydrocephalus. Z Kinderchir 41(Suppl 1): 38–41
44. Sulaiman A, Ismail H (1998) Pattern of electroencephalographic abnormalities in children with hydrocephalus. Childs Nerv Syst 14:124–126
45. Talwar D, Baldwin M, Horbatt C (1995) Epilepsy in children with meningomyelocele. Pediatr Neurol 13: 29–32
46. Veggiotti P, Beccaria F, Papalia G, Termine C, Piazza F, Lanzi G (1998) Continuous spikes and waves during sleep in children with shunted hydrocephalus. Childs Nerv Syst 14:188–194
47. Venes J, Deuser R (1987) Epilepsy following ventricular shunt placement. J Neurosurg 66:154–155

Part III

Complications of Intrathecal Shunts-Endoscopic Treatment

Introduction: The Changed Epidemiology of CSF Shunt Complications, Failures Versus Complications

19

Mehmet Saim Kazan and Ethem Taner Göksu

Contents

19.1 **Introduction** 263

19.2 **Indications of Neuroendoscopy** 264

19.3 **Prevention of Complications of Neuroendoscopic Interventions** 264

Conclusion 265

References 266

19.1 Introduction

Even today, the management of hydrocephalus is the subject of continuing debate in the neurosurgery community. Numerous studies have reported on treatment options, outcomes, and complications of different management strategies for hydrocephalus and on the accumulation of a large amount of data on the use of extrathecal shunt systems, their complications, and management, which currently represent one of the two major approaches in the field of neurosurgery [13, 35]. As a result of technological advances, endoscopic methods are increasingly being used in the treatment of hydrocephalus, leading to a change in the nature of complications.

It is not uncommon that ventricular shunt systems widely used for hydrocephalus management may present with complications associated with a variety of signs and symptoms. Major complications of shunt systems include mechanical problems such as shunt obstruction, malposition, migration, disconnection, or fractures; overdrainage problems such as subdural hematoma, slit ventricle syndrome, or post-shunt craniosynostosis; infective complications; and abdominal complications occurring with VP shunts [14, 31, 39, 45, 46]. Also, cardiac complications have been reported with the use of VA shunts [26, 49]. These complications require at least one surgical intervention, which may lead to significant morbidity and mortality [15]. The reported risk of shunt failure within the first 2 years following

M.S. Kazan, MD (✉) • E.T. Göksu, MD
Department of Neurosurgery, Akdeniz University Faculty of Medicine, Antalya, Turkey
e-mail: skazan@akdeniz.edu.tr; ethemgoksu@akdeniz.edu.tr

C. Di Rocco et al. (eds.), *Complications of CSF Shunting in Hydrocephalus: Prevention, Identification, and Management*, DOI 10.1007/978-3-319-09961-3_19,

implantation is 50 %, with another retrospective study reporting functionality in only 19 % of the shunts 12 years after the initial shunt procedure [13, 39]. Advances in endoscopic technology have led to a new era in the management of hydrocephalus, allowing independency of the patient from CSF shunts while resulting in a shift from shunt-related complications to endoscopy-related complications, although the latter having low occurrence.

19.2 Indications of Neuroendoscopy

Currently, major uses for neuroendoscopy include the following:

1. Creating alternative CSF circulation pathways (third ventriculostomy) [34]
2. Restoring normal CSF flow (endoscopic aqueductoplasty, septostomy, and foraminoplasty) [3, 12, 17, 29, 41, 48]
3. Reducing CSF production (coagulation of the choroid plexus) [33, 40]
4. Creating intercompartmental connections in complex multiloculated hydrocephalus [4, 30, 44]

A better understanding of the current status of neuroendoscopic interventions for hydrocephalus and their complications requires a historical perspective on the evolution of these techniques. In 1910, the first neurosurgical endoscopic intervention and the first endoscopic cauterization of the choroid plexus were accomplished by L'Espinasse. He accomplished choroid plexus ablation by using a rigid cystoscope in two children with hydrocephalus. One patient died postoperatively, but the other was successfully treated. The event received little attention and passed almost unnoticed [1, 15]. In 1922, Walter Dandy performed a lamina terminalis fenestration through craniotomy for the treatment of hydrocephalus, describing the third ventriculostomy approach. Dandy also performed an endoscopic choroid plexectomy after a previously reported experience in performing open choroid plexectomy on four patients. The attempt to perform the endoscopic choroid plexectomy was unsuccessful, and he did not attempt any further on such cases [1]. Shortly after, in 1923, Mixter penetrated the floor of the third ventricle using a urologic endoscope, pioneering the use of endoscopic third ventriculostomy. In 1936, Stookey and Scarff and, in 1951, Scarff described their own approaches for third ventriculostomy. The technical limitations of that period such as poor magnification and illumination conditions had inevitably led to perceptions of difficulty and unreliability. The morbidity and perioperative mortality rates were high [1, 15]. In 1970, Scarff reviewed all available series of endoscopic choroid plexus cauterization for the treatment of hydrocephalus. Of 95 patients so treated, 14 (15 %) had died, whereas 52 (60 %) had initial successful results [40]. During the 1970s and 1980s, a number of different third ventriculostomy techniques with open or closed approaches were described. Among these studies, the Toronto experience reported by Hoffmann, which described the use of percutaneous third ventriculostomy technique for the treatment of obstructive hydrocephalus, deserved special notice [20, 21]. The overall success rate was about 53 %. Operative mortality was 10.3 % with the open method and 3.5 % with the percutaneous technique. Hoffman concluded that percutaneous third ventriculostomy is a less invasive and effective means of treating noncommunicating hydrocephalus [21]. Following the advances in optic systems after the 1990s and availability of detailed neuroradiological imaging, endoscopic interventions have become more frequent.

19.3 Prevention of Complications of Neuroendoscopic Interventions

Minimizing the complications of neuroendoscopic interventions requires a good knowledge of the intervention-related anatomy as well as the use of appropriate neuroradiological imaging studies tailored individually according to the needs of the patient [5, 28, 34, 37, 41]. Initial recognition and tracing of the choroid plexus within the lateral ventricle leads us to the third ventricle through the foramina of Monro. Thus, if direct visualization of the foramina of Monro cannot be

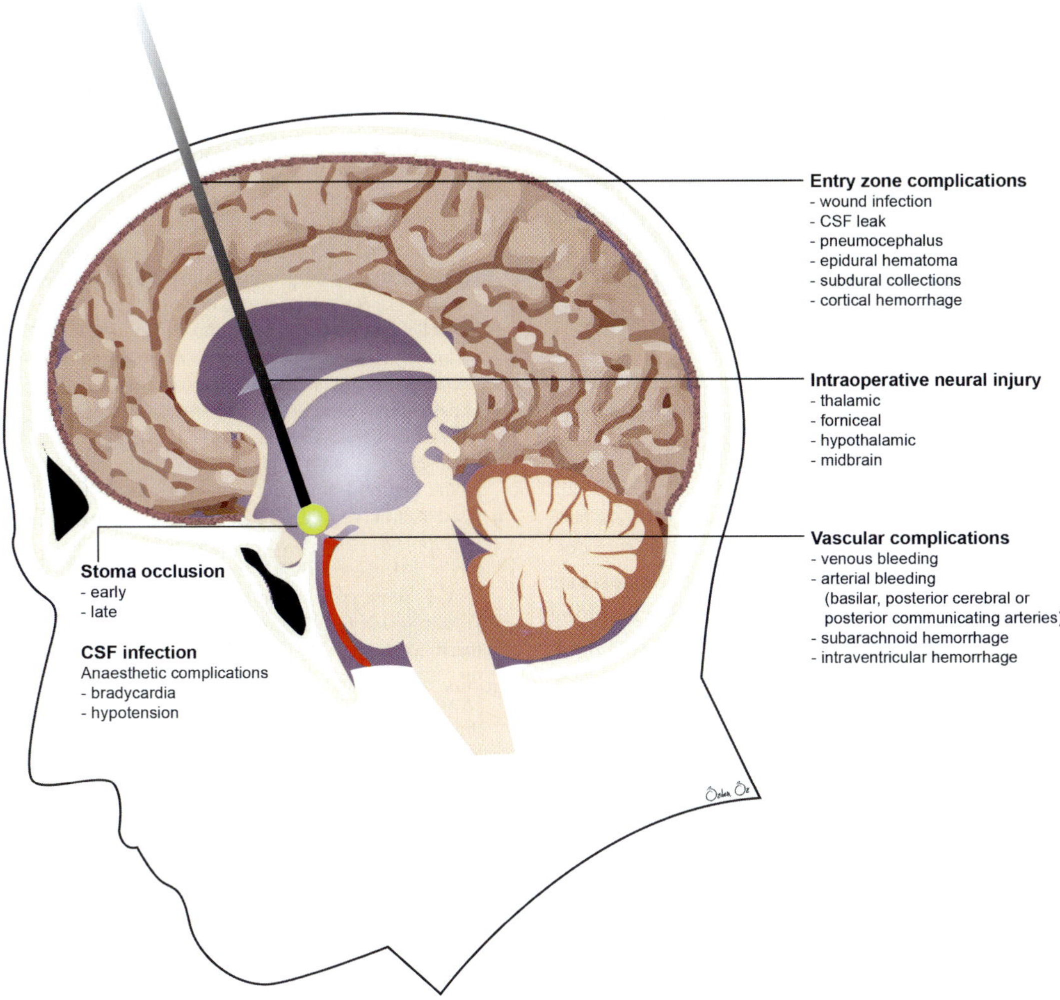

Fig. 19.1 Schematic drawing of complications of endoscopic third ventriculostomy

possible with initial endoscopy, the choroid plexus provides reliable guidance for the ventricular anatomy even in cases of distorted anatomy, such as spina bifida. Other anatomical structures that should certainly be recognized during endoscopic ventriculostomy include the fornix, hypothalamus, third ventricular floor, and Lillequist's membrane. Furthermore, each stage of the endoscopic ventriculostomy including the manipulation of the endoscope tip, dissection or balloon dilatation at the floor of the third ventricle, and irrigation with physiological saline or Ringer's lactate solution requires a certain level of expertise [1, 10, 15, 32, 36–38]. Inadequate surgical technique may lead to a wide spectrum of complications ranging from intraoperative acute hydrocephalus due to blockade and continuous irrigation at the level of the foramina of Monro, to hypothalamic injury at the floor of the third ventricle and endocrine disturbances, and to catastrophic complications such as injury of the basilar artery and/or its branches (Fig. 19.1) [2, 6, 7, 9, 11, 16, 18, 19, 22–25, 27, 42, 43, 47].

Conclusion

In conclusion, endoscopic third ventriculostomy, as an alternative to conventional ventriculoperitoneal or ventriculoatrial shunting, is a firmly established treatment for hydrocephalus, and it has yielded a higher success rate with lower morbidity and mortality than earlier methods of third ventriculostomy. Results of endoscopic third ventriculostomy are most closely associated with the etiology of hydrocephalus encountered as well as with the clinical and radiographic features of the individual patient [23]. High success rates have been reported for patients with aqueduct stenosis. Lower success rates have been reported for patients with hydrocephalus from other causes, such as postinfection, posthemorrhage, or myelomeningocele, and for patients with previous ventricular shunt failure [8, 24]. Although endoscopy seems to be performed with ease in general, it can be difficult and hazardous in certain situations. Intraoperative complications due to injury to anatomical structures resulting from inappropriate surgical technique or inadequate knowledge of anatomy, and early or late postoperative complications such as infections, CSF fistula, pneumocephalus, subdural hematoma, or re-closure of an opened orifice will be discussed in the following chapters.

References

1. Abbott R (2004) History of neuroendoscopy. Neurosurg Clin N Am 15:1–7
2. Abtin K (1998) Basilar artery perforation as a complication of endoscopic third ventriculostomy. Pediatr Neurosurg 28(1):35–41
3. Aldana PR, Kestle JRW, Brockmeyer DL, Walker ML (2003) Results of endoscopic septal fenestration in the treatment of isolated ventricular hydrocephalus. Pediatr Neurosurg 38:286–294
4. Andresen M, Juhler M (2012) Multiloculated hydrocephalus: a review of current problems in classification and treatment. Childs Nerv Syst 28:357–362
5. Aquilina K, Pople IK, Sacree J, Carter MR, Edwards RJ (2012) The constant flow ventricular infusion test: a simple and useful study in the diagnosis of third ventriculostomy failure. J Neurosurg 116:445–452
6. Basaldella L, Fiorindi A, Sammartino F, De Caro R, Longatti P (2013) Third ventriculostomy site as a neuroreceptorial area. Childs Nerv Syst. doi:10.1007/sw00381-013-2289-z
7. Baykan N, Isbir O, Gerçek A, Dağçınar A, Özek MM (2005) Ten years of experience with pediatric neuroendoscopic third ventriculostomy. Features and perioperative complications of 210 cases. J Neurosurg Anesthesiol 17:33–37
8. Boschert J, Hellwig D, Krauss JK (2003) Endoscopic third ventriculostomy for shunt dysfunction in occlusive hydrocephalus: long-term follow up and review. J Neurosurg 98:1032–1039
9. Bouras T, Sgouros S (2012) Complications of endoscopic third ventriculostomy: a systematic review. Acta Neurochir Suppl 113:149–153
10. Brockmeyer D (2004) Techniques of endoscopic third ventriculostomy. Neurosurg Clin N Am 15:51–59
11. Cinalli G, Sainte-Rose C, Chumas P, Zerah M, Brunelle F, Lot G, Pierre-Kahn A, Renier D (1999) Failure of third ventriculostomy in the treatment of aqueductal stenosis in children. J Neurosurg 90:448–454
12. Cinalli G, Spennato P, Savarese L, Ruggiero C, Alberti F, Cuomo L, Cianciulli E, Maggi G (2006) Endoscopic aqueductoplasty and placement of a stent in the cerebral aqueduct in the management of isolated fourth ventricle in children. J Neurosurg 104 (1 Suppl):21–27
13. Drake JM, Kestle JRW, Milner R, Cinalli G, Boop F, Piatt J, Hainess S, Schiff SJ, Cochrane DD, Steinbok P, MacNeil N (1998) Randomized trial of cerebrospinal fluid shunt valve design in pediatric hydrocephalus. Neurosurgery 43:294–305
14. Drake JM, Kulkarni AV, Kestle J (2009) Endoscopic third ventriculostomy versus ventriculoperitoneal shunt in pediatric patients: a decision analysis. Childs Nerv Syst 25:467–472
15. Enchev Y, Oi S (2008) Historical trends of neuroendoscopic surgical techniques in the treatment of hydrocephalus. Neurosurg Rev 31:249–262
16. Fukuhara T, Voster SJ, Luciano MG (2000) Risk factors for failure of endoscopic third ventriculostomy for obstructive hydrocephalus. Neurosurgery 46:1100–1111
17. Gangemi M, Maiuri F, Donati PA, Signorelli F, Basile D (1999) Endoscopic surgery for monoventricular hydrocephalus. Surg Neurol 52:246–250
18. Hader WJ, Drake J, Cochrane D, Sparrow O, Johnson ES, Kestle J (2002) Death after late failure of third ventriculostomy in children. Report of three cases. J Neurosurg 97:211–215
19. Hellwig D, Giordano M, Kappus C (2013) Redo third ventriculostomy. World Neurosurg. doi:10.1016/j.wneu.2012.02.006
20. Hoffman HJ (1976) The advantages of percutaneous third ventriculostomy over other forms of surgical treatment for infantile obstructive hydrocephalus. In: Morley TP (ed) Current controversies in neurosurgery. WB Saunders, Philadelphia, pp 691–703
21. Hoffman HJ, Harwood-Nash D, Gilday DL (1980) Percutaneous third ventriculostomy in the management of non-communicating hydrocephalus. Neurosurgery 7:313–321
22. Hopf NJ, Grunert P, Fries G, Resch KDM, Perneczky A (1999) Endoscopic third ventriculostomy: outcome analysis of 100 consecutive procedures. Neurosurgery 44:795–806

23. Iantosca MR, Hader WJ, Drake JM (2004) Results of endoscopic third ventriculostomy. Neurosurg Clin N Am 15:67–75
24. Kadrian D, van Gelder J, Florida D, Jones R, Vonaou M, Teo C, Stening W, Kwok B (2005) Long-term reliability of endoscopic third ventriculostomy. Neurosurgery 56: 1271–1278
25. Kehler U, Regelsberger J, Gliemroth J (2003) The mechanism of fornix lesions in 3rd ventriculostomy. Minim Invasive Neurosurg 46(4):202–204
26. Kluge S, Bauman HJ, Regelsberger J, Kehler U, Gliemroth J, Koziej B, Klose H, Meyer A (2010) Pulmonary hypertension after ventriculoatrial shunt implantation. J Neurosurg 113(6):1279–1283
27. Kurschel S, Ono S, Oi S (2007) risk reduction of subdural collections following endoscopic third ventriculostomy. Childs Nerv Syst 23(5):521–526
28. Lindert EJV, Beems T, Grotenhuis JA (2006) The role of different imaging modalities: is MRI a conditio sine qua non for ETV? Childs Nerv Syst 22:1529–1536
29. Mohanty A (2003) Endoscopic third ventriculostomy with cystoventricular stent placement in the management of Dandy-Walker malformation: technical case report of three patients. Neurosurgery 53:1223–1229
30. Oi S, Abbott R (2004) Loculated ventricles and isolated compartments in hydrocephalus: their pathophysiology and the efficacy of neuroendoscopic surgery. Neurosurg Clin N Am 15:77–87
31. Oi S, Matsumoto S (1985) Slit ventricles as a cause of isolated ventricles after shunting. Childs Nerv Syst 1:189–193
32. Oka K, Yamamoto M, Nonaka T, Tomonaga M (1996) The significance of artificial cerebrospinal fluid as perfusate and endoneurosurgery. Neurosurgery 38:733–736
33. Pople IK, Ettles D (1995) The role of endoscopic choroid plexus coagulation in the management of hydrocephalus. Neurosurgery 36:698–702
34. Rekate HL (2004) Selecting patients for endoscopic third ventriculostomy. Neurosurg Clin N Am 15:39–49
35. Ribaupierre S, Rilliet B, Vernet O, Regli L, Villemure JG (2007) Third ventriculostomy vs ventriculoperitoneal shunt in pediatric obstructive hydrocephalus: results from a Swiss series and literature review. Childs Nerv Syst 23:527–533
36. Romero L, Ros B, Ibanez G, Rius F, Gonzalez L, Arraez MA (2014) Endoscopic third ventriculostomy: can we predict success during surgery? Neurosurg Rev 37(1):89–97
37. Ros B, Romero L, Ibanez G, Iglesias S, Rius F, Perez S, Arraez MA (2012) Success criteria in pediatric neuroendoscopic procedures. Proposal for classification of results after 67 operations. Childs Nerv Syst 28:691–697
38. Roth J, Constantini S (2012) Selective use of intra-catheter endoscopic-assisted ventricular catheter placement: indications and outcome. Childs Nerv Syst 28:1163–1169
39. Sainte-Rose C, Piatt JH, Renier D, Pierre-Kahn A, Hirsch JF, Hoffman HJ, Humpreys RP, Hendrick EB (1991) Mechanical complications in shunts. Pediatr Neurosurg 17:2–9
40. Scarff J (1970) The treatment of nonobstructive (communicating) hydrocephalus by endoscopic cauterization of the choroid plexus. J Neurosurg 33:1–18
41. Schroeder HWS, Gaab MR (1999) Endoscopic aqueductoplasty: technique and results. Neurosurgery 45:508–518
42. Schoeder HW, Niendorf WR, Gaab MR (2002) Complications of endoscopic third ventriculostomy. J Neurosurg 96:1032–1040
43. Schroeder HWS, Schweim C, Schweim KH, Gaab MR (2000) Analysis of aqueductal cerebrospinal fluid flow after endoscopic aqueductoplasty by using cine phase-contrast magnetic resonance imaging. J Neurosurg 93:237–244
44. Schulz M, Bohner G, Knaus H, Haberl H, Thomale U-W (2010) Navigated endoscopic surgery for multiloculated hydrocephalus in children. J Neurosurg Pediatr 5:434–442
45. Stone JJ, Walker CT, Jacobson M, Philips V, Silberstein HJ (2013) Revision rate of pediatric ventriculoperitoneal shunts after 15 years. J Neurosurg Pediatr 11(1):15–19
46. Surchev JK, Georkiev KD, Enchev Y, Avramov RS (2002) Ventriculoperitoneal shunt in children – our 14-year experience. Childs Nerv Syst 18:259 (abstr)
47. Walker ML (2004) Complications of third ventriculostomy. Neurosurg Clin N Am 15:61–66
48. Wong TT, Lee LS (2000) Membranous occlusion of the foramen Monro following ventriculoperitoneal shunt insertion: a role for endoscopic foraminoplasty. Childs Nerv Syst 16:213–217
49. Yavuz C, Demirtas S, Calıskan A, Kamasak K, Karahan O, Guclu O, Yazıcı S, Mavitas B (2013) Reasons, procedures, and outcomes in ventriculoatrial shunts: a single-center experience. Surg Neurol Int 4:10. doi:10.4103/152-7806

Iatrogenic and Infectious Complications

20

David A. Chesler and George I. Jallo

Contents

20.1 **Overview** ... 269

20.2 **Techniques for the Endoscopic Treatment of Hydrocephalus** ... 270

20.3 **Iatrogenic Complications in Endoscopic Surgery** ... 271

20.4 **Avoidance of Complications** ... 272

Conclusions ... 274

References ... 274

D.A. Chesler, MD PhD • G.I. Jallo, MD (✉)
Division of Pediatric Neurosurgery,
The Johns Hopkins Hospital,
600 N Wolfe St, Phipps 579,
Baltimore, MD 21287, USA
e-mail: dchesle2@jhmi.edu; gjallo1@jhmi.edu

20.1 Overview

The use of neuroendoscopy in the treatment of hydrocephalus is a well-recognized part of the neurosurgeon's armamentarium. The technique of neuroendoscopy, and thereby the treatment of intraventricular pathologies such as hydrocephalus, has its origins with Antonin Desormeaux, whom is credited with the invention of the first endoscope in the 1850s; its first clinical application was in the removal of a urethral papilloma [1–3]. Subsequent to this feat, refinements in the design of the endoscope allowed for refinement of cystoscopy and ureteroscopy by urologists; these improvements included the incorporation of internal lighting and refined prismatic optics as demonstrated in the Nitze-Leiter cystoscope [4]. It was not until 1910 when a urologist from Chicago by the name of Victor Darwin Lespinasse performed the first known neuroendoscopic procedures, utilizing a urethroscope; he treated two children by fulgurating the choroid plexus of the lateral ventricles [3, 5]. Though Lespinasse was first credited with the endoscopic treatment of hydrocephalus, Walter Dandy and William Mixter are considered by many to be the predominant influences of neuroendoscopy and modern intraventricular endoscopic surgery.

Intraventricular endoscopy in the treatment of hydrocephalus is an invaluable tool in the modern neurosurgeon's armamentarium. Whereas traditional shunting techniques rely upon the diversion of cerebrospinal fluid (CSF) to primarily

C. Di Rocco et al. (eds.), *Complications of CSF Shunting in Hydrocephalus: Prevention, Identification, and Management*, DOI 10.1007/978-3-319-09961-3_20,

extra-axial locations (e.g., the pleura, the peritoneal cavity, the cardiac atrium) utilizing synthetic tubing in conjunction with mechanical valves, a technique fraught with the risk of subjecting patients to numerous future surgical procedures as well as infections due to indwelling foreign materials, neuroendoscopy provides a method by which alternative, intra-axial pathways for CSF outflow may be created, potentially providing durable treatment for hydrocephalus, avoiding the need for retained foreign material(s) in the majority of instances.

While successes using these techniques have been widely published, and even championed as potentially providing long-term shunt independence in the properly selected patient, the incidence, prevalence, and significance of iatrogenic complications as well as infection are sparsely discussed in the literature and have been largely limited to isolated case reports [6–13].

In this chapter, we will discuss the iatrogenic and infectious complications of neuroendoscopy in the treatment of hydrocephalus, paying particular attention to the relevant anatomy and considerations, with the aim of aiding in complication avoidance by the practicing clinician.

20.2 Techniques for the Endoscopic Treatment of Hydrocephalus

While a number of intraventricular techniques for the endoscopic treatment of hydrocephalus have been described, we will limit our discussion to those most likely to be employed by the majority of neurosurgeons; the nuances of these techniques will be discussed in more detail in the relevant chapters.

First described by William Mixter in 1923, the endoscopic third ventriculostomy (ETV) is the most commonly utilized endoscopic technique to treat obstructive hydrocephalus arising from pathologies distal to the floor of the third ventricle [3, 14, 15]. Through a transcortical approach via the lateral ventricle and subsequently the foramen of Monro, the floor of the third ventricle is directly visualized and then fenestrated using a rigid instrument such as an endoscopic forceps, Bugbee monopolar wire, or a 3- or 4-french Fogarty balloon creating a direct communication with the prepontine cistern. In some instances, this ETV may be paired with cauterization of the choroid plexus (CPC) to further reduce CSF production [16–19]. Primarily used for CSF diversion in the setting of obstructive hydrocephalus due to congenital aqueductal stenosis, this procedure also finds use in the treatment of CSF outflow obstruction secondary to neoplasms in the posterior fossa [20, 21]. As an alternative to the fenestration of the floor of the third ventricle as performed in the typical ETV, fenestration of the lamina terminalis can be considered if the anatomy is found to be unfavorable for ETV [22].

As an alternative to the ETV, a direct aqueductoplasty with or without stenting can be used to address short segment stenosis and/or membranous obstruction of the aqueduct of sylvius [22–25]. As with the ETV, the more common technique uses a transcortical approach to the third ventricle via the lateral ventricle through the foramen of Monro. In the case of an aqueductoplasty, a more anterior entry point is used to provide a slightly more posterior trajectory through the foramen of Monro to facilitate visualization of the aqueduct and allow the passage of an endoscope through the aqueduct of sylvius. After cannulation of the aqueduct, a 3-french Fogarty balloon is used to gently dilate the stricture or perforate the web causing obstruction. In cases where there is isolated enlargement of the fourth ventricle or the supratentorial ventricular anatomy is not compatible with approaching the aqueduct, a retrograde approach can be utilized whereby the fourth ventricle is directly visualized by endoscopy and the aqueduct is entered inferiorly [22, 25].

For instances in which unilateral obstruction of the foramen of Monro leads to ipsilateral trapping and enlargement of a lateral ventricle, a septostomy can be undertaken to provide a communication for CSF between the trapped ventricle and the contralateral, patent foramen of Monro [22, 26]. As with the previously described procedures, a transcortical approach is used to cannulate the lateral ventricle and an endoscope is used to visualize the ventricle. The septum pellucidum is then identified and fenestrated in a fashion similar to that used for an endoscopic third ventriculostomy.

20.3 Iatrogenic Complications in Endoscopic Surgery

Although the per-case risk of endoscopic procedures for hydrocephalus are considered to be higher compared with shunt-related procedures, the fact that a successful endoscopic procedure frees a patient from shunt dependence makes the lifetime risk potentially lower. The overall rate of complication in neuroendoscopic procedures for hydrocephalus is considered to be low, with reported incidences ranging from 0 to 20 %. In considering complications there are those that are clinically insignificant (e.g., an asymptomatic contusion) and those that are clinically significant (e.g., forniceal injury with memory loss), those that are considered unavoidable (e.g., failure from restenosis or occlusion of a fenestration), and those that are felt to be avoidable (hypothalamic dysfunction from overly aggressive dilation of a fenestration) (Table 20.1) [6, 7, 13, 27]. Ultimately, some of these complications may be unavoidable; however, recognition of them as well as their suspected cause may limit their frequency.

Table 20.1 Summary of reported complications with endoscopic intraventricular surgery [6–13, 27–29]

Procedure	Complication
Third ventriculostomy	CNIII or VI injury
	CSF leak
	Extra-axial hematoma or hygroma
	Failure to improve hydrocephalus
	Hemiparesis
	Herniation
	Hypothalamic or hypophyseal dysfunction (diabetes insipidus, amenorrhea, change in appetite)
	Hypothermia
	Infection/meningitis
	Intraventricular hemorrhage
	Memory loss
	Seizure
	Compromised short-term memory
	Subarachnoid hemorrhage/vascular injury
Aqueductoplasty	CSF leak
	Dysconjugate eye movements
	Extra-axial hemorrhage or hygroma
	Herniation
	Hypothermia
	Infection/meningitis
	Intraventricular hemorrhage
	Seizure
	Compromised short-term memory
Septostomy	CSF leak
	Extra-axial hematoma or hygroma
	Herniation
	Hypothermia
	Infection/meningitis
	Seizure

Several series have been published focusing on the incidence of complications in endoscopic procedures [6–13, 27–29]. In their series of 173 endoscopic procedures in 152 patients, Teo et al. experienced 33 complications (19 %). Complications were divided into clinically insignificant (13 %) and clinically significant events (7.5 %). Clinically insignificant cases were noted to extend the length of hospital stay by 0.4 days. In evaluating the rate of complication by type of procedure, Teo et al. noted that the highest incidence was seen with aqueductoplasty. Experience was also noted to be an important contributing factor with a higher incidence of clinically insignificant complications occurring early on the first author's experience; interestingly, the rate of significant complications remained constant [6].

In comparison, Schroeder et al. published their experience with 193 endoscopic third ventriculostomy procedures in 188 patients, and a 12 % complication rate was noted. Complications were defined as lethal (1 %), resulting in permanent deficit (1.6 %), transient deficit (7.8 %), or causing intraoperative difficulties, which did not cause patient harm (4.7 %). Two mortalities (1 %) were reported in this series as the result of septic multi-organ failure stemming from a superficial wound infection in one instance and a fatal subarachnoid hemorrhage due to avulsion of a basilar perforating artery by inflation of a Fogarty balloon in the other. Consistent with Teo et al., Schroeder et al. found that the incidence of complications decreased with experience [6, 8]. In contrast however, Schroeder et al. noted a decrease in all types of complications as the authors gained experience [8]. Beems et al. and Cinalli et al. have reported similar results to both Teo et al. and Schroeder et al. with 1.6 and 13.8 % incidences of complications, respectively, reported [30, 31].

Infection is an infrequent complication of endoscopic surgery with an incidence of 0–5 % reported [6–13, 27–29]. In many cases, infections are limited to superficial wound infections; however, given the direct cannulation of the ventricular system during these procedures, meningitis/ventriculitis with its resultant risk of permanent disability or mortality is a possibility.

As mentioned above, one mortality secondary to septic multi-organ failure was reported originating with a wound infection [8].

20.4 Avoidance of Complications

Avoidance or minimization of complications in the endoscopic treatment of hydrocephalus, like any other surgical procedure, requires the operator to understand the intricacies of the relevant anatomy, the steps of the procedure to be performed, and the advantages as well as limitations of the instruments to chosen for use.

Beginning with the layout of the operating theatre, the location of the surgical bed, the surgical assistants, the surgical equipment and instruments, and the monitors must be considered. It is important to ensure that the surgeon is able to comfortably work about the patient's head while simultaneously visualizing the endoscopic view via monitors without placing themselves in an uncomfortable or disadvantageous position. Concurrent with this, the assistant must be able to follow the progression of the procedure while being able to aid the surgeon without spatially interfering with the operator's tasks.

In positioning the patient, the operator must choose in such a way as to take into consideration that which will facilitate visualization of the surgical objective but also maximize the ergonomic advantage for the surgeon. This includes the height of the bed, how the patient's head is angled or rotated, as well as how the patient's head is supported (donut on bed versus horseshoe versus pin fixation). When choosing how to position the patient's head, the approach and site of the burrhole to be used must also be considered. The goal in this instance is in understanding the objectives of the surgery, choosing a burrhole location that provides a trajectory allowing the operator to maximize visualization of the target structures and simultaneously minimizing the scope's movement and avoiding unnecessary pressure on sensitive structures. Large, sweeping motions of the endoscope while within the ventricle should be avoided as these can cause direct injury to the traversed cortex as well as the structures that reside in the blind spot of the endoscope such as the blood vessels or the fornices [6, 27, 32, 33].

The surgeon should ensure that the appropriate instruments needed are present in the operating theatre and functioning appropriately. Time should be taken to ensure the endoscope camera is aligned properly to help with maintaining surgical orientation; the surgeon must also ensure that the optics of the endoscope provide for adequate image quality and the light source is sufficiently bright before beginning a procedure. Further, the surgeon must determine if the appropriately sized instruments are present. Consider, for example, the case of an ETV. How extensively is the foramen of Monro dilated? Is the endoscope chosen of adequate diameter to traverse the foramen safely? Attempting to traverse the foramen of Monro with an inappropriately large endoscope places the fornix and thalamus at risk for injury, as well as the associated vascular structures such as the choroid plexus, septal vein, and caudate vein. Is the angle of the endoscopic optics (e.g., 0°, 12°, or 30° scope) appropriate to allow simultaneous visualization of the appropriate structures and working instruments to pass down the working channel?

Continuing with the example of an ETV, how and where is the operator anticipating fenestration of the floor of the third ventricle? At risk with this maneuver are the thalamus and hypothalamus laterally, mammillary bodies, corticospinal tracts, and the remainder of the brain stem posteriorly, the infundibulum and optic apparatus anteriorly, and the oculomotor nerve as well as the basilar artery with its associated arterial branches beyond the ventricular floor. Ideally, a point in the midline, halfway between the infundibular recess and mammillary bodies, should be chosen to minimize injury to the adjacent structures (particularly the hypothalamus, infundibulum, and brain stem structures). Blunt fenestration using a Fogarty balloon or Bugbee wire may reduce the risk of a vascular injury but alternatively may increase the risk of hypothalamic injury [27]. Alternatively sharp fenestration utilizing a closed dissection forceps, a bipolar cautery, or a contact laser is thought to reduce the risk of hypothalamic injury associated with traction upon the floor of the third ventricle but in turn may increase the risk of injury to the vascular structures and cranial nerves deep to the ventricular floor, or result in thermal injury to surrounding tissues [6, 7, 27, 28].

Along these same lines, when performing an aqueductoplasty, choosing the adequate scope size and optic angle is essential not only for passing the foramen of Monro but also for visualizing the outlet to the aqueduct of Sylvius. Further, when dilating or stenting the aqueduct, the size of the balloon to be used, along with the amount of liquid or air used to inflate the balloon, and the outer diameter of the stent to be placed must be carefully considered. The tectum, comprising the roof of the aqueduct, is exquisitely sensitive to pressure, and the resultant injury to extraocular gaze, particularly vertical gaze, can be easily encountered [23–25, 27, 31, 34].

Hypothermia and herniation syndromes can in most cases be avoided by paying attention to intraoperative irrigation. In addition to general measures such as controlling room temperature and utilizing warming devices such as warming blankets, the judicious use of irrigation, which has been pre-warmed to approximate body temperature, can reduce the incidence of hypothermia in most cases. The risk of herniation can be reduced through limiting the volume of irrigation used and, more importantly, ensuring that an exit for irrigation is available (e.g., an open *AND* unused working channel on the endoscope, or alternatively an adequate room between the inner wall of the cannula/working sheath and the outer wall of the endoscope itself) [6, 27].

To reduce infection rates, meticulous attention to cleansing and surgical preparation of the operative site must be adhered to along with proper draping and adherence to accepted sterile operative techniques. Concurrently, perioperative antibiotics consisting of a second-generation or newer cephalosporin or other appropriate antibiotic with adequate coverage of skin flora with quick infusion times should be selected and administered within 30 min of surgical incision [35, 36].

Conclusions

The endoscopic treatment of hydrocephalus provides the potential for a shunt-free existence in the appropriately selected patient. Though the rate of complication is considered higher on a per-case basis compared with shunt-based therapies, the majority of endoscopic cases are a one-time procedure, therefore having an overall lower risk of adverse outcome. It is clear however, based on reports evaluating complication rates, that endoscopic techniques possess a particularly steep learning curve [6, 8–13, 27, 31]. Experience and therefore knowledge of complications and their causes are thought to be critical in reducing the frequency of complications associated with these procedures.

Learning from the experience of others, laboratory training including cadaveric and computerized simulations of surgeries, and extensive preparation with attention to detail may all contribute to reducing iatrogenic and infectious complications in the endoscopic treatment of hydrocephalus.

References

1. Abbott R (2004) History of neuroendoscopy. Neurosurg Clin N Am 15:1–7
2. Hsu W, Li KW, Bookland M, Jallo GI (2009) Keyhole to the brain: Walter Dandy and neuroendoscopy. J Neurosurg Pediatr 3:439–442
3. Schmitt PJ, Jane JJA (2012) A lesson in history: the evolution of endoscopic third ventriculostomy. Neurosurg Focus 33:E11
4. Herr HW (2006) Max Nitze, the cystoscope and urology. J Urol 176:1313–1316
5. Walker ML (2001) History of ventriculostomy. Neurosurg Clin N Am 12:101–110, viii
6. Teo C, Rahman S, Boop FA, Cherny B (1996) Complications of endoscopic neurosurgery. Childs Nerv Syst 12:248–253; discussion 253
7. Abtin K, Thompson BG, Walker ML (1998) Basilar artery perforation as a complication of endoscopic third ventriculostomy. Pediatr Neurosurg 28:35–41
8. Schroeder HWS, Niendorf W-R, Gaab MR (2002) Complications of endoscopic third ventriculostomy. J Neurosurg 96:1032–1040
9. Schroeder HWS, Oertel J, Gaab MR (2004) Incidence of complications in neuroendoscopic surgery – Springer. Childs Nerv Syst 20:878–883
10. Navarro R, Gil-Parra R, Reitman AJ, Olavarria G (2006) Endoscopic third ventriculostomy in children: early and late complications and their avoidance – Springer. Childs Nerv Syst 22:506–513
11. Dusick JR, McArthur DL, Bergsneider M (2008) Success and complication rates of endoscopic third ventriculostomy for adult hydrocephalus: a series of 108 patients. Surg Neurol 69:5–15
12. Erşahin Y, Arslan D (2008) Complications of endoscopic third ventriculostomy. Childs Nerv Syst 24: 943–948
13. Bouras T, Sgouros S (2011) Complications of endoscopic third ventriculostomy. J Neurosurg Pediatr 7: 643–649
14. Mixter W (1923) Ventriculoscopy and puncture of the floor of the third ventricle: preliminary report of a case. Boston Med Surg J 188:277–278
15. Jallo GI, Kothbauer KF, Abbott IR (2005) Endoscopic third ventriculostomy. Neurosurg Focus 19:E11
16. Warf BC (2005) Comparison of endoscopic third ventriculostomy alone and combined with choroid plexus cauterization in infants younger than 1 year of age: a prospective study in 550 African children. J Neurosurg 103:475–481
17. Warf BC, Kulkarni AV (2010) Intraoperative assessment of cerebral aqueduct patency and cisternal scarring: impact on success of endoscopic third ventriculostomy in 403 African children. J Neurosurg Pediatr 5:204–209
18. Warf BC (2013) The impact of combined endoscopic third ventriculostomy and choroid plexus cauterization on the management of pediatric hydrocephalus in developing countries. World Neurosurg 79:S23. e13–25
19. Warf BC, Tracy S, Mugamba J (2012) Long-term outcome for endoscopic third ventriculostomy alone or in combination with choroid plexus cauterization for congenital aqueductal stenosis in African infants. J Neurosurg Pediatr 10:108–111
20. Ruggiero C, Cinalli G, Spennato P, Aliberti F (2004) Endoscopic third ventriculostomy in the treatment of hydrocephalus in posterior fossa tumors in children – Springer. Childs Nerv Syst 20:828–833
21. Fritsch MJ, Doerner L, Kienke S, Mehdorn HM (2005) Hydrocephalus in children with posterior fossa tumors: role of endoscopic third ventriculostomy. J Neurosurg Pediatr 103:40–42
22. Schroeder HWS, Oertel J, Gaab MR (2007) Endoscopic treatment of cerebrospinal fluid pathway obstructions. Neurosurgery 60:44–52
23. Schroeder HW, Gaab MR (1999) Endoscopic aqueductoplasty: technique and results. Neurosurgery 45:508–515; discussion 515–508
24. Teo C, Burson T, Misra S (1999) Endoscopic treatment of the trapped fourth ventricle. Neurosurgery 44:1257–1261; discussion 1261–1252
25. Sansone JM, Iskandar BJ (2005) Endoscopic cerebral aqueductoplasty: a trans—fourth ventricle approach. J Neurosurg 103:388–392

26. Hongo K, Morota N, Watabe T, Isobe M, Nakagawa H (2001) Giant basilar bifurcation aneurysm presenting as a third ventricular mass with unilateral obstructive hydrocephalus: case report. J Clin Neurosci 8:51–54
27. Yadav Y, Kher Y, Parihar V (2013) Complication avoidance and its management in endoscopic neurosurgery. Neurol India 61:217
28. McLaughlin MR, Wahlig JB, Kaufmann AM, Albright AL (1997) Traumatic basilar aneurysm after endoscopic third ventriculostomy: case report. Neurosurgery 41:1400–1403; discussion 1403–1404
29. Oumar S, Sergio B, Valérie L-C, Martin D, Franck-Emmanuel R (2010) Endoscopic third ventriculostomy: outcome analysis in 368 procedures. J Neurosurg Pediatr 5:68–74
30. Beems T, Grotenhuis JA (2004) Long-term complications and definition of failure of neuroendoscopic procedures – Springer. Childs Nerv Syst 20:868–877
31. Cinalli G, Spennato P, Savarese L, Ruggiero C, Aliberti F, Cuomo L, Cianciulli E, Maggi G (2006) Endoscopic aqueductoplasty and placement of a stent in the cerebral aqueduct in the management of isolated fourth ventricle in children. J Neurosurg 104:21–27
32. Chen F, Chen T, Nakaji P (2013) Adjustment of the endoscopic third ventriculostomy entry point based on the anatomical relationship between coronal and sagittal sutures. J Neurosurg 118:510–513
33. Bonanni R, Carlesimo GA, Caltagirone C (2004) Amnesia following endoscopic third ventriculostomy: a single case study. Eur Neurol 51:118–120
34. Erşahin Y (2006) Endoscopic aqueductoplasty. Childs Nerv Syst 23:143–150
35. Bratzler DW, Houck PM (2005) Antimicrobial prophylaxis for surgery: an advisory statement from the National Surgical Infection Prevention Project. Am J Surg 189:395–404
36. Steinberg JP, Braun BI, Hellinger WC, Kusek L, Bozikis MR, Bush AJ, Dellinger EP, Burke JP, Simmons B, Kritchevsky SB (2009) Timing of antimicrobial prophylaxis and the risk of surgical site infections. Ann Surg 250:10–16

CSF Fistulae as a Complication Due to Insufficient Correction of Altered CSF Dynamics

21

Jogi V. Pattisapu

Contents

21.1 **Objectives** 277
21.2 **Introduction** 277
21.3 **Symptoms** 278
21.4 **Imaging** 278
21.5 **Discussion** 279
21.6 **Conclusion** 281
21.7 **Questions** 281
References 282

J.V. Pattisapu, MD, FAAP, FACS, FAANS (L)
Pediatric Neurosurgery, University of Central Florida, College of Medicine, Orlando, FL, USA
e-mail: JPattisapu@Ped-Neurosurgery.com; Jogi.Pattisapu@UCF.edu

21.1 Objectives

This chapter will outline issues related to cerebrospinal fluid (CSF) dynamics in patients with hydrocephalus. Presenting symptoms and related factors, necessary diagnostic tests, and clinical thinking in treating patients presenting with such conditions will be reviewed. Potential avoidable complications will be discussed.

21.2 Introduction

Several factors are important in maintaining ideal CSF dynamics within the cranial compartment. Constant CSF production, pulsatility from blood flow, normal circulation, and absorption at the proper pressure are necessary to maintain central nervous system (CNS) structure and function. Abnormalities of spinal fluid dynamics often lead to hydrocephalus, and little is known regarding CSF mechanisms or potential reserves in causing diseases.

Common situations associated with abnormal CSF dynamics include imbalance of fluid production or absorption, spinal fluid fistulae, or altered anatomy such as macrocephaly/microcephaly. Increased intracranial pressure (ICP) due to hydrocephalus may lead to CSF leak as described by Clark et al. or due to idiopathic intracranial hypertension (IIH), as noted by Schlosser [3, 29]. Patients with low ICP may sometimes present with similar symptoms suggestive of increased pressure, prompting shunt insertion as a treatment.

C. Di Rocco et al. (eds.), *Complications of CSF Shunting in Hydrocephalus: Prevention, Identification, and Management*, DOI 10.1007/978-3-319-09961-3_21,

Intracranial hypotension may result from a traumatic dural tear, after a lumbar puncture or a persistent CSF leak from chronic increased ICP [4, 7]. This condition may occur due to persistent fluid leakage after inadequate dural repair or after ventricular shunt insertion with excessive fluid drainage and siphoning phenomenon. Spontaneous cases of low ICP have been reported, caused by a variety of conditions such as dehydration, uremia, metabolic coma, or after thoracic surgery [21, 33].

Intracranial hypotension may result from alterations obesity, empty sella syndrome, or other causes affecting structure or pressure. Altered CSF dynamics may lead to intracranial hypotension associated with ventriculomegaly, a condition referred to as "low-pressure hydrocephalus," and Bannister et al. described disappointing outcomes after shunting in eight such children with low pressures ("boggy brain"), recommending increasing EVD output using the "subzero" method to improve brain elastance [2]. This concept was further advanced by Foltz to treat "zero pressure hydrocephalus," wherein patients lose the brain turgor [9].

The exact incidence of chronic CSF leak or spontaneous intracranial hypotension is unknown, although an estimate of 1–50,000 is suggested and related to chronic increased ICP, trauma, or postpartum status [26, 27]. Additionally, longstanding intracranial hypertension presumably leads to chronic CSF escape via small dural lacunae or areas of membrane weakness [15].

21.3 Symptoms

A delicate balance is maintained within the intact skull and the contents in its limited space require pressure-volume homeostasis. Alterations of ICP due to CSF production and absorption often lead to a variety of symptoms such as headaches, visual changes, cranial nerve findings, or mental changes. The most common symptom of intracranial hypotension is postural headache, sometimes associated with neck pain, nausea, and vomiting [1, 28]. The headache is associated with activity and often resolves spontaneously or with rest and hydration.

In certain situations, symptoms caused by intracranial hypotension (often associated with postural headaches) are difficult to differentiate with those associated with increased ICP. Photophobia, tinnitus, and difficulty with concentration are secondary symptoms often seen in patients with intracranial hypotension and may be mistaken for signs of increasing ICP, prompting shunt insertion as a treatment for alleviation of symptoms.

Lethargy is often noted in patients with persistent CSF leak and intracranial hypotension, due to constant traction or pressure on dural structures. Although the exact mechanism is unknown, EEG abnormalities such as diffuse nonspecific slowing or status epilepticus have been reported [10]. Some patients exhibit visual obscurations or concentration difficulty that may be related to chronic headaches although it is unclear if cortical dysfunction or other specific phenomenon may be related to this finding [12].

Gait abnormalities are also noted in patients experiencing low intracranial pressure such as normal pressure hydrocephalus (NPH) [17, 27] This finding may be related to fiber stretch over distended ventricles or global cortical dysfunction with malaise due to chronic headaches. Although no particular pattern of gait abnormality is noted with low ICP, signs of radiculopathy and numbness are sometimes noted.

21.4 Imaging

Imaging of spontaneous CSF leaks is well described in the literature using CT scan with intrathecal dye or contrasted MRI studies [30] (Fig. 21.1). CSF fistulae may be seen in cases of trauma, empty sella syndrome, postpartum situations, or other conditions where patients present with symptoms of intracranial hypotension [14]. In many cases, dural thickening and enhancement associated with mild ventricular enlargement is noted, and in some cases, empty sella syndrome is described [31]. Temporal pits or other small areas of enhancement are sometimes seen with dural openings or brain herniation suggestive of a focal CSF leakage [26].

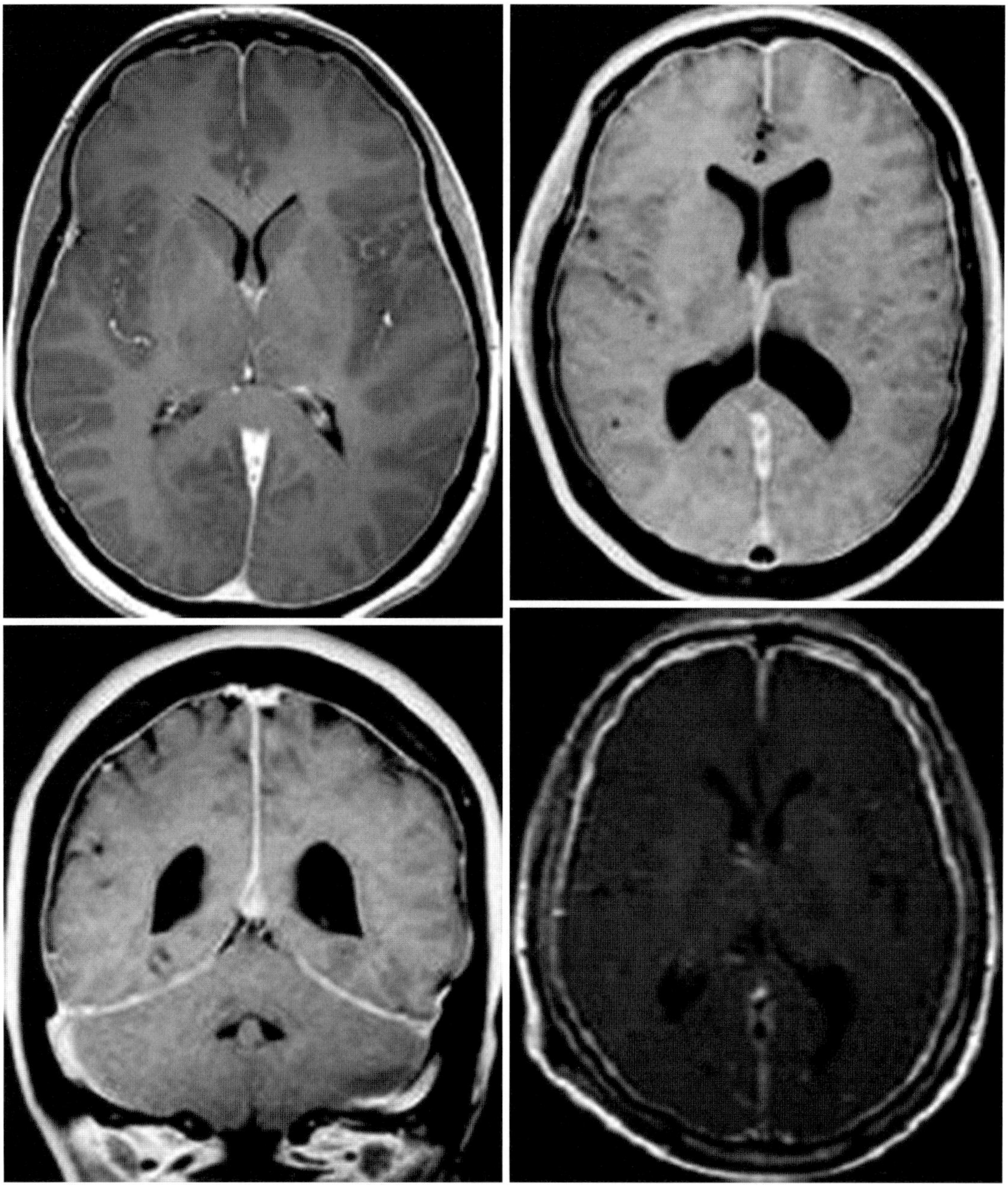

Fig. 21.1 Contrasted MRI images of dural enhancement in cases of intracranial hypotension

21.5 Discussion

Any abnormality that offsets the delicate intracranial pressure-volume balance can lead to symptoms. Altered CSF dynamics due to fluid drainage from functioning shunts affects brain function in many ways, sometimes causing symptoms suggestive of intermittent malfunction. Lowered intracranial pressure changes CSF output resistance and in some situations, overdrainage may cause collapse of the ventricles with associated symptoms of shunt malfunction.

Implantation of a shunt device establishes a more physiologic CSF circulation phenomenon, where resistance to CSF outflow is affected, end-plateau pressure and baseline pressures are altered, and compensatory reserve is improved [23]. Shunting often drains large volumes of fluid due to decreased resistance, leading to a temporary over-drainage phenomenon in some cases. Naturally, this impact on pressure-volume relationship is an important factor in symptom causation.

CSF leak leads to intracranial hypotension and diminished brain turgor such as NPH due to decreased spinal fluid volume rather than decreased pressure [6, 26–28]. Major issues associated with shunting in patients with CSF leak include decreased brain turgor or further worsening low ICP symptoms [9, 8, 22, 25].

The dural opening does not completely seal in some cases after shunting, maintaining a potential avenue for organisms or air entry, increasing the risk of subsequent infection or tension pneumocephalus [24]. Studies suggest that persistent CSF leak after shunt surgery has a very high incidence of infection, which is a major concern for any neurosurgeon who must diligently observe for spinal fluid leakage at the surgical site [13, 16]. Often, aggressive measures to revise/replace the shunt mechanism are warranted since a negative pressure situation may allow air to enter the cranial cavity [11]. In cases of traumatic CSF leak, the dual tear often causes a ball valve phenomenon, which becomes an avenue of air entry into the cranium.

Patients undergoing tethered cord release may develop persistent CSF leak, leading to shunt malfunction [32]. Although the exact mechanism is unknown, it is possible that a delicate balance in CSF dynamics is upset, or blood products in the spinal fluid occlude a functioning shunt. Another possibility is collapse or coaptation of the ventricular walls due to CSF loss during surgery, leading to temporary shunt malfunction. It is possible that a vicious cycle of persistent CSF leak leads to shunt malfunction or an improperly opening shunt causes increased pressure causing a persistent leak at the site of tethered cord release.

Most shunts function as like on-off mechanisms with altering flow rates and intracranial pressures during the day. Although evidence is lacking on how CSF dynamics are affected after shunting, it is interesting and perhaps beneficial to identify its role during hydrocephalus management. Typically, the opening and closing at various pressures does not fully replicate physiologic responses, sometimes mimicking symptoms of intermittent malfunction (Czosnyka [5, 23]). Although improvements in spinal fluid dynamics may not be observed in imaging or clinical observations, resistance to CSF outflow (RCSF) decreases with a functioning shunt, which improves the vasogenic components of the ICP waveform (such as the respiratory, pulse, and B waves) [34]. It is unclear if antisiphon devices function as expected to completely correct this phenomenon, although recent advances inflow-regulated valve mechanisms have decreased the overall revision rates.

It is known that abnormal intra-abdominal pressures caused by constipation may lead to transient shunt malfunction. CSF dynamics affecting CSF flow rates are altered in these situations as the rising intra-abdominal pressure offsets ventricle-to-abdomen pressure gradient [18]. Two pediatric cases were reported of temporary ventriculoperitoneal shunt malfunction with increased ICP. These children spontaneously improved after the constipation was resolved, and a similar description was previously offered by others [19].

Treatment of aqueductal stenosis by endoscopic third ventriculostomy versus VP shunt insertion is a frequent dilemma, and identification of certain parameters may facilitate the decision process. Oi and Di Rocco offered novel ideas regarding CSF dynamics explaining why endoscopic third ventriculostomy does not fully correct the symptoms in approximately 1/3 of infants, suggesting improperly developed "minor pathways" that maybe necessary in adulthood [20]. This "evolution theory in CSF dynamics" may suggest newer mechanisms of normal circulation and CSF absorption pathways within the cranial cavity. The authors proposed five stages of CSF dynamics during maturation, with the last two stages developing postnatally. The "minor pathway" of CSF absorption via the extra-arachnoid sites plays a significant role soon after birth until the first year of life, and the "major pathway" begins to take effect at approximately 6 months. This overlap between the two pathways may explain some of the reasons why our initial attempts at third ventriculostomy may not be as successful.

During the later stages of development, increased ICP due to shunt malfunction may require these "minor" (extra-arachnoid) pathways, which in some situations are no longer available in an acute situation. However, certain patients maintain these "minor" CSF absorption pathways that can be recruited as necessary during periods of intermittent shunt malfunction or as a buffer during periods of excess need [20]. Identification of such factors may offer a better understanding to guide attempts at correcting abnormal CSF dynamics.

Patients with CSF fistulae have altered intracranial fluid dynamics and the approaches to correct them require individual consideration. For example, some patients undergo shunt insertion as a primary treatment rather than a procedure to control the CSF leak; however, a direct attack at the site of CSF leak is more appropriate than CSF diversion (which again affects overall pressure-volume balance). Local treatment of CSF fistula may be accomplished by various methods, but symptoms often persist in patients with increased intracranial hypertension, if the fluid leakage occurred as a vent to diminish the pressure.

Persistent CSF fistulae with functioning shunt systems may develop entry of air or organisms into the cranial cavity due to the relative negative pressure. Postoperative pneumocephalus sometimes occurs after shunt insertion in patients with an occult CSF leak, and management of patients with hydrocephalus is more difficult if associated with infection, pneumocephalus, or persistent symptoms of low intracranial pressure [16].

21.6 Conclusion

This chapter reviewed issues related to CSF dynamics in patients with hydrocephalus. Presenting symptoms and related factors, clinical thinking, and imaging studies useful in treating patients and potential avoidable complications were discussed.

Intracranial CSF dynamics are complex and significantly altered in patients with hydrocephalus, spinal fluid fistulae, and after shunt insertion. Pressure-volume relationships, resistance to CSF outflow, and pulsatility with changes in the wave forms are known features which create a delicate balance leading to various symptoms that are difficult to attribute to a particular phenomenon. Together, they offer some insight into the mechanics and interplay between the various parameters affecting these patients, and further study is warranted to provide a more complete understanding of these mechanisms.

21.7 Questions

1. Describe the relationship between hydrocephalus and CSF fistulae?
   A. CSF fistulae may develop in hydrocephalic patients due to chronic increased intracranial pressure (ICP) with gradual thinning of dura and erosion, causing fluid leakage.
2. Which symptoms might warrant consideration of combined existence of these two issues?
   A. Although many symptoms are frequently seen in both conditions, postural headaches are often noted in patients with intracranial hypotension (others such as visual disturbances or mental focusing issues and cranial nerve findings may occur in both situations).
3. What are the altered CSF dynamics in patients with fluid leaks?
   A. Many patients experience low-pressure symptoms due to chronic CSF leaks, causing traction on meninges and cranial nerves while in the upright position. Often complaints of postural headache, difficulty with concentration, visual changes, or back pain are reported.
4. What are some potential issues/complications of shunting in patients with CSF fistulae?
   A. Decreased intracranial pressure symptoms may lead to air entry into the cranial cavity, leading to pneumocephalus or infection. In

some cases, gradual decrease in flow via the shunt system may cause shunt failure.

5. How can complications be avoided/minimized in patients with CSF fistulae requiring shunting?
   A. By vigilant observation and constant monitoring of patients with potential CSF leaks, the surgeon should identify and treat the cause of CSF leak prior to shunt implantation. In some cases, temporary drainage may be necessary to control the situation until a more permanent approach can be used. Any CSF leak from a postoperative site should be addressed immediately so as to minimize the risk of a shunt infection.

References

1. Angelo F, Giuseppe M, Eliana M, Luisa C, Gennaro B (2011) Spontaneous intracranial hypotension: diagnostic and therapeutic implications in neurosurgical practice. Neurol Sci 32(Suppl 3):S287–S290
2. Bannister CM (1972) A report of eight patients with low pressure hydrocephalus treated by C.S.F. Diversion with disappointing results. Acta Neurochir (Wien) 27(1):11–15
3. Clark D, Bullock P, Hui T, Firth J (1994) Benign intracranial hypertension: a cause of CSF rhinorrhoea. J Neurol Neurosurg Psychiatry 57(7):847–849
4. Cohen-Gadol AA (2009) Acute ventriculoperitoneal shunt malfunction following opening of the spinal subarachnoid space. Childs Nerv Syst 25(5):599–600
5. Czosnyka M, Czosnyka Z, Momjian S, Pickard JD (2004) Cerebrospinal fluid dynamics. Physiol Meas 25(5):R51–R76
6. De Bonis P, Mangiola A, Pompucci A, Formisano R, Mattogno P, Anile C (2013) CSF dynamics analysis in patients with post-traumatic ventriculomegaly. Clin Neurol Neurosurg 115(1):49–53
7. Dias MS, Li V, Pollina J (1999) Low-pressure shunt 'malfunction' following lumbar puncture in children with shunted obstructive hydrocephalus. Pediatr Neurosurg 30(3):146–150
8. Filippidis AS, Kalani MY, Nakaji P, Rekate HL (2011) Negative-pressure and low-pressure hydrocephalus: the role of cerebrospinal fluid leaks resulting from surgical approaches to the cranial base. J Neurosurg 115(5):1031–1037
9. Foltz EL, Blanks J, Meyer R (1994) Hydrocephalus: the zero ICP ventricle shunt (ZIPS) to control gravity shunt flow. A clinical study in 56 patients. Childs Nerv Syst 10(1):43–48
10. Hedna VS, Kumar A, Miller B, Bidari S, Salardini A, Waters MF, Hella M, Valenstein E, Eisenschenk S (2014) Intracranial hypotension masquerading as nonconvulsive status epilepticus: report of 3 cases. J Neurosurg 120(3):624–627
11. Honeybul S, Bala A (2006) Delayed pneumocephalus following shunting for hydrocephalus. J Clin Neurosci 13(9):939–942
12. Hong M, Shah GV, Adams KM, Turner RS, Foster NL (2002) Spontaneous intracranial hypotension causing reversible frontotemporal dementia. Neurology 58(8): 1285–1287
13. Jeelani NU, Kulkarni AV, Desilva P, Thompson DN, Hayward RD (2009) Postoperative cerebrospinal fluid wound leakage as a predictor of shunt infection: a prospective analysis of 205 cases. Clinical article. J Neurosurg Pediatr 4(2):166–169
14. JosÈ G-U, Luis L, Avelino P, Gonzalo B (1999) Spontaneous cerebrospinal fluid fistulae associated with empty sellae: surgical treatment and long-term results. Neurosurgery 45(4):766–773
15. Kenning TJ, Willcox TO, Artz GJ, Schiffmacher P, Farrell CJ, Evans JJ (2012) Surgical management of temporal meningoencephaloceles, cerebrospinal fluid leaks, and intracranial hypertension: treatment paradigm and outcomes. Neurosurg Focus 32(6):E6
16. Kulkarni AV, Drake JM, Lamberti-Pasculli M (2001) Cerebrospinal fluid shunt infection: a prospective study of risk factors. J Neurosurg 94(2):195–201
17. Marmarou A, Bergsneider M, Relkin N, Klinge P, Black PM (2005) Development of guidelines for idiopathic normal-pressure hydrocephalus: introduction. Neurosurgery 57(3 Suppl):S1–S3; discussion ii–v
18. Martinez-Lage JF, Martos-Tello JM, Ros-de-San Pedro J, Almagro MJ (2008) Severe constipation: an under-appreciated cause of VP shunt malfunction: a case-based update. Childs Nerv Syst 24(4):431–435
19. Muzumdar D, Ventureyra EC (2007) Transient ventriculoperitoneal shunt malfunction after chronic constipation: case report and review of literature. Childs Nerv Syst 23(4):455–458
20. Oi S, Di Rocco C (2006) Proposal of evolution theory in cerebrospinal fluid dynamics and minor pathway hydrocephalus in developing immature brain. Childs Nerv Syst 22(7):662–669
21. Paldino M, Mogilner AY, Tenner MS (2003) Intracranial hypotension syndrome: a comprehensive review. Neurosurg Focus 15(6):ECP2
22. Pang D, Altschuler E (1994) Low-pressure hydrocephalic state and viscoelastic alterations in the brain. Neurosurgery 35(4):643–655; discussion 655–656
23. Petrella G, Czosnyka M, Keong N, Pickard JD, Czosnyka Z (2008) How does CSF dynamics change after shunting? Acta Neurol Scand 118(3):182–188
24. Pitts LH, Wilson CB, Dedo HH, Weyand R (1975) Pneumocephalus following ventriculoperitoneal shunt. Case report. J Neurosurg 43(5):631–633
25. Rekate HL (1994) The usefulness of mathematical modeling in hydrocephalus research. Childs Nerv Syst 10(1):13–18
26. Schievink WI (2013) Novel neuroimaging modalities in the evaluation of spontaneous cerebrospinal fluid leaks. Curr Neurol Neurosci Rep 13(7):358

27. Schievink WI, Maya MM, Louy C, Moser FG, Sloninsky L (2013) Spontaneous intracranial hypotension in childhood and adolescence. J Pediatr 163(2):504–510
28. Schievink WI, Schwartz MS, Maya MM, Moser FG, Rozen TD (2012) Lack of causal association between spontaneous intracranial hypotension and cranial cerebrospinal fluid leaks. J Neurosurg 116(4): 749–754
29. Schlosser RJ, Wilensky EM, Grady MS, Bolger WE (2003) Elevated intracranial pressures in spontaneous cerebrospinal fluid leaks. Am J Rhinol 17(4):191–195
30. Schuknecht B, Simmen D, Briner HR, Holzmann D (2008) Nontraumatic skull base defects with spontaneous CSF rhinorrhea and arachnoid herniation: imaging findings and correlation with endoscopic sinus surgery in 27 patients. AJNR Am J Neuroradiol 29(3):542–549
31. Shetty PG, Shroff MM, Fatterpekar GM, Sahani DV, Kirtane MV (2000) A retrospective analysis of spontaneous sphenoid sinus fistula: MR and CT findings. AJNR Am J Neuroradiol 21(2):337–342
32. Tubbs RS, Pugh J, Acakpo-Satchivi L, Wellons JC 3rd, Blount JP, Oakes WJ (2009) Acute ventriculoperitoneal shunt malfunction following opening of the spinal subarachnoid space: a case series. Childs Nerv Syst 25(5):599–600; discussion 601–605
33. Wang EW, Vandergrift WA 3rd, Schlosser RJ (2011) Spontaneous CSF leaks. Otolaryngol Clin North Am 44(4):845–856, vii
34. Weerakkody RA, Czosnyka M, Schuhmann MU, Schmidt E, Keong N, Santarius T, Pickard JD, Czosnyka Z (2011) Clinical assessment of cerebrospinal fluid dynamics in hydrocephalus. Guide to interpretation based on observational study. Acta Neurol Scand 124(2):85–98

22 Subdural Collections: Hygroma and Haematoma

Miguel Gelabert-González, Eduardo Aran-Echabe, and Ramón Serramito-García

Contents

22.1 **Introduction** 285
22.2 **Subdural Collections After Ventricular Shunting** 286
22.2.1 Subdural Hygroma After Ventricular Shunting 286
22.2.2 Subdural Haematomas After Ventricular Shunting 289
22.3 **Subdural Collections Following Neuroendoscopic Procedures** 290
22.3.1 Subdural CSF Hygromas Following Neuroendoscopic Procedures........... 291
22.3.2 Subdural Haematomas Following Neuroendoscopic Procedures........... 293
22.3.3 Infectious Subdural Collections After Hydrocephalus Surgery 295
22.4 **Subdural Collections After Treatment of Arachnoid Cyst** 295
22.5 **Other Extra-axial Collections After Hydrocephalus Treatment** 296
References 298

M. Gelabert-González, MD (✉)
E. Aran-Echabe, MD • R. Serramito-García, MD
Neurosurgical Service, Clinic Hospital of Santiago de Compostela, Santiago de Compostela, Spain

Department of Surgery (Neurosurgery), University of Santiago de Compostela, San Francisco 1, 15705 Santiago de Compostela, Spain
e-mail: miguel.gelabert@usc.es; eduardo.aran.echabe@sergas.es; ramon.serramito.garcia@sergas.es

22.1 Introduction

Hydrocephalus is not a single pathologic entity nor is a simple well-defined disease process. It represents a diverse group of clinical situations sharing a common feature of increased intracranial pressure (ICP) resulting from an imbalance of cerebrospinal fluid (CSF) formation and absorption. The overall incidence of hydrocephalus in the general population is unknown, because this common neurosurgical condition is associated with other congenital or acquired disorders [31].

Excluding a minority of cases that may benefit from drug treatment, the best treatment of hydrocephalus, both in child and in adults, is surgery. Currently we have three major surgical treatment options: (a) ventricular shunting using a peritoneal or atrial diversion, (b) lumboperitoneal shunts, and (c) endoscopic techniques, fundamentally endoscopic third ventriculostomy. Other obsolete techniques, such as the Torkildsen procedure, are of minor importance.

The surgical treatment of hydrocephalus is one of the most commonly performed procedures in modern paediatric neurosurgical practice, and cerebrospinal fluid shunting constitutes the main means of treatment for hydrocephalus, independently of the site of obstruction compared with third ventriculostomy. Cerebrospinal fluid shunting is one of the most important procedures in the neurosurgical armamentarium, exceeding any other cranial operation in the number of lives saved and neurological function preserved.

C. Di Rocco et al. (eds.), *Complications of CSF Shunting in Hydrocephalus: Prevention, Identification, and Management*, DOI 10.1007/978-3-319-09961-3_22,

However, the operation continues to be associated with a series of well-known complications, being the most frequent mechanical and infectious.

Complications due to insufficient correction of the altered cerebrospinal fluid dynamics include (a) subdural collections of cerebrospinal fluid, (b) blood collections (acute or chronic subdural haematomas) and (c) infectious collections (empyema).

22.2 Subdural Collections After Ventricular Shunting

Subdural collections arise in the dural border cell (DBC) layer, a loose cellular layer devoid of intercellular collagen and tight junctions, located between two firm meningeal layers: the dura mater wired with abundant intercellular collagen on one side and the arachnoid matter with cells anchored to a basal membrane and clamped together with tight junctions on the other [16]. Undulated fibroblasts of the DBC layer may extend for considerable distance parallel to flat axes of the meninges and form a layer several cell-process thick. These cells frequently appear sinuous and may present interdigitations.

The pathophysiological mechanism of this disorder is based on an early and rapid reduction in ventricular size that may result in the collapse of the brain with the subsequent accumulation of surrounding fluid. However, the exact mechanism underlying this condition is controversial, i.e., at times it may be motivated by low intracranial pressure that facilitates the arachnoid pulling away from the inner dura mater through small tears that could filter CSF. This subdural CSF may cause separation of the arachnoid and dura mater due to increased pressure in the subdural space. An alternative hypothesis proposes that increased permeability of the intracranial vessels may occur in cases of a head injury.

22.2.1 Subdural Hygroma After Ventricular Shunting

A common clinical scenario for the development of extra-axial fluid collection is shunt insertion for large ventricles in older children. As the ventricle decreases in size, the brain/CSF volume decreases in the cranial vault, allowing for space to develop in the subdural compartment. The incidence of subdural hygroma after shunt insertion ranges from 1 to 10 % [27]. In the randomized Shunt Design Trial, extra-axial fluid collections in children were observed in 12 of 344 (3.4 %) patients, but they were unrelated to the aetiology of hydrocephalus [8].

Most of subdural effusions are asymptomatic, particularly in older children and adults, and their diagnosis is made through imaging controls with computed tomography (CT) or magnetic resonance imaging (MRI). When the collections become symptomatic in young children with an open skull, increased pressure in the subdural space may result in a full fontanel and in rapid enlargement of head size accompanied by vomiting and lethargy, whereas in older patients headache, behavioural disorders and not infrequently focal signs such as motor or language alterations.

CT or MRI imaging reveals the presence of a unilateral crescent-shaped hypodensity over the cerebral convexity in most cases. A bilateral presentation may occur on other occasions with symmetrical effusions in most cases (Fig. 22.1).

The treatment options for children or adults with extra-axial fluid collections include surgical treatment in symptomatic cases or observation in asymptomatic patients. In the former therapeutic options comprise serial percutaneous drainage, burr hole fluid drainage with or without a closed external system, fluid shunting to the peritoneum or other cavities and craniectomy with fluid evacuation [24]. In all cases shunt occlusion/ligation is recommended to raise intraventricular pressure thereby reducing the pressure difference between the subdural and intraventricular compartments.

Several treatment options for the management of these patients have been proposed [3] that resulted in:

(a) Resolution without treatment: 85 % of subdural hygromas resolved spontaneously and resolution was greater and faster in younger patients.
(b) Resolution by surgical drainage and shunt removal: though a good solution in Carmel et al.'s experience patients needed re-shunting.
(c) Resolution by increasing the valve pressure with or without fluid drainage. This was the

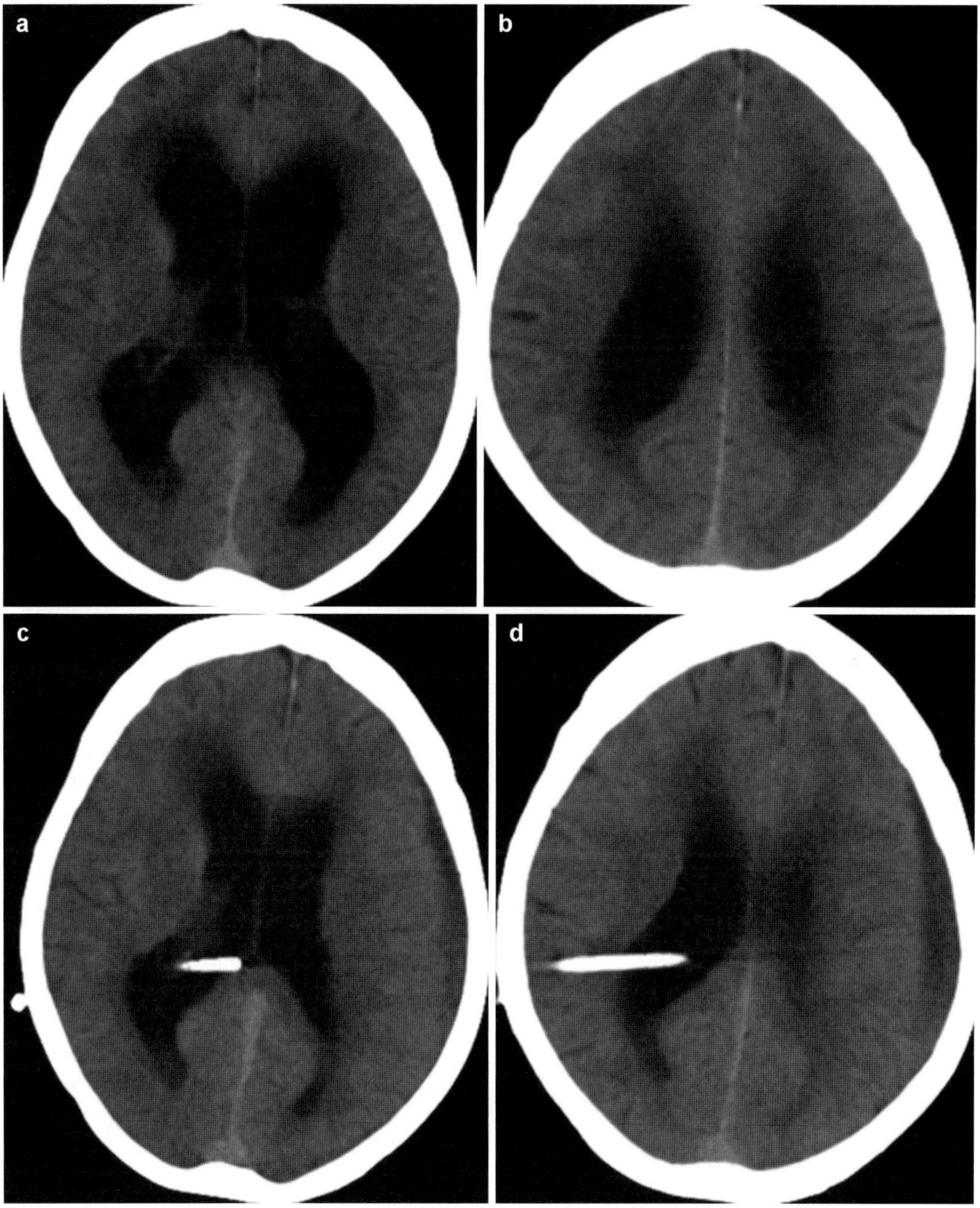

Fig. 22.1 Normal pressure hydrocephalus: (**a**) CT at diagnosis. (**b–d**) CT showing the emergence of a left subdural hygroma at 3 months after shunting

most efficacious treatment. If the patient has a programmable valve, the opening pressure should be increased, whereas in fixed pressure shunts, the valve must be replaced with a higher-pressure device. If valve replacement is not tolerated, evacuation of the hygroma may be necessary (Fig. 22.2).

The key criterion for the prevention of subdural collections is the correct choice of shunt. Though most authors claim programmable valves not only reduced the incidence of subdural hygromas significantly by altering the pressure, other authors assert that programmable valves do not influence the incidence of subdural fluid collections as compared to fixed-pressure valves [44]. Siphoning is inherent to any differential-pressure valve system, which allows for sudden ventricle decompression and in turn for development of a subdural hygroma. A further explanation for subdural hygroma formation is that surgeons fail to programme the valve properly. Data from the Dutch normal-pressure hydrocephalus study found that subdural effusions occurred in 71 % of patients treated with a low-pressure shunt and in 34 % of patients with a medium-pressure shunt system [2]. The benefits of adjustable shunts are further reinforced in a report by Zemack and Romner [46], who concluded that non-invasive

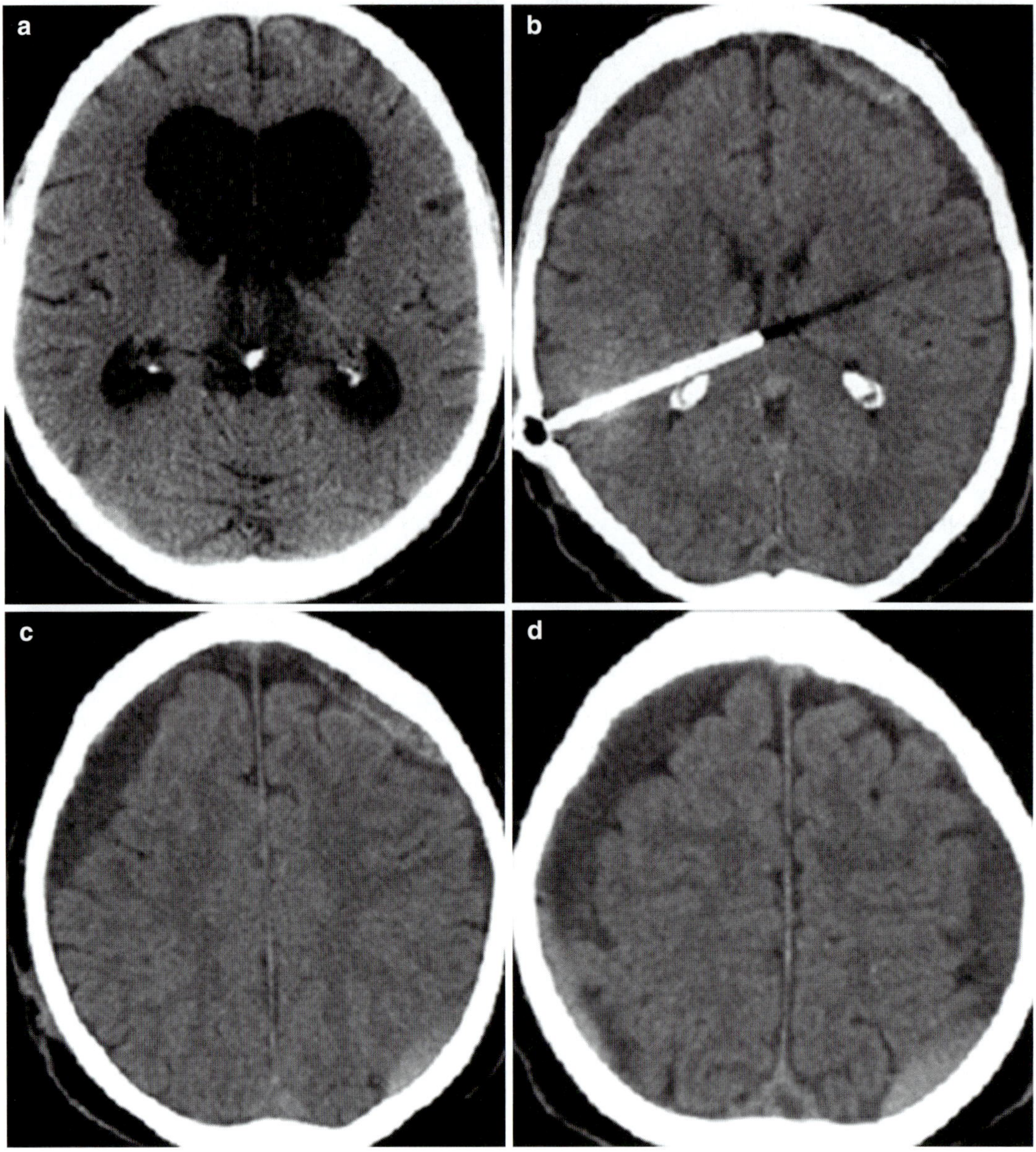

Fig. 22.2 Hydrocephalus after idiopathic subarachnoid haemorrhage. CT cuts showing (**a**) haemorrhage at admission, (**b**) ventricular dilatation 1 month after the haemorrhage and (**c**–**e**) appearance of left subdural hygromas and right subdural hematoma after shunting. (**f**) One month after raising the valve pressure at 1 month

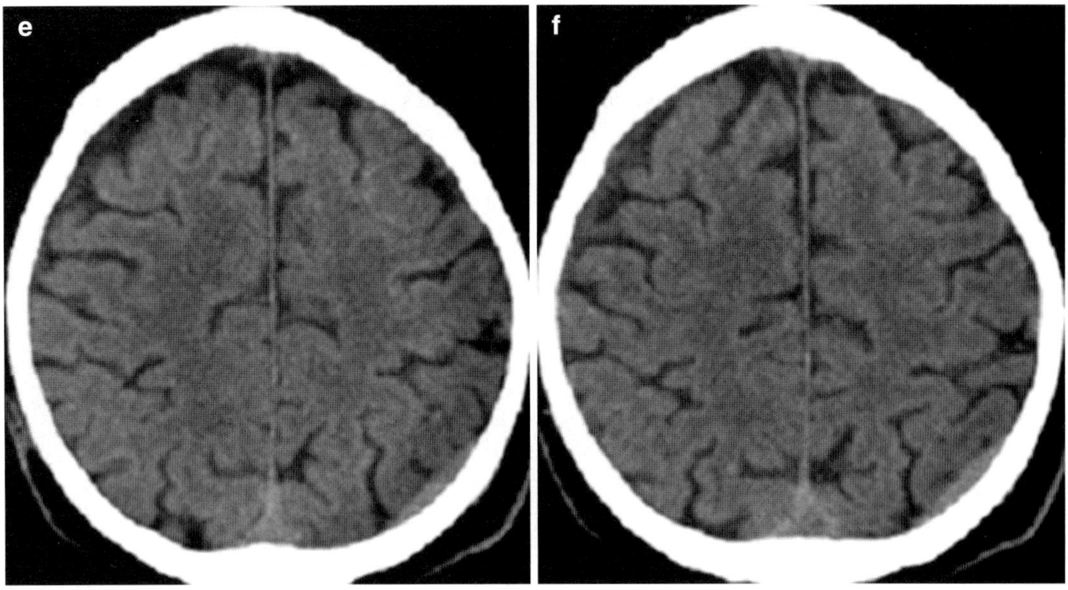

Fig. 22.2 (continued)

shunt adjustment improved outcomes for patients with normal pressure hydrocephalus (NPH) after reporting a 5-year survival rate of 80.2 % for adjustable shunts, with good to excellent outcomes observed in 78.1 % of people with idiopathic NPH.

22.2.2 Subdural Haematomas After Ventricular Shunting

The incidence of subdural haematomas related to hydrocephalus treatment varied considerably in early published reports (from 4.5 to 21 %), but this figure has fallen sharply to 4–5 % as CT scans have become a routine procedure in the follow-up of shunt patients. Though most subdural haematomas appearing after hydrocephalus treatment, regardless of the technique employed, are chronic with subacute evolution, acute subdural haematoma cases have also been reported [17].

Pathogenesis is probably no different for subdural haematoma formation of any aetiology, but the negative ventricular pressure produced by the shunting drainage appears to be an important additional predisposing factor [29, 38].

In a series of 1,000 CSDH (age 12–100 years) operated over a 22-year period, only six cases (0.6 %) had a previously implanted ventriculoperitoneal shunt [14]. However, the true incidence of CSDH after shunting is unknown.

Samuelson et al. [34] pointed out that patients with NPH were found to be particularly susceptible to subdural haematomas formation following ventricular shunt placement, in contrast to the lower incidence of SDH development following high-pressure hydrocephalus treatment.

In most instances subdural haematomas in shunted patients do not cause specific symptomatology (i.e., headache, confusion, lethargy and vomiting are the most common symptoms, being focal neurologic deficits unusual), which is identical for non-functioning shunts.

When the haematomas are symptomatic, they require surgical treatment (burr hole or craniotomy) depending on the type of haematoma (chronic or acute) and often shunt ligation to prevent reaccumulation or SDH expansion.

However, the most crucial factor for preventing this complication is the use of an adjustable valve. This type of shunt not only enables the nonsurgical increase of valve settings to prevent subdural effusions but also offers the added benefit of high-pressure drainage to aid subdural haematoma treatment (Fig. 22.3).

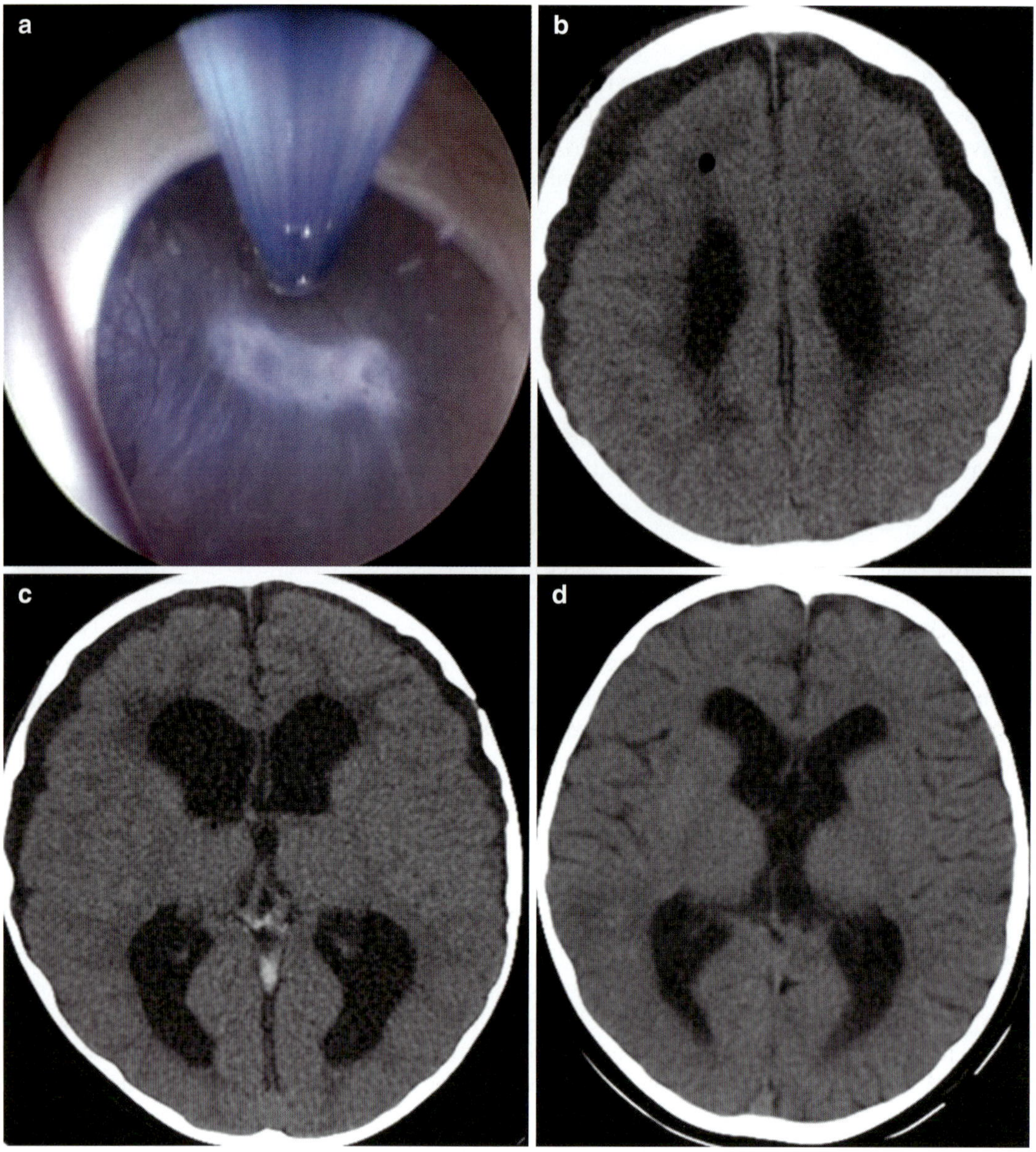

Fig. 22.3 Posttraumatic hydrocephalus: (**a**) CT scan at diagnosis. (**b–d**) Chronic subdural hematoma on the right hemisphere 2 months after shunting; there was no evidence of a head injury

22.3 Subdural Collections Following Neuroendoscopic Procedures

Endoscopic third ventriculostomy (ETV) has become a popular treatment particularly for cases of obstructive hydrocephalus though it may be used for the management of several conditions such as colloid cysts, fenestration of arachnoid cyst, etc. [12].

The main advantage of treating hydrocephalus by a third ventriculostomy is the avoidance of a diversionary cerebrospinal fluid shunt, thereby sparing the patient the distress and the risks of further surgery due to shunt complications. This procedure offers advantages but entails certain drawbacks, i.e., intra-and post-operative complications. The technical problems and complications of ETV have been well documented such as adverse effects on the cardiovascular system, injury of the fornix with memory deficits, hypothalamic dysfunction, and injury to the basilar artery or cranial nerves ([7, 41]).

22.3.1 Subdural CSF Hygromas Following Neuroendoscopic Procedures

Subdural effusion is a rare complication that is probably more frequent than reported in the literature [43]. Following ETV, ipsilateral, contralateral or bilateral subdural effusions may occur, primarily on the operated side or on both sides, but rarely they occur on the contralateral side. In adults, subdural fluid accumulations after ETV have been described as a rare complication accounting for less than 2 % in most series. Peretta et al. [32] described two subdural hygromas in 355 ETV (0.6 %), Jones et al. [18] reported two subdural hygromas in 101 ETV (2 %), Schroeder et al. [35] observed three cases of subdural collections in 188 ETV (1.5 %) and de Ribaupierre et al. [5] found a higher rate of hygroma after ETV in infants and children (3 of 24 cases; 12.5 %).

Hygroma after ETV in young infants may be an under-reported phenomenon for two main reasons: patients may be asymptomatic post-operatively and delayed growth of the effusion/s after several days experience spontaneous regression in most cases. Wiewrodt et al. [43] pointed out that subdural hygromas after ETV have been reported to be far less frequent in young infants (under 3 years) than in older children. Whether there is a higher risk for the development of hygromas in the very first months of life as opposed to infants beyond age 1 year remains unclear with an age distribution analogous to ETV failure rate, decreasing later over the first 12 months [43].

A further aspect of post-operative subdural collections after ETV is gender, showing a clear predominance of boys over girls [20, 35]. The presumed pathophysiology is that CSF forces its way through the frontal cerebral tract toward the overlying subdural space as a newly created "normal" pathway. In addition, the absorptive mechanisms need time to mature in this age, so CSF naturally tries to escape through the least resistant pathway [10]. The cortical mantle may also collapse due to excessive and abrupt loss of CSF during the procedure which in turn would enlarge the space between the dura mater and the brain [32, 41, 43].

The complication is also more common in children owing to coexistent macrocephaly and to what some authors have termed "craniocerebral disproportion" in cases with long-standing significant ventricular dilatation and thin cortical mantle. In contrast, older children and adults are predisposed to subdural hygroma as the brain has been stretched for many years and no longer have the ability to expand after ETV due to the loss of the viscoelastic properties of the brain [20].

A further explanation is that ETV decreases the volume of the lateral and third ventricles due to the CSF outflow from the ventricles to the subarachnoid cisterns, but CSF absorption fails to increase as rapidly, resulting in an increase in the CSF subarachnoid space. Therefore, after long-standing obstructive hydrocephalus, the absorption pathways may not be adequate [22, 43].

In many cases, subdural collections are asymptomatic and are only diagnosed by imaging studies performed after the procedure. In symptomatic cases, clinical manifestations include nausea, vomiting, headache and decrease in the level of consciousness. Hygromas may appear several days or weeks after ventriculostomy, and this could be due to the fact that initially they are regarded to be an asymptomatic collection of CSF in the subdural space [43] (Figs. 22.4 and 22.5).

Most subdural hygromas after ventriculocisternostomy are asymptomatic. Clinical and radiological surveillance of patients is recommended although they resolve spontaneously. When symptomatic, hygromas can be treated with drainage of the subdural space using a burr hole or a twist drill, and only if the collection relapses should a permanent subduro-peritoneal shunt be considered [23].

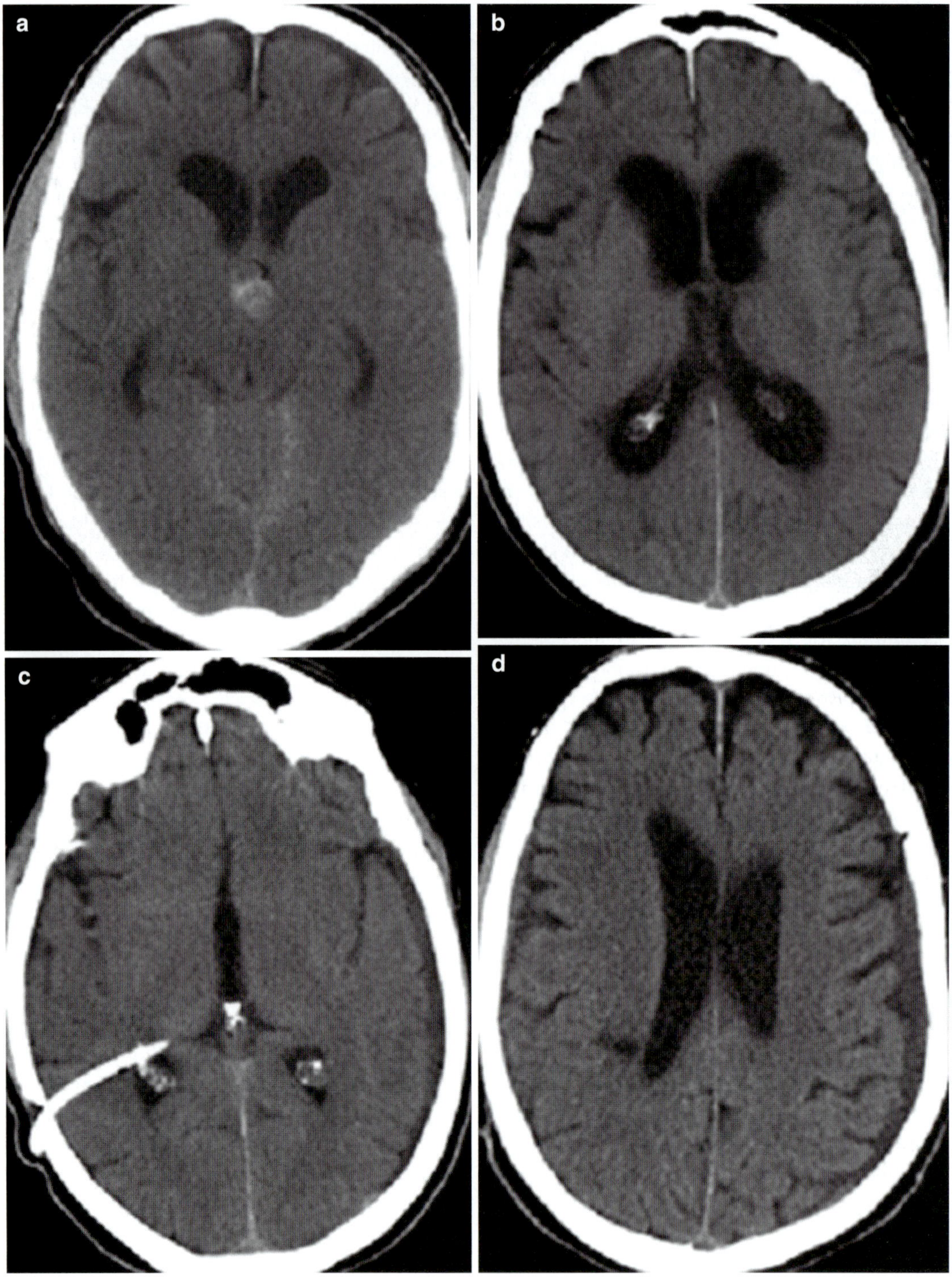

Fig. 22.4 Normal pressure hydrocephalus treated with an adjustable valve. (**a**) CT at diagnosis. (**b–d**) Emergence of a chronic subdural hematoma after a minor head injury. (**e**, **f**) CT after increasing the valve pressure

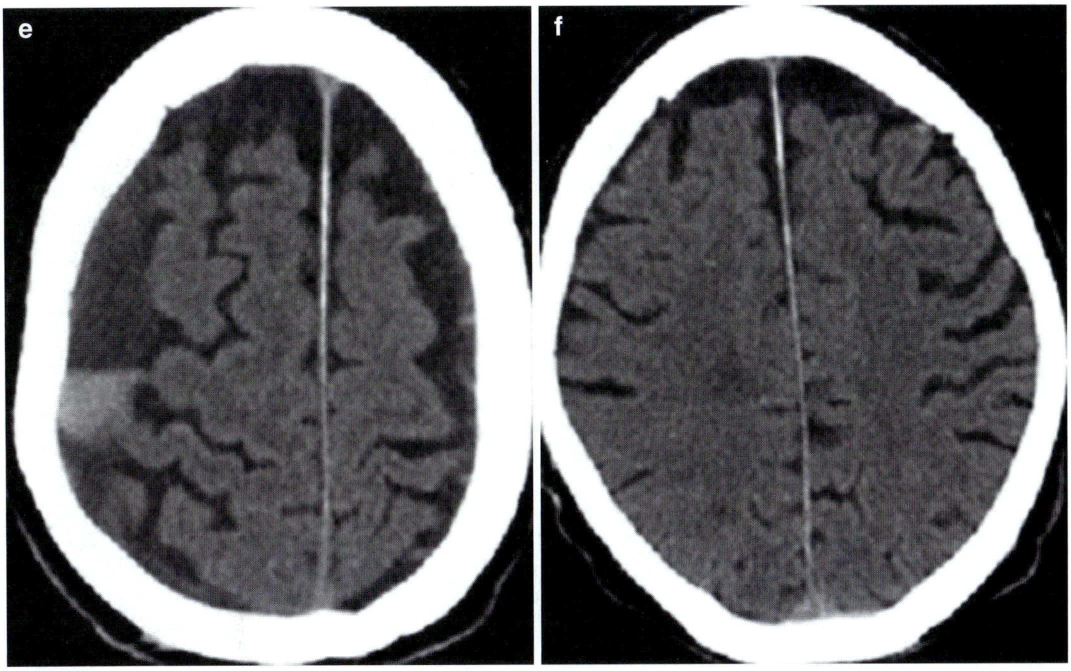

Fig. 22.4 (continued)

As for prevention, tapping the ventricle with a thin brain needle ensures a small cortical puncture that is just large enough (not larger than necessary) to allow the insertion of the endoscope without causing displacement of the underlying brain [40, 43]. The diameter of the endoscope probably influences the occurrence of hygroma after ETV as a large cortical orifice in the presence of large ventricles may cause the passage of CSF from the ventricles to the subdural space. Some authors reported that covering the endoscopy tract with fibrin glue after completion of ETV and using haemostatic sealant agents decrease the incidence of subdural collections. Sgaramella et al. [37] recommend to rigorously control both the amount of Ringer's solution used for flushing and the escape of CSF during ETV and to quickly close the wound as soon as the endoscope is withdrawn.

In patients with large ventricles and a thin cortical mantle, a rapid outflow of ventricular CSF during the procedure should be avoided [30]. Other authors stress that this complication can be prevented by re-expanding the ventricles with Ringer's solution before removing the endoscope sheath from the lateral ventricle to avoid the collapse of the brain and to seal the cortical hole with a piece of gel foam [20, 26].

22.3.2 Subdural Haematomas Following Neuroendoscopic Procedures

Subdural haematoma is a rare complication of ETV with only a few cases reported up to the present day [4, 37, 39]. Though most subdural bleeding occurs on the operated side, contralateral or bilateral haematomas have also been reported [1, 37]. In a recent paper, a case of subdural haematoma after endoscopic ventriculostomy in a 21-year-old man was reported, and in the review of the literature, only another five cases with this complication were found in adults, of which two cases (33.3 %) were contralateral and one bilateral [39] (Table 22.1).

Several hypotheses have been proposed for explaining the occurrence of subdural haematomas even though its physiopathology remains elusive. Schroeder et al. [35] suggested that large cortical punctures in patients with large

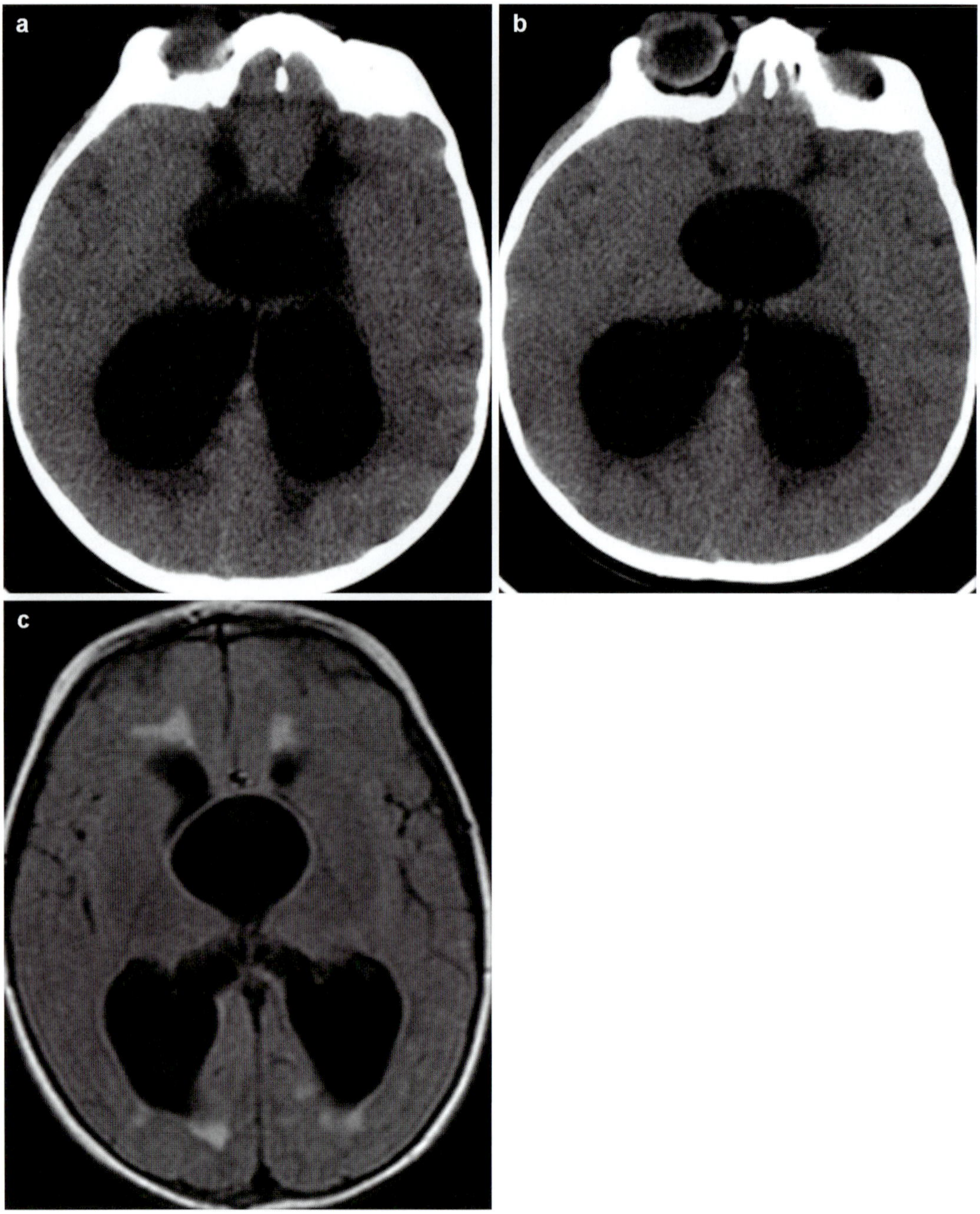

Fig. 22.5 Three-year-old child with an arachnoid cyst. (**a**, **b**) CT at diagnosis. (**c**) MRI (T1) at diagnosis

ventricles may lead to CSF accumulation in the subdural space causing subdural haematoma, firstly via a subdural hygroma and then by venous bleeding. Mohanty et al. [30] have suggested that the ventricles collapse with the sudden reduction of pressure occurring in a short period of time and that bleeding in the cortical veins may lead to subdural collection between the dura and the brain during CSF drainage. In long-standing triventricular hydrocephalus,

Table 22.1 Adult chronic subdural collections and endoscopic third ventriculostomy

Author	Age and sex	Aetiology of hydrocephalus	Localization	Symptomatology	Treatment
Beni-Adani et al.	20 y, M	Obstructive	Ipsilateral	Asymptomatic	Burr hole
Sgaramella et al.	69 y, M	Obstructive	Contralateral	Asymptomatic	Evacuated
Kim et al.	51 y, M	Obstructive	Bilateral	Headache	Bilateral burr hole
Kamel et al.	16 y, M	Obstructive	Ipsilateral	Gait disturbance and headache	Craniotomy
Civelek et al.	42 y, M	Obstructive	Contralateral	Headache	Burr hole
Tekin et al.	21 y, M	Obstructive	Ipsilateral	Headache	Burr hole

M male, *y* year

ventriculostomy creates a new CSF pathway which can cause sudden changes in the CSF regulation system. Although the endoscopic third ventriculostomy results in a decrease of the lateral and third ventricular volumes as CSF flows from the ventricles into the subarachnoid cistern, the CSF absorption rate does not increase as rapidly and this results in an increase in the CSF subarachnoid space [22]. When a CSF collection persists in the subdural space for more than a few weeks, it may induce migration or proliferation of inflammatory cells derived from the dural border cells, resulting in a layer of fibroblasts along the dura mater that develop into the outer membrane of the haematoma. Moreover, delayed reabsorption of subdural effusions is likely to result in haemorrhage into the subdural fluid due to either tearing of bridging veins or bleeding from the neomembrane [20, 23].

These subdural haematomas are always symptomatic with headache and decreasing levels of consciousness, and contrary to what happens with hygromas, they always require burr hole surgery or a craniotomy since there is no spontaneous resolution. Prognosis is good with total recovery in all reported cases.

22.3.3 Infectious Subdural Collections After Hydrocephalus Surgery

Subdural empyema is a rare occurrence resulting most commonly from a secondary spread of a sinus infection via the valveless veins of the diploe connecting intracranial and extracranial structures. Less frequently, empyema is the result of surgical contamination of the subdural space following subdural hygroma or haematoma evacuation.

Subdural empyema following ventriculoperitoneal shunting is extremely rare and only a few cases have been reported, the first being documented in a child with congenital hydrocephalus treated with a ventriculoperitoneal shunt who presented with fever, vomiting and seizures. After removal of the infected shunt, a CT scan detected a right extra-axial collection, with an enhancing border. A culture of fluid recovered from the subdural empyema yielded *Enterobacter cloacae* [6].

Subdural empyema is usually diagnosed in the first days or weeks after shunting; however, in one case the infectious collection developed 9 years after inserting a ventriculoperitoneal shunt [21].

Treatment includes craniotomy for empyema evacuation, shunt removal, antibiotic therapy for 4–6 weeks and, once the infection has been resolved, a new valve implant.

22.4 Subdural Collections After Treatment of Arachnoid Cyst

Arachnoid cyst (AC) is a frequent pathological condition accounting for 1 % of all intracranial lesions, with an estimated incidence of 0.5–2.6 %. The optimal treatment for symptomatic ACs remains controversial. Cyst-peritoneal (CP) shunt placement is believed to be a safe and effective surgical therapy for symptomatic ACs in children allowing rapid symptom relief and cyst reduction, especially in younger children [47]. At first glance, CP shunting appears as a safe and practical procedure with which most neurosurgeons are familiar. However, placement of a CP shunt creates dependency of the patient on a mechanical device, which is known to be fraught of multiple complications, and diverse manifestations of excessive valve functioning occurred in 18 % of hydrocephalic patients [28]. The presentation of subdural or epidural collections after CP shunting is rare. In our experience, of 49 children treated with a CP shunt, no case of extra-axial collections after shunting was found after 1-year follow-up [15]. When present in symptomatic patients, replacement with a higher pressure valve may be necessary, whereas in patients with adjustable valves, the solution simply entails increasing the valve closing pressure.

Neuroendoscopy has become the procedure of choice for the treatment of intracranial arachnoid cyst as it maintains the basic surgical strategy of marsupialization without the invasiveness of open craniotomy while avoiding the complications caused by shunt treatment [9].

The development of a subdural hygroma appears frequently associated with the endoscopic treatment of arachnoid cysts, but in most cases asymptomatic hygromas are observed in the imaging studies carried out within the first week after endoscopy. Most of these hygromas resolve spontaneously and do not require surgical treatment (Figs. 22.5 and 22.6). During convexity cyst surgery, the cyst is directly penetrated through the dura, so there is no cerebral mantle behaving as a stopper to the outlet of CSF. However, in midline cysts it is necessary to cross the brain, which underscores the importance of adapting the endoscope as closely as possible to the thickness of the cerebral puncture.

22.5 Other Extra-axial Collections After Hydrocephalus Treatment

Epidural haematomas are a rare complication of ventricular shunting procedures and only few cases have been reported in the literature [13]. These haematomas occurred mostly in young and middle age patients and usually appeared distant from the site of the burr hole with a predilection for the anterior half of the cranial vault [45]. Most haematomas appear on the shunt side, but some contralateral cases have also been reported [33].

A possible hypothesis for explaining extradural haematoma formation after shunting is the occurrence of traction forces over the middle meningeal artery and its branches (weekly adhered to the inner table of the skull) that follow the collapse of the brain tissue [25]. Alternatively, in a case of a child with congenital factor X deficiency and a huge extradural haematoma after shunting, Fujimoto et al. [11] suggested that the reduction of intracranial pressure resulted in the detachment of the dura mater from the inner table of the skull followed by minor venous bleeding from emissary veins or from the dural vessels that are abundant in children. Moreover, the dura mater is less adherent to the skull in children than in adults, and it is easily detached particularly in the convexity region of the skull. Other authors have proposed that in some patients, the skull-dura adhesions may be less significant than the dura-arachnoid adhesions, which would contribute to the collapse of the dura mater along with the brain parenchyma after over-shunting, favouring the appearance of extradural haematomas [36].

The treatment of choice for extradural haematoma is craniotomy, with a sufficient large bone flap for drainage and for achieving complete haemostasis. Prophylactic methods that should be considered against the re-accumulation of blood after evacuation of the haematoma are the placement of a higher pressure valve, closing the valve system, refilling and inflating the ventricular system with isotonic solution [11].

Lumboperitoneal shunts are widely used for CSF diversion, especially in patients with communicating hydrocephalus. Lumboperitoneal shunting does not require cerebral puncture, so the risk of intracranial complications is minimal and results in fewer clinical complications than the placement of ventriculoperitoneal shunts [19]. The development of extra-axial haematomas

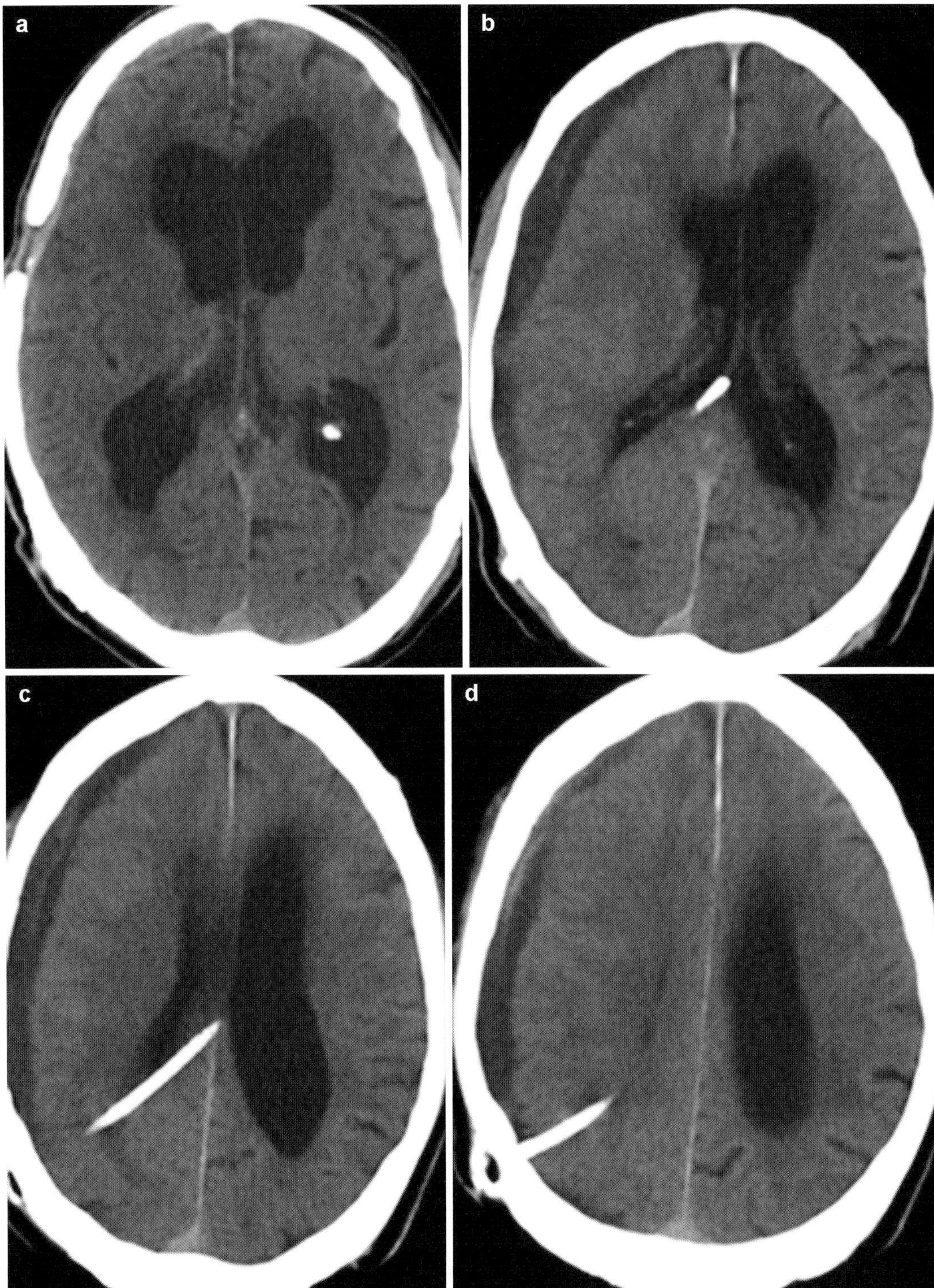

Fig. 22.6 Same patient of Fig. 22.4. (**a**) Performing an endoscopic fenestration. (**b**, **c**) CT at 48 h after endoscopic fenestration showing bilateral subdural hygroma. (**d**) CT at 4 weeks after surgery showing resolution of the subdural hygroma

is thus a quite rare complication and only a few cases have been reported in the literature. Lumbar CSF drainage may result in a reduction of CSF volume with a corresponding fall in intracranial pressure. Overdrainage of CSF during surgery may lead to the production of an intracranial haematoma [42].

Acknowledgements The authors thank Romen Das Gupta for assistance in preparing the manuscript.

References

1. Beni-Adani L, Siomin V, Segev Y, Beni S, Constantini S (2000) Increasing chronic subdural hematoma after endoscopic III ventriculostomy. Childs Nerv Syst 16:402–405
2. Boon AJ, Tans JT, Delwel EJ et al (1998) Dutch normal-pressure hydrocephalus study: randomized comparison of low-and medium-pressure shunts. J Neurosurg 88:490–495
3. Carmel PW, Albright AL, Adelson PD et al (1999) Incidence and management of subdural hematoma/hygroma with variable-and fixed-pressure differential valves: a randomized, controlled study of programmable compared with conventional valves. Neurosurg Focus 7(4):e7
4. Civelek E, Cansever T, Karasu A et al (2007) Chronic subdural hematoma after endoscopic third ventriculostomy: case report. Turk Neurosurg 17:289–293
5. de Ribaupierre S, Rilliet B, Vernet O et al (2007) Third ventriculostomy vs ventriculoperitoneal shunt in pediatric obstructive hydrocephalus: results from a Swiss series and literature review. Childs Nerv Syst 23:527–533
6. Dickerman RD, Piatt JH, Hsu F, Frank EH (1999) Subdural empyema complicating cerebrospinal fluid shunt infection. Pediatr Neurosurg 30:310–311
7. Di Rocco C, Massimi L, Tamburrini G (2006) Shunts vs endoscopic third ventriculostomy in infants: are there different types and/or rates of complications? A review. Childs Nerv Syst 22:1573–1589
8. Drake JM, Kestle JR, Milner R et al (1998) Randomized trial of cerebrospinal fluid shunt valve design in pediatric hydrocephalus. Neurosurgery 43:294–303
9. El-Ghandour NMF (2013) Endoscopic treatment of quadrigeminal arachnoid cysts in children. J Neurosurg Pediatr 12:521–528
10. Freudenstein D, Wagner A, Ern U et al (2002) Subdural hygroma as a complication of endoscopic neurosurgery. Neurol Med Chir 42:554–559
11. Fujimoto Y, Aguiar PH, Carneiro JDA et al (1999) Spontaneous epidural hematoma following a shunt in an infant with congenital factor X deficiency. Neurosurg Rev 22:226–229
12. Furlanetti LL, Santos MV, de Oliveira RS (2013) Neuroendoscopic surgery in children: an analysis of 200 consecutive procedures. Arq Neuropsiquiatr 71:165–170
13. Gelabert-González M, Bollar A, Garcia A et al (1987) Epidural hematoma as a complication of ventrículo-peritoneal shunt. Present of a new case and literature review. Rev Neurol XV(76):189–191
14. Gelabert-González M, Iglesias-Pais M, García-Allut A et al (2005) Chronic subdural hematoma: surgical treatment and outcome in 1000 cases. Clin Neurol Neurosurg 107:223–229
15. Gelabert-González M (2011) Cisto-peritoneal shunt in the surgical treatment of intracranial arachnoid cysts: an analysis of 49 cases. Arch Argent Pediatr 53:357–361
16. Haines DE, Harkey HL, al-Mefty O (1993) The "subdural space" a new look at an outdated concept. Neurosurgery 32:111–120
17. Hayes J, Roguski M, Riesenburger R (2012) Rapid resolution of an acute subdural hematoma by increasing the shunt valve pressure in a 63-year-old man with normal-pressure hydrocephalus with a ventriculoperitoneal shunt: a case report and literature review. J Med Case Rep 6:393
18. Jones RFC, Kwok BCT, Stening WA et al (1994) The current status of endoscopic third ventriculostomy in the management of non-communicating hydrocephalus. Minim Invasive Neurosurg 37:28–36
19. Kamiryo T, Hamada J, Fuwa I et al (2003) Acute subdural hematoma after lumboperitoneal shunt placement in patients with normal pressure hydrocephalus. Four case reports. Neurol Med Chir (Tokyo) 43:197–200
20. Kamel MH, Murphy M, Aquilina K et al (2006) Subdural haemorrhage following endoscopic third ventriculostomy. A rare complication. Acta Neurochir (Wien) 148:591–593
21. Kasliwal MK, Sinha S, Kumar R et al (2009) Giant hemicranial calcified subdural empyema-unusual complication following ventriculoperitoneal shunt insertion. Indian J Pediatr 76:651–652
22. Kim BS, Jallo GI, Kothbauer K, Abbott IR (2004) Chronic subdural hematoma as a complication of endoscopic third ventriculostomy. Surg Neurol 62:64–68
23. Lee KM (1998) The pathogenesis and clinical significance of traumatic subdural hygroma. Brain Inj 12:595–603
24. Litofsky NS, Raffel C, McComb JG (1992) Management of symptomatic chronic extra-axial fluid collections in pediatric patients. Neurosurgery 31: 445–450
25. Louzada PR, Requjo PR, Viana M et al (2012) Bilateral extradural haematoma after acute ventricular over-drainage. Brain Inj 26:95–100
26. Maeda Y, Inamura T, Morioka T et al (2000) Hemorrhagic subdural effusions complicating and

endoscopic III ventriculostomy. Childs Nerv Syst 16:312–314
27. Martínez-Lage JF, Pérez-Espejo MA, Almagro MJ et al (2005) Syndromes of overdrainage of ventricular shunting in childhood hydrocephalus. Neurocirugia (Astur) 16:124–133
28. Martínez-Lage JF, Ruíz-Espejo AM, Almagro MJ et al (2009) CSF overdrainage in shunted intracranial arachnoid cysts: a series and review. Childs Nerv Syst 25:1061–1069
29. McCullough DC, Fox JL (1974) Negative intracranial pressure hydrocephalus in adults with shunts and its relationship to the production of subdural hematoma. J Neurosurg 40:372–375
30. Mohanty A, Anandh B, Reddy MS et al (1997) Contralateral massive acute subdural collection after endoscopic third ventriculostomy: a case report. Minim Invasive Neurosurg 40:59–61
31. Pattisapu JV (2001) Etiology and clinical course of hydrocephalus. Neurosurg Clin N Am 12:651–659
32. Peretta P, Ragazzi P, Galarza M et al (2006) Complications and pitfalls of neuroendoscopic surgery in children. J Neurosurg 105(3 Suppl):187–193
33. Power D, Ali-Khan F, Drage M (1999) Contralateral extradural haematoma after insertion of a programmable-valve ventriculoperitoneal shunt. J R Soc Med 92:360–361
34. Samuelson S, Long DM, Chou SN (1972) Subdural hematoma as a complication of shunting procedures for normal pressure hydrocephalus. J Neurosurg 37:548–551
35. Schroeder HWS, Niendorf WR, Gaab MR (2002) Complications of endoscopic third ventriculostomy. J Neurosurg 96:1032–1040
36. Seyithanoglu H, Guzey FK, Emel E et al (2010) Chronic ossified epidural hematoma after ventriculoperitoneal shunt insertion: a case report. Turk Neurosurg 20: 519–523
37. Sgaramella E, Castelli G, Sotgiu S (2004) Chronic subdural collection after endoscopic third ventriculostomy. Acta Neurochir 146:529–530
38. Sternbach GL (2005) Subdural hematoma in a shunted patient. J Emerg Med 29:483–484
39. Tekin T, Colak A, Kutlay M et al (2012) Chronic subdural hematoma after endoscopic third ventriculostomy: a case report and literature review. Turk Neurosurg 22: 119–122
40. Teo C, Rahman S, Boop FA, Cherny B (1996) Complication of endoscopic neurosurgery. Childs Nerv Syst 12:248–253
41. Teo C (2004) Complications of endoscopic third ventriculostomy. In: Cinalli G, Maixner WJ, Sainte-Rose C (eds) Pediatric hydrocephalus. Springer, Milano, pp 411–420
42. Wang VY, Barbaro NM, Lawton MT et al (2007) Complications of lumboperitoneal shunts. Neurosurgery 60:1045–1049
43. Wiewrodt D, Schumacher R, Wagner W (2008) Hygromas after endoscopic third ventriculostomy in the first year of life: incidence, management and outcome in a series of 34 patients. Childs Nerv Syst 24:57–63
44. Xu H, Wang ZX, Liu F et al (2013) Programmable shunt valves for the treatment of hydrocephalus: a systematic review. Eur J Paediatr Neurol 17:454–461
45. Yue CP, Mann KS (1985) Chronic epidural haematoma: a rare complication of ventriculo-peritoneal shunt. J Neurol Neurosurg Psychiatry 48:953–955
46. Zemack G, Romner B (2002) Adjustable valves in normal-pressure hydrocephalus: a retrospective study of 218 patients. Neurosurgery 51:1392–1401
47. Zhang B, Zhang Y, Ma Z (2012) Long-term results of cystoperitoneal shunt placement for the treatment of arachnoid cyst in children. J Neurosurg Pediatr 10: 302–305

Complications Related to Endoscopic Fenestration in Loculated Hydrocephalus

23

Yoshua Esquenazi and David I. Sandberg

Contents

23.1 **Introduction** 301
23.2 **Etiology and Pathophysiology** 301
23.3 **Diagnosis** 302
23.4 **Treatment Options** 303
23.5 **Shunting** 304
23.6 **Endoscopic Management** 304
23.7 **Craniotomy for Fenestrations** 305
Conclusions 305
References 306

Y. Esquenazi, MD • D.I. Sandberg, MD (✉)
Departments of Neurosurgery and Pediatric Surgery, Children's Memorial Hermann Hospital, and Mischer Neuroscience Institute, University of Texas Health Science Center at Houston, 6431 Fannin Street, Suite 5.144, Houston, TX 77030, USA
e-mail: David.I.Sandberg@uth.tmc.edu

23.1 Introduction

Loculated hydrocephalus (LH) occurs when multiple cerebrospinal fluid (CSF)-filled compartments form in the brain that do not communicate with the ventricles or with one another. These compartments are separated by septations and can progressively enlarge. The etiology of LH can vary, but it has been described in association with intraventricular hemorrhage, birth trauma, central nervous system infections, and tumors [7, 10, 11, 13, 16, 21, 23]. Neurosurgical management of patents with this condition can be extremely challenging, and outcomes are often poor despite multiple procedures. Treatment options include placement of multiple shunt systems [12], fenestration of the septations via endoscopy [8, 14, 17–19, 24, 26] or craniotomy [16, 22], or a combination of these methods. The goal of treatment is to restore communication among the isolated CSF-filled compartments in order to treat patient's symptoms, normalize intracranial pressure, and avoid complex shunt systems with multiple shunt catheters. In this chapter we review the etiology, pathophysiology, diagnosis, and management strategies for patients suffering from this condition.

23.2 Etiology and Pathophysiology

The etiology of LH can vary, but is most often associated with neonatal bacterial meningitis and intraventricular hemorrhage [2, 7, 11, 13, 23]. LH

C. Di Rocco et al. (eds.), *Complications of CSF Shunting in Hydrocephalus: Prevention, Identification, and Management*, DOI 10.1007/978-3-319-09961-3_23,

has also been described in association with birth trauma and tumors [10]. Predisposing factors for this condition include low birth weight, premature birth, perinatal complications, and congenital CNS malformations [27]. Major advances in neonatal intensive care have enabled the survival of low-birth-weight infants who are prone to the consequences of prematurity such as infections and intraventricular hemorrhage (IVH). Meningitis caused by gram-negative organisms appears to be particularly associated with subsequent development of LH [11, 13]. LH can also occur in patients with IVH in the absence of CNS infection [7]. Since many patients with LH have both a history of IVH and CNS infection in the setting of prematurity, it is often difficult to determine which of these factors played a dominant role in the pathogenesis of the condition [22]. The septations that give rise to the loculations are likely to represent the organization of intraventricular exudate and debris produced by ventriculitis. The inflammatory response at the ependymal surface is thought to encourage proliferation of subependymal glial tissue in which exudate and debris organize to form fibroglial webs. Disruption of the overlying ependymal lining leads to the emergence of tufts that serve as a nidus for the formation of septations that span the ventricles. These septations alter the ventricular anatomy and disrupt the normal flow of CSF, creating entrapped compartments that progressively dilate and cause elevated intracranial pressure and associated symptoms [16]. Septations can create artificial divisions within a single ventricular cavity and/or occlude the foramen of Monro, the cerebral aqueduct, and the fourth ventricular outlets [11]. Common findings in LH are ventricular dilatation and compartmentalization by membranes, which appear filmy and translucent and may vary in thickness. Microscopically, the septations are formed by fibroglial elements with polymorphonuclear cells [23].

23.3 Diagnosis

Preoperative radiological evaluation plays a crucial role in planning the best treatment strategy and minimizing the number of surgical procedures in patients with LH. Although radiographic examinations can provide morphological definition of the ventricular anatomy, accurate assessment of the CSF flow and the sites of obstruction can be challenging. Multiple imaging modalities have been used over the past few decades for the assessment of patients with hydrocephalus. One of the most important factors in the evaluation of patients with LH is to select an imaging modality that will demonstrate all possible obstructive pathological processes throughout the CSF pathways [5].

Ultrasound (US) provides useful information about the ventricles in the first 12–18 months of life, while the anterior fontanel is still open and can be used as a bedside screening test. The size and shape of the lateral ventricles is easily visualized, but the third and fourth ventricular anatomy is not easily assessed. Its quality is user-dependent and the reproducibility of US is not high [4].

Computed tomography (CT) is easily available, fast and reliable, and shunt catheters are better visualized on CT than on other imaging modalities. However, CT does not provide any information about CSF flow dynamics. Moreover, limitation of exposure to ionizing radiation is an important concern in children such as those with LH who typically require multiple imaging studies throughout their childhood [4]. Therefore, the use of CT in the management of patients with LH is limited.

Magnetic resonance imaging (MRI) is the examination of choice, as it provides the most detailed assessment of ventricular anatomy and the best view of loculated CSF compartments as well as the thickness of septations separating these compartments (Fig. 23.1). Previously, T1-weighted and especially T2-weighted sequences were the most commonly utilized sequences in the radiographic management of patients with LH. Currently, newer MRI sequences that provide additional information about the CSF pathways and sites of obstruction with better detail have emerged. The absence or presence of hemorrhage and related membranes in the cisterns is useful when planning endoscopic approaches, and the use of hemosiderin-sensitive sequences such as gradient echo (GRE) T2 or susceptibility weighted imaging (SWI) can

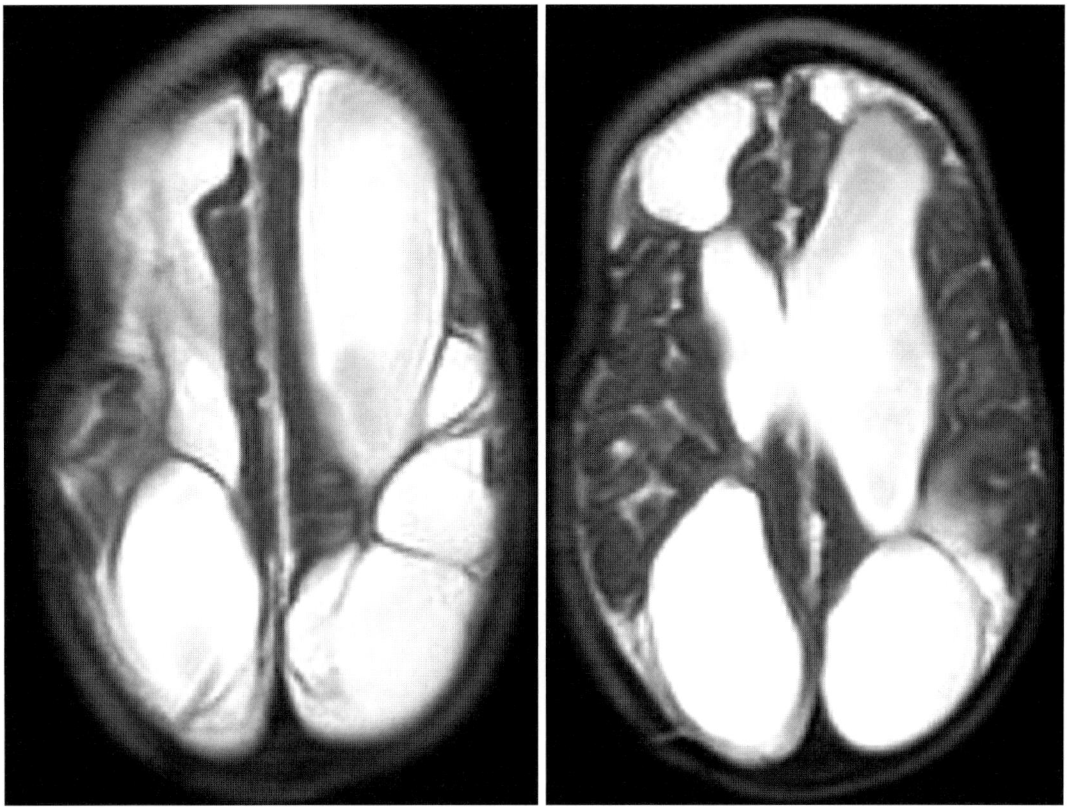

Fig. 23.1 Axial T2-weighted MRI showing multiple loculations in a 7-month-old patient with hydrocephalus caused by intraventricular hydrocephalus associated with prematurity as well as likely meningitis. The patient has already required four surgeries within the first 7 months of life: reservoir placement, endoscopic fenestration of LH with third ventriculostomy and choroid plexus coagulation, shunt placement, and shunt revision

be helpful. Three-dimensional constructive interference in the steady state (3D CISS) provides optimal morphological images and fine anatomic details about CSF pathways and has been proven to be superior to conventional MRI in the demonstration of thin membranes, especially in the posterior cranial fossa and cisternal spaces [1, 3]. 3D CISS is valuable for both preoperative decision-making and postoperative evaluation [3]. However, 3D CISS is prone to artifact and requires extensive scanning time [9].

Computer tomography-based ventriculography can provide functional data about CSF flow but offers poor spatial resolution and multiplanar imaging capability, and its use is limited by exposure to radiation. Magnetic resonance ventriculography has the advantages of avoiding ionizing radiation, the capability of direct multiplanar imaging, and absence of bony artifact with high spatial and contrast resolution [9]. Overall, MRI is the single best imaging modality to yield both anatomical and functional information. A more sophisticated MRI approach with various MRI sequences and administration of intravenous gadolinium to rule out infection are recommended [4]. Utilizing both morphological and functional data can greatly assist in guiding appropriate surgical management of patients with LH.

23.4 Treatment Options

The primary goal of treatment for patients with LH is to alleviate symptoms caused by enlarging, loculated CSF compartments. Ideally, this goal is accomplished in a way that maximizes communication between CSF compartments and enables adequate CSF circulation with one shunt catheter or, occasionally, without any shunt catheters. Fenestration procedures enable fewer shunt catheters and therefore fewer opportunities for obstruction, disconnection, and infection. Moreover, fewer shunt catheters enable easier identification of the source of presenting signs and symptoms in the setting of a symptomatic patient with a shunt malfunction. Fenestration can usually be accomplished endoscopically, as described below, but craniotomy is an option for patients with thick membranes and very complicated anatomy. Many patients with LH will require several or many procedures over the course of their childhood, which will include shunting procedures and fenestration procedures, either open or endoscopic. Given the complexity of LH, treatment options must be individualized and carefully planned to minimize both complications and the requirement for additional treatments [27].

23.5 Shunting

Most patients with LH, regardless of fenestration procedures, will require a CSF diverting shunt. The rate of shunt malfunction in patients with LH is very high. Nida and Haines [16] and Lewis et al. [15] reported a median of 2.75 and 3.04 shunt revisions per year, respectively, in their series. Prior to the advent of modern neuroendoscopy, many patients with LH had multiple shunt catheters placed into different loculated compartments. When patients with multiple shunt catheters present with new symptoms, it is often difficult to assess exactly what needs to be done surgically to alleviate these symptoms. Many patients with LH are significantly developmentally delayed, making diagnosis of clinically significant shunt malfunction challenging at baseline, and shunt taps in the setting of multiple shunt systems can be practically difficult and misleading [22]. Moreover, shunt infections require multiple incisions for removal of all potentially colonized hardware. Fenestration of loculated CSF compartments via endoscopic techniques, open craniotomy, or a combination of these to reduce the number of required shunt catheters as much as possible is currently recommended.

23.6 Endoscopic Management

Recent advances in endoscopy such as improvements in optic design, bright cold-light sources, and small-diameter rigid and flexible endoscopes have expanded the use of neuroendoscopy in the management of intraventricular pathology and LH [26]. Many authors have reported that endoscopic procedures may reduce shunt revision rates in patients with LH [6, 15, 25, 26]. The main advantages of endoscopic fenestration over craniotomy include its limited invasiveness as well as a shorter recovery period [15]. Carefully planned endosopic approaches enable wide access to loculated CSF compartments bilaterally via a single small incision and burr hole [24]. Fenestrations should be as wide as possible to ensure durability. When fenestrations are small, there is a high incidence of early reclosure due to the low-pressure differential across cyst walls and the inflammatory origin of the disease [26, 27]. Fenestrations can be enlarged with forceps, scissors, Fogarty balloons, or a combination of these instruments [27].

When performing endoscopic fenestrations, the surgeon must carefully evaluate structures on the other side of the wall being fenestrated, as it can be easy to lose anatomic orientation in these sometimes challenging cases. Once the fenestration has been completed, the endoscope should be advanced through it to inspect structures beyond the fenestrated wall. Challenges of endoscopic procedures in the management of LH include the distorted anatomy as a result of prior hemorrhages, infections, or congenital malformations. Shifts in the anatomy as a result of the cyst fenestration and CSF drainage can also be challenging as cysts typically lack landmarks. Therefore, the integration of neuronavigation to aid in preoperative planning and intraoperative orientation and the use of navigated endoscopy and intraoperative MR imaging have become increasingly popular [19, 24]. Ultrasound can

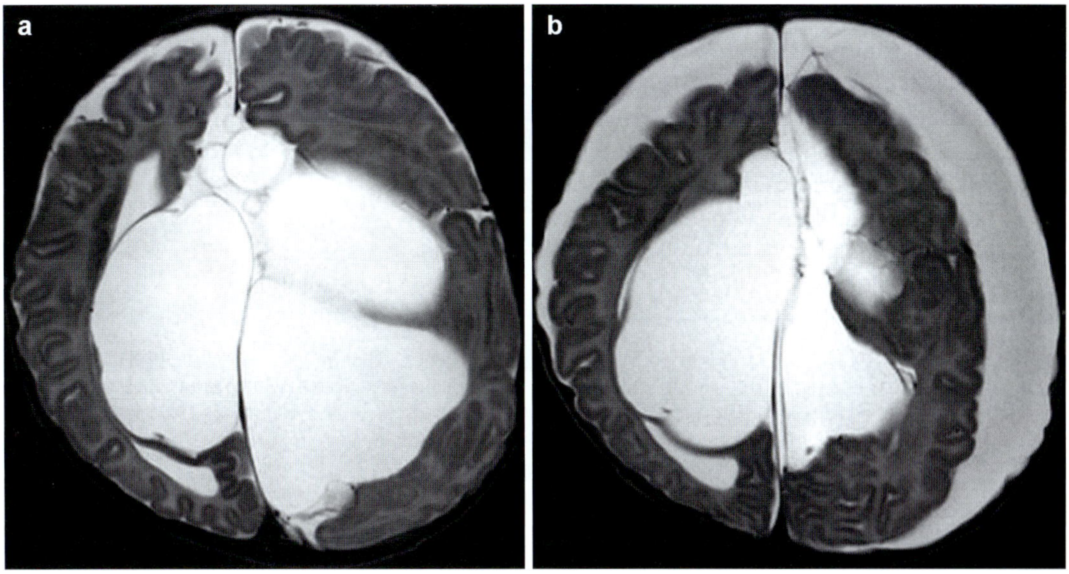

Fig. 23.2 (**a**) Preoperative axial T2-weighted MRI in a 4-month-old patient with hydrocephalus associated with a likely in utero CSF infection. (**b**) Postoperative MRI after endoscopic cyst fenestration. Some loculated compartments now communicate, but new subdural CSF compartments are visualized

also be utilized in real time to aid with endoscopic fenestrations, especially in infants with open fontanelles. While ultrasound image resolution is less than MRI, ultrasound has the advantage of providing real-time special orientation of loculated CSF compartments.

Despite technical success with endoscopic fenestrations, the majority of patients with LH require repeat endoscopic fenestrations and/or shunting procedures. Postoperative images may demonstrate decrease in some CSF compartments but increased size of other compartments and/or new subdural CSF collections (Fig. 23.2a, b).

23.7 Craniotomy for Fenestrations

There are limited published reports describing craniotomy for fenestration of intraventricular septations in the management of LH [16, 20, 22, 27]. The operating microscope enables a wider and deeper field of view than current endoscopic technology and allows for a broader range of microsurgical instruments to be utilized. Thus, craniotomy for microscopic fenestration may facilitate better visualization of compartments and membranes and wider fenestration of septations. Bleeding is much easier to control with standard techniques under the operating microscope than with endoscopy, during which a small amount of bleeding can significantly hamper visualization. Disadvantages of this technique include a larger skin incision, requirement for a craniotomy, and longer operating room times. In many instances the craniotomy is performed simultaneously with a shunt revision, and only a small extension of the existing shunt incision is typically required [22]. In a prior report of craniotomy for fenestration of LH [22], there were no new neurologic deficits as a consequence of the procedure. This, however, can be difficult to truly assess since the majority of patients in the series were severely developmentally delayed.

Conclusions

Although treatment options for patients with LH have expanded over the years as a result of advances in imaging modalities and less invasive surgical techniques, this condition continues to be one of the most challenging diseases in pediatric neurosurgery practice. Outcomes remain disappointing, as the majority of patients ultimately have a very poor quality of life and are physically and cognitively impaired despite neurosurgical interventions. Treatment goals need to be carefully defined to minimize the overall number of neurosurgical procedures and provide the best possible outcome for each patient.

References

1. Aleman J, Jokura H, Higano S, Akabane A, Shirane R, Yoshimoto T (2001) Value of constructive interference in steady-state three-dimensional, Fourier transformation magnetic resonance imaging for the neuroendoscopic treatment of hydrocephalus and intracranial cysts. Neurosurgery 48(6):1291–1295; discussion 1295–1296
2. Brown LW, Zimmerman RA, Bilaniuk LT (1979) Polycystic brain disease complicating neonatal meningitis: documentation of evolution by computed tomography. J Pediatr 94(5):757–759
3. Dincer A, Kohan S, Ozek MM (2009) Is all "communicating" hydrocephalus really communicating? Prospective study on the value of 3D-constructive interference in steady state sequence at 3 T. AJNR Am J Neuroradiol 30(10):1898–1906
4. Dincer A, Ozek MM (2011) Radiologic evaluation of pediatric hydrocephalus. Childs Nerv Syst 27(10):1543–1562
5. Dincer A, Yildiz E, Kohan S, Memet Ozek M (2011) Analysis of endoscopic third ventriculostomy patency by MRI: value of different pulse sequences, the sequence parameters, and the imaging planes for investigation of flow void. Childs Nerv Syst 27(1):127–135
6. El-Ghandour NM (2013) Endoscopic cyst fenestration in the treatment of uniloculated hydrocephalus in children. J Neurosurg Pediatr 11(4):402–409
7. Eller TW, Pasternak JF (1985) Isolated ventricles following intraventricular hemorrhage. J Neurosurg 62(3):357–362
8. Fritsch MJ, Mehdorn M (2002) Endoscopic intraventricular surgery for treatment of hydrocephalus and loculated CSF space in children less than one year of age. Pediatr Neurosurg 36(4):183–188
9. Gandhoke GS, Frassanito P, Chandra N, Ojha BK, Singh A (2013) Role of magnetic resonance ventriculography in multiloculated hydrocephalus. J Neurosurg Pediatr 11(6):697–703
10. Handler LC, Wright MG (1978) Postmeningitic hydrocephalus in infancy. Ventriculography with special reference to ventricular septa. Neuroradiology 16:31–35
11. Jamjoom AB, Mohammed AA, al-Boukai A, Jamjoom ZA, Rahman N, Jamjoom HT (1996) Multiloculated hydrocephalus related to cerebrospinal fluid shunt infection. Acta Neurochir 138(6):714–719
12. Kaiser G (1986) The value of multiple shunt systems in the treatment of nontumoral infantile hydrocephalus. Childs Nerv Syst 2(4):200–205
13. Kalsbeck JE, DeSousa AL, Kleiman MB, Goodman JM, Franken EA (1980) Compartmentalization of the cerebral ventricles as a sequela of neonatal meningitis. J Neurosurg 52(4):547–552
14. Kleinhaus S, Germann R, Sheran M, Shapiro K, Boley SJ (1982) A role for endoscopy in the placement of ventriculoperitoneal shunts. Surg Neurol 18(3):179–180
15. Lewis AI, Keiper GL Jr, Crone KR (1995) Endoscopic treatment of loculated hydrocephalus. J Neurosurg 82(5):780–785
16. Nida TY, Haines SJ (1993) Multiloculated hydrocephalus: craniotomy and fenestration of intraventricular septations. J Neurosurg 78(1):70–76
17. Nowoslawska E, Polis L, Kaniewska D, Mikolajczyk W, Krawczyk J, Szymanski W, Zakrzewski K, Podciechowska J (2003) Effectiveness of neuroendoscopic procedures in the treatment of complex compartmentalized hydrocephalus in children. Childs Nerv Syst 19(9):659–665
18. Oi S, Hidaka M, Honda Y, Togo K, Shinoda M, Shimoda M, Tsugane R, Sato O (1999) Neuroendoscopic surgery for specific forms of hydrocephalus. Childs Nerv Syst 15(1):56–68
19. Paraskevopoulos D, Biyani N, Constantini S, Beni-Adani L (2011) Combined intraoperative magnetic resonance imaging and navigated neuroendoscopy in children with multicompartmental hydrocephalus and complex cysts: a feasibility study. J Neurosurg Pediatr 8(3):279–288
20. Rhoton AL Jr, Gomez MR (1972) Conversion of multilocular hydrocephalus to unilocular. Case report. J Neurosurg 36(3):348–350
21. Salmon JH (1970) Isolated unilateral hydrocephalus following ventriculoatrial shunt. J Neurosurg 32(2):219–226
22. Sandberg DI, McComb JG, Krieger MD (2005) Craniotomy for fenestration of multiloculated hydrocephalus in pediatric patients. Neurosurgery 57 (1 Suppl):100–106; discussion 100–106
23. Schultz P, Leeds NE (1973) Intraventricular septations complicating neonatal meningitis. J Neurosurg 38(5):620–626
24. Schulz M, Bohner G, Knaus H, Haberl H, Thomale UW (2010) Navigated endoscopic surgery for multiloculated hydrocephalus in children. J Neurosurg Pediatr 5(5):434–442
25. Spennato P, Cinalli G, Ruggiero C, Aliberti F, Trischitta V, Cianciulli E, Maggi G (2007) Neuroendoscopic treatment of multiloculated hydrocephalus in children. J Neurosurg 106(1 Suppl):29–35
26. Teo C, Kadrian D, Hayhurst C (2013) Endoscopic management of complex hydrocephalus. World Neurosurg 79(2 Suppl):S21.e1–7
27. Zuccaro G, Ramos JG (2011) Multiloculated hydrocephalus. Childs Nerv Syst 27(10):1609–1619

Late Failures

24

Federico Di Rocco

Contents

24.1	**Introduction**	307
24.2	**Late Complication: Occlusion of the Stoma**	308
24.2.1	Risks Factors	308
24.2.2	Clinical Course	309
24.3	**Radiological Follow-Up**	310
24.4	**Risk Prevention**	311
24.5	**Other Late Complications**	311
References		311

F. Di Rocco, MD, PhD
Pediatric Neurosurgery, Necker Hospital,
149 rue de Sèvres, Paris 75015, France
e-mail: federico.dirocco@nck.aphp.fr

24.1 Introduction

Though life-threatening complications may occur during endoscopic procedures [17], the endoscopy-related mortality and permanent morbidity are usually low in large series (0.6 and 4.4 %, respectively, in Schroeder et al. series on 344 endoscopic procedures [30]). However, the rate of complications is extremely variable in the literature, going from 0 to 20 % and most of the papers dealing with this subject are anecdotic case reports or coming from the same institutions and authors [4, 26, 27, 29, 30].

The evaluation of complications related to neuroendoscopy is also complicated by the fact that they depend on the type of neuroendoscopic procedure: endoscopic third ventriculostomy (ETV) or septa fenestrations intracranial cyst fenestration, endoscopic biopsy for intraventricular lesions, or endoscopic tumor removal [3, 11]. All these procedures in fact carry a specific risk of morbidity [1, 3, 4, 7, 11, 15, 23–26, 31–34].

Complications can be further subdivided according to the impact they have on the outcome (transient vs. permanent or symptomatic vs. asymptomatic) or on the grounds of their occurrence (during the operation, in the immediate postoperative period, or in the late postoperative phases).

Herein, we have reviewed the recent literature on the complications according to their time of occurrence and/or clinical recognition focusing on late complications.

However, a clear definition of the early and late failure is lacking [20]. Some authors have

C. Di Rocco et al. (eds.), *Complications of CSF Shunting in Hydrocephalus: Prevention, Identification, and Management*, DOI 10.1007/978-3-319-09961-3_24,

considered that any failure occurring within 6 months after the endoscopic procedure should be considered as early [22].

This distinction has its importance since the mechanisms of the ETV failure differ substantially between the immediate postoperative period (mainly technical failure or inappropriate indication) and the late period (closure of a previously patent stoma).

Such simple distinction based on the time of occurrence has some limitations. In fact, a delayed recognition of an early occurring complication is always possible [2], thus falsely considering it has a late complication. Conversely, the recognition that a clinical deterioration is due to a late closure of a stoma may be also difficult. This is especially true in case of rapid and fatal evolution such in case of sudden death occurring several years after an ETV that might not be recognized as a late failure. Moreover, some patients may be lost during follow-up, making thus the analysis of long-term complications difficult.

24.2 Late Complication: Occlusion of the Stoma

Late complications of endoscopic procedures are mainly represented by the delayed reocclusion of the stoma with the risk of symptom recurrence. Several cases of reocclusion have been reported in the literature especially in case of ETV [5, 6, 11]. Reocclusion may occur early (i.e., within the first weeks after surgery) or in a delayed manner, that is, after several months to years.

Such delayed failure after an initially successful ETV remains an uncommon event (3.4 % in Erşahin et al. series with a mean delay of 105 weeks [12]). Late failure occurring after 6 or 7 years has been reported [5, 6, 10, 20, 22]. Late ETV dysfunction is substantially less frequent than extrathecal CSF shunt dysfunction [20].

24.2.1 Risks Factors

The occurrence of a late occlusion of the stoma seems to depend on two main factors: the quality of the stoma opening and the etiopathogenesis of the underlying hydrocephalus.

The quality of the opening of the stoma is considered to be actually a key factor for the early failure. However, depending on the onset of the clinical signs of recurrence, such failure of the procedure may become overt only after several weeks.

The risk of delayed closure depends also on the etiology of the hydrocephalus.

Reocclusion can occur in hydrocephalus due to all etiologies [20]: malformative, tumoral, infective, etc. But its occurrence seems to vary according to the different subtypes. It is in fact well known that ETV is more effective in pure aqueductal stenosis compared to posthemorrhagic or postinfective hydrocephalus. Similarly, the risk of a delayed closure of a previously patent stoma will differ according to the etiology of the hydrocephalus. The risk of a late ETV failure seems, for instance, higher in multiloculated postinfective hydrocephalus compared to intrinsic aqueductal stenosis. Late ETV failure might occur also in cases of hydrocephalus related to PFT despite a removal of the tumor itself and its risk varies according to the histology of the tumor (more common in posterior fossa ependymomas or medulloblastomas, for instance, than posterior fossa pilocytic astrocytomas) and extension of the removal (more common in low-grade brain stem tumors).

In our series of 141 successful ETV for posterior fossa tumors, a late failure was found in 14 children (10 % of the cases) at a 44.7-month follow-up. Six of them responded to a second endoscopic procedure, whereas in the remaining eight children, a ventriculoperitoneal shunt was implanted. The histologies were low-grade brain stem tumors, ependymomas, and recurring medulloblastoma.

The importance of the histological type is also confirmed by the differences in recurrence rates between hydrocephalus related to pineal lesion and to tectal plate lesions.

In fact, in our experience at Necker Enfants Malades, whereas in tectal plate lesions a secondary closure was found in up to 40 % of the cases, its occurrence was observed in only 26 % of ETV for hydrocephalus associated to pineal lesions and pineal tumors (Figs. 24.1, 24.2, 24.3, and 24.4).

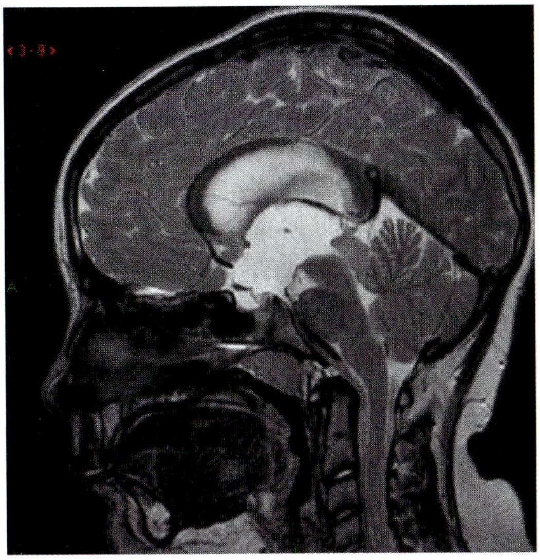

Fig. 24.1 Magnetic resonance imaging showing a hydrocephalus related to a tectal plate lesion. The patient presented with signs of increased ICP, nystagmus, and ataxia

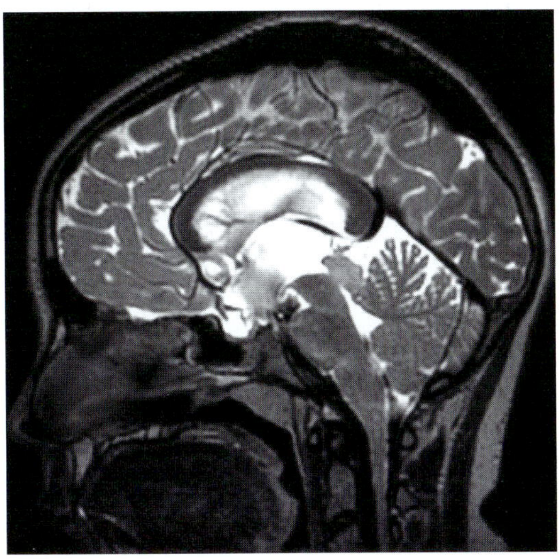

Fig. 24.2 Magnetic resonance (MR) imaging 6 months after an endoscopic third ventriculostomy. The patient was asymptomatic. The MR shows the reduction of the ventricular size, the enlargement of subarachnoid spaces, and a flow void signal at the floor of the third ventricle

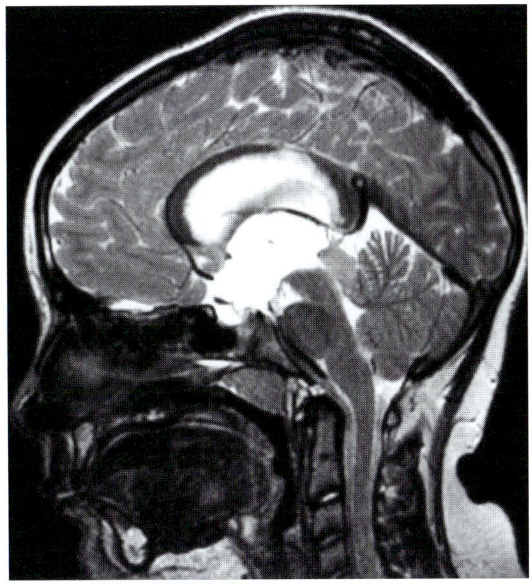

Fig. 24.3 One year after surgery, the patient is hospitalized for an acute symptom recurrence. The magnetic resonance imaging shows a ventricular dilatation with reduction of the subarachnoid spaces and disappearance of the flow void artifact. No change in the tectal lesion was found

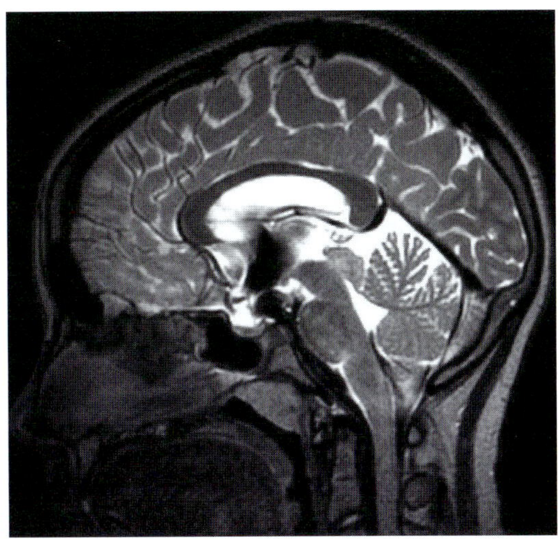

Fig. 24.4 After a redo of the endoscopic third ventriculostomy, the magnetic resonance control shows the reduction in size of the ventricles associated with the enlargement of the subarachnoid spaces and a flow void signal. The clinical status was normalized

24.2.2 Clinical Course

In some cases, the late closure may be recognized by a progressive clinical deterioration and symptom recurrence. In others, a rapid clinical deterioration can occur that needs to be promptly diagnosed.

The rapidity of onset of the clinical manifestations in case of closure of a patent stoma might depend according to some authors on the pathogenesis of the hydrocephalus [20]. The rapidity of

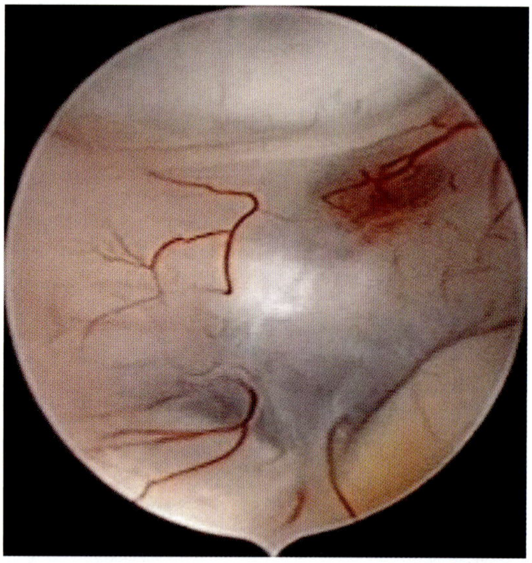

Fig. 24.5 Preoperative endoscopic image showing the scar tissue closing the third ventricle floor stoma

onset of the clinical manifestations of the hydrocephalus before the ETV was performed would suggest the rapidity of the manifestations at the time of ETV failure [20]. However, because of the paucity of the reported cases, such correlation is difficult to assess and remains speculative.

Cases of delayed sudden death after a functional ETV have also been reported [10, 16, 20]. Patients in whom an autopsy or repeated ETV were performed were found to have an occluded ETV [5, 10, 35] usually by a new membrane or scar (Fig. 24.5) and rarely by a clot or tumoral extension [13, 20, 21].

Because of the potential consequences of the raised hypertension, education of patients and their families about the risk of a late closure is of paramount importance to allow for a rapid management with a timely intervention. In fact, a repeated ETV is generally effective to restore the stoma and allow a symptom resolution.

A similar information that the one is given to the patients having an extrathecal CSF shunt device (i.e., of hardware dysfunction) and his or her family, should be given after an ETV even if there is no hardware implanted, in order to recognize any delayed ETV failure on time.

Similarly, a late closure can occur in other endoscopic procedures: cystostomies may close, with consequent cyst enlargement and symptom recurrence (2/23 in Tamburrini et al. series [32]). Large fenestrations in the cyst wall are often necessary to avoid cyst recurrence [14]. The opening of the cyst in the ventricles and in the cisterns (ventriculo-cysto-cisternostomy) may reduce such risk of secondary closure [8].

24.3 Radiological Follow-Up

Radiological follow-up is recommended in order to monitor the effectiveness of the endoscopic procedure.

A diminished ventricular volume, an increase in pericerebral CSF, a flow void signal through the stoma, as well as a modification of the ventricular shape are the main radiological criteria to assess on postoperative MR [13, 14, 19, 28]. However, the ventricular volume might remain enlarged in the postoperative imaging so that persisting ventriculomegaly should not be considered necessarily a failure of the procedure [14, 19].

Though after a successful ETV even if the ventricular volume might reduce only slightly, other radiological criteria can allow to confirm the patency of the stoma and efficacy of the surgical procedure.

On MR imaging, the CSF motion through the stoma can be assessed. A flow void signal is present at the level of the third ventricle floor that has lost its downward convexity due to the supratentorial/infratentorial pressure gradient.

The presence of the flow void signal is correlated to the patency of the stoma and success of the ETV. Conversely, its disappearance at a control MR may be considered as a marker of the closure of the stoma.

Another main criterion to assess on postoperative MR imaging is the enlargement of the subarachnoid spaces. This enlargement usually occurs in the first postoperative weeks and correlates with the patency of the stoma. In case of occlusion of the ETV, the subarachnoid spaces tend to reduce in size [9].

These radiological criteria should be monitored regularly because, in case of ETV closure, their modification might precede the occurrence of the clinical manifestations allowing an early recognition of the ETV dysfunction and a prompt management.

The recommended duration of such radiological follow-up is still debated, but the occurrence of late closures after several years suggests that more than 8–10 years follow-up should be performed.

24.4 Risk Prevention

Whereas early failure might be prevented by a proper indication and technique, no prevention of late ETV failure is known. In some centers, at the end of the endoscopic procedure, a ventricular reservoir (i.e., Ommaya or Rickheim) is implanted as a routine in order to have the possibility to draw some CSF in case of acute ETV dysfunction [20, 22]. However, the actual utility of such implant has not been proven. Indeed, other centers question its utility. Such system might not be patent or correctly in place when needed, that is, at the time of the ETV failure because of the large delay that might exist between the ETV procedure and its potential failure. Moreover, leaving an implanted device increases significantly the risks of infection.

24.5 Other Late Complications

Some cases of late morbidity such as the occurrence of chronic subdural hematomas or of neuropsychological disturbances have also been reported in the literature [2, 18]. These should be considered in many cases as a delayed recognition of an early complication of the surgical procedure itself more than an actual late complication.

References

1. Beems T, Grotenhuis JA (2004) Long-term complications and definition of failure of neuroendoscopic procedures. Childs Nerv Syst 20(11–12):868–877
2. Benabarre A, Ibáñez J, Boget T, Obiols J, Martínez-Aran A, Vieta E (2001) Neuropsychological and psychiatric complications in endoscopic third ventriculostomy: a clinical case report. J Neurol Neurosurg Psychiatry 71(2):268–271
3. Cappabianca P, Cinalli G, Gangemi M, Brunori A, Cavallo LM, de Divitiis E, Decq P, Delitala A, Di Rocco F, Frazee J, Godano U, Grotenhuis A, Longatti P, Mascari C, Nishihara T, Oi S, Rekate H, Schroeder HW, Souweidane MM, Spennato P, Tamburrini G, Teo C, Warf B, Zymberg ST (2008) Application of neuroendoscopy to intraventricular lesions. Neurosurgery 62(Suppl 2):575–597
4. Cinalli G, Spennato P, Ruggiero C, Aliberti F, Trischitta V, Buonocore MC, Cianciulli E, Maggi G (2007) Complications following endoscopic intracranial procedures in children. Childs Nerv Syst 23(6):633–644
5. Cinalli G, Sainte-Rose C, Chumas P, Zerah M, Brunelle F, Lot G, Pierre-Kahn A, Renier D (1999) Failure of third ventriculostomy in the treatment of aqueductal stenosis in children. J Neurosurg 90(3):448–454
6. Cinalli G, Sainte-Rose C, Chumas P, Zerah M, Brunelle F, Lot G, Pierre-Kahn A, Renier D (1999) Failure of third ventriculostomy in the treatment of aqueductal stenosis in children. Neurosurg Focus 6(4):e3
7. Di Rocco C, Massimi L, Tamburrini G (2006) Shunts vs endoscopic third ventriculostomy in infants: are there different types and/or rates of complications? A review. Childs Nerv Syst 22(12):1573–1589
8. Di Rocco F, Yoshino M, Oi S (2005) Neuroendoscopic transventricular ventriculocystostomy in treatment for intracranial cysts. J Neurosurg 103(1 Suppl):54–60
9. Di Rocco F, Grevent D, Drake JM, Boddaert N, Puget S, Roujeau T, Blauwblomme T, Zerah M, Brunelle F, Sainte-Rose C (2012) Changes in intracranial CSF distribution after ETV. Childs Nerv Syst 28(7):997–1002
10. Drake J, Chumas P, Kestle J, Pierre-Kahn A, Vinchon M, Brown J, Pollack IF, Arai H (2006) Late rapid deterioration after endoscopic third ventriculostomy: additional cases and review of the literature. J Neurosurg 105(2 Suppl):118–126
11. Enchev Y, Oi S (2008) Historical trends of neuroendoscopic surgical techniques in the treatment of hydrocephalus. Neurosurg Rev 31(3):249–262
12. Erşahin Y, Arslan D (2008) Complications of endoscopic third ventriculostomy. Childs Nerv Syst 24(8):943–948
13. Fukuhara T, Luciano MG, Kowalski RJ (2002) Clinical features of third ventriculostomy failures classified by fenestration patency. Surg Neurol 58(2):102–110
14. Gangemi M, Maiuri F, Colella G, Sardo L (1999) Endoscopic surgery for intracranial cerebrospinal fluid cyst malformations. Neurosurg Focus 6(4):e6
15. Goumnerova LC, Frim DM (1997) Treatment of hydrocephalus with third ventriculocisternostomy: outcome and CSF flow patterns. Pediatr Neurosurg 27(3):149–152
16. Hader WJ, Drake J, Cochrane D, Sparrow O, Johnson ES, Kestle J (2002) Death after late failure of third ventriculostomy in children. Report of three cases. J Neurosurg 97(1):211–215

17. Handler MH, Abbott R, Lee M (1994) A near-fatal complication of endoscopic third ventriculostomy: case report. Neurosurgery 35(3):525–527; discussion 527–528
18. Kim BS, Jallo GI, Kothbauer K, Abbott IR (2004) Chronic subdural hematoma as a complication of endoscopic third ventriculostomy. Surg Neurol 62(1): 64–68
19. Kulkarni AV, Drake JM, Armstrong DC, Dirks PB (2000) Imaging correlates of successful endoscopic third ventriculostomy. J Neurosurg 92(6):915–919
20. Lipina R, Palecek T, Reguli S, Kovarova M (2007) Death in consequence of late failure of endoscopic third ventriculostomy. Childs Nerv Syst 23(7): 815–819
21. Massimi L, Tamburrini G, Caldarelli M, Di Rocco F, Federica N, Di Rocco C (2006) Late closure of the stoma by spreading of a periaqueductal glioma: an unusual failure of endoscopic third ventriculostomy. Case report. J Neurosurg 104(3 Suppl):197–201
22. Navarro R, Gil-Parra R, Reitman AJ, Olavarria G, Grant JA, Tomita T (2006) Endoscopic third ventriculostomy in children: early and late complications and their avoidance. Childs Nerv Syst 22(5):506–513
23. Oi S, Abbott R (2004) Loculated ventricles and isolated compartments in hydrocephalus: their pathophysiology and the efficacy of neuroendoscopic surgery. Neurosurg Clin N Am 15(1):77–87
24. Oi S, Shibata M, Tominaga J, Honda Y, Shinoda M, Takei F, Tsugane R, Matsuzawa K, Sato O (2000) Efficacy of neuroendoscopic procedures in minimally invasive preferential management of pineal region tumors: a prospective study. J Neurosurg 93(2): 245–253
25. Oi S, Hidaka M, Honda Y, Togo K, Shinoda M, Shimoda M, Tsugane R, Sato O (1999) Neuroendoscopic surgery for specific forms of hydrocephalus. Childs Nerv Syst 15(1):56–68
26. Oertel J, Baldauf J, Schroeder HW, Gaab MR (2009) Endoscopic options in children: experience with 134 procedures. J Neurosurg Pediatr 3:81–89
27. Peretta P, Ragazzi P, Galarza M, Genitori L, Giordano F, Mussa F, Cinalli G (2006) Complications and pitfalls of neuroendoscopic surgery in children. J Neurosurg 105(3 Suppl):187–193
28. Preul C, Hübsch T, Lindner D, Tittgemeyer M (2006) Assessment of ventricular reconfiguration after third ventriculostomy: what does shape analysis provide in addition to volumetry? AJNR Am J Neuroradiol 27(3):689–693
29. Schroeder HW, Niendorf WR, Gaab MR (2002) Complications of endoscopic third ventriculostomy. J Neurosurg 96(6):1032–1040
30. Schroeder HW, Oertel J, Gaab MR (2004) Incidence of complications in neuroendoscopic surgery. Childs Nerv Syst 20(11–12):878–883
31. Siomin V, Cinalli G, Grotenhuis A, Golash A, Oi S, Kothbauer K, Weiner H, Roth J, Beni-Adani L, Pierre-Kahn A, Takahashi Y, Mallucci C, Abbott R, Wisoff J, Constantini S (2002) Endoscopic third ventriculostomy in patients with cerebrospinal fluid infection and/or hemorrhage. J Neurosurg 97(3):519–524
32. Tamburrini G, D'Angelo L, Paternoster G, Massimi L, Caldarelli M, Di Rocco C (2007) Endoscopic management of intra and paraventricular CSF cysts. Childs Nerv Syst 23(6):645–651
33. Teo C, Jones R (1996) Management of hydrocephalus by endoscopic third ventriculostomy in patients with myelomeningocele. Pediatr Neurosurg 25(2):57–63
34. Teo C (1999) Complete endoscopic removal of colloid cysts: issues of safety and efficacy. Neurosurg Focus 6(4):e9
35. Wellons JC 3rd, Tubbs RS, Banks JT, Grabb B, Blount JP, Oakes WJ, Grabb PA (2002) Long-term control of hydrocephalus via endoscopic third ventriculostomy in children with tectal plate gliomas. Neurosurgery 51(1):63–67

Index

A

Abdominal complications
  ascites, 66–67
  CSF pseudocyst, 65–66
  inguinal hernia and hydrocele, 66
  visceral–intestinal perforation, 66–68
Abdominal pseudocyst, 188, 191–192, 254
Acquired cranio-cerebral disproportion (ACCD)
  brain, 236–237
  clinical features, 235
  congenital hydrocephalus, 242
  cranial vault, 242, 244
  features, CSF overdrainage, 235
  intracranial pressure, 234
  overdrainage, 236
  skull, 237–238
  ventricular dilation, 234
Acute–subacute complications
  catheter malposition and migration, 47–50
  complications in ETV, 55
  disconnection and breakage, 47
  loculation, 50–52
  overdrainage and slit ventricle syndrome, 50–52
  shunt infection, 45–6
  shunt obstruction, 46–7
  subcutaneous CSF collections and fistulas, 52–55
Adjustable valves, 112, 162–163, 169, 171, 173
Antibiotic-impregnated shunts, 8
Antisiphon devices, 121–122, 124–125, 169–170
Antisiphon valves (ASV), 125
Aqueductoplasty, 270–271, 273
Arachnoid-cyst shunting, 14–15, 100
Arrested hydrocephalus, 15
Atrial erosion, 181
Atrial shunts
  cardiac tamponade, 181–182
  endocarditis, 181
  pulmonary thromboembolism and consequences, 178–180
  shunt nephritis, 182–183
  thrombosis, 180–181
Atrial thrombosis, 178, 180–181
Atriovenous thrombosis, 180

B

Bioglide® catheter, 135
Bladder perforation, 194–195
Bowel perforation, 95, 100
  description, 193
  diagnosis, 193–194
  fibrosis, 193
  laparotomy, 193
  pathophysiology and risk factors, 193
  prognosis, 194
  serious vascular damage, 193
  spring-coiled catheters, 193
  treatment, 194
B-waves, 163, 170

C

Calcification
  dystrophic, 130
  metastatic, 130
Cardiac tamponade, 181–182, 184, 224–225
Catheter disconnection, 205
Catheter fracture, 113
Catheter malposition, 205–206
Catheter migration, 205
CCD. *See* Cranio-cerebral disproportion (CCD)
Chiari type I malformation, 240
Choroid plexus cauterization, 9
Cine phase-contrast (PC) MRI, 40–41
Clinical manifestations, CSF shunt complications
  CSF draining systems, types, 16
  epilepsy, 27
  functional complications, 24–25
  hemorrhage, 25–27
  hydrocephalus and shunt problems, 13–14
  of shunt failure (*see* Shunt failure)
  shunt infection, 23–24
  shunt malfunction and complications, 16
  shunt structure, 15–16
Closure, patent stoma, 309
Cognitive outcome, 7
Compensated hydrocephalus, 15
Complications
  atrial shunts (*see* Atrial shunts)
  avoidance, 272–273

C. Di Rocco et al. (eds.), *Complications of CSF Shunting in Hydrocephalus: Prevention, Identification, and Management*, DOI 10.1007/978-3-319-09961-3,

Complications (*cont.*)
cardiac, 263
causes of shunt failure, 3–4
CCD (*see* Cranio-cerebral disproportion (CCD))
clinical improvement, iNPH, 166
clinical manifestations (*see* Clinical manifestations, CSF shunt complications)
definition, 16
device (*see* Shunt device)
due to altered CSF dynamics, CSF fistulae (*see* CSF fistulae)
endoscopic fenestration (*see* Loculated hydrocephalus (LH))
epilepsy (*see* Epilepsy)
extrathecal CSF shunts
due to age, 79
due to design, 79
due to material, 78
due to miscellaneous causes, 79
factors associated, 4
heterogeneity, 4–5
iatrogenic (*see* Iatrogenic complications)
impact, evaluation, 5
insufficient correction, altered CSFdynamics, 286
long-term neurodevelopmental outcomes, 149
mechanical complications, shunts (*see* Mechanical complications)
mortality, 164–165
neuroendoscopy, 264–265
overdrainage, 169
patients with iNPH, 163
pleural shunt (*see* Pleural shunt)
posthemorrhagic hydrocephalus (*see* Posthemorrhagic hydrocephalus)
postinflammatory hydrocephalus (*see* Postinflammatory hydrocephalus)
rate, LP shunt, 204, 206
selected measures, 9
shunt systems, 263
VPS (*see* Ventriculoperitoneal shunts (VPS))
VSGS, 152, 155
Continuous spikes and waves during slow sleep (CSWS), 254–255
Conventional radiography (shunt series), 34–36
Cortical bleeding, 26–27
Cortical malformation, 253
Cranio-cerebral disproportion (CCD), 25
ACCD (*see* Acquired cranio-cerebral disproportion (ACCD))
calvarial expansion, 242, 244
craniosynostosis, 242–243
definition, 233
diagnosis, 238–240
lumbo-peritoneal shunting, 241
prevention, 240–241
surgical approaches, 241
and SVS, 234–235
Craniosynostosis, 56–7
Craniotomy, fenestrations, 305
CSF absorption (R_{out}) values, 161–162
CSF diversion, 227–228, 230
CSF draining systems, 16
CSF dynamics, 245, 277, 281
CSF fistulae
altered CSF dynamics, 279
CSF dynamics, abnormalities, 277
CSF leak, 280–281
endoscopic third ventriculostomy, 280
imaging, 278–279
implantation of a shunt device, 280
incidence of chronic CSF, 278
intra-abdominal pressures, 280
intracranial CSF dynamics, 281
intracranial hypotension, 278, 280
"minor" (extra-arachnoid) pathways, 281
over-drainage phenomenon, 280
resistance to CSF outflow (RCSF), 280
symptoms, 278
CSF leak, 207, 230, 271, 280–281
CSF production, 270
CSWS. *See* Continuous spikes and waves during slow sleep (CSWS)

D
Degradation process
biopolymers, 131
distal catheter fracture, 132
silicone catheter, 131
VP and VA shunts, 131–132
Device, CSF shunting
basic hydrodynamics, 110
catheter characteristics, 112–115
patient factors
CSF outflow, 115
CSF red cell count or protein levels, 116
low CSF compliance ('brittle ventricles'), 115–116
post-meningitic hydrocephalus, 115
pre-term babies, 115
risk of subdural haematoma, 115
slit-ventricle syndrome (SVS), 115
types of valves (*see* Shunt valves)
Diagnosis, CSF shunting
computerized tomography (CT), 37–38
conventional radiography (shunt series)
causes of shunt failure, 34
disconnections of VP shunt mechanism, 34–35
ectopic position, shunt catheters, 34
radiation dose, 36
magnetic resonance imaging (MRI)
cine phase-contrast (PC) MRI, 40–41
conventional sequences, 38–40
3D-CISS, 39–40
modern programmable valves, 37
ventricular dilatation, 37
radionuclide shunt studies, 41
ultrasounds, 36–37

Differential pressure valves
ball-in-cone valve, 111
diaphragm valves, 111
mitre valves, 111
slit valves, 111
Discitis, 205
Disconnection of shunt component, 34–35, 137
Dislocation of shunt component
definition, 134
distal catheter
forceful rotation or flexion–extension movements, 136
"iatrogenic" theory, 135–136
laparoscopic-assisted technique, 135
migration of lumboperitoneal shunt catheter, 136–137
migration of distal tube, 136
myelomeningoceles (MMC), 136
in peritoneal cavity, 135
retrograde migration, 136
spontaneous knot formation, 135
spring-coiled catheters, 136
"transperitoneal" dislocations, 135
management
antibiotics, 138
endoscopic third ventriculostomy (ETV), 137
endovascular methods, 138
neuroendoscopy, 137
shunt taps, 137
presentation, 137
proximal catheter, 134–135
Distal obstruction, 61–62

E
Economic cost, 8
Effusions, 121–122
Endocarditis, 178, 181
Endoscope/Endoscopy
challenges, 304
fenestrations, 304
hydrocephalus treatment, 270–271
iatrogenic complications, 271–272
modern neurosurgeon's armamentarium, 269
mortality and permanent morbidity, 307
Nitze–Leiter cystoscope, 269
origins, 269
shunting procedures, 305
Endoscopic third ventriculostomy (ETV), 9, 13, 42, 125, 290–291, 307
complications, 55, 265
description, 270
hydrocephalic patients, 227
late ETV failure, 308
PHH, 153, 155
pseudocysts, 192
Epidural hematomas, 27
Epilepsy, 7
hemispherectomy procedures, 256–257
hydrocephalus (*see* Hydrocephalic patient)
incidence, 248
long-term follow-up retrospective study, 254
mental/physical disability, 256
related to CSF shunting, 27
seizures development, 248
Epileptic seizure, 248, 251–254, 256
ETV. *See* Endoscopic third ventriculostomy (ETV)
External hydrocephalus, 14
External ventricular drainage (EVD), 16, 82
Extra-axial fluid or blood collections, 296–298
benign CSF collections (effusions), 120–121
formation of subdural effusions, 121
iatrogenic normal pressure hydrocephalus (iNPH), 121
incidence of subdural hematoma, 121
management
antisiphon device, preventing overdrainage, 122
drainage, 122
follow-up with CT, 122
higher resistance, 122
subdural hematoma, 122–123
siphoning, 121
Extra-axial haematoma
bilateral subdural hygroma, 296–298
craniotomy, 296
lumboperitoneal shunts, 296
Extracerebral fluid collections
arachnoid cysts, 86–88
benign pericerebral collections, 86–87
brain atrophy, 86
initial stages of communicating hydrocephalus, 86
leptomeningeal seeding of tumors, 86
posttraumatic and postinfectious subdural collections, 86
Extracranial complications, 59
complications related to shunt variants, 64–65
disconnection and fracture of the shunt, 60–61
distal obstruction, 61–62
fibrothorax, 64
hydrothorax (pleural effusion), 62–64
pneumothorax and subcutaneous emphysema, 62
shunt misplacement, 59–60
thromboembolic disease and pulmonary arterial hypertension, 65
tricuspid valve pathology, 65
Extrathecal CSF shunts
features, 76
indications, 77–78
types
lumboperitoneal (LP) shunts, 75–76
ventriculoatrial (VA) shunts, 76
ventriculo-gallbladder shunts (VGS), 76–77
ventriculoperitoneal shunts, 76–77
ventriculopleural shunts, 76
ventriculoureteric shunt (VUS), 76
unavoidable complications
due to age, 79
due to design, 79
due to material, 78
due to miscellaneous causes, 79

F

Fibrothorax, 64, 221–222
Flow-regulated valves, 110–111
Focal EEG changes, 255–256
Fogarty balloon, 270, 272–273
Foramen of Monro, 270, 273
Fracture of shunt component
  epidemiology, 129–130
  implanted material
    calcification, 130
    degradation and altered physical properties, 131–132
    immune response, 131
    polysiloxanes (silicon rubber), 130
  material selection and importance of hardware
    antibiotic-impregnated shunt catheters, 133
    catheters with barium, 133
    Mini–Holter valve, 133
    number of shunt components, 133
    polyurethane, 132–133
    tubular or round-bodied valves, 133
  surgical technique
    burr-hole site, 134
    monofilament sutures, 134
    proximal obstruction, 134
    surgical knots, 134
Functional complications
  hyperdrainage
    cranial sutures or iatrogenic craniosynostosis, 125
    extra-axial fluid or blood collections, 120–123
    historical review, 119–120
    incidence, 120
    siphoning effect, 120
    slit ventricle (*see* Slit ventricle syndrome (SVS/SLVS))
  overdrainage, clinical features, 25
  underdrainage, clinical manifestations, 24–25

G

Gastrointestinal perforation, 205
Gravitational devices
  adjustable valves, 162
  antisiphon, 169–171
  medium and high-pressure valves, 169
Gravitational valves, 111–112

H

Haematoma(s), 119, 121–123
  contralateral or bilateral, 293
  CSF accumulation, 294
  endoscopic third ventriculostomy, 293, 295
  incidence, 289
  normal pressure hydrocephalus, 291–293
  pathogenesis, 289
  posttraumatic hydrocephalus, 289–290
  reaccumulation or SDH expansion, 289
  subdural, 27, 43
  symptomatic, 289
Headaches, 25
Health-related QOL, 6
Hemorrhage
  abdominal, 205
  cortical bleeding, 26–27
  epidural hematomas, 27
  intraventricular hemorrhage, 25–26
  subdural hematomas, 27
Heterogeneity, 4–5
Hydrocele, 207
Hydrocephalic patient
  diagnosis, 248
  EEG changes, 254–256
  epilepsy, 257
  etiology, 249–250
  hemispherectomy procedures, 256–257
  incidence ratio, 247
  intracranial shunting procedure, 250–251
  shunting (*see* Shunting procedure)
  treatment options, 257
Hydrocephalus
  active or passive, 15
  adult normal pressure, 84
  apparent clinically arrested, 85
  arachnoid cysts, 14–15
  arrested, 15
  asymptomatic pediatric ventriculomegaly, 83–84
  compensated, 15
  complications, shunt systems, 263
  and CSF shunt revisions, 14
  endoscopic treatment, 270–271
  etiology, 7, 14–15
  ETV, 266, 290–291
  external, 14
  extracerebral fluid collections, initial stages, 86
  ICP monitoring or hydrodynamic tests, 15
  incidence ratio, 14, 247
  intelligence quotients (IQ), 7
  low-pressure, 278
  management strategies, 263
  multiloculated, 100
  neonatal and infantile
    ETV and CSF shunting, 83
    intracranial pressure (ICP), 83
    measurements of head circumference (HC), 82–83
    in myelomeningocele patients, 83
    posthemorrhagic hydrocephalus, 83
  NPH, 15
  pathophysiology, 14
  pediatric normal pressure, 83
  posttraumatic hydrocephalus *vs.* brain atrophy, 84
  reocclusion, 308
  scope and CSF shunt revisions, 14
  and shunt problems, 13–14
  societal impact, 8
  success rates, 266
  surgery, infectious subdural collections, 295
  surgical treatment, 285
  temporal occurrence, 15
  treatment, 3, 187, 296–298
  uncompensated hydrocephalus, 15

ventricular shunts, 33, 41–42
VPL shunting, 215
Hydrocephalus outcome questionnaire (HOQ), 7
Hydrostatic pressure (p), 110, 120
Hydrothorax (pleural effusion), 96, 99
lung atelectasis, 63
pleural effusion, 63–64
ventriculopleural (VPL) shunting, 62–63
Hygroma(s)
after ETV, 291
"craniocerebral disproportion," 291
CT or MRI imaging, 286
extra-axial fluid collections, 286
incidence, 286
normal pressure hydrocephalus, 286–289, 291–293
prevention, 287–288, 293
re-expanding the ventricles, 293
siphoning, 288
subdural effusion, 291
symptomatic cases, 291
treatment options, 286–287
ventriculocisternostomy, 291
Hyperdrainage. *See* Overdrainage

I
Iatrogenesis. *See also* Iatrogenic complications
description, 82
in diagnostic procedures
CT and MRI, 89–90
ICP measurement, 88–9
reservoir pumping, 88
of shunt infection, 89–90
shuntogram, 89
shunt series, 89
shunt Tap, 88
ultrasonography, 89
in diverse indications and distal draining locations
arachnoid-cyst shunting, 100
lumboperitoneal (LP) shunting, 99
subduroperitoneal shunting, 100
ventriculoatrial shunting, 98–99
ventriculogallbladder shunting, 99
ventriculopleural (VPL) shunting, 99
ventriculosubgaleal shunting, 99
ventriculoureteral shunting, 99
Iatrogenic complications, 271–272
antisiphon devices, 97
burr hole, 92
Dandy–Walker cyst, 100–101
dural opening, 92
external ventricular drainage (EVD), 82
extracerebral fluid collections, 86–88
follow-up, education, and continuity of care, 102
hydrocephalus, 82–85
iatrogenesis, 88–90, 98–100
iatrogenic failure ("friendly fire"), 82
in-line filters, 97
local anesthetics, 91
medical-device-associated complications, 82
patient position, 91
peritoneal access, 95
posterior fossa cysts, 100–101
preparations for surgery, 90–91
principles, 82
programmable valves, 101
reservoirs, 96
rupture, disconnection, and migration, 96
shunt infection, 102
shunt parts, losure, and wound dressing, connection, 97
skin incisions, 92
skin preparation, 91
trapped fourth ventricle, 100–101
tunneling and subcutaneous passage, distal catheter, 95–96
valves, 96–97
ventricular catheter insertion-related pitfalls, 92–94
VP-shunt-related complications, 82
Iatrogenic craniosynostosis, 125
Idiopathic NPH (iNPH)
acute respiratory infection, 163–164
clinical diagnosis, 161
clinical improvement and complications, 166
continuous ICP and CSF dynamics studies, 161
CT scans, 165
management, 160–161
mortality and complication rates, 164
pathological cause, 160
patients, after surgery, 160
physiopathology, 160
suspect, 160
SVASONA study, 169
treatment, 172
valve selection, 162
Ileus, 205
Immune response, 131
Indications, extrathecal CSF shunts
increased intracranial pressure (ICP), 77
NPH, 77
occlusive hydrocephalus, 77
in premature infants, 77
radiologic imaging, 77
radionuclide cisternogram, 78
transfontanellar craniosonography, 77
Infective complications
clinical presentation
neonates, 144
repeated malfunctions, 143–144
Staphylococcus aureus infections, 143
Staphylococcus epidermidis, 144
diagnostic studies
imaging studies, 144
recurrent shunt malfunctions, 144
routine blood tests, 144
shunt tap, 144
epidemiology and risk factors, 142
pathogens
anaerobic organisms, 142–143
coagulase-negative staphylococci, 143
non-bacterial shunt infections, 143
prevention, 146

Infective complications (*cont.*)
- "shunt infection," definition, 141
- treatment and outcome
  - optimal duration of antibiotic therapy, 145
  - removal of the shunt, 145

Inguinal hernia and hydrocele, 66
Intelligence quotients (IQ), 7
Intra-abdominal pressure (IAP), 110, 171–172
Intracranial complications, 46
- acute–subacute complications
  - catheter malposition and migration, 47, 50–51
  - complications in ETV, 55
  - disconnection and breakage, 47, 49–50
  - loculation, 52, 54–55
  - overdrainage and slit ventricle syndrome, 50–52
  - shunt infection, 45–6
  - shunt obstruction, 46–7
  - subcutaneous CSF collections and fistulas, 52–53, 55
- chronic complications
  - acquired cranioencephalic disproportion, 57
  - craniosynostosis, 56–7
  - meningeal fibrosis, 57
  - perishunt encephalomalacia, 57–59
  - periventricular leukomalacia, 57–59
  - pneumocephalus, 57–59
  - trapping of the fourth ventricle, 57–59

Intracranial hemorrhage, 253–254
Intracranial hypotension, 206, 251, 254, 278
Intracranial pressure (ICP), 163, 167–168, 171
- hydrodynamic tests, 15
- monitoring, 84, 150, 160, 162, 173
- values, 120

Intraventricular hemorrhage (IVH), 25–26, 43, 227, 229, 302
Intraventricular pressure (IVP), 110
IVH. *See* Intraventricular hemorrhage (IVH)

L

Late failures
- definition, 308
- occlusion of the stoma
  - clinical course, 309–310
  - risks factors, 308–309
- radiological follow-up, 310–311
- risk prevention, 311

Length of stay, hospital, 5–6
Lifetime years of potential life lost (LYPLL), 8
Loculated hydrocephalus (LH)
- craniotomy for fenestrations, 305
- diagnosis
  - computed tomography (CT), 302
  - CT-based ventriculography, 303
  - 3D CISS, 303
  - magnetic resonance imaging (MRI), 302–303
  - preoperative radiological evaluation, 302
  - ultrasound (US), 302
- endoscopic management, 304–305
- etiology and pathophysiology, 301–302
- fenestration procedures, 304
- neurosurgical management, 301
- shunting, 304
- treatment options, 304

Loculations, 52, 54–55
LOVA (long-standing overt ventriculomegaly of adults), 84
Lumboperitoneal (LP) shunt, 16, 75–76, 99
- back pain, 205
- complications postlumboperitoneal shunt, 205
- CSF leakage, 207
- IIH, 203
- indication, 203–204
- infection, 207
- leading surgical treatment, 203
- mechanical failure, 205–206
- mechanical-induced pain, 207
- NPH, 203
- obstruction, 204
- overdrainage, 206–207
- polyethylene catheters, 204
- pregnancy, 207–208
- publication report, 204
- radiculopathy, 205
- reported complications, 205–206
- silastic catheters, 204
- spinal deformities, 207

M

Magnetic resonance imaging (MRI)
- cine phase-contrast (PC) MRI, 40–41
- conventional sequences, 38–39
- 3D-CISS, 39–40

Mechanical complications
- dislocation
  - distal catheter, 135–137
  - management, 137–138
  - presentation, 137
  - proximal catheter, 134–135
- fracture
  - epidemiology, 129–130
  - implanted material, 130–132
  - material selection and hardware, 132–133
  - surgical technique, 133–134

Meningeal fibrosis, 57
Meningitis, 141, 205, 207, 302
Mental disability, 256
Migration of shunt catheter, 133–136, 152, 179, 183–184
Misplacement, 183–184
Myelopathy, 207

N

Neuroendoscopic procedures
- complications, 264–265
- endoscopic third ventriculostomy (ETV), 290–291
- indications, 264
- infectious subdural collections, 295
- subdural CSF hygromas, 291–293
- subdural haematomas, 293–295

Neuroimaging
abdominal complications, 65–68
extracranial complications, 59–65
imaging appearance, 41–42
imaging techniques, 34–41
intracranial complications, 45–59
postoperative complications after shunt placement, 43–45
Normal pressure hydrocephalus (NPH), 9, 14–15, 41
after shunting, 163–164
CBF reduction, 160
characterization, 159
CSF malabsorption, 160
diagnose, 161–162
Gait abnormalities, 160
gravitational devices and antisiphon, 169–171
idiopathic, 112
iNPH (*see* Idiopathic NPH (iNPH))
intra-abdominal pressure, 171–172
mortality and complication rates, 164–165
near-zero shunt infection rate, 165–167
overdrainage, 167–169
patients management, 160
rapid eye movement, 160
sophisticated diagnostic tests, 159–160
treatment, 160–161, 172–173
valve selection, 162–163
worsening, 172
NPH scale, 163–164

O
Optic nerve fenestration (ONF), 203
Overdrainage, 167–169, 235–237
chronic, 50–52
clinical features, 25–26
complications
cranial sutures, 125
definition, 119
extra-axial fluid or blood collections, 120–123
historical review, 119–120
iatrogenic craniosynostosis, 125
slit ventricle syndrome, 123–125
diagnosis, 52
LP shunt, 206–207
slit ventricle syndrome, 51, 53
subdural hygromas or hematomas, 50

P
Parenchymal hemorrhage, 43
Pediatric normal pressure
normal pressure hydrocephalus (NPH), 83
occult hydrocephalus, 83
Perishunt encephalomalacia, 57–59
Peritoneal shunts
abdominal metastasis, 197
abdominal wall perforation, 196–197
bladder perforation, 194–195
bowel perforation and anal extrusion, 193–194
catheter placement
gallbladder, 198–200
laparoscopy, 197–198
mortality and morbidity, 200
omental bursa, 198
peritoneal adhesions, 198
shunt nephropathy, 197
thromboembolism, 197
ventriculo-gallbladder shunt, 199
ventriculopleural diversion, 198
VOB shunting, 198
complications, 187–188
epidemiology, 188
intestinal volvulus, 196
migration, 195–196
nonfunctional abdominal complications, catheters, 188–189
pseudocyst, 190–192
sterile ascites, 189–190
ventriculoperitoneal shunting, 187
Peritonitis, 205, 207
Periventricular leukomalacia, 57–59
Physical disability, 256
Pleural effusion
age-related event, 213
antisiphon device, 218
bacterial invasion, 221
cerebrospinal fluid, 224
identification and management, 218–220
inflammatory process, 223
prevention, 218
VPL shunts, 217–218
Pleural shunt
cardiac tamponade, 224–225
cerebrospinal fluid galactorrhea, 224
chest radiograph, 214–215
complications rate, 215
costal nerve, 214
disconnection and coiling, 223
effusions, empyema, and fibrothorax
fibrotic changes, 218
fluid collection, 217
identification and management, 218–222
prevention, 218
hydrothorax, 213
migration, 222–223
overdrainage, 222
pneumothorax and subcutaneous emphysema, 216–217
proximal and distal obstructions, 223
scalp incision, 214
transdiaphragmatic route, 215
tumor spread, 224
ventricular catheter, 214
VPL shunting, 213–214
Pneumocephalus, 43–45, 57–59
Pneumoencephalus, 205
Pneumothorax
definition, 216
identification, 216
management, 217
prevention, 216
and subcutaneous emphysema, 62, 95, 99

Poiseuille's law, 115
Polyethylene catheters, 204
Posthemorrhagic hydrocephalus (PHH)
  adjunctive therapies, 153
  and complications, 150–152
  intraventricular hemorrhage, 149
  pathophysiology, 150
  ventriculoperitoneal shunt, 149
Postinflammatory hydrocephalus (PIH)
  and complications, 154–155
  ETV, 154
  long-term outcomes, 155
  pathophysiologic mechanisms, 153
  pathophysiology, 154
Postoperative complications, after shunt placement, 43
  appearance of ventricular collapse, 45
  intraventricular hemorrhage, 43
  occurrence of subarachnoid hemorrhage, 45
  parenchymal hemorrhage, 43
  pneumocephalus, 43, 45
  subdural hematomas or hygromas, 43
Preterm delivery, 208
Programmable valves, 96, 101, 112
Pseudocysts
  abdominal cerebrospinal fluid, 190
  allergic reactions, 191
  antisilicone antibodies, 191
  bacterial infection, 190
  description, 190
  diagnosis, 191
  ethylene oxide (ETO), 191
  ETV, 192
  formation, 61–62
  laboratory tests, 191–192
  peritoneal catheter, 192
  predisposing factors, 190
  silicone elastomers and gels, 191
  symptoms, 191
  treatment, 192
Pseudomeningocele, 207
Pulmonar embolus, 205
Pulmonary arterial hypertension, 65
Pulmonary embolization, 178, 181
Pulmonary hypertension, 178–180

Q

Quality-adjusted life years (QALY), 8
Quality of life (QOL)
  disease-specific measures, 7
  generic SF-36 instrument, 6
  health-related, 6
  Hydrocephalus Outcome Questionnaire (HOQ), 7
  individual's, 6

R

Radiculopathy, 205, 207
Radionuclide shunt studies, 41
Raised intracranial pressure, 251, 254
Retrograde ventriculo jugular shunt (RVJ), 229
Retrograde ventriculo sinus shunt (RVS), 229

S

Seizure, 207, 256
Septations-craniotomy, 305
Septicemia, 178, 183
SF-36, 6
Sharp wave activity, 256
Shunt(s)
  calcification, 130
  complications (*see* Peritoneal shunts)
  CSF, 213
  failure, 33, 59
  location, 252
  malfunction, 33–34, 234, 236
  misplacement, 59–60
  nephritis, 144, 182–183
  neuroimaging (*see* Neuroimaging)
  revision, 234, 252
  VAS, 213
  VPL (*see* Ventriculopleural (VPL) shunting)
  VPS, 213
Shunt catheter characteristics
  material properties
    anti-microbial catheters, 114
    biopolymers, 113
    calcified or degraded catheter tubing, 113
    dystrophic calcification, 113
    modern shunt catheter tubing, 112–113
    platinum-and barium-coated silicon catheters, 113–114
    polymer breakdown, 113
  outflow mechanism, 115
  physical properties, 114–115
  valve complex
    Hakim valve (Codman), 114
    round-bodied valves (Orbis-Sigma), or burr-hole valve, 114
Shunt device, 235–236, 238, 240
  basic hydrodynamics, 110
  catheter characteristics, 112–115
  patient factors, 115–116
  types of valves (*see* Shunt valves)
Shunted hydrocephalus, 250, 255–256
Shunt failure
  age, risk factor
    chronic and subtle clinical features, 19
    in neonates and infants, 18, 20
    non-NPH and NPH hydrocephalus, 19
    in older children and adults, 18–21
    shunt infection, 19, 21
    symptoms and signs, 19–21
    technique of fontanel palpation, 18, 20
  causes, 4
  definition, 16
  diagnosis
    clinical history, 27
    monitoring of intracranial pressure, 28

neuroimaging studies, 28
physical examination, 27
pumping of valve reservoir, 28
shunt tap, 28
tension of fontanel, 27
ventricular pressure, 28–29
early *vs.* late shunt failures, 20
malfunction in draining spaces, 22–23
of mechanical failures
detachment of ventricular catheters, 17–18
distal catheters of VA valves, 17
obstruction of the distal catheter, 17, 19
proximal catheters, 17, 19
mortality, 5
role of hydrocephalus etiology, 20–21
of shunt failure, 16–17
Shunt infections, 102, 253
clinical manifestations
infection prophylaxis, 23
in peritoneal shunts (VP or LP), 23–24
risk factors, 23
surgical techniques, 23
symptoms, 23
ventricular, 23
clinical signs, 46
definition, 141
epidemiology and risk factors, 142
ETV procedure, 46
incidence, 45
mortality rates, 6
pathogens in late infection, 46
premature neonates, 4
skin bacteria, 45–46
ventriculitis, 46
in VP shunts, 46
Shunting procedure
epilepsy development, 250–251
epileptic seizure, 254
hydrocephalic patient
cortical malformation, 253
epileptic seizure, 254
hyponatremic seizure, 254
infection, 253
intracranial hemorrhage, 253–254
intracranial hypotension, 254
location, 252
malfunction, 252–253
revisions, 252
SLVS, 253
surgery, patient's age and sex, 251
Shunt malfunction, 129–130, 134, 252–253, 279–280
definition, 16
in draining spaces
lumboperitoneal shunts, 22
subdural-peritoneal shunts, 22–23
ventriculoatrial shunts, 22
ventriculo-gallbladder shunts, 22
ventriculoperitoneal shunts, 22
ventriculopleural valves, 22
ventriculo-subgaleal shunts, 23
Shunt obstruction
after shunt placement, 46–7
clinical presentation, 47
imaging, 47–48
proximal catheter obstruction, 47
ventricular catheter obstruction, 47
Shunt structure
antisiphon device, 15
components, 15–16
pumping devices or reservoirs, 15
unishunt, 15
Shunt valves
adjustable or 'programmable' valves, 112
complex, 114–115
differential pressure valves, 111
flow-regulated valves, 110–111
gravitational valves, 111–112
selection, 109
Silastic catheters, 204
Silicone allergy, 78
"Siliconomas," 78
Siphoning effect, 120–121, 124–125
Slit ventricle syndrome (SVS/SLVS), 25, 50–53, 83, 233–234, 253, 256
collapse of the lateral ventricles, 123
definition, 123
incidence, 124
intermittent proximal catheter obstruction, 123
medical treatment, 124
overdrainage, 124
pathophysiological events, 124
position-dependent symptoms, 123
subgroups, 124
surgical treatment
antisiphon valves (ASV), 125
endoscopic third ventriculostomy (ETV), 125
resistant SVS, 125
shunt revision, 125
subtemporal craniectomy, 124–125
Societal impact
in developed world, 8–9
in developing world, 9
healthcare costs, 8
quality of life, 8
shunted hydrocephalus, 7–8
Spinal deformities, 207
Sterile ascites, 189–190
Subacute bacterial endocarditis, 144
Subarachnoid hemorrhage, 207
Subcutaneous emphysema, 62
Subdural collections: hygroma and haematoma
after treatment of arachnoid cyst
arachnoid cyst (AC), 295
cyst-peritoneal (CP) shunt placement, 295–296
neuroendoscopy, 296
after ventricular shunting
dural border cell (DBC) layer, 286
pathophysiological mechanism, 286
subdural haematomas, 289–290
subdural hygroma, 286–289

Subdural collections: hygroma and haematoma (*cont.*)
  extra-axial collections, 296–298
  following neuroendoscopic procedures
    infectious subdural collections, 295
    subdural CSF hygromas, 291–293
    subdural haematomas, 293–295
  hydrocephalus, 285
Subdural effusion, 291
Subdural empyema, 295
Subduroperitoneal shunting, 100
Subtemporal craniectomy, 124–125
"Subzero" method, 278
Sudden death, 308, 310
Syringomyelia, 205, 207

T
TBM. *See* Tubercular meningitis (TBM)
Temporal occurrence, 15
Thoracic empyema
  bacterial invasion, 221
  description, 221
  intrapleural complication, 219
  management, 221
Three-dimensional constructive interference in the steady state (3D-CISS), 39–40, 303
Thromboembolic disease, 65
Tonsilar herniation, 206
Tricuspid valve pathology, 65
Tubercular meningitis (TBM), 227
Tumoral hydrocephalus, 21

U
Ultrasounds, 36–37
Uncompensated hydrocephalus, 15
Underdrainage, 163, 169–170, 172
  isolated fourth ventricle, 25
  siphoning-retarding devices or flow-controlled valves, 25

V
Valued years of potential life lost (VYPLL), 8
Valve's opening pressure (OPV), 110
Venous sinus thrombosis, 207
Ventricular catheter, 214
  cannulation, 92
  intracranial migration and retention, 92–93
  intraparenchymal hemorrhage, 94
  intraventricular hemorrhage in shunt revision, 93–94
  misplacement, 92–93
  selection, 92
Ventricular drainage (ventriculostomy), 142, 146
Ventricular shunts
  anatomy, 41–42
  catheters, 41–42
  programmable shunts, 42
  VA shunts, 42
  VP shunting, 42
Ventriculoatrial (VA) shunting, 16, 42, 76, 98–99
Ventriculoatrial shunts (VAS), 22, 98–99, 177, 213, 220, 227, 230
Ventriculocholecysto (VC) shunt, 228–229
Ventriculo-gallbladder (VGB) shunting, 16, 99
Ventriculo-gallbladder shunts (VGS), 76–77
Ventriculo-omental bursa (VOB) shunting, 198
Ventriculoperitoneal (VP) shunting, 3, 16, 42, 187
  evolution, 230
  hydrocephalic patients, 227
Ventriculoperitoneal shunts (VPS), 77
  misplacement/migration, distal catheter, 183–184
  septicemia, 183
Ventriculopleural (VPL) shunting, 62–63, 76, 99
  drainage, 213
  hydrocephalus, 215
  insertion technique, 214
  patients follow-up, 222
  pleural fluid collection, 217
  pneumothorax, 215
  transdiaphragmatic migration, 222–223
Ventriculosinus shunts, 229–230
Ventriculosubgaleal (VSG) shunt, 99, 151–152, 155, 228–229
Ventriculoureteral shunting, 99, 230
Ventriculoureteric shunt (VUS), 76
Visceral–intestinal perforation, 66–68

W
Wound dehiscence, 207

Y
Years of potential life lost (YPLL), 8
Years of potential productivity lost (YPPL), 8

Printing and Binding: Stürtz GmbH, Würzburg